Psychosocial
Occupational
Therapy:
A Clinical Practice

Psychosocial Occupational Therapy:
A Clinical Practice

Second Edition

Elizabeth Cara, PhD, OTR/L, MFT
Associate Professor, San Jose State University
San Jose, California

Anne MacRae, PhD, OTR/L
Professor, San Jose State University
San Jose, California

THOMSON

DELMAR LEARNING   Australia   Canada   Mexico   Singapore   Spain   United Kingdom   United States

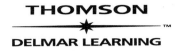

THOMSON
™
DELMAR LEARNING

Psychosocial Occupational Therapy: A Clinical Practice, 2nd Edition

by Elizabeth Cara, PhD, OTR/L, MFT and Anne MacRae, PhD, OTR/L

Vice President,
Health Care Business Unit:
William Brottmiller

Executive Director:
Cathy L. Esperti

Acquisitions Editor:
Kalen Conerly

Developmental Editor:
Juliet Byington

Editorial Assistant:
James Duncan

Marketing Director:
Jennifer McAvey

Marketing Coordinator:
Chris Manion

Art and Design Specialist:
Connie Lundberg-Watkins

Production Coordinator:
John Mickelbank

Project Editor:
Daniel Branagh

Library of Congress Cataloging-in-Publication Data

Cara, Elizabeth.
    [Psychosocial occupational therapy in clinical practice]
    Psychosocial occupational therapy : a clinical practice / Elizabeth Cara and Anne MacRae.—2nd ed.
        p. cm.
    Rev. ed. of: Psychosocial occupational therapy in clinical practice. © 1998.
    Includes bibliographical references and index.
    ISBN 13: 9781-4018-1232-4 (alk. paper)
    ISBN 10: 1-4018-1232-5 (alk. paper)
    1. Occupational therapy.
    2. Mentally ill—Rehabilitation.
    I. MacRae, Anne.   I. Title.
    RC487.C36 2005
    616.89'165—dc22
                                    2004013041

NOTICE TO THE READER

Contents

Preface to the Second Edition

Introduction

It seems that the six years since we wrote the first edition of this text have passed quickly. Our initial goal was to write a book directed to students and entry-level practitioners in mental health to fill what we felt was a large gap in occupational therapy psychiatric and psychosocial information and expertise. From the many comments we have received since then, we believe that our text was instrumental in interesting occupational therapy students in mental health practice and in assisting beginning psychosocial occupational therapists to enhance and deepen their practice. Comments we have received also tell us it was a valuable asset for experienced clinicians. Having completed what we felt was our original intention to illuminate the practice of mental health occupational therapy, our desire for this edition was to expand the content of the book to continue to appeal to both experienced and novice occupational therapists and to be more inclusive of current occupational therapy practice, particularly practice areas that are not considered strictly psychiatric but include primarily psychosocial interventions. For example, there is a new part titled "Mental Health with Physical Disorders," with chapters covering such topics as adjustment, brain injury, and pain management. Also, we have included new chapters on assessment as well as methods and interpersonal strategies that are relevant for a variety of populations and settings. We have always advocated for the view of occupational therapy (OT) as a generalist profession and hope that the new chapters will assist occupational therapists in many practice specialties to embrace the psychosocial nature of our profession.

Organization of the Text

In addition to adding new material, we have also reorganized the previous parts of the text to be more inclusive of a general occupational therapy practice that reflects occupational therapy's long-standing value placed on treating the whole person. Also, they more accurately reflect our field's contemporary domain of practice, which emphasizes the role of the person in context engaging in occupation. In addition, the parts of the book mirror the general trend in psychiatry and mental health to intervene more aggressively using medicine and assessments, to evaluate and treat more briefly, to focus on function, and to use community settings. Thus the book is divided into parts on the mental health context, theoretical concepts, diagnosis and dysfunction, mental health across the lifespan, mental health with physical disorders, occupational therapy intervention in mental health, expanded roles for OT in mental health, and clinically related roles.

Each part now includes a brief explanation of the chapters that are contained in that part. Each chapter follows the same format, which includes key terms, case illustrations, summaries, review questions, references, and suggested reading. The key terms aid the reader in quickly understanding the main ideas in the chapter as well as alerting him or her to the language of mental health and psychiatry. The case illustrations have been universally praised by students, academics, and practitioners for making the ideas come alive and, more important, assisting the reader in understanding mental health clients and practice outside of the textbook. End-of-chapter summaries integrate the information in each chapter as well as aid the reader in remembering what is important. Review questions provide the same assistance as the summaries, but in a much deeper way. If the reader thinks about and answers the questions, she or he will be assured that everything that the chapter has to offer has been learned. For students the questions may serve as an assessment of how much they have learned from each chapter while for clinicians the questions may offer an expanded way of thinking about their practice. The extensive references and suggested reading not only tell the reader where to go for additional current information on each topic, but together they offer the latest research concerning each topic and suggest how the research has been applied in practice.

New to This Edition

The Occupational Therapy Practice Framework (2002) has guided much of this second edition's reorganization. In addition, all chapter authors were asked to reflect on the current trends of professional globalization and accountability in clinical practice. As a result, the reader will find a great increase in citations of international literature and evidence-based research.

To be inclusive, we have added a total of six new chapters, revised most of the earlier edition's chapters, and deleted a few chapters. Many elements of deleted chapters can be found in either revised or new chapters, but the material is restructured to better meet the needs of clinicians and students. For example, our original edition included a chapter on the occupational therapy process. However, since our first edition the occupational therapy domain and practice document has more specifically spelled out the occupational therapy domain. Therefore, we have included chapters with more specific information on the environment and culture, evaluation and assessment, and methods and interpersonal strategies.

Another example of this restructuring is the deletion of the first edition's chapter on occupational therapy models. The literature on OT models of practice has proliferated over the last six years and we simply could not do justice to each model within the confines of this book. Instead, the reader will find a greater emphasis on models of practice in each clinical chapter and a new focus on understanding the history and philosophy of the profession as well as the contexts in which we practice. We strongly urge the reader to also use primary sources on the several excellent models of practice that can be found in the OT literature. In addition to deleting the chapters on OT models and OT process, we also deleted the chapters on psychiatric issues in HIV infection and dissociative disorders. Both of these disorders obviously still exist; however, knowledge of HIV infection has become more known worldwide and less of a focus in psychiatry, and dissociative disorders are equally less likely to be a focus in psychiatry. Also, as we stated previously, the new chapters regarding physical disability, brain disorders, and pain management reflect the generalist nature of current occupational therapy practice to include general psychosocial as well as specific psychiatric issues.

In this edition there is an increased emphasis on mental health across the lifespan. The developmental and life stage issues of children, adolescents, and older adults are now addressed in three distinct chapters. We have also added two new appendixes. The first provides a brief overview of psychopharmacology to the occupational therapist. Although information on medication can be found in a variety of sources, the focus is on the information that is most important for the occupational therapist. While there is more than enough information to warrant a chapter on the subject, a decision was made to include this information as an appendix to highlight the significance of psychopharmacology with all of the clinical chapters. We recommend that you refer to the appendix often when reading other chapters in the book. The second appendix on resources is a compilation of Web sites relevant to psychosocial occupational therapy. The proliferation of such sites in the last six years has been astounding but can also be confusing. Our intention in providing these resources is to encourage both students and practicing occupational therapists to use these resources—therapists especially for continuing education and as opportunities for educating clients and their families.

For educators using this textbook in the classroom, an Instructor's Manual is now available to accompany the second edition. We believe that this new tool will greatly assist instructors to comfortably use our text and thus to facilitate lively classes. This Instructor's Manual begins with a section titled "Theory-Based Instruction for Occupational Therapy Curriculum" that provides instructors with the basis of constructivist and cognitive learning theories as a starting point for thinking about classroom instruction. Other sections provide practical information on how to build a syllabus, assess student progress, teach, use technology in instruction, and give assignments. The Instructor's Manual also provides instructional materials to accompany the text, such as learning activities, review questions and answers, supplemental references and resources, as well as handouts that can be photocopied and used in classes.

While these various changes have been made we have expanded some areas that were universally praised by students, practitioners, educators, and researchers. For example, we have included even more case studies and illustrations and evidence-based knowledge, and we believe we have preserved the ease of reading style of the first edition.

As we did in the first edition, we sincerely believe that working in mental health and with psychosocial concepts is interesting, exciting, and satisfying work, and we hope that students and practitioners will continue to benefit from this clinically oriented text. We also hope that students, academics, and practitioners will continue to send us their comments. Enjoy the adventure!

Elizabeth Cara, PhD, OTR/L, MFT
edcara@casa.sjsu.edu

Anne MacRae, PhD, OTR/L
amacrae@email.sjsu.edu

Reference

Occupational therapy practice framework: Domain and process (2002). *American Journal of Occupational Therapy, 56,* 609–639.

Preface to the First Edition

In 1954, Wade and Franciscus wrote:

> The attitude of the occupational therapist toward the mental disease and the approach which he makes to the patient determine to a great extent the quality of the therapy he administers and the results he obtains. Opportunities for the development of a therapeutic approach and a healthy mental attitude toward this group of patients should hold the highest priority in the educational plan of the student therapist. (p. 77)

This is not an outdated notion but rather the principle that guides our teaching and clinical work. It is our hope that through the chapters of this book, the occupational therapy student and the practicing occupational therapist will develop or enhance not only their knowledge of mental health care, but also their respect for, and understanding of, people with mental illness.

Health care—specifically, mental health care—is a dynamic field, with new ideas being introduced and old ones being discarded at sometimes unpredictable rates. This is one of the inherent problems in writing a textbook on this topic. The editors and contributing authors have made every effort to provide the most up-to-date information available, but it is up to the readers to study with a critical view and supplement the information as appropriate.

As of the writing of this text, there were several unresolved issues that are addressed in individual chapters and one controversy that applies to all the chapters: the use of terminology. What is the best word to describe the role of the person receiving services or treatment? This may seem like a relatively simple, even trivial, issue, but it is not. A word can be a label with subtle emotional, often derogatory, meanings attached to it. If one doubts the power of a label, consider that it was not long ago that terms such as *idiot* and *moron* were considered accurate medical terminology. Finding the best word to describe the people involved in a therapeutic relationship has been an ongoing debate for some time, and it is unlikely to be resolved with a simple answer.

It is the editors' opinion that finding a single, universal term for this role is not possible at this time. Rather, the term's meaning does, and should, vary depending on the setting where treatment is given as well as the philosophy guiding the treatment. For example, the term *patient* still seems appropriate when discussing people hospitalized for acute disorders. *Client* is the preferred term for a person accessing ongoing contractual services, such as those found in the case management relationship. Currently, the term *consumer* seems to be favored, as it implies that the receivers of service have freedom of choice and control over their own lives. However, no one term is ideal, and the reader should be aware of the limitations of language. For example, when using the term *consumer*, one needs to ask, "What exactly is being consumed?" If the person is clearly using a specific service, such as a prevocational assessment package, then the term makes sense, but in ongoing supportive services, the most valuable commodity offered is the therapeutic relationship (and, obviously, the therapist is not for consumption). The term *participant* would be more accurate in such a relationship, but since it is not a widely used or recognized term, it may be confusing when used in documentation. In summary, the reader is cautioned about the limitations of language and encouraged to think about the nuances of terms and be particularly aware of their context. Although labels are sometimes necessary for the sake of clarity, it is recommended that every effort be made to maintain human dignity and identity by using such terms as *person* or *individual* whenever possible.

Another controversial use of terminology applies to all the chapters of this book. What is the best word to describe the specific area of service that we are targeting? As with words applied to people, words used to describe a specific arena in which we practice can have subtle meanings attached to them. For some time the term *psychosocial* has been applied very broadly in occupational therapy practice. *The Random House College Dictionary* (1973) defines psychosocial as "pertaining to or caused by both psychological and social factors." It is a useful term that implies treating the psyche, or mind, and social factors, as distinguished somehow from bodily, physical factors (though we all recognize how mind and body, as embedded in a social context, are interconnected and that you cannot possibly treat one without treating the other).

However, *psychosocial* could be applied to everyone, whether able or disabled in body and/or mind. A term that more specifically elucidates and distinguishes this text is *psychiatry*, "the practice or the science of treating mental disorders" (*Random House College Dictionary*, 1973). "Mental disorders" encompasses psychosocial causes and problems; however, the term is even richer, encompassing biology, chemistry, cognition and perception, linguistic, interpersonal, environmental, and cultural factors and the manifestations of each. Although the techniques discussed in the chapters are directed toward the amelioration of "psyche," or mental, problems as they manifest in the social or interpersonal realm, the techniques are applied specifically in the treatment of mental disorders.

Again, it is our opinion that there is not yet one universal term that adequately describes our practice. Instead, the term will vary throughout chapters; *mental health, mental health arena, psychiatric,* and *psychosocial* are used somewhat interchangeably according to each author's bias. The reader is encouraged to think about the various terms in the continuing quest to clarify practice in the mental health arena and, hopefully, to discover a universal term that does justice to our complex treatment for mental disorders.

In the past two decades, different models of occupational therapy have been delineated and expanded on. There has also been a focus on developing assessments specifically for occupational therapy. The historical roots of our profession have vibrantly infused and broadened our sense of ourselves as professionals. We recognize the importance of models, assessments, and history; however, the purpose of this text is to fill what we perceive as a gap in the information for the clinician practicing in mental health. It is intended to inform students and beginning therapists of the basic and rich forms of occupational therapy that are practiced in mental health. We have included overviews of theories, evaluation and treatment, and the occupational therapy process, but our primary purpose is not theoretical but rather clinical. We aim to provide sound information regarding treatment specifically for practice in psychiatry. To that end we employed clinicians as chapter authors and encouraged them to discuss what they actually do in their practice. We also provided an understanding of mental disorders, as they are currently defined in the *Diagnostic and Statistical Manual of Mental Disorders, Fourth Edition (DSM-IV)* (APA, 1994). Our goal is to provide students and beginning clinicians with information they will need to adequately practice as psychiatric occupational therapy clinicians.

Because we wanted the text to be clinical in its focus and, therefore, encouraged our chapter authors to write about their practice, we have allowed for differing styles and opinions. In fact, throughout the book you may find that the authors disagree. You may also realize that some chapters vary in depth or breadth of scope or focus, either more on understanding a disorder or more on providing treatment. The chapters include a resource list and also a list of suggested reading. For example, Chapter 21, on vocational programming, encourages a psychosocial community approach, whereas Chapter 1, on personal effects of mental illness, focuses on family and national support groups. All chapters include case illustrations, some of which are brief illustrations of particular points made in the chapter while others are long illustrations of treatment. We have allowed for a variety of authorship styles, which, we think, appeals to our various readers' styles and helps to enhance learning.

Information on treatment for one population in one chapter can easily translate into treatment for another population. For example, the relaxation exercises for anxiety disorders described in Chapter 8 can also be helpful for many other people, particularly those with agitated depression, personality disorders, or HIV, due to the symptoms of anxiety that they may experience. In fact, due to the recent explosion of information concerning stress in everyday life, there are probably very few people who would not find them beneficial. Hopefully, readers can extrapolate and adapt treatment suggestions for various populations and settings.

You will find that the length of chapters varies depending on how much information is in the literature. For example, Chapter 7, on mood disorders, is shorter than Chapter 8, on anxiety disorders. There is much information, particularly in occupational therapy, about depression, but less about generalized anxiety disorder. We encourage you to be analytical in your reading, to interact with the material in a critical way, and to freely use this volume as a base from which to create your clinical practice.

We do not know what the mental health arena will look like in the near future. It is changing rapidly and being strongly influenced by managed care. Treatment is becoming more acute and is being dictated by cost-efficiency, while at the same time it seems that more people are in need of services. In this book, we have attempted to provide a broad base of information that includes what we know of "mental disease" and its treatment through occupational therapy to date. This text provides the infrastructure on which daily life in psychiatric occupational therapy exists. We believe that this knowledge will not change but rather can only be added to, and we invite the reader to take this underlying structure and build on it.

Sustaining Professional Identity in Mental Health—Personal Paths

We often hear comments predicting the demise of psychiatric occupational therapy, but occupational therapists are a diverse group of people in a multifaceted profession. The occupational therapy (OT) philosophy and process is not fully articulated in the literature; however, despite diverse paths into the field and in practice, there are common threads of a belief system that is enculturated in the profession. Historically, this belief system was not separate from the practice in mental health, and we believe it will sustain our unique contribution in the psychosocial arena.

Throughout the text we present case illustrations to make concepts, ideas, and people with various diagnoses and problems "come alive" and, hopefully, be remembered. In keeping with that, and in the wish that psychosocial occupational therapists and practitioners could be sustaining mentors, we present here some case illustrations of people's personal paths into the profession, excerpted from personal statements they provided. We highlight the interests, joys, rewards, and challenges of occupational therapists who work in mental health. While these therapists represent the vast differences of our paths, it is also clear that there is a unifying passion and an identity. It is our hope that the passion infuses this text, and that threads of a common belief system and identity will be recognized throughout. The first two are our own.

LIZ CARA

College Faculty, San Jose, CA
I graduated from college with a BA in history, moved to Pennsylvania, and began working in business. Although I was very successful, becoming a manager by the age of 24, I felt that administration was dry and that I was not doing anything to benefit people. I literally went to the library and researched careers. Health care careers matched my requirements—working with and benefiting people, available jobs, and the flexibility to move to other states and countries.

I had never heard of occupational therapy until a physiatrist (an MD who specializes in physical rehabilitation) steered me to it. I talked with people from several departments at the University of Pennsylvania before enrolling, but it seemed that the occupational therapists were the most animated, lively, interesting people, and they discussed their job as if it were fun.

OT school offered me a combination of learning that I loved—science, psychology, and crafts. I thought then and still do that it is the perfect course; it integrated all of the things I want to know about. I originally wanted to work with people with arthritis, but during my fieldwork, I realized that I really liked the opportunity for creativity, unpredictability, and up-close relationships in mental health. I looked forward to the nonsameness of every day and I felt that indeed, I had an effect on people.

Since entering the field, I have had the opportunity to work in a variety of settings and roles on both coasts; with teenagers on an inpatient locked unit, at an inpatient psychiatric facility exclusively for women, at one of the oldest private psychiatric hospitals that based treatment on moral treatment. Also, my experience in community settings includes developing an agency known as Community Vocational Enterprises, specializing in vocational rehabilitation for people with serious mental illness, working in a clubhouse model program called Townehouse Creative Living Center, and coordinating vocational treatment for a large community residential organization.

Practicing occupational therapy in the mental health area has fit who I am as a person. It satisfies my values, particularly my very deep belief that the essence of life is relationship. I am thrilled that I now have the opportunity to be an educator and continue to impart my knowledge and values.

ANNE MacRAE

College Faculty, San Jose, CA
My first degree was in education, and although I loved teaching (and still do!), I felt there was something else I wanted to do. I spent several years exploring possibilities, taking courses, and working as a program leader in a recreation center for people with disabilities, and developed a special fascination for the workings of the brain. I found that cognitive, affective, and perceptual dysfunctions were evident in a wide variety of developmental, physical, and psychiatric conditions but I was still resistant to pursuing a medically oriented career. I also

wanted to pursue my creative, artistic, and social interests that seemingly didn't fit into a health care profession. A friend of mine who is a physical therapist told me about OT and said it would be a perfect match for me. She was right! I returned to graduate school for a master's degree in occupational therapy and I never regretted that choice.

My first couple of years in practice, I worked in the home health care arena. This experience led me to the strong belief that mental health is essential to address in any treatment plan. The primary diagnostic categories seen in home health care are cardiovascular, neurological, orthopedic, and oncologic, but I often felt that the real issues behind dysfunction were more related to problems with adjustment, depression, substance abuse, and various cognitive and perceptual dysfunctions.

As part of my teaching responsibilities, I currently supervise an on-campus occupational therapy mental health clinic, which allows me a wonderful blend of clinical practice, teaching, and supervision. In addition, I maintain a limited practice at San Francisco General Hospital, a large county facility serving a very diverse and often disenfranchised population. Most of the clients that I see in both of these settings have serious and persistent mental illnesses. I consider this group to be one of the most stigmatized in the Western world. Consequently, a necessary part of my work is being involved in community education to increase awareness about the plight of people with mental illness.

JUDY PRITCHETT

Clinical director and program developer, community outreach agency, New York City

I was very interested in schizophrenia because I had relatives with that disorder, but my first occupational exposure to mental illness was as a mental health aide in a day treatment center. It became apparent to me that the activities done at this center—crafts, cooking, outings, artwork, and clerical groups—were more meaningful and therapeutic than the group or individual talking therapies. After two years working for this program in the Riverdale Mental Health Association, I decided to go to graduate school for a degree in occupational therapy.

I had felt strongly that I always wanted to work in mental health, but somehow my first job out of OT school was in a school for multiply handicapped children. In this setting I clearly saw the relevance of sensory integration theory and perceptual motor development, and could relate this information easily to the processing deficits seen with schizophrenia. I also developed programs related to sex education and career exploration which are examples of what I think is OT at its best: focusing on areas of human occupation that are in themselves important and meaningful while developing specific competencies and providing activities that improve psychosocial adjustment in many other ways, including improved self-esteem, reality testing, and social skills.

For the last 10 years I worked at Project Reachout, a program for the mentally ill homeless population. I liked this setting most of all, because it allowed me to have fun addressing a serious social problem and because I could see people who had been outcasts become part of a community which we created and which in turn connected them to a broader community from which they had become estranged. We enabled them to learn the skills they lacked in order to make this connection, and we enabled them to access and value the supports they needed in order to stay connected.

ANITA MARYE NELSON

Clinician & program developer, home health agency, Colorado Springs
I was originally a COTA (certified occupational therapy assistant) in the military, and a "die hard" physical disabilities clinician with little or no interest in practicing in mental health. After a job relocation, I was reassigned to work in mental health. The organization at that base was such that the OTRs (occupational therapists, registered) treated clients with physical disabilities and the COTAs treated those with psychiatric disabilities. Actually, it was a negative experience because I didn't feel competent. But the experience did lead me to pursue further education.

I returned to school to become an OTR and developed an appreciation for the generalist perspective of occupational therapy and a greater understanding of the underlying theory. My psychiatric internship at the Kettering Medical Center in Ohio opened my eyes to the richness of mental health OT. This experience was positive because of excellent role modeling, communication, and supervision.

My present practice is in home care where the primary caseload consists of clients needing physical rehabilitation. When the agency decided to expand to include a psychiatric caseload, they initially did not consider including occupational therapy, but at my persuasion, OT has been made an integral part of the mental health team. Home care provides me the opportunity to work in an interdisciplinary team, in a real-life setting, with a mixed caseload that allows me to put the generalist OT concepts into practice.

SUSAN LANG

Private practice, San Francisco
I was initially attracted to the physical disabilities area of OT because it seemed more organized, concrete, and easier to follow. I was especially interested in neuroanatomy and that interest has persisted. But my internship in physical dysfunction was very negative—I almost left OT altogether. Fortunately, my internship experience in psychiatry was extremely positive, and I ended up being hired there afterward. Langley Porter Institute is part of a large teaching hospital at the University of California Medical Center in San Francisco. It was a very supportive learning environment that used an excellent multidisciplinary approach. It was here that I felt I was able to develop my expertise and my skills. But this was also my most "traditional" job setting.

Another unique setting in which I worked was the Indian Hospital in Santa Fe, New Mexico. It was an incredible experience for me because I have always been fascinated by cross-cultural issues, but it was also here that I think I became most aware of what clients had to offer me, rather than the other way around. In this setting, there was a bit of irony in that I was using nonverbal interventions among a cultural group whom I consider to be masters at nonverbal communication.

My respect for the diversity of clients and what they bring to the therapeutic relationship led me to my favorite treatment arena, which is private practice. Most occupational therapists who engage in private practice do so through the use of contracts with particular agencies. Another way to do private practice is to provide direct services to clients. There are limitations in reimbursement but I prefer this approach because it allows me the greatest autonomy and flexibility.

Mental health care has changed so much that occupational therapists have become more central; in terms of the overall goals of mental health, the whole functional arena has become central to treatment. Although the problems in mental health care are very real, I have no doubt that we have a valuable service to offer and there are many avenues for occupational therapists in mental health to explore and pursue.

VIRGINIA STOEFFEL

College Faculty, Milwaukee, WI

I wanted to be an occupational therapist since I was 13. At that time my mother had cancer and indeed died. One of my sisters was hospitalized with major depression and a suicide attempt. I was aware that people had feelings around illness. My perception was that people might be able to deal with their feelings through activities.

I was shaped by and formed by my supervisor on my level I fieldwork. She told me that I had very good interpersonal skills, even more advanced than those expected of level II students; she urged me to develop my skills in mental health. I also benefited from an excellent professor in mental health. She knew how to bring out the best in me—she felt that I was self-actualized!

I was hired onto a pilot project for those with substance abuse. This broadened into addictive disorders, such as eating disorders. This began a long and fruitful career as the program developed into long-term, outpatient, wellness, and prevention programs. I was fortunate to move into different management jobs. Eventually I worked on a research program implementing cognitive behavioral programs for people, and I realized how substance abuse interfered with people carrying out performance roles.

I am sustained in my career because I am continually amazed at the strengths and resiliency people bring with them. I have always been interested in what makes people tick, what drives them, and I have good observation and interpersonal skills. I know how to be human with people; that includes being flexible, adaptive, open, vulnerable to others, confident in myself. People have remarked that I pay attention to them.

What is rewarding? to see that people can make changes in a supportive and trusting, consistent relationship. It makes me really aware, too, as a parent what needs to be done and how to be with my family, and how to keep myself grounded.

I want to say that I don't see psychosocial practice as a dying art. What we have to offer is a package that helps people best in a fairly economical way—they get the most bang for their buck by having an occupational therapist as part of their health care system.

It is not uncommon for people to enter occupational therapy as a second career, or not to know at first their choice of an OT practice area. One of the themes of these illustrations is that people often think that they want to practice in a different area, until they discover mental heath. Although they may not be able to articulate exactly how mental health captured them, the choice to practice is not necessarily a conscious decision, of the head only, but clearly includes an unconscious process of the heart. One of the themes is the significance of key people in our lives or role models who help us discover our paths, whether serendipitous or logical. This is especially important during clinical internships, a concept that is further elaborated in Chapter 23.

Another theme of these vignettes is the idea that occupational therapy is a career that, while not without its challenges, can provide deep personal satisfaction, and that there is a shared belief in the efficacy and practicality of what we do. All of the occupational therapists interviewed worked at one time or another in what would be considered traditional settings. They also explored and developed programs in nontraditional settings—community agencies, schools, outreach programs, homeless shelters, university-based collaborative programs, private practice, clubhouse model programs, and home health care agencies. This diversity in occupational therapy practice settings sometimes makes it difficult to define our scope, but it also provides us with remarkable flexibility. The generalist nature of occupational therapy practice provides opportunities in a broadly described mental health arena, even within the tremendous changes going on in health care delivery today. Chapter 13 and all of Part V address diverse and nontraditional practice settings in psychosocial practice.

A theme touched on by the illustrators is becoming aware of mental illness and psychosocial problems in relatives' lives. This awareness may develop into a desire to be an occupational therapist who can assist others in daily occupations or into an understanding and interpersonal facility in working with people with mental illnesses. This theme is discussed from the family viewpoint in Chapter 1.

"Creativity," "unpredictability," "flexibility," "nonsameness," "have fun"—all describe the work of occupational therapy in psychiatry. Although there are no specific chapters that address these intangible and more elusive qualities, all the chapter authors were asked to convey what they felt was unique, important, and perhaps not written about in their personal clinical experience, and these terms were their answers.

In the prefatory illustrations, a theme of relationship, an awareness of what clients have to offer in a reciprocal connection, and a yen for knowledge of what is happening to a person, is evident throughout. People speak of being interested in what makes others tick, being able to support them in their daily lives, being accepting and embracing the whole person for where and who she or he is. At the same time they speak of being interested in neurology and in special conditions and sustaining that interest throughout their careers. We hope the reader will recognize that these themes are implicit in all of the chapters of the book.

Although we can specify certain themes through different paths, we are still not able to state definitively what attracts a person to the practice of occupational therapy in the mental health arena. We believe that this is as it should be in a diverse, eclectic profession in which beliefs are historically based on complex and broad concepts of adaptation and occupation. We also believe it's as it should be because diverse practitioners create their practice in mental health even as they practice this occupation daily in varied contexts.

We hope that this text will evoke a desire to know more about this rich field and the people in it, and we hope that you will follow the spirit of these occupational therapist case illustrations and practice with seriousness, passion, fun, intelligence, clarity, and creativity.

References

American Psychiatric Association. (1994). *Diagnostic and Statistical Manual of Mental Disorders* (4th ed.). Washington, DC: Author.

Wade, B., & Franciscus, M. L. (1954). Occupational therapy for the mentally ill. In H. Willard & C. Spackman, *Principles of occupational therapy* (2nd ed., pp. 76–116). Philadelphia: Lippincott.

About the Authors

Liz Cara is an associate professor at San Jose State University, where she has taught psychosocial, research, and other courses to graduates and undergraduates in the on-campus and distance program since 1990. Prior to education, she worked as an occupational therapist in mental health for approximately 20 years. She has worked in a variety of settings with both adolescents and adults, created and developed groups and new programs, and consulted for organizations. She has a doctorate in clinical psychology from the first APA-accredited distance program, a marriage and family therapy license in California, and experience in infant-parent and adult psychotherapy. Her current research interests include fieldwork education and training, psychoanalytic relational theories, and life history or psychobiography specializing in the lives and works of the primatologist and occupational therapist, Dian Fossey, and the artist, Georgia O'Keeffe. She is also learning more than she imagined about the foster and adoption process since she and her partner recently adopted Cynthia and Lisa, siblings who are 10 and 11. She remains active by continuing to practice Iyengar yoga, working out with weights, and cross country skiing and hoping that she can get back into tennis and running. She is an avid football and baseball fan, loyal to the teams of her youth, the San Francisco 49'ers and Giants.

Anne MacRae is a professor and postprofessional program director at San Jose State University in California, where she has taught a myriad of different courses since 1983. In addition to courses in theory and practice, from both a psychosocial and generalist perspective, as well as courses in cultural diversity, she has supervised the campus-based psychosocial occupational therapy clinic for 20 years. Her other clinical experience includes inpatient acute psychiatry, partial hospitalization programs, and home health care. She is also a recipient of multiple Fulbright Fellowships and engages in international consultation about occupational therapy and mental health care. She holds degrees in education and human science in addition to occupational therapy. Her current research and scholarly interests include cultural diversity, phenomenology, client-centered models of practice, environmental issues in intervention, collaborative models of treatment, community mental health, and functional deficits of psychiatric symptoms. She lives in San Francisco surrounded by an incredibly talented group of musicians and artists (who happen to be her children, Nora and Malcolm, and husband, Joseph) as well as a host of other living creatures (among them, dogs, chickens, fish, turtles, and others) who provide love, fun and entertainment. Her hobbies include crafts, swimming, and travel, but at top of the list for relaxation is a good mystery novel!

Contributors

Michael Alessandri, PhD
Director and Clinical Associate Professor
University of Miami, FL

Eileen S. Auerbach, MS, OTR/L
Senior Occupational Therapist
Mission Multicultural Assertive Community Team (Mission ACT)
Chair, Psychiatric Occupational Therapy Action Coalition of Northern
    California (POTAC)
San Francisco, CA

Nancy Cooper, MS, OTR/L
Occupational Therapist
Harborview Mental Health Services
Seattle, WA

Jane Dressler, MS, OTR, JD
Attorney
Private Practice
San Francisco, CA

Susan Haiman, MPS, OTR/L, FAOTA
Assistant Professor
Occupational Therapy
Philadelphia University School of Science and Health
Philadelphia, PA

Glenda Jeong, PhD, MA, OTR/L
Ph.D. in Intuition & Energy Medicine
Private Wellness Practice for children and adults
San Francisco, CA

William L. Lambert, OTR/L
Occupational Therapist
First Hospital, Wyoming Valley
Kingston, PA

Vivian Banish Levitt, OTR/L, ATR-BC, LFMT
Licensed Occupational Therapist
Licensed Marriage and Family Therapist
Board Certified Art Therapist
Stanford Hospital and Clinics
Palo Alto, CA
Faculty Notre Dame de Namur University
Belmont, CA

Carole Calkins McCune, MA, LMFT
Diplomat, American Psychotherapy Association
Past President, NAMI-Santa Clara County
Member, Mental Health Commission El Dorado County
Private Practice in Diamond Springs, CA

Penelope A. Moyers, EdD, OTR, FAOTA
Professor and Dean
School of Occupational Therapy
Indianapolis, IN

Heidi McHugh Pendleton, PhD, OTR/L, FAOTA
Associate Professor, Occupational Therapy
San Jose State University
San Jose, CA

Shawn C. Phipps, MS, OTR/L
Acting Supervisor I
Rancho Los Amigos National Rehabilitation Center
Department of Occupational Therapy and Recreation Therapy
Downey, CA
Instructor of Clinical Occupational Therapy
California State University, Dominguez Hills

Deborah B. Pitts, MBA, OTR/L, CPRP
Clinical Faculty

Department of Occupational Science and Occupational Therapy
University of Southern California
Los Angeles, CA

Barbara Rodrigues, MS, OTR/L
Lead OTR/Program Supervisor
Dominican Hospital-Behavioral Health Unit
Santa Cruz, CA

Sharon Roth, RN, BSN, MA
Secretary, Board of Directors, NAMI-California
Past President, NAMI-Santa Clara County
Mental Health Board of Santa Clara County
Santa Clara Valley Chapter Bay Area Critical Incident Stress (Debriefing)
    Management Team
San Mateo, CA

Winifred Schultz-Krohn, PhD, OTR/L, BCP, FAOTA
Associate Professor of Occupational Therapy
San Jose State University
San Jose, CA

Kathleen Barker Schwartz, EdD, OTR/L, FAOTA
Professor and Graduate Coordinator
Occupational Therapy
San Jose State University
San Jose, CA

Marti Southam, PhD, OTR/L
Associate Professor
Occupational Therapy
San Jose State University
San Jose, CA

Fred Snively, BS, OTR/L
Senior Occupational Therapist
California Medical Facility
Vacaville, CA

Virginia C. Stoffel, MS, OTR, FAOTA
Associate Professor and Coordinator, Graduate Program Occupational
    Therapy
Core Leader and Scientist, Center for Addiction and Behavioral Health
    Research
University of Wisconsin-Milwaukee
Milwaukee, WI

The Mental Health Context

The understanding of context in relationship to occupational therapy is paramount in being able to provide effective and meaningful intervention. The two chapters included in part I set the stage for the remainder of the book by addressing cultural, physical, social, personal, and temporal contexts, the relationships between these contexts, and the implications for psychosocial occupational therapy.

The first chapter is written from the perspective of family members and describes their experiences and their perspectives on individuals with mental illness. This background is especially important for occupational therapists who have little or no exposure to the mental health system or to people with mental illness. This includes novice clinicians and students as well as occupational therapists who may be changing their practice area to mental health. The information in this chapter is also helpful for experienced mental health occupational therapists to refocus their interventions. It is only through understanding the client's and family's life experiences that the occupational therapist can be truly client-centered.

The second chapter addresses several different contexts through the concepts of environment and culture. The emphasis is on how these contexts specifically relate to occupational performance of people with mental illness. However, the psychosocial concerns discussed in this chapter are applicable to occupational therapy in all settings with all populations.

The Client and Family Experience of Mental Illness

Sharon Roth, RN, BSN, MA

Carole Calkins McCune, LMFT

Key Terms

National Alliance for the Mentally
   Ill (NAMI)
client-driven services
competency model
consumer empowerment

consumers' movement
decompensation
schizophrenogenic mother
self-help
treatment team

Chapter Outline

Introduction

In recent years there has been an increased emphasis on hearing the clients' and their families' personal stories (Molineux & Rickard, 2003). Understanding these personal experiences is the cornerstone for providing client-centered intervention (Beer, 2003; Mattingly & Lawlor, 2003; Pollock & McColl, 1998).

    This chapter was developed from firsthand accounts and experiences of serious and persistent mental illness. While material has been changed to protect confidentiality, the case vignettes found throughout the chapter reflect universal experiences of both individuals with serious mental illness and their family members, who are equally affected. Both authors have personal experience as parents—and one also as a sibling—of individuals with serious mental illness. Perceptions of serious mental illness vary from individual to individual among those who have contact with it. Figure 1-1 offers some of the many impressions that serious mental illness imprints on those who deal with it.

THE FAMILY PERSPECTIVE—WHO IS THE CLIENT?

We generally think of the person with a mental illness as the client. However, mental illness reaches beyond the individual, affecting the other family members and the person's significant relationships. Because so much focus falls on the symptoms or behaviors of the ill family member, the (increasing) needs of the family are generally minimized or overlooked. Considering the severe disruption that accompanies mental illness, it is amazing how many families have been able to cope without the benefit of professional help or education.

    The illness often comes on so suddenly that the family is caught off guard. This results in confusion, fear, denial, isolation, and a myriad of responses, as one might expect when a loved one becomes ill and there is little information given as to the cause. At other times, there is a gradual change in the individual that is difficult to understand, which, in adolescents, is often thought to be teenage rebellion. Sometimes the change in the individual is complicated by substance abuse, which may evoke other family responses. Unless a diagnosis is made, support and education are provided, and the family is included in the consultation about treatment and care, relief may be denied the family, yet often treatment is not sought for months or even years.

Mental Illness—What's It Like?

It: is emotionally and physically painful.
is frustrating.
is confusing.
is costly.
makes you poor and unable to pay bills.
means you are overly dependent on others.
is time consuming.
means you're angry at yourself and others.
means you hate yourself and others.
means you don't trust yourself.
is a lot of hard work.
means losing control.
means feeling guilty.
means being lonely.
means you are often a failure.
means you are treated differently from "normal" people.
means people won't let you be normal.

Mothers:
feel judged before I'm known, and stigmatized.
feel outraged and silenced at the same time—outraged by being blamed again, silenced by the fact that if I express my rage at this new person who blames me, it will be used against me as proof that I am unstable.
feel healed and able to move ahead.
sometimes get overwhelmed.
feel such pain for her/him. It is so unfair.
believe she has a right to take her own life if that is what she decides and feel sad.
believe I will never give up hoping for a cure.

Fathers:
I feel devastated by knowing my child has this illness.
The stress is getting to me.
I'm damned bewildered and confused. I don't know where to go or what to do.
I worry that he will end up on the streets or in jail.
We often fight about what is best to do. This illness is dividing us.

Siblings:
I'm afraid it will happen to me someday—or to my children, if I have any.
I love my brother but resent him and the time he takes.
I don't feel I can talk about my problems to my parents, they have so much to worry about already.
I learned to not feel guilty that she got the illness and not me.
I became a social worker.

(continues)

Figure 1-1. A Sampling of Impressions of Mental Illness from Philadelphia Community Access

Psychiatrist:
> I am expected to "cure" my patients, but sometimes I truly don't know what else to do.
>
> I'm afraid I'll be sued.
>
> I'm isolated, there is so little coordination with other programs.

Social Worker:
> I feel effective when I can help a client tap into his or her talents and strengths.
>
> There are not enough resources.
>
> I feel let down by my client's failures.
>
> I like the challenge and enjoy many of my clients, though the work is difficult.

Emergency Worker:
> I feel frustrated when I can't do what I feel is the best for the client.
>
> All I ever see is people in crisis; I never get to see improvement.
>
> Sometimes there are no doctors, beds, or meds available; what should I do then?
>
> A lot of crisis situations could be averted, but family members wait until the last minute.
>
> At times I deal with other people's mistakes.

Figure 1-1.   (continued)

Until that time, the family members may be at odds with one another about what is really wrong and how to respond to the individual's puzzling behaviors. They begin to experience a totally new set of relationships as exacted by the effects of the illness and their lack of understanding about what to do. When this happens, the family members, or each of the members in differing ways, may need their own professional intervention. In addition, for parents, the fear of having done something to cause this in a son or daughter is often reinforced by insensitive treatment professionals who do not interact with the parents in a positive or empathic manner. Some therapists even continue to believe in the concept of the **schizophrenogenic mother**. This old theory has been refuted but still lingers in outdated textbooks and can be heard in discussions by uninformed professionals, as described in the following illustration.

CASE ILLUSTRATION: Missed Diagnosis and the Family Impact

One parent remembers her son at 11 years of age. He had been on medication for attention deficit disorder for five years without improvement. As he reached puberty, his pediatrician stated that the mother was neurotic and that if she simply left the boy alone and stopped worrying, he would outgrow the behaviors. By 12 years of age, he was already using street drugs and committing petty theft, for which he was arrested. He spent the next six years in the criminal jus-

tice system. When he was 18 years of age, his probation officer observed that there was something wrong with the boy and referred him for assessment. The diagnosis was schizophrenia. The mother states that she felt a profound sense of relief in knowing that the mental illness she had suspected for years had finally been confirmed and would now be treated.

Discussion

One can certainly understand the need for a mother coping with the long-standing difficult behavior of her child to benefit from an early referral. To label her neurotic hardly addresses the stresses of her situation. It is more likely that this mother was depressed, overanxious, and aware of the risk of having her marriage fail. In addition, other siblings might have been equally affected and in need of some treatment interventions. In fact, the entire family would probably have benefited from occasional therapy in the course of dealing with such traumatic issues as having a child who abused drugs and alcohol, committed theft, and was incarcerated, and for managing the resultant feelings of guilt and stigma. Early intervention has been found to make a tremendous difference in the outcome of treatment. It decreases the frequency of relapse and hospitalization as well as encourages compliance with medication (Pharoah & Streiner, 2002).

Family Roles

In healthy families, there are roles and rules that typically define how each member behaves. The parents provide the basic needs of food, clothing, and shelter; give guidelines for behavior; and offer nurturance and support during difficult times in their children's development. How these basic needs are provided and how roles are assigned may differ from one culture to another. In most cultures in the United States, the children are expected to abide by the rules, while being given opportunities to learn by experience. When a member becomes ill, consultation within the family is the usual first step. If this is unsuccessful, the family may look outside to paraprofessionals, teachers, clergy, or health care providers. For most cultures this is not easy, as there is a great deal of shame and blame related to mental problems. Ideally, a careful assessment is made with the family fully involved in the process; and a diagnosis is then given, along with treatment plans, a prognosis, and referrals for services. Everyone is helped to understand the illness and course of treatment, including the expected outcome.

Few families deal with mental illness easily. The family roles may be changed for a number of reasons, but lack of information and poor guidelines for coping are the major reasons why problems occur. Even the most well-adjusted family will be forced to adapt. If they do this through gaining information and education about how best to deal with the ill member, they will become a successfully coping family. For example, their roles may shift as members take on new responsibilities, resulting in parents becoming more involved with the ill member due to increased behavioral demands. Other changes will include finding support from other families, losing friends who cannot cope or are frightened by the ill member, getting time off from work to deal with crises, and finding ways to maintain stable relationships with each of the other members.

Siblings will be faced with fears of becoming ill, too. They also must face the stigma of having a brother or sister who is "crazy." It is not only the person with mental illness who is stigmatized by society, but family members as well. A study conducted by Oestman and Kjellin (2002) showed that a majority of family members experienced stigma by association. In addition, siblings receive less attention from their parents because of the demands of the ill member. Coping involves giving up a lot without getting angry. There is often confusion as to what is the illness and what is simply bad manners, so that expectations of the ill member are sometimes unrealistic. Later, as the family members learn more about managing mental illness, they may feel guilty about earlier demands they made and may even worry that their emotional reactions may have caused the individual to get worse (Bernheim, Lewine, & Beale, 1982).

Crisis and the Family

Because of their close proximity and long history with the individual, family members are more likely than **treatment team** members to recognize an individual's decompensating mental health. The signs of **decompensation**, as described by Meinhardt (1988), are listed in Table 1-1. Families are encouraged to watch for these signs and be able to report them; conversely, clinicians are encouraged to listen to the families' stories in order to understand the current crisis.

Mentally ill persons have crises that are often difficult to predict and manage. Moreover, people respond to crisis differently. Certainly, mental illness can represent a crisis for a family. What is important to remember is that the ideal family

Table 1-1. Signs of Decompensation

Early symptoms	Middle symptoms	Late symptoms
Mood shifts	Drops usual routine	Extreme change in behavior
Poor concentration	Develops erratic sleep pattern	
Preoccupation		Assaultive or destructive
Mild depression	Stops caring for self	
Fears	Loses interest in almost everything	Suicidal thoughts or actions
Altered sleep patterns		
Change in appetite	Depression deepens	Requires hospital stay
Loss of energy	Denial or poor insight	
Withdrawal into isolation	Stops taking medications	

Source: Meinhardt (1988).

response to the crisis of mental illness is rarely the typical response. Figure 1-2 provides guidelines for families to reduce and prepare for the incidence of crisis. While each experience may differ from one family or individual to another, there are some things that families can do.

People are not taught how to be a family. Each partner brings unique experiences to the marriage. Hopefully, these are shared and blended as the couple evolves into a family. Both partners bring strengths and weaknesses to the new unit. It is critical for the professional to assess the family from two perspectives, as individuals and as a group. The strengths, coping skills, typical defenses, responses to past crisis, personality variables, cultural backgrounds, stages in the life cycle, levels of education, understanding and acceptance of mental illness, and levels of personal guilt and feelings of stigma are only a few of the areas to be assessed (Marsh, 1993). It is of utmost importance to take care of each member of the family so that

1. Get to know the members of the treatment team. Know how to contact them for regular questions as well as in emergencies, and how to alert them to increased symptoms.
2. Keep a journal, using a loose leaf notebook. Section it into Health History, Psychiatric History, Medications, Placements, What Works and What Makes Things Worse, Resources. Add any other sections you personally feel are important.
3. Document what is most successful in the journal. This might be having only one or two visitors for dinner rather than a party.
4. Rely on experience with the mentally ill person to tell you when there is subtle, but significant change that might indicate future problems.
5. Do not argue with someone who is mentally ill. It is better to state your thoughts in simple language and then "back off" to allow time for the message to sink in. Keep calm and in control, using a lowered voice.
6. Give the individual time to calm down if upset. Suggest a walk, a nap, listening to music in another part of the house.
7. Call for help if the situation begins to get out of hand. This may be to another family member, or someone on the treatment team. It may also be to the police.
8. Invite a local police officer to your home to meet the ill family member and to get some history regarding past problems and potential help you might need. Establishing a relationship of cooperation and trust may avoid unnecessary stress if they are needed in the future.
9. Don't slip into denial about what is happening. Delaying an intervention may only make things worse. Whenever possible, discuss your concerns with the ill member.
10. Remember that when your family member is becoming out of control, he or she needs you to be in control.

Figure 1-2. Crisis Management Guidelines

they remain healthy and can serve as a continued support to the ill member. The rules on learning to take care of oneself can increase each family member's tolerance for the stress and salvage the family's caring relationship.

As the clinician encourages the family members to develop internal resources, both individually and as a group, they will become more independent, capable, resourceful, and, most of all, accepting of mental illness as a fact of life for them. Crisis management becomes a part of this. No family wants to be in a state of crises all the time, so there is great motivation to learn to reduce the incidence of crises.

Guiding the family from the present situation to healthy coping should be a goal for the clinician. The family can be an important support system for the ill family member. Generally, there are many strengths that can be reinforced among individual members. New roles can be defined that balance the burden, and opportunities to grieve can be provided. Mental illness is a loss—a great loss to the individual, but also a loss to the relatives and friends who lose the person they knew to the effects of the illness.

RESPONSES TO MENTAL ILLNESS

The Individual

What is it like to be mentally ill? The following illustrations include examples of how mental illness has affected individuals differently. Among the responses there are basic categories that emerge: denial, blame, substance use/abuse, isolation, suicidal ideation, and fear. All these areas can benefit from treatment. The most difficult is denial, because if the individual refuses to acknowledge that something is wrong, there is little chance of beginning treatment unless he or she is committed or incarcerated. Even then, if the client refuses treatment, there are laws that prevent it. Clients' rights are strongly protected to the extent that they can refuse treatment to the point that they are a danger to themselves and/or others.

Denial is a common reaction for anyone facing a serious health, social, or personal crisis, and compliance with treatment recommendations is a universal issue in health care. However, the nature of mental illness itself complicates the issue because the often-found symptoms of poor insight and distorted thought processes compound the denial.

CASE ILLUSTRATIONS: Personal Experiences of Mental Illness

- *My family seemed to be a pretty intense bunch—my parents alternated between being very loving toward each other and arguing loudly. I grew up feeling different from most of the people around me. Later, I was diagnosed as having bipolar illness.*
- *I started using drugs and alcohol as a teenager. I always thought that caused me to become mentally ill. Now I know it was more complicated than that. I used drugs to be like everyone else, but it also made me feel better. I didn't*

hear the voices as much. The drugs I take now help with that, too, but I don't like the other ways they make me feel.

- *I have schizophrenia. I guess I'll never find a girlfriend and I'd like to have someone to be close to, to hug.*

- *My family says I have mental illness. But I think I have special powers. I can hear things they can't. Like the traffic outside sometimes has hidden messages in the noise the tires make on the road. Or the music I listen to can do that. Sometimes it tells me bad things, over and over, like, "You're no good, you're no good." Then I feel worthless and want to die. That can be scary.*

- *I hate this illness. It is so hard. And there is nothing I can do about it. Sometimes I just want to die and get it over. The only reason I don't kill myself is because I believe I'll have to come back and live this life all over again if I commit suicide, and I couldn't stand that.*

Once in treatment, the individual must deal with other issues, of which the most common is compliance with medications. Because of the many side effects, medications are often a problem. (See Appendix A for further discussion of medication.) Helping the individual to experience the benefits during the early stages of treatment is difficult because during this phase, the medications are still being tried to see what benefits they provide. It may take months or years to find the best combination for the presenting symptoms. In addition, the diagnosis may not be clearly understood due to the symptoms' complexity.

Some individuals will continue to use alcohol or other substances in spite of being told they should not. Even when they know that this can be extremely dangerous, the addiction is often too great for them to manage. This presents problems in terms of what issues should be given priority. Generally, it is thought that unless the substance abuse is controlled, there is little that one can do about the mental illness. However, more proactive models of practice now incorporate treatment modalities for both substance abuse and mental illness as needed. Getting them into 12-step programs will be difficult if there is also a denial about being mentally ill (see Chapter 10 on substance abuse). These individuals often are seen in homeless shelters or on the streets. They present a great challenge for the treatment professionals as well as the family.

Once the ill person is on medications and stable, other symptoms may present. One of these is isolation. This may be due to a paranoid fear that is not based on reality or to chronic symptoms such as poor motivation. It is very difficult for people on major tranquilizers to get up and out of bed. Depression has a similar effect. The social world collapses and friends are lost. People remember having had a much different life before the illness, but cannot regain it. The resulting sense of loss is great. With it comes a fear of what the future holds. How will they live on limited resources? Where will they go and whom can they trust? Sometimes suicide looks like the best alternative.

There are many questions that face a person with a mental illness. They form the tip of an iceberg that contains a myriad of devastating realities for the individual. Some of these realities are too painful to accept. Moving from disability to ability will surely be an important focus of treatment, as discussed in the following illustration.

CASE ILLUSTRATION: Moving from Disability to Ability

It wasn't until I accepted all of the labels as being conditions that I have (not who I am) that I could begin to get well. I started reading up on manic depression and attending AA [Alcoholics Anonymous] meetings. I took charge of my own wellness. Doctors and therapists weren't going to heal me (though some have been invaluable). Medication alone couldn't do it either. Until I felt the need to remain clean and sober for myself and to stay on medication and monitor my own symptoms, I did not improve. Today, I haven't been hospitalized for five years. I have remarried, have one of my children living with me, and see the other regularly. I have been working full-time for four years, and I accept who I am in a way that I was never able to before.

Discussion

Moving to ability meant acceptance of having a disease, learning about it, remaining clean and sober, and generally "taking charge" of one's own life.

Family Members

Emotions reported by relatives coping with ill family members have been described as including feelings of anxiety, anger, frustration, depression, exhaustion, and helplessness. There are both objective and subjective burdens. *Objective* refers to the demands of the illness on the family; *subjective* refers to the personal suffering of each member due to having a family member with mental illness (Marsh, 1993). The objective burden is substantial and well documented (see, e.g., Hatfield & Lefley, 1993; Marsh, 1993).

Denial is usually a first reaction. One parent can remember hoping that her son was "on drugs" so that he would be better when he stopped using. This same reaction is often stated time and again in the "Caring and Sharing" support groups, sponsored by the **National Alliance for the Mentally Ill (NAMI).** Friends who do not understand the ramifications of the illness believe that the proper discipline of the behaviors would stop them. This makes it difficult to differentiate between denial and stigma. Either one is the product of a basic lack of education about mental illness.

Grief comes after acceptance of the diagnosis and with the realization that the hopes and dreams one had for one's child are no longer possible. The individual has grown and developed into someone who may physically appear the same but has changed dramatically in personality and behavior, often leaving the family mourning the loss of what might have been. This is further complicated during any remissions or periods of stabilization, when there may be the hope that a cure has been effected. The family is thrown back into the grieving process with each subsequent episode. Unlike grief from death, this grieving process can be as cyclic as the illness, undergoing no resolution. It will be important to work with the family to develop coping skills and an understanding of this process (Bernheim & Lehman, 1985).

Guilt can be as devastating as any of the other emotions. To believe that one has caused the mental illness in a loved one can make the family burden even greater. Without education about the possible genetic and viral causes of mental illness, each family member may think it was caused by something he or she said or did to the ill person. Mothers are especially vulnerable to this situation, which in the past was the main focus of blame, especially by professionals. The term *schizophrenogenic mother*, coined in the early 1950s, refers to a parenting style that is cold, rejecting, distant, aloof, and yet dominating. This might also be the style of the father, but the mother was the primary target because of the relatively longer time the children spent with the nonworking mother in those days. In addition, siblings who feel thankfulness that they did not get the disease often experience a form of survivor guilt.

Questions asked of family members by insensitive clinicians, such as, "What did you do to cause this break?" or "What was going on at home?" contribute to the guilt. The family must be aided in understanding that they were responding to bizarre behavior and did the best they could. They did not cause the illness. A genetic predisposition may have been present, and for some, the symptoms simply manifest themselves when an environmental stressor was introduced, such as the death of a parent, experimental drug use, a heavy work or school schedule, moving from home, or the breakup of a relationship. Only more research will allow a true understanding of this process.

Fear can destroy a family. For example, the siblings may fear that they will become ill, too. A very real physical fear can also exist because the ill relative may be frightening and sometimes threatening. A study conducted by Vaddadi, Gilleard, and Fryer (2002) indicated that a significant number of family members and caregivers of those with mental illness experience verbal and physical abuse. Often parents relate that they are afraid of their children because of the anger displayed. Many families have used restraining orders to control the angry mentally ill member from attacking them. One mother was forced to use a gun in self-defense when her son ran toward her in anger. She fired the gun to stop him and accidentally killed him, causing a tragedy no parent should have to experience.

While those with a mental illness are no more violent than the normal population, the family is often the target of their anger. There are any number of reasons for their rage and frustration. The ill member may be aware that the siblings are getting on with their lives while he or she is, in effect, on a treadmill, or even becoming worse. They may feel that the parents should be giving them money or material goods and are out of touch with reality. Their symptoms may result in cognitive impairment and poor judgment affecting their relationships with family members. The frustration and anger expressed by the ill person can be very frightening to the family and creates an added burden.

Diminished socialization from the stigma and embarrassment evoked by an ill relative affects the entire family. Large family get-togethers become a thing of the past, either because of the behavior of the ill person and avoidance of other family members or because of protective feelings for that person. Family holiday celebrations become too difficult for siblings and their friends or extended family and, over a period of time, may even cease to happen. "Can we take a chance and invite the Joneses to the wedding, or will their mentally ill son be too disruptive?" "Will the stress of attempting to control my behavior be too much and cause an embarrassing episode?" "How can a family be included when one of the members always causes embarrassment or chaos?" Typically, the entire family will become excluded from the social events.

CONFLICTS

The confidentiality of client information and the involvement of the family in treatment decisions does, at times, create conflict between families and the mental health system. The following sections describe some of the issues related to these conflicts as perceived by family members.

Confidentiality Issues

A mother recently expressed her frustration with the health care system because her adult son, who resides with her, was hospitalized after he stopped taking his medication and decompensated. When she called the hospital she could not get confirmation that he was there, due to confidentiality laws in her state. (Each state has such laws, which vary somewhat but effectively protect the adult psychiatric client from any information being given out without his or her express written consent.) The mother, as the primary caregiver, was not informed about medication changes, treatment, or discharge plans. The son was over 18 years of age; thus, the treatment professionals were bound by the laws of confidentiality. There had been no release-of-information form signed by the son to give permission to talk with his mother. She asked that they do this, but it did not happen until she and her husband went to the hospital with the forms and made the request in person. Even then, it was only with the son's persistence that the forms were signed.

The confidentiality laws are so protective of individual rights that they can interfere with continuity of care. When the family caregivers are not included, the continuity of care is greatly diminished. Often the family has the best record of effective medications and treatment over the years and can be invaluable as a resource in the treatment planning. It is seldom likely that ill persons can give accurate information at times when they have decompensated. Records are not conveyed easily from one place to another, so medications are often changed or interrupted, delaying stabilization. Often the parent or another family caregiver—who may be the only person who knows what works—is the last person asked because of the confidentiality laws.

Many family members now understand the law and have found ways of sharing information in times of crisis that will not violate the rules of confidentiality or the rights of the ill individual. In particular, families are permitted to share information with professionals even though the professional is not permitted to share information with them. Providing a history of the course of the illness and a list of helpful medications can aid in the treatment. Many professionals recognize the value of the family as a part of the treatment team. Sometimes everyone can work through a case manager who has a signed release form on file.

Treatment Issues

Information about medications can be critical to the timely care of a client, but past history about experiences with medication is often necessary in order to prescribe the most useful drug or prevent serious complications. One family member may explain: "We know that our son is extremely sensitive to certain medications. There is one in particular that has immediate, extreme side effects. One of the reasons our son refuses medications is the fear of experiencing these side effects again." Without the family input, this individual is at risk of being given a medication that has had poor results in the past, thus further reinforcing the belief that medicines are bad.

In addition, there may be other kinds of family information that can be helpful. For example, one family told of their son relapsing for seemingly no apparent reason. On further inquiry, the mother suggested that the death of his grandfather and, six months later, the death of one of the family dogs were the triggering events that caused the man to become confused and stop taking prescribed medications. She stated that he showed no emotion and was unable to cry or mourn. Obviously there was sadness, but it was unexpressed, and his inability to know how to deal with the deaths was a critical factor in the relapse.

Many treating professionals want to hear about the significant events that are stressors for their clients, but the time constraints of managed care often do not permit this. This man's doctor had no way of knowing about the deaths without the parents sharing that information. Because the man had schizophrenia, he was not considered a good candidate for insight-oriented therapy and was not being seen by a therapist who might have discussed these losses with him (see Chapter 6 on schizophrenia). People with psychosis are often discounted when it comes to therapy needs, even as it relates to the normal events for which one might be expected to have difficulty in coping. By regular check-ins with the family, such stressors can be identified and worked through.

Another treatment issue is the value of having the family monitor any medication side effects while the individual is living at home. It is important that the family understand the medications, their use, possible side effects, and what to do if there are problems. Education generally covers this, but the family that is excluded from treatment will not be given this information, as is shown in the next case illustration.

CASE ILLUSTRATION: Family and Medication Management

One mother remembers how her son visited for the weekend. After noticing him becoming increasingly agitated and confused, she called his residential facility to report her observations and was told that the cause was probably the reduced dosage of medicine he was on. His medications had been decreased the day before he was to go home, yet the family was not advised of this. The mother just remembers that she was terrified that there would be a crisis again and the police would need to be called. Her anxiety could have been avoided had the family been told about the reduced medications.

There are, of course, times when the ill individual does not wish to have the family involved. This presents additional problems for the continuity of care. One of the recent outcomes of grass-roots support is the **consumers' movement.** The voice of the mentally ill grows stronger as more individuals come "out of the closet" to speak of their experiences and complain about treatment. This has resulted in **client-driven services** in most states, such as California, New York, and Minnesota. As the individual with a mental illness gains a voice in his or her own care, the family may be less involved. This presents a problem when there is a crisis because it is helpful to have all members of the support/treatment team involved in the intervention. Establishing healthy relationships prior to a crisis will help maintain involvement.

Education and careful mediation between members by the health professional are important. After establishing a trusting relationship among members, setting rules and roles about communication may be possible, with contracts written about how this will work. A treatment team that includes all the caregivers and the individual with the mental illness can generally work out solutions to potential problems and include the perspective of both the mentally ill family member and the family. The **consumer empowerment** office and the **self-help** movement are of great assistance in this area. With the advent of newer, improved medications we see less side effects and better results for many. Consumers can now participate in self-help and consumer empowerment and many can now return to the workforce.

INVOLVEMENT OF FAMILY IN THE TREATMENT REGIME

Because of the prevailing attitude toward parents, and especially mothers, during the 1950s and 1960s, families of the seriously mentally ill were generally considered dysfunctional. When psychiatric hospitals were closed in the early 1960s, people with mental illness were forced into communities across the nation. The result was an increase of persons in other institutions, such as nursing homes and the criminal justice system (Talbot, 1988), more homeless (Bachrach, 1988), and more families taking in a mentally ill son or daughter.

Recent research showing that many mental illnesses are neurobiological diseases with a genetic base has gone far in changing the attitudes of professionals toward parents. Today, there is less blaming, more openness, and a greater willingness to work with families. Advocacy work by the NAMI has also helped to change attitudes toward families with a mentally ill member.

NAMI support groups began to spring up across the country 25 years ago. At one time, there was a new group forming every 15 minutes. Families were so hungry for information and help in dealing with mental illness. The stigma that kept these diseases in the closet came under attack as conferences and workshops sprang up. Mental illness still carries tremendous stigma, but with families receiving grass-roots support, the pain and suffering are being reduced. One outcome of this is the inclusion of the family on the treatment team. The typical treatment team has many different players and each has a role in contributing to the care of the individual with a mental illness, including the mentally ill individual (Woolis, 1992). Throughout this text, the concept of team is discussed. Depending on the setting, the disciplines represented may vary, but it is always optimum to include both the client and interested family when possible.

Family Education

Often the family members have been so immersed in meeting one crisis after another that they have had little or no information about the illness itself. If they have been given a diagnosis, they will usually make every effort to learn about the disorder. It is not unusual for health professionals to provide a list of reading material for family members, but the most important help is information presented in a clear format with an opportunity for questions and answers. This is provided in classes and workshops across the country. Mental health professionals who offer these classes generally are impressed with the level of insight, interest, and commitment on the part of the families in attendance. The authors' own experience in working with family support groups confirms this.

The course outline generally follows a historical perspective of mental illness, including myths, diagnostic criteria for mood disorders, thought disorders and anxiety disorders, treatment therapies in common usage, medications and side effects, legal aspects, community supports, symptom management, and communication skill building. Often a support group will evolve from these courses, providing ongoing information sharing among members and consultation with the mental health professional. NAMI will continue the successful "caring and sharing" or support groups that have been ongoing. NAMI also offers a 12-week educational program called Family-to-Family. The reception of this program has been almost overwhelming. New programs are being started that will train consumers to present a program to fellow consumers. They are tentatively named Peer-to-Peer, Living with Schizophrenia and Other Mental Illnesses, or NAMI Cares.

One of the most important outcomes of these courses and workshops is a growing appreciation of the family in coping with difficult to treat symptoms. This has resulted in a paradigm shift away from blame and pathologizing the family. Instead, the family is seen as competent and capable. A study conducted by Doornbos (1996) concluded that "although the families of the mentally ill have significantly more stressors than normative families, they have clear strengths relative to family coping and the family health subconcepts of adaptability and conflict management" (p. 214). Given the tools, family members can be excellent team partners. The **competency model** (Marsh, 1993) offers many advantages.

While this model has long been used in education, when applied to the mentally ill, it offers a more positive approach for working with the family. Accordingly, the mental health professional focuses on competencies and competence deficits rather than on functional and dysfunctional family systems. In other words, it is not what the family is doing wrong, but what it is doing right, in spite of the illness.

Four areas have been identified as important for families to accomplish. The mental health professional will appreciate the family's growth and development as the members gain experience and ability in these areas. (These areas are described in Figure 1-3.) The family has adaptational attributes that can be operationalized to cope with mental illness. This provides a good framework for working with and understanding the family and can facilitate alliances between families and professionals. It is empowering and allows family members to actively acquire greater competency in coping with the mentally ill individual.

Two important aspects of adaptation are learning effective communication skills and creating a supportive environment. Both have usually been skewed due to the family members' responses to the symptoms of the illness. It is important to assess how the family has changed as a result of trying to cope with these symptoms. Often, one discovers a very guarded atmosphere where everyone fears they will upset the mentally ill individual. They may be rendered speechless and help-

Cognitive Attributes
- Understanding of the illness and treatment as well as a solid knowledge of community resources.
- Understanding the prognosis and having realistic expectations.
- Being able to adapt to the demands of the illness.

Behavioral Attributes
- Communication skills including conflict resolution, problem solving, and assertiveness.
- Stress management and behavior management.

Emotional Attributes
- Maintaining a stable emotional climate and mature defenses within the family.
- Resolving the emotional burden of mental illness in the family.

Social Attributes
- Achieving a normal balance of activities for all family members.
- Use of support networks, both formal and informal, and friendships.
- Developing outside interests and activities.
- Collaboration with professionals.
- Becoming advocates in the community.

Figure 1-3. Competency Model

less by such fear. In other families, there is a great deal of disagreement as to what is wrong and how to deal with the ill person. One parent may think the other is being too lenient, while siblings may be jealous of so much attention being given to the mentally ill member. Arguing may result, throwing the household into a constant state of agitation and stress.

Much has been written about communication with mentally disabled people. One parent stated her guide as, "Say it in five words or less." This had gotten her by for the most part. Figure 1-4 suggests other ways in which families can learn to communicate more effectively. The suggestions are also helpful for health care professionals, particularly when the individual is in the acute stages of illness or the early stages of treatment. Knowing what to say in a difficult situation is critical to feeling competent about being in control and able to avoid an argument or crisis.

By helping the family members to see how the illness has caused changes in themselves in response to the symptoms, they can begin to learn new ways to cope. Establishing a supportive environment that is not overly stimulating will be important if the ill member is to live at home. This may not be possible, in which case the family will need to learn of other options, such as residential programs. Adapting may require being able to accept some of the symptoms, such as

---

It is often helpful to use the following guidelines when communicating to someone with a mental illness.

1. Keep it simple—when confused or hearing voices, it is difficult to discriminate and understand what is being said. Also, if feeling depressed it takes a real effort to listen if the message is too complex.
2. Repeat if necessary—sometimes the message is not heard completely and needs repeating. Also, asking to repeat it may help to know if the listener really heard you.
3. Give only one message at a time. If you ask too many questions, or say too many things, it will further confuse the individual.
4. Speak slowly and calmly. How you deliver the message often determines how it is received.
5. Don't argue over delusions. Don't agree, either. Simply state you don't have the same view and change the subject.
6. Remember you are talking to someone who may have difficulty understanding. Be patient and empathic. Don't talk down. You are speaking to another adult, not a child.
7. Speak with respect. Self-esteem is important in getting cooperation and understanding. You can have a role in assuring improved self-esteem gained from a satisfying communication that is respectful.
8. Be solution oriented, not problem oriented.
9. Know when to terminate the conversation and leave—or stay, and enjoy a quiet nonverbal communication with your loved one.

Figure 1-4.   Effective Communication

delusions, hallucinations, or poor motivation. For example, it is hard to watch someone struggle while hearing voices, but the family can learn ways to reduce the stimuli that tend to increase auditory hallucinations. Being able to have realistic expectations of the mentally ill member regarding family activities, family burdens, and changed family roles will be important to explore.

Much of this exploration will be directly related to how the ill individual responds to treatment. Do the family members understand the treatment and any possible limitations? Do they know the risks versus benefits of medications? Are they aware that there is no cure and, for many, no return to their former life? Have they had enough experience with the illness to be able to predict causes and effects? This is very important if the family is to have some measure of control over the illness and be able to communicate to the professionals about what has happened in the past or may happen in the future.

The family members are the historians. They know by a look or a remark when something is not right and an individual is changing for the worse. They have been living with the illness and can be of critical importance in preventing a crisis. By listening to their alerts, mental health professionals can save precious resources of time and money by responding in a timely manner to the individual's changing status.

A supportive environment is very important to the ill relative's recovery and continued stabilization. It is also critical for the caregiver. Sensitivity to the tension and stress on the family are important factors to consider when creating an environment that meets the needs of both. Ultimately, this may mean that the family cannot have the ill person live at home. However, if they do decide to have the ill member live with them, family caregivers can be taught to:

• Keep things calm and quiet
• Create a predictable schedule
• Use words carefully
• Support growth of confidence and self-esteem
• Help the ill person come to terms with the illness
• Come to terms with their own changed lives

THE PROFESSIONAL WORKING WITH FAMILIES

The exhaustion known to professionals as "burnout" is also likely to be felt by families and caretakers of people with persistent mental illness. The burden of day-to-day demands and sacrifices of families and caregivers is well documented (Doornbos, 2002; Obloy & Hutcheson, 2002; Rose, Mallinson, & Walton-Moss, 2002; Stengard, 2002). By helping families cope, develop realistic expectations, talk about their experiences privately or in a group, and deal with stigma, the professional can reduce the potential for burnout. The simple act of cooperating and sharing information includes rather than excludes the family. Developing trust with family members will establish a collaborative interaction that can improve the timeliness of interventions and reduce hospitalizations (Bernheim & Lehman, 1985).

The professional must develop empathy for the family caregiver. By understanding the burden that mental illness places on the family, the professional can offer sincere assistance for coping, thus helping the family to continue as the caregiver. One of the most important aspects of this process is establishing a balance between the ill person's needs and those of the other family members. As the latter gain education and experience in managing and coping with the symptoms and behaviors of the ill person, they will find more time to spend on themselves. It is important that they avoid becoming burned out or overstressed. Figure 1-5 provides guidelines for managing the inevitable increase in stress. The ability to find humor and have a life apart from the role of caregiver are important aspects of this process (Dearth, Labenski, Mott, & Pellegrini, 1986).

Stress management classes are given all over the country, but families often do not realize the tremendous amount of stress they undergo on a day-to-day basis. Offering simple stress management exercises can greatly relieve them. The following list provides guidelines for managing the inevitable stress involved in being a caregiver.

1. Learn a simple breathing exercise that can be used whenever stressors increase.
2. Join a support group and attend one meeting a month for support and one meeting a month for education.
3. Identify a member or two from your support group that can be available when you need to "check in" with someone.
4. Offer to volunteer in your local organization. As you give, you learn that you are not alone and helping others often makes one feel better about oneself.
5. Find a place in your home or garden that can be your special retreat, even for a few minutes a day. Use it to remind yourself that you deserve a moment of peace away from the stress. If you can, visualize that place and the feelings of calm you have when you are there, at other times during the day when you cannot be physically present in your retreat area.
6. Get regular exercise, eat regular meals that are balanced, and get plenty of rest. You need to take care of yourself before you can care for others.
7. Find your spiritual core. Somewhere, regardless of religion or culture, there is a place in all of us where we have our center of understanding and acceptance of ourselves. If you find this in church or temple, then maintain your connection to this support.
8. What other ways do you know that reduce your stress? Make a list and hang it where you can be reminded of them.

Figure 1-5.   Stress Management Guidelines

Family caregivers also need exercise, rest, regular and healthy meals, and time to socialize and play. Parents need time for intimacy, and everyone needs privacy. Paying attention to a family environment that provides for these needs will go a long way toward preventing burnout and reducing tension and stress.

The emotional response that the family members experience in adapting to their relative's illness needs to be recognized as normal. Providing encouragement to talk about their feelings and start taking care of themselves is of primary importance. Through education they can gain a better understanding of mental illness, and through sharing experiences they can learn that they are not the only family with these problems and concerns. This will promote growth and compassion among the family members both toward their ill relative and toward each other.

THE ROLE OF OCCUPATIONAL THERAPY

Throughout this book there are multiple discussions of occupational therapy intervention. These discussions are for the most part appropriately focused on the individual receiving services. However, the definition of "client" in the Occupational Therapy Practice Framework (2002) is expanded to include individuals who are involved in supporting the primary client, such as family, and also groups or populations relative to the individual, such as organizations or community groups.

Hospitals and other institutions traditionally have family visiting hours in the evenings when the majority of the therapy staff is not present. The rationale for this was that valuable therapy time would not be in competition with family visits. However, the result is that there is very little interaction between therapists and family members, who therefore often do not understand the services being provided to their family members.

The growth of community-based practice and a growing awareness of family roles in treatment have increased the inclusion of the greater community in practice. Occupational therapists' adopting a broad definition of the "client" must create opportunities to advocate and educate both the family and the community at large.

ADVOCACY AND SUPPORT NETWORKING

Stigma has brought many individuals together in the fight for acceptance and self-esteem. Recently, a number of famous persons have been identified as having a mental illness and becoming successful in spite of their disabilities, including Abraham Lincoln, Ludwig van Beethoven, Patty Duke, Ernest Hemingway, Leo Tolstoy, Tennessee Williams, Dan Rather, and Carrie Fischer. Reducing stigma has helped to strengthen the determination among the mentally disabled to fight for better treatment, parity in benefits for other health problems, and rights as consumers through a grievance process.

A number of consumer, family, and community groups have arisen directly from the community mental health system. Many are actively engaged in changing the way treatment is provided, improving expedient access to care, developing housing and housing support programs, seeking increased funding, fighting for parity through legislation, advocating client rights and equal entitlements under the Americans with Disabilities Act, the federal legislation that guaranteed equal civil rights to individuals with disabilities, and any number of issues and concerns that surface at the local and national levels. Some of these organizations are listed in Appendix B.

Summary

The effects of mental illness reach far beyond the afflicted individual. They touch the family, friends, and caregivers as well. How the symptoms are managed depends to a great degree on the amount of information provided by the mental health professional. In addition, the cultural perspective will often dictate the level of shame and stigma that must be overcome and how treatment will be provided.

The stress of coping with a persistent, serious mental illness can create challenging problems to be addressed by the treatment professionals. Including all support members in treatment has proven helpful, especially with the current general reduction in resources. Sometimes the genetic aspect of mental illness is evidenced in families, and more than one member has symptoms that are difficult to understand and accept. This may cause roles to change and communication to be strained and ineffective. Some of the emotions that must be dealt with are guilt, shame, fear, denial, grief, isolation, depression, and anger. Confidentiality laws complicate open discussion about the ill family member, and as a result, treatment plans must include methods to assure all members of the treatment team be included at times of crisis and in planning for intervention and prevention.

The family offers a resource to monitor changes in symptoms, provide history, support treatment goals, and assist with housing and the regular taking of medication. It also provides an important social network for the ill individual. Support groups such as NAMI have promoted advocacy and education about mental illness. Education of both the family and the individual has improved understanding of the effects of the illness on both. Classes on stress management, understanding helpful responses to symptoms, improving socialization skills, and generally preventing burnout have allowed family members to return to fulfilling personal goals and achieving an improved quality of life.

Consumer groups have likewise provided a safe means to come forward for many individuals who have been too ashamed or afraid to admit they have a mental illness. As advocacy and support networks grow and as more and more famous personalities share their own perspectives of living with a mental illness, stigma will be reduced for both the individuals and the families. The caring professional who can adapt to working with the family as a resource and respect the mentally ill individual as potentially rehabilitatable, will come to appreciate the tremendous strengths and determination of those they serve.

The only true enemy is mental illness . . . not one another.

Review Questions

1. What are the effects of mental illness on the family?
2. How are family roles and rules changed by mental illness?
3. What are some points to remember for improving communications within the family?
4. Who are the members of a treatment team and what are their roles?
5. How can inclusion of the family enhance the treatment team?

References

Bachrach, L. L. (1988). The homeless mentally ill. In W. W. Menninger & G. T. Hannah (Eds.), *The chronic mental patient II* (pp. 65–91). Washington, DC: American Psychiatric Press.

Beer, D. (2003). The illness and disability experience from an individual perspective. In E. Crepeau, E. Cohn, & B. Schell (Eds.), *Willard and Spackman's occupational therapy*. Philadelphia: Lippincott Williams & Wilkins.

Bernheim, K., & Lehman, A. (1985). *Working with families of the mentally ill*. New York: Norton.

Bernheim, R., Lewine, R., & Beale, C. (1982). *The caring family: Living with chronic mental illness*. Chicago: Contemporary.

Dearth, N., Labenski, B., Mott, M. E., & Pellegrini, L. (1986). *Families helping families: Living with schizophrenia*. New York: Norton.

Doornbos, M. (1996). The strengths of families coping with serious mental illness. *Archives of Psychiatric Nursing, 10*(4), 214–220.

Doornbos, M. (2002). Predicting family health in families of young adults with severe mental illness. *Journal of Family Nursing, 8*(3), 241–263.

Hatfield, A., & Lefley, H. (1993). *Surviving mental illness: Stress, coping and adaptation*. New York: Guilford.

Marsh, D. (1993). *Families and mental illness: New directions in professional practice*. Westport, CT: Praeger.

Mattingly, C., & Lawlor, M. (2003). The illness and disability experience from a family perspective. In E. Crepeau, E. Cohn, & B. Schell (Eds.), *Willard and Spackman's occupational therapy*. Philadelphia: Lippincott Williams & Wilkins.

Meinhardt, K. (1988). *Early symptoms recognition workshop*. Workshop presented to Santa Clara County Mental Health Department, San Jose, CA.

Molineux, M., & Rickard, W. (2003). Storied approaches to understanding occupation. *Journal of Occupational Science, 10*(1), 52–60.

Obloy, C., & Hutcheson, S. (2002). Planned lifetime assistance network: A new service model with promising results. *Psychiatric Rehabilitation Journal, 25*(4), 409–412.

Oestman, M., & Kjellin, L. (2002). Stigma by association: Psychological factors in relatives of people with mental illness. *British Journal of Psychiatry, 18*(6), 494–498.

Occupational Therapy Practice Framework: Domain and Process. (2002). *American Journal of Occupational Therapy, 56*(6), 614–639.

Pharoah, F. M., Mari, J. J., & Streiner, D. (2002). Family intervention for schizophrenia (Cochrane Review). In *The Cochrane Library*, 3. Oxford: Update Software.

Pollock, N., & McColl, M. A. (1998). Assessment in client-centered occupational therapy. In M. Law (Ed.), *Client Centered Therapy*. Thorofare, NJ: Slack.

Rose, L., Mallinson, R. K., & Walton-Moss, B. (2002). A grounded theory of families responding to mental illness. *Western Journal of Nursing Research, 24*(5), 516–536.

Stengard, E. (2002). Caregiving types and psychosocial well-being of caregivers of people with mental illness in Finland. *Psychiatric Rehabilitation Journal, 26*(2), 154–164.

Talbot, J. A. (1988). The chronic adult mentally ill: What do we now know, and why aren't we implementing what we know? In W. W. Menninger & G. T. Hanna (Eds.), *The chronic mental patient II* (pp. 1–29). Washington, DC: American Psychiatric Press.

Vaddadi, K. S., Gilleard, C., & Fryer, H. (2002). Abuse of carers by relatives with severe mental illness. *International Journal of Social Psychiatry, 48*(2), 149–155.

Woolis, R. (1992). *When someone you know has a mental illness: A handbook for family, friends, and caregivers.* New York: Tarcher/Perigee.

Suggested Reading

Andreasen, N. (1984). *The broken brain: The biological revolution in psychiatry.* New York: Harper & Row.

Andreasen, N. (2001). *Conquering mental illness in the era of the genome.* New York: Oxford University Press.

Cooney, C. (1986). *Don't blame the music.* New York: Putnam.

Duke, P., & Turan, K. (1987). *Call me Anna.* New York: Bantam.

Fieve, R. E. (1975). *Mood swing.* New York: Bantam.

Fuller Torrey, E. (2001). *Surviving schizophrenia: A manual for families, consumers, and providers* (4th ed.). New York: Harper Trade.

Heriot, J., & Polinger, E. (Eds.). (2002). *The use of personal narratives in the helping professions: A teaching casebook.* Binghamton, NY: Haworth.

Hyland, B. (1987). *The girl with the crazy brother.* Danbury, CT: Franklin Watts.

Isaac, R., & Armat, V. (1990). *Madness in the streets: How psychiatry and the law abandoned the mentally ill.* New York: Free Press.

Johnson, J. (1988). *Hidden victims: An eight-stage healing process for families and friends of the mentally ill.* New York: Doubleday.

Lefley, H. P. (1996). *Family caregiving in mental illness.* Thousand Oaks, CA: Sage.

Marsh, D. T. (1998). *Serious mental illness and the family.* New York: Wiley.

Papolos, D., & Papolos, J. (1987). *Overcoming depression.* New York: Harper & Row.

Sheehan, S. (1983). *Is there no place on earth for me?* New York: Random House.

Walsh, M. (1986). *Schizophrenia: Straight talk for families and friends.* New York: William Morrow.

Environmental and Cultural Considerations

Anne MacRae, PhD, OTR/L

Key Terms

allopathic
Ayurvedic
cultural blindness
culture-bound syndromes
Feng-Shui
least restrictive environment
Monochronic (M-time)

moxibustion
Polychronic (P-time)
polyculturalism
proxemics
TM/CAM
universal design

Chapter Outline

Introduction

"Context (including physical, social, personal, spiritual, temporal, and virtual) refers to a variety of interrelated conditions within and surrounding the client that influence performance" (Occupational Therapy Practice Framework, 2002, p. 623). Contextual factors "represent the complete background of an individual's life and living. They include environmental factors and personal factors that may have an effect on the individual with a health condition" (WHO, 2001, p. 16). This chapter is organized using the concepts of environment and culture, while recognizing that these concepts are interrelated with all of the contextual areas outlined by the American Occupational Therapy Association (AOTA) and the World Health Organization (WHO). Environmental and cultural considerations have unique implications for mental health as occupational therapists (OTs) work together with their clients toward the goal of "ecological well being" (Wilcock, 1998, p. 107).

ENVIRONMENT

The role of environment in health is of critical importance in all of the health care disciplines and is discussed in both clinical and theoretical terms throughout the scholarly literature. Recently, environmental considerations for health have also been a focus for many non-health related disciplines, such as architecture, as well as becoming a prominent theme in the popular literature. Although occupational therapists have always been and will continue to be involved in adapting existing environments, there is now a trend toward **univeral design**, which "is defined as the design of products and environments to be usable by all people, to the greatest extent possible, without adaptation or specialized design" (Christophersen, 2002, p. 13). The benefits of universal design are in its ultimate cost-effectiveness and reduction of stigma often associated with adapted environments for people with disabilities. Occupational therapists are urged to increase their awareness and use of universal design, as it "contributes to a person's health and well-being by facilitating participation in life's occupations in the areas of self-care, productivity and leisure" (Canadian Association of Occupational Therapists, 2003, p. 1). The move toward universal design has gained momentum throughout the world in the past decade but nowhere is it more evident than in Norway, where the Norwegian State Housing Bank has created incentives and projects geared toward the inclusion of universal design in the curricula of "architects, planners, designers, engineers, occupational therapists and craftsmen" (Christophersen, 2002, p. 7).

Well-developed universal design concepts are not limited to the physical needs of individuals but also take into account the personal, social, emotional, and cognitive contexts of the inhabitants, which all have particular significance for people with mental illness. For example, one of the principles of universal design is "simple and intuitive use," meaning designs that accommodate an individual's cognitive and linguistic skills as well as level of education and experience. Appliances with unfamiliar or complicated components may add to the confusion or agitation of a client, which ultimately will affect her or his ability to function in the environment. Another principle of universal design is "tolerance for error," meaning that the "design minimizes hazards and adverse consequences of accidental or unintended actions" (Christophersen, 2002, p. 14). Clients with poor judgment, impulsivity, or memory deficits may experience burns, electrical shock, or trauma through interaction with poorly designed elements in the built environment.

Interest in such philosophies as **Feng-Shui**, a Chinese art form that is concerned with how energies of the environment interact with individuals and their dwellings, has greatly increased as people strive to attain an emotional and spiritual balance in fast-paced and stressful environments (Wong, 1996). Although it is a specific cultural practice, Feng-Shui and universal design both propose simplifying the environment. This is in direct contrast to the often cluttered and chaotic physical environments in which people with mental illness may live. Social, particularly economic, realities may limit the ability to create an optimal environment, but even small changes may assist people with mental illness in feeling more calm, safe, and organized.

The Natural and Built Environment

Universal design primarily refers to the built environment (created by human beings). Experiencing the natural environment, however, has widespread appeal and is seen by many people as a critical element of mental health. A walk on the beach, in a park, or in woodlands may provide relaxation and stress reduction as well as a mechanism for the development of healthy hobbies and leisure pursuits. For some individuals, the natural environment is crucial in establishing a meditative or reflective state of mind. As elements of nature seem to be particularly important in developing a healthful environment, there has been an increased interest in combining the natural world with the built environment. For example, the role of gardens and animals in a balanced environment is the topic of many studies related to health care (Perrins-Margalis, Rugletic, Schepis, Stepanski, & Walsh, 2000; Barker & Dawson, 1998; Cole & Gawlinski, 2000).

Hammon, Kellegrew, and Jaffe, (2000) concluded that pet ownership can be a meaningful and significant occupation and studies on the use of animals in conjunction with occupational therapy have demonstrated improved social interac-

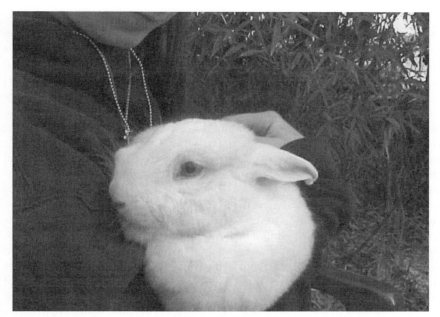

Figure 2-1.   The Soft Fur of a Rabbit Providing Comfort

tion among clients (Fick, 1993; Roenke & Mulligan, 1998). Figure 2-1 is an example of the potential calming and nurturing effects of interaction with an animal.

Animals and plants are often used by occupational therapists to facilitate nurturing and a sense of connectedness as well as help develop the roles and responsibilities of daily living. Appendix B includes resources for information on horticulture and pet therapy that may assist the occupational therapist in designing adjunctive interventions or enhanced environments. However, animals and plants should not be viewed as a panacea for all dysfunction nor are they a replacement for comprehensive occupational therapy. Plants and animals may provide a mechanism for achieving or enhancing therapeutic outcomes, but occupational therapists must use their clinical judgment and skill in activity and environmental analysis to determine the specific uses, benefits, and risks for particular clients. Included in such an analysis is the determination of personal and cultural attitudes, as well as the risk of infection, injury, or allergic reactions.

Occupational Therapy and the Environment

"A unique concept within client-centered occupational therapy is the acknowledgment that clients are not divorced from the environments and community in which they live, work and play" (Law & Mills, 1998, p. 15). That occupation occurs in a context appears to be obvious, and it has always been embedded in the thinking of occupational therapy. However, in recent years renewed emphasis on the role of the environment has been found in the occupational therapy literature

(Creek, 1997; Hagedorn, 2001; Kielhofner, 1995; Rowles, 2003; Schade & Schultz, 1992; Schwartzberg, 2002). There are also several conceptual or practice models in occupational therapy that specifically address the role of the environment in occupational performance and that can be used to promote overall mental and physical well-being. Among them are the Person-Environment-Occupational Performance Model (Christiansen & Baum, 1997); the Ecology of Human Performance Model (Dunn, Brown, & McGuigan, 1994); and the Person-Environment Occupation Model (Law, Cooper, Strong, Steward, Rigby, & Letts, 1996).

In terms of practice, the most obvious environmental role of the occupational therapist is related to architectural barriers and adapting the physical environment for increased accessibility. However, this practice primarily focuses on people with physical disabilities when, in fact, occupational therapy has much to offer in environmental adaptation for those with mental illness. One of the hallmarks of Claudia Allen's cognitive disability theory (1985) is that the environment or the tasks within an environment must be adapted to meet the cognitive level of the client in order for that client to function at her or his best. By using the Allen's Cognitive Levels (ACL) assessment, a therapist can determine what kind of structure and environmental cues are needed to engage the client in task completion. The occupational therapists' role when applying the cognitive disabilities theory is that the focus is more on changing the task or environment rather than the person. Assessing a client's level of cognitive function and the ability to predict how well the client will be able to care for himself or herself is valuable information for the entire treatment team in determining discharge environments and appropriate aftercare needs.

Brown (2001) suggests using the Adult Sensory Profile Assessment to determine with the client the optimum environment for her or his sensory processing preferences. This assessment is based on Dunn's Model of Sensory Processing, "which describes the intersection of neurological threshold and behavioral responses resulting in the following four quadrants: sensory sensitivity, sensation avoiding, low registration and sensation seeking" (Brown, 2001, p. 115). Sensory processing deficits are very common in serious mental illness (see Chapter 6 on schizophrenia for further discussion) and are probably more common in the general population than generally recognized. Therefore, this assessment provides valuable information in determining optimum environments and needed adaptation. Although occupational therapists have made important contributions to the understanding and evaluation of the physical, cognitive, and sensory aspects of the environment, further research needs to be done on addressing the environment in its totality. This includes all components of occupational performance (motor, sensory, cognitive, emotional, and spiritual) as they relate to the environment.

Mental Health Treatment Environments

Mental health occupational therapy is provided in a wide variety of treatment settings. Among the most common are inpatient hospitals with both locked and unlocked units, outpatient clinics, day treatment programs, and partial hospital-ization programs. In addition, occupational therapists specializing in mental health are developing programs in many so-called "nontraditional" sites, includ-ing home health care, vocational and community programs, jails and prisons, homeless shelters, and private practices. Many of these sites are discussed in chapters throughout this book, and, although divergent in appearance, they are all appropriate venues for occupational therapy services. It is common practice in mental health to attempt to treat a client in the **least restrictive environment,** meaning the environment with the optimum balance of individual freedoms and supervision for the client to function. However, as discussed throughout this chapter, there are many variables in the optimum environment for function; restrictions are simply among them.

Regardless of the treatment setting, and in many cases despite some of the limitations of the treatment setting, occupational therapists place great impor-tance on the environment in the occupational therapy (OT) process. This has been documented since the early writings of the profession. In 1954, Wade and Franciscus stated the following:

An orderly, well-kept, attractive unit is good mental hygiene in itself and is important for the morale of patient and therapist alike. It gives to the patient a feeling of order and direction rather than one of chaos and indi-rection. All supplies and equipment should have a given place in which to be kept when not in use, and the therapist must assume the responsibili-ty of seeing that each item is returned to its proper place, not merely pushed aside in a heap on a shelf until it is impossible to locate desired items as they are needed. In addition, a working area need not be drab and depressing, for with ingenuity, some inexpensive material and paint, any room can be made inviting and attractive, and many patients would enjoy working on a project, taking pride in the end result. These latter considerations are an important part of the therapist's responsibility in creating a therapeutic atmosphere. (p. 83)

The atmosphere created in a clinic or other institutional setting is indeed impor-tant to the overall safety, health, and comfort of clients. However, as client-centered practice and other health care trends move occupational therapists more into the homes and communities of clients, therapists must use their considerable skill in adaptation of various environments and their creativity to problem-solve and compensate for the immutable limitations of any given environment.

The Institutional and Clinic Environment

There has been extensive documentation on the particularly negative effects of institutional environments (Chou, Lu, & Chang, 2001; Topf, 2000) where the expense, space limitations, and the necessity of medical procedures as well as security limit the amount of environmental adaptation that is actually pos-sible. However, within these environments, a separate space (clinic) is usually designated for OT that can be therapeutically altered to enhance function and comfort. Indeed, hospitalized clients often view the OT clinic as an oasis.

CASE ILLUSTRATION: Mrs. Vigar—The Safety and Comfort of the OT Clinic

Mrs. Vigar is a 57-year-old housewife diagnosed with major depression and hospitalized in a locked psychiatric unit because of severe suicidal ideation. Initially, Mrs. Vigar refused to leave her room, even though she was quite agitated by the noise of her roommate and the proximity to the nurses' station. The occupational therapist was able to coax her out of her room for a short visit to the OT clinic for a cup of tea. The following day, the therapist once again escorted Mrs. Vigar to the clinic and invited her to look at the artwork on the walls and engaged her in the task of watering the plants. Mrs. Vigar attended clinic regularly thereafter, sometimes engaging in clinic activity, other times simply observing. However, she never missed a session and the nursing staff reported that she was less agitated during and after OT.

Discussion

The OT clinic environment was arranged to provide a sense of comfort, familiarity, and safety as well as a balance of sensory stimulation. This had a direct impact on Mrs. Vigar's sense of control and symptom reduction.

An OT clinic should be a warm, inviting, and safe place. All aspects of the individual client's humanity should be recognized and acknowledged. What may seem like trivial details on the surface can greatly affect the overall "feel" of the clinic. For example, it is optimum if fresh water is available at all times in the clinic. This is a gesture of courtesy, and a desire to have clients in the clinic feel comfortable. It is also an acknowledgment of the problems of dehydration and "dry mouth" commonly found in people on psychotropic medication. It is, therefore, a tool to educate clients about symptom and side effect management, as well as role-modeling healthy nutritional habits. (See Appendix A for further discussion of medication side effects.)

Determining the level of sensory stimulation in the clinic can be difficult, especially regarding auditory stimulation. People have very different thresholds of tolerance to sound. For some individuals, it is necessary to have a quiet room for them to engage in any task. It is especially important for the therapist to provide a quiet place for some clients to retreat to if other clients are engaging in a particularly noisy activity. On the other hand, sound (as in music), if used judiciously, can enhance the therapeutic effect of an activity and the clinic environment. "Music can facilitate mood changes, alter states of awareness, modify one's consciousness and increase affective response. Music can be effectively used to shift a person's attention, soothe agitation and as an aid with visualization techniques" (MacRae, 1992, p. 275).

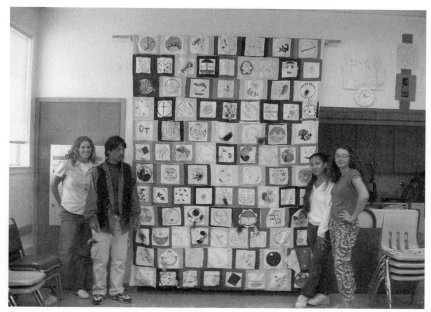

Figure 2-2.   Group Quilt Project at San Jose State University Clinic

The visual representations found in a clinic ideally are pleasant and calming but, most important, they should have some personal meaning for the clients. For example, Figure 2-2 shows the mandala quilt that is displayed in the San Jose State University (SJSU) Occupational Therapy Clinic. Each individual square of this quilt consists of the expressive artwork of a client or an OT student enrolled in the campus clinic course. Returning clients often look for their contribution and new clients have not only enjoyed its aesthetics but have become motivated by its presence to contribute to other long-term projects for the clinic environment.

There are many advantages to creating a therapeutic environment within an institutional or clinical setting. It may be especially important for acute care where the primary goal is stabilization, but it is also important for any client who has experienced repeated failures in life and needs to develop a sense of mastery and competency. However, there are also several drawbacks to the clinical environment. The client's home and community environment may be substantially different than the created OT clinic, therefore, functional assessment may not be reliable. Performance that occurs in the controlled clinical environment may not carry over to "real-world" situations or be indicative of a client's actual performance in a community environment (Hoppes, Davis, & Thompson, 2003). A study conducted by Jacobshagen (1990) concluded that interruption in activity performance significantly decreased both the satisfaction with and performance of the activity. A well-ordered clinic may limit interruptions but the living situations of many clients remain chaotic. Assessments conducted in a clinical environment often represent the clients' potential for community functioning, but may not represent actual performance.

CASE ILLUSTRATION: Uyen—Performance in Community

Uyen is a 24-year-old woman with a 4-month-old baby. Her parents expressed concern about her ability to care for the child and took her to a psychiatrist. She was diagnosed as having obsessive compulsive disorder and was referred to an assertive community treatment program in the community. Several functional assessments were completed to document her skills and abilities. Treatment initially consisted of role-playing various living skills for the purpose of providing practice in managing her anxiety. The occupational therapist felt that she was ready to try these skills in the community and accompanied her on a trip to the store. Uyen was able to negotiate the market effectively until she arrived at the checkout counter, where she dropped her intended purchases and ran from the building. She later told the OT that the man at the counter scratched under his arm and she "knew" that the germs would be given to her and her baby and make them sick.

Discussion

While Uyen was successful in carrying out simulated living skills in the safety of the clinical environment with a therapist that she trusted, it is not possible to account for the behavior of all individuals or the levels of stimulation in the community at large. In order to master the necessary living skills needed for parenting, Uyen will need further intervention in the community with the goal of developing coping skills for environments that she cannot change.

The Community and Home Environment

Ideally, a therapist can continue to follow a client into a different environment or at the very least be in communication with the therapist who will follow the client in the community. Skills learned in a clinic require practice in the community and can best be integrated by feedback, encouragement, and modification from the occupational therapist. For example, a young man with a goal of productive employment may have developed a resume, problem-solved job seeking strategies with the clinic-based OT, and even role-played various interview strategies. Nevertheless, he may experience failure in his first community attempt. Follow-up in the community is essential for successful completion of goals, and without the support of a community-based therapist, an initial failure may persuade the client not to try again.

A study conducted by Nelson, Hall, and Walsh-Bowers (1998) showed "that the number of living companions, housing concerns, and having a private room all significantly predicted different dimensions of community adaptation" (p. 57). (Further discussion of housing issues can be found in Chapter 22 on case management). As critical as the physical and sensory environment is to overall functioning, the community-based occupational therapist must also look at the many complex realities of community living, including such variables as social stratification and poverty (Blais, 1997; Hartery & Gahagan, 1998). For example, students in the SJSU clinic frequently address the issue of money management in their treatment plans. While it is true that the poor judgment and impulsivity found in many psychiatric disorders may lead to poor money management skills, students are often surprised to discover how limited the financial entitlements, if they exist at all, are for their clients. Money management implies that the individual has funds to actually manage. Even taking into account the often limited budgets of clients, skills learned in the clinic do not account for the many community variables of budgeting, including the greatly increased opportunities for careless spending and the vulnerability of many clients to financial exploitation.

Another variable in the community is the level of comfort the client feels. Unfortunately, stigma and violence against people with mental illness are very real phenomena. Therefore, fears voiced by mental health clients in the community are often based on actual negative experiences, not on paranoid delusions, and have a significant impact on independent living. For example, fear of harm or ridicule is often a major factor in clients' poor performances in negotiating public transportation. Occupational therapists have vital roles to play in both clinical and institutional environments as well as in the community. OTs understand the limitations of any environment and creatively problem-solve to either change the environment or assist the client in developing coping strategies to negotiate the environment. "People are never independent of their environment but learn how to adapt to it, or adapt it to themselves, to satisfy their needs" (Creek, 1997 p. 101).

Environmental Analysis and Adaptation

As interest in therapeutic environments increases, the occupational therapy profession has responded with several theoretical and practical models for understanding and analyzing the environment. Hagedorn (2000) proposes a microanalysis involving the "5 Cs" of content, convenience, comfort, cues, and communication. Another useful environmental analysis tool is the Environment-Independence Interaction Scale (EIIS) developed by Dunn, Brown, and Youngstrom (2003), designed to "provide an easy and effective method for capturing contextual factors to facilitate consideration of all factors that might contribute to positive rehabilitation outcomes" (p. 253). Table 2-1 outlines environmental analysis and adaptation using body functions and contexts as organizational modifiers. However, this table is specific to the concerns of mental health and is therefore not inclusive of all body functions and structures identified by the World Health Organization's *International Classification of Function* (ICF) and the Occupational Therapy Practice Framework. For example, all environmental adaptations, regardless of the current health status of the individuals within the environment, should take into account the muscular-skeletal requirements for optimal health such as ergonomically correct furniture. In addition there are other body function concerns that may apply to people with mental illness. For

Table 2-1.   Environmental Analysis and Adaptation

Client Factors (Body Functions)	Environmental Analysis	Examples of Adaptation
Mental Functions	Organization Safety Cues	Supplies organized in an orderly and familiar way, instructions provided at the cognitive level for individual clients. Potential safety hazards removed or placed under controlled access.
Sensory Functions	Light Auditory and visual stimulation Safety	Adequate light for task. Opportunities or multisensory stimulation. Auditory and visual stimulation balanced to prevent sensory overload. Safety features in place to prevent injury.

Context	Environmental Analysis	Examples of Adaptation
Cultural	Symbolic representations Beliefs Expression	Evidence of sensitivity to potential diversity or specific cultural groups. Opportunities for multimodel cultural expression. Respect for diversity of values is evident.
Physical	Space requirements Accessibility Ergonomics Outside space Natural objects Water, air, food Supplies and tools for occupational tasks	Accessible supplies. Sufficient outside and inside space for engagement in occupation. Ergonomically correct furniture. Ventilation. Access to restrooms and areas for clean-up. Access to food and water.
Social	Opportunities for interaction Observable support Roles and routines Inclusion	Opportunity for spontaneous interaction. Facilitates group involvement and inclusion in all activities. Supports the development of meaningful roles as well as healthy routines and habits.
Personal	Personal representation Expression	A climate that supports freedom of choice and individual diversity. Offers a wide range of modalities and potential expressive and functional occupations.
Spiritual	Reflection Meaning Symbolic representation Expression Sacred objects	Iconic representations (pictures, altars, etc.) that are representative and acceptable to the individual or the group. Space provided that is conducive to reflection, meditation, or prayer.

(continues)

Context	Environmental Analysis	Examples of Adaptation
Temporal	Age-stage-appropriate Orientation	Relevant and meaningful age-appropriate artwork and decorations. Additions of calendars, clocks, seasonal displays.
Virtual	Communication access as appropriate	Computer access as well as training and supervision as needed to ensure personal safety.

Table 2-1. (continued)

example, clients with cardiac dysfunction including general deconditioning, commonly found in people with serious mental illness, may need adaptations, such as energy-conserving design, to improve physical fitness or as compensation for physical limitations. Another example would be environmental adaptations for a client with mental illness and a metabolic disorder such as diabetes. People with diabetes are more prone to infection and the inadequate healing of wounds. Coupled with the poor judgment often found in individuals with mental illness, this creates increased risks that may be compensated for by special attention to potential injury-causing hazards. These concerns are partially addressed through the principles of universal design previously discussed. However, environmental adaptation addresses the specific needs and desires of an individual rather than the needs of a community, as is the focus of universal design.

Occupational therapists have a unique philosophy and set of skills to not only analyze the totality of an environment but also to create new environments or to adapt existing ones. These skills have been underutilized in the mental health arena and should be part of the daily repertoire of clinical skills in mental health (Dressler & MacRae, 1998).

CULTURE

Culture is a conscious and unconscious internal process of identification with overt manifestations of traditions, beliefs, and values, often involving the use of objects, which create meaning and guide human beings in organizing their lives. It is probably obvious that this definition reflects the values of an occupational therapist. But all definitions of culture reflect the specific situation and environment being addressed. "There is not a single definition of culture, and all too often definitions tend to omit salient aspects of culture or are too general to have any real meaning" (Spector, 2004, p. 9). The AOTA defines the context of culture as "customs, beliefs, activity patterns, behavior standards, and expectations accepted by the society of which the individual is a member" (Occupational Therapy Practice Framework, 2002, p. 623). Although the AOTA definition provides parameters for culturally sensitive occupational therapy intervention, it lacks an explanation of the purpose of culture, which is to create meaning, develop or enhance personal as well as role identity, and provide structure and organization to our daily lives. All of these themes have been embedded in the thinking of occupational therapy since its inception, which leads to the conclusion that cultural considerations must be a part of competent OT practice for a diverse population.

Culture and Health Care

There has been much recent effort devoted to understanding health and illness in a cultural context and to research the role of traditional medicine as well as complementary and alternative medicine **(TM/CAM)** in providing adequate health care for the world's population. The literature is inconsistent in the use of the terms *traditional, alternative,* and *complementary,* therefore, some definitions are in order. Traditional medicine simply means the tradition or approach that is primarily used within one's culture. In the dominant culture of the United States, **allopathic** or Western medicine is traditional (also called the medical model), whereas in India, the traditional medical system is **Ayurvedic.** This ancient health care system (approximately 4,000 years old) is closely related to Chinese medicine and is primarily based on using elements of nature, including diet and herbs (Spector, 2004).

Alternative practices are health care techniques and approaches that are not typically viewed as compatible with Western medicine but may or may not be viable health care options (*instead of* Western medicine). Complementary health care practices are those that can be used in conjunction with Western medicine but fall outside of the traditional domain of the allopathic system. Whether a particular practice should be considered alternative or complementary often depends on the attitudes and knowledge of the health care provider and the client rather than on any inherent quality of the practice. It is becoming more common to find physicians and other health care providers willing to work in conjunction with an alternative/complementary practitioner and, perhaps most important, willing to work with their clients, the consumers, for health promotion and awareness. This pluralistic wellness model is both client-oriented and holistic. Hopefully, consumers and health professionals alike will nurture this trend.

There are several alternative and complementary practices that have become so popular they are now considered somewhat mainstream. These include chiropractic, homeopathy, various bodywork, movement, and message techniques, as well as the use of diet and herbs. Some of these practices have ancient cultural histories while others are more recent. As our population changes, the mixture of these beliefs becomes profound. Given that the majority of people throughout the world now use some form of nonallopathic treatment either in isolation or in conjunction with Western medicine (WHO, 2002), occupational therapists are likely to encounter unfamiliar practices in their work and may misinterpret their observations. For example, **moxibustion** and cupping are healing rituals based on the traditional Chinese medicine principles of heat and cold. These techniques as well as the Vietnamese ritual of coining, or rubbing the body with a coin for the treatment of colds and flu, tend to leave marks on the body that have been misconstrued as evidence of abuse. Although these practices, like many others, can be potentially dangerous if administered incorrectly, they have been in use for a very long time and there is ample evidence that when properly administered, such techniques do no permanent harm and may have positive psychological as well as physical effects. In order for occupational therapists to provide the optimal interventions for their clients, it is imperative that clinicians continue to expand their knowledge base of TM/CAM and to determine its importance in the individual client's life.

Although there has been some growing disillusionment with allopathic medicine, people in Western society tend to be either very skeptical of TM/CAM or uncritically embracing of nonallopathic approaches. The World Health Organization (WHO) has addressed this issue through the WHO TM/CAM strategy document (2002), which aims to assist countries in developing national policies for evaluation and regulation of TM/CAM practices, create an evidence base, determine the safety of practices, and ensure the affordability and availability of TM/CAM throughout the world.

Culture and Mental Health

Cultural awareness is necessary for the delivery of all quality health care, but it has particular significance for the mental health field because of the very nature of practice. Concepts of normal and abnormal behavior are the basis for psychiatric diagnosis. Normality, however, can differ cross-culturally. What is normal to one can be abnormal to another. Since the concept of normality is undoubtedly value laden, the issue of culture must be addressed not only in the treatment process but in the evaluation and diagnostic process as well. There have been recent efforts to identify manifestations of mental illness unique to a particular cultural group, such as the **culture-bound syndromes** described in the *Diagnostic and Statistical Manual,* 4th Edition, Text Revised (*DSM-IV-TR*) (APA, 2000). However, further work is needed to increase the understanding of the role of culture in mental illness. The *DSM-IV-TR* currently identifies 25 such culture-bound syndromes that are considered to be among the best studied. One such syndrome is "ataque de nervios," which is a sense of being out of control, where the person may exhibit verbal or physical aggression, uncontrollable crying, shouting, and sometimes fainting, and dissociative experiences. This condition is commonly recognized among the Caribbean Latino population as well as other Latino groups around the world. Another culture-bound syndrome is "Shenjing shuairuo." This condition, found in China and among other traditional Chinese populations, is characterized by fatigue and irritability as well as various physical complaints including headaches and stomachaches. Individuals who experience either of these culture-bound syndromes may or may not also meet the *DSM-IV-TR* criteria for an anxiety or mood disorder. However, the conditions are unique and it cannot be assumed that they are synonymous with the Western view of psychopathology. Whether or not a clinician acknowledges these syndromes as distinct conditions, it is important to understand the perspective of the client, as he or she may use these terms to explain his or her experiences.

Cultural Identification

The most common method of cultural identification is race or ethnicity. This is partially because there are usually easily recognized and observable features.

Although ethnicity can certainly be a part of culture, it is not synonymous with culture. Identification of culture with ethnicity alone does not represent the many interrelated facets of culture such as gender, socioeconomics, age, and geographic location. Cultural identity may also be linked to chosen or inherent lifestyles based on personal choice, disability, or sexual orientation. This broad-based view of culture encompasses much human diversity and not all authors in occupational therapy agree with the use of such broad definitions (McGruger, 2003). The concern is that the over-identification of culture tends to simplify complex phenomena and promote stereotyping by categorizing groups of people. This criticism is well justified and care must be taken to not assume that an individual will always represent or agree with all aspects of a designated culture. One of the hallmark traits of culture is that it is dynamic and so are the individuals within a culture. Nevertheless, this chapter uses a broad-based view of culture to expose the reader to the depths of human diversity and because there are groups of people who self-identify with this broad view of a culture.

In our complex society, influenced by many events, some people may feel "cultureless," while others identify themselves as members of several cultures (i.e., African American, gay, Christian, occupational therapist, etc.) This **polyculturalism** gives rise to a situation where some people feel cultural conflicts within themselves, let alone with their neighbors. The clinical significance of either a lack of cultural identity or a conflicted cultural identity is profound. Stress, guilt, poor self-esteem and self-concept, and lack of support are all contributing factors to poor health. For example, a woman who has immigrated to the United States from a traditional Islamic culture may want to be a part of the working and social world of American women but feels conflicted about her role. She may also lose the emotional support of her family for choices they view as rebellious. Another example is a young man from a fundamentalist Christian family coming to grips with an emerging homosexual identity. For some individuals, "coming out" or acknowledging an identity as a gay man would mean a conscious rejection of familial or religious culture. Unless other support networks are available, the individual may feel cultureless or disconnected from any group. For others, especially those who continue to cherish some parts of their cultural upbringing, there are unresolved conflicts regarding morals, lifestyle, and acceptance that can lead to guilt, shame, and poor self-esteem.

As society becomes more polycultural, there must be greater sophistication in how cultures are identified. The first question is often why we need cultural identification at all. It is clear that the concept of culture, especially as it pertains to race or ethnicity, has often been used to marginalize and stereotype certain groups of people, and several erroneous conclusions have been drawn from research on ethnicity. However, simply choosing not to recognize differences in people is a form of **cultural blindness**. In a more naive era than the present, many well-meaning people felt that "everybody is the same" and we shouldn't even acknowledge the differences. Unfortunately, what this often meant was "I will accept you looking different if you think and act like me." Cultural blindness today takes many forms, including some public officials who are supporting the dismantlement of equalization policies such as affirmative action legislation. Even in the scholarly literature, there are suggestions that the concept and definitions of "multiculturalism" are too limited and need to be broadened to include a global multinational, postethnic perspective. While such melding and equalization may someday become reality, it seems that we have a long way to go in embracing the world's diversity. As long as racism and discrimination exist, a concerted effort to understand, not ignore, differences is needed. The "melting pot" mythos of the United States is an example of cultural blindness. In more recent research and popular thinking, retaining a unique cultural perspective has more benefits than drawbacks. A more positive metaphor is to think of society as a "tossed salad," with many different ingredients maintaining their unique flavor while contributing to the whole.

Culturally Appropriate Language

The literature and teachings regarding culturally appropriate language tend to agree that terms used to denote cultural groups or practices must be sensitive and devoid of negative connotations. Of course, terms that are used in a derogatory and mean-spirited way are offensive and unacceptable; however, the designation of which terms they might be is more difficult than one might think. There are geographical, generational, situational, and personal differences in one's choice of terms. For example, depending on a person's age and where she or he grew up, one might identify themselves as Negro/Black/African American/or Person of Color. Another example is how to designate people who speak Spanish as their primary language or people who originate from Spanish-speaking countries. In the eastern United States, the term *Hispanic* is most commonly used (geographical difference), whereas, in the West, the term *Latino* or *Latina* (gender difference) is more common. To further complicate these identifications, some people who originate from the countries so designated may have no European (Spanish) background at all and are members of the indigenous populations of Mexico, Central America, or South America. Another scenario is that people may be the ancestors of Africans or American slaves (as is the case in several of the Spanish-speaking Caribbean islands). This became a controversial issue in the development of the 2000 U.S. Census as the authors struggled with various classification schemes. Still another example, in Canada the preferred term for indigenous people is *First Nation.* To some people the designation of "tribal" is considered archaic and offensive. However, in many parts of the United States, the word *tribal* is used with pride (regional difference). There are still "tribal" councils that have political authority on reservations and "tribal" ceremonies that are conducted, sometimes for members of the group only, other times for the larger community. The designation *Indian* to mean Native Americans (rather than East Indian) is usually considered to be derogatory (at least by Caucasians!). However, the term is used frequently by tribal political activists. Some tribal members report that the term *Native American* is an artificial distinction coined to assuage the guilt of white liberals (personal difference). There is also quite a bit of debate going on among American Indian groups about the value of being

There are times when using a cultural or ethnic term is necessary for the preciseness of a particular topic in conversation. However, sometimes the use of qualifiers is its own form of bias. In a client-centered practice it is important to not define a person by a label (Black, Latino, etc.).

Make an attempt to identify a person as she or he wants to be identified, keeping in mind the generational, geographic, situational, and personal differences affecting choice of terms. (Don't make assumptions—ask!)

Be sensitive to different cultural standards of speech, including rate of speech (fast or slow), acceptable volume, use of silence, appropriate response time, and order of speakers (amount of deference, acceptance of interruptions, or simultaneous multiple speakers).

Be aware of use of time and acknowledgment of relationships. Clients may need to establish a social relationship prior to a professional relationship, which may not be viewed as "productive" time by the therapist.

Be aware of posture and body language. Familiarize yourself with culturally acceptable use of eye contact, proximity of speakers, and hand gestures.

Figure 2-3. Guidelines for Cross-Cultural Communication

identified only by one's tribe or nation (i.e., Mohawk, Pomo, etc.). Although this is probably more precise and acknowledges the differences between the groups, it can also weaken their unity when addressing political and social issues (situational difference).

Culturally sensitive or what is commonly called "politically correct," or PC, terminology is an attempt to eliminate or reduce bias and stereotypes. However, it does nothing to solve the underlying problem of why stigma developed in the first place. Attitudinal differences may not be significantly affected by a change in terminology. Sometimes the concern about not offending anyone becomes so complicated that conversation simply shuts down. That is the worst possible scenario for culturally competent health care. Figure 2-3 lists guidelines for cross-cultural communication that can be used in any clinical or community environment.

Communication

Both nonverbal and verbal communication can vary in style and this is at least partially culturally determined. In the northeastern United States, there is a strong value placed on direct, assertive communication. Sometimes this value is taken to the point where all other styles of communication are considered to be pathologic. However, there are many cultures where either aggressive or passive communication styles are the norm and "American"-style communication is either not respected or is considered offensive. Clinicians must sometimes adjust their style to the client's and adjust their expectations of the client. This becomes particularly difficult when the demands of the environment do not match the cultural background of the individual.

CASE ILLUSTRATION: The Passivity of Oi Ling

Oi Ling is a 19-year-old college student being treated for major depression in an interdisciplinary outpatient treatment program. One of the regular weekly groups is on the topic of assertive communication. The social worker and the occupational therapist who co-lead the group encourage her to speak up and coach her in both nonverbal and verbal techniques for assertive communication. The clinical documentation reflects little change in Oi Ling's demeanor or affect.

Discussion

While passivity may be a symptom of depression, many cultures value silence and expect people, especially women, to be quiet and deferential, particularly to their elders. It is up to the team and Oi Ling together to decide whether this group is appropriate for her. If her home or community environment does not value assertive "Westernized" style of communication, there is little benefit to be derived from participation in this group and it is very unlikely that any meaningful change would occur. The social worker and occupational therapist should avoid pathologizing behavior that is acceptable in the context of the client's life.

On the other hand, if Oi Ling needs to function within a school, work, or community environment that expects assertiveness, then an open discussion about the topic should be pursued. The leaders of an assertive communication group need to assess the relevance of the topic in all clients' lives and help them identify what, if any, benefits would be gained from participating in the group. If Oi Ling sees the lack of assertiveness as a problem in her daily life, then participation is appropriate. However, the group leaders need to be aware that Oi Ling may be experiencing polyculturalism, living in two cultural worlds, and may need to develop further strategies for dealing with inherent conflicts.

Communication is often thought of merely in terms of language. Although this is a critical component of communication, it is not the sum total, nor in many cases, is it even the most important or reliable means of communication. Nonverbal communication, including body language and gestures, often carries more meaning and is more readily understandable. But this is assuming that one knows the meaning of the nonverbal communication for a particular culture. Even when people are competent linguists, misunderstandings can and do occur because of poorly understood nonverbal communication.

Occupational therapists by tradition are "doers" and do not overly rely on verbal communication. However, all clinicians require practice in both using and accurately reading nonverbal messages as well as understanding the context of verbal language. Table 2-2 provides several clinical examples highlighting the linguistic challenges between a therapist and a client.

Obviously, people who do not share a common language or dialect will have serious limitations in communication. It is certainly in the best interest of the professional to be fluent in more than one language. (In large, culturally diverse

Table 2-2. Communication in Context

Clients	Example	Comment
Individuals who are monolingual are often treated in settings that do not routinely use their primary language.	A Spanish-speaking person being treated in an English-speaking clinic.	The use of translators/interpreters is highly recommended but cannot take the place of direct clinician interaction with the client for building rapport; therefore, nonverbal communication is essential.
Individuals who may be bi- or multilingual may be treated in a setting that does not routinely use their primary language.	A Cantonese-speaking person known to have learned English as an adult and uses English when needed in routine community tasks.	During times of stress, such as might occur during interactions with any authority figures (i.e., health care providers or police), it is typical for an individual to revert to the use of primary language and have difficulty with recently acquired language.
Individuals may speak the same primary language as the health care provider but use a colloquial form of the language not shared by the clinician.	An African American urban youth may have difficulty explaining personal experiences in terms understandable to the clinician and may resent the expectation to use "standard" English.	It is NOT acceptable for the clinician to attempt to use the colloquial form of the language if it is not part of her or his cultural identity. Rather than building rapport, this attempt will more likely be seen as ridicule.
Individuals may have limited or nonexistent language usage secondary to a perceived social climate.	Situations that may induce fear, suspicion, or paranoia such as a recent arrest, political refugee status, or other concerns for personal safety.	Clinicians need to take care not to over-pathologize behavior that in fact may be appropriate to the context.

urban areas, linguistic ability often becomes a factor in hiring policies.) However, it is not sufficient to simply know the words or the grammar because all language occurs within a cultural context. This leads to a practice dilemma for monolingual therapists. Assuming there is someone available who does know the language of the client (family member or friend, another professional, another client), the question is whether an interpreter or a translator is needed. Words are often used interchangeably but they are really very different. A translator will be able to provide the words as closely rendered in English as possible, often leaving out the words that cannot be translated. An interpreter takes into account the cultural meanings of the words and applies them to the concepts of the other language. Many health care providers prefer translation, because it allows the professional to interpret the meaning within the health care context. There is always a concern that the interpreter will inadvertently withhold valuable information because of widely different cultural contexts and values. However, literal translations often fall very short of providing the occupational therapist with the whole story. In a profession that prides itself on client-centeredness, which implies hearing the client's story, translation alone is usually insufficient. Taking the time to learn other languages may be more than individual occupational therapists can realistically be expected to do. However, OTs should strive to become cultural interpreters themselves or learn to work closely with interpreters and translators so as not to miss the nuances of the languages encountered.

CASE ILLUSTRATION: The OT and Cultural Interpretation

Mary is an American occupational therapist working in Central America. She knows some Spanish but not the indigenous dialect spoken here. Several of her clients insist on calling her "Doctor." Each time she feels an ethical responsibility to correct him or her, stating, "No, I'm the OT, not the doctor." The clients look puzzled but drop the subject.

Discussion

It could be that the clients don't know the role of the various health professionals, but more likely the problem lies in the literal translation of the language. In most countries throughout the world, there is a word or words for "healer" that often gets translated as "doctor." The culture may not have the rigid regulations (years of schooling, licenses, etc.) that Americans assume entitles one to be called "Doctor," but they do understand and respect the role of healers. These individuals would not feel comfortable using their native word for healer (curandera, santeria, shaman) because clearly the OT is not one of them.

Values and Social Relationships

Closely tied to communication is the process of relationship development, the values and attitudes regarding relationships, and the concept of social space. How one interacts with others is largely environmentally and culturally determined. Embedded in one's culture are beliefs and attitudes regarding spirituality, family structure, gender roles, and health care. All of these affect relationships, choice of activity, and preferred environment.

Proxemics, a term coined by E. T. Hall (1966), is an aspect of culture that refers to people's use and comfort with personal and social space. For example, in some cultures it is acceptable and expected to touch frequently and to stand very close together in a conversation. However, in other cultures, this closeness would feel intrusive. Therapists must be aware of the cultural value of proxemics in their clients and adjust their interactions accordingly. It may not be possible to have

advanced knowledge of this particular cultural trait, but an occupational therapist with strong observation skills will take cues from the client and adapt to his or
her sense of proximity. In mental health service, this becomes difficult because
there are many space-related behaviors that are part of psychopathology. For
example, someone who is experiencing paranoia or who has sensory processing
problems may not want to have anyone near, let alone touching, her or him. Conversely, a person with a brain injury or psychotic disorder may lose sense of personal boundaries and act impulsively with touch. He or she will often not be able
to pick up the subtle social cues that the behavior is inappropriate or is uncomfortable for another person. Each situation is unique, but the OT who has an
understanding of cultural traits such as proxemics will be less likely to over-
pathologize behavior simply because it is different from his or her own.

Cultural values regarding relationships and space vary tremendously and must
be taken into account when planning any aspect of intervention. For example,
grooming in European-American culture is considered a private activity usually
undertaken in the morning time in one's bedroom or bathroom. But in some cultures, such as among Latina women, grooming can be a very social activity, where
helping each other with hair styles and makeup is considered highly desirable
(Dillard, Andonian, Flores, Lai, MacRae, & Shakir, 1992). It is the responsibility
of occupational therapists to educate themselves about the particular values and
relationship styles of the cultural groups who may be the recipients of OT services.
The degree of privacy is only one of several important values that must be considered in OT practice. Table 2-3 lists other common cultural values and provides
examples and suggestions for the clinician.

Time Sense

Although the importance of temporality has long been recognized in the OT literature, it must be acknowledged that particularly in the profession's early writings, the view of temporality was firmly embedded in Western society's concept
of time. In the current Occupational Therapy Practice Framework (2002), temporality is considered a context and consists of "stages in life, time of day, time of
year, duration" (p. 623). However, this view of temporality does not take into
account the vastly different time sense or perception that is partially mediated in
individuals by their culture. Some cultures value a future orientation, while others are firmly grounded in the present or past.

People in poverty tend to have a present sense of time, meaning that the day-
to-day issues or crises must take priority over future plans; therefore, goal setting
may be difficult. This is consistent with Maslow's hierarchy of needs (see Chapter
4 for further discussion of this theory), which explains that physiological and
safety needs must be met before other needs. It is not realistic to think about self-
actualization, aesthetics, or even esteem needs when you don't know where your
next meal is coming from. Since health care providers will typically be in a higher
socioeconomic bracket than many of their clients, it is critical that an awareness
of the effects of poverty on time sense be developed. This increased awareness

Table 2-3. Cultural Values

Cultural Value	Comments and Suggestions
Formality	Specific knowledge of a particular culture's value of formality will help clinicians decide how to introduce themselves, plan for treatment, address the client, and explain their role. For example, in some societies it is expected to arrange appointments with another family member and be granted permission to proceed, while in others the informality of arriving without notice is perfectly acceptable. Some cultures expect the use of formal titles, while others would see this type of communication as cold and distant.
Individuality	The emphasis in American culture and health care is to meet the needs of the individual. However, many cultures around the world value the needs and health of the family, or even the whole community, above the individual. When planning treatment, the OT should be cognizant of who else, besides the individual client, should be involved. It may include immediate or extended family as well as other members of the community.
Independence	Independence is highly valued in Western, particularly dominant American culture. It is also highly emphasized within the professional culture of occupational therapy. However, in many cultures, caregiving is a strong and noble value and there is no shame in having to be cared for. For some cultures, wanting a client to be independent is seen as selfish because family members would not be taking their expected responsibility to care for the person.
Locus of Control	Many people around the world believe that what happens to them is out of their control. Either a greater spiritual power is in control or "things just happen." People with an external locus of control may not be willing to make a large investment (emotionally, financially or otherwise) to change the course of their health. Occupational therapists tend to hold the value of internal locus of control and usually attempt to "empower" their clients to take both responsibility and control of their lives. The downside of this approach is that clients may feel guilt, shame, denial, or personal responsibility for their illness.
Authority	Respect for authority is common in many cultures. As occupational therapy moves more toward a client-centered approach, it is important to consider that many clients expect the therapist to be the expert and to know what's best for them. They may not feel comfortable in expressing their personal goals.

will help occupational therapists negotiate realistic and manageable goals for their clients in poverty.

Hall (1976) suggests that the perception of time is not an inborn trait but rather determined by the culture or society. He classified time sense as being either **Monochronic (M-time)** or **Polychronic (P-time).** M-time societies view time as linear and rely on implicit or explicit scheduling. People in M-time societies also tend to view time as a commodity, as a thing that can be saved or lost, spent or wasted, squandered or managed (Peloquin, 1991). However, P-time cultures do not share the same time values. P-time tends to be cyclical and unscheduled, typically a natural rhythm where several things can happen at once and is not controlled by human beings.

Treating a client with a different time sense is one of the most frustrating aspects of working cross-culturally. Part of the frustration stems from not being aware that different time senses even exist. A culturally competent therapist first determines if the client's time sense is culturally different than what would be expected in the treatment setting or dominant culture. Otherwise, it is possible to erroneously assume a pathology or dysfunction that does not exist within the individual's cultural world.

CASE ILLUSTRATION: Mr. Maliu's Perception of Time

Mr. Maliu recently arrived in the United States from a small village in Samoa. He now lives with his brother's family, who arranged for his migration because they felt that he could receive better care in the United States for his long-standing mental illness. His brother arranged for an initial evaluation at a county mental health office that also operates a day treatment center on site. Mr. Maliu arrived two hours late for his initial appointment and was asked to reschedule for another time. He was considerably late for the second appointment as well; however, the interviewing team, consisting of a psychiatrist, a social worker, and an occupational therapist, was able to accommodate him. He was accepted into the program but told that he would have to arrive on time to remain in the treatment group. He immediately established a pattern of late arrival to the group. Therefore, the treatment team is considering discharging him and referring him to outreach case management only. The conclusion of the treatment team is that he is perhaps too ill to benefit from the program at this time. Furthermore, his behavior is disruptive to the rest of the group.

Discussion

Time-related behaviors such as those displayed by Mr. Maliu may be due to symptoms of serious mental illness such as disorganization, disorientation, or avolition. (See Chapter 5 for description of symptoms.) However, care must be taken to avoid pathologizing behaviors that may be culturally appropriate. First and foremost, an understanding of the meaning of time to the client is essential to determine if Mr. Maliu's behavior is related to his illness or not. If it is determined that his time sense is consistent with his cultural background and lifestyle, the treatment team has several options. It may indeed be in the client's and the group's best interest for him to receive individual treatment or case management initially. However, another approach would be to involve the family in a discussion of the norms, expectations, and benefits of group participation. If the client and his family saw the group treatment as desirable, then strategies, such as telephone reminders and schedules or pairing him with a travel partner from the group, could be developed to help Mr. Maliu adapt to the environment's expected time sense. Still another option open to the team is to simply let Mr. Maliu attend the program with late arrival. Often clients are more tolerant of flexible time schedules than professionals and his late arrival may not be as disruptive as the team assumes.

In order for occupational therapists to provide culturally competent treatment to a diverse population it is essential that the profession's beliefs about time be explored. Occupational therapy originally developed in an M-time society. Specifically, the middle- and upper-class values of the northeastern United States at the turn of the century greatly affected the development of occupational therapy as a profession (See Chapter 3 for further discussion of the foundations of OT.) However, in today's multicultural environment and with the growth of the profession around the world, occupational therapists must adapt to include, or at least recognize, the values of other societies. There are many implications for treatment when the therapist has a different time sense than the person receiving services. The trends toward managed care and increased productivity in the workplace have placed a high value on a minute increment therapy model, in which quantity of therapy minutes is equated with quality of intervention. This trend must somehow be reconciled with the trends toward incorporating multicultural and individual client perspectives and needs.

Culturally Competent OT Practice

Guidelines for culturally competent occupational therapy began to emerge in the literature in the early 1990s (Dillard, Andonian, Flores, Lai, MacRae, & Shakir, 1992) and continue to be a topic of discussion in the current literature (MacDonald, 1998; Harris, 2000). Although several definitions of cultural competence have been introduced, all of them go beyond the simple acquisition of knowledge and skills to discuss the necessity for interpersonal skills and attitudes such as self-reflection, flexibility, acceptance of differences, and lifelong learning. Wells and Black (2000) suggest that occupational therapists construct a plan for competency that includes evaluating one's personal values and beliefs, identifying support in the environment, developing resources, and establishing specific personal goals.

As world demographics continue to shift toward a diverse society and occupational therapy strives to be increasingly client-centered, it is necessary that every occupational therapist develop a myriad of interventions that can acknowledge, honor, and address the complex cultural backgrounds of clients. Choices of occupations, including styles and approaches to activities of daily living, work habits, hobbies, and recreation, as well as the practice of rituals and traditions are all representative of one's culture and must be individually tailored to the client or client group. Throughout this book the illustrations and examples are designed to represent the diversity of occupational therapy clients. An aware occupational therapist creatively addresses culture in treatment; however, culturally appropriate assessment provides different challenges.

The cultural sensitivity of standardized assessments continues to be a controversial subject and many formal evaluation tools have such significant bias that their use with culturally diverse populations is questionable (Polgar, 2003). Even the informal tools and interview protocols commonly used in occupational therapy rarely adequately address the cultural background of the client. Table 2-4 provides a format for a culturally based interview and observation. This structure allows the therapist to understand the client's values and beliefs as well as cultural style, in addition to the personal meaning of the individual's culture.

Table 2-4. Cross-Cultural Initial Interview and Observation

Name:

Setting (Context):

Cultural Identity	*Observations*
Where were you born?	Apparent cultural identity (features, dress, icons, etc.)
How long have you lived here?	
Do you identify with a specific culture?	
Do you identify with a specific religion?	

Communication	*Observations*
What is your preferred language?	Use of Silence:
	Appropriate ____ Not Appropriate ____
	Comments:
If you have something important to discuss with your family, how would you approach them?	Use of Nonverbal Communication (e.g., hand movement, eye movement, entire body movement, gestures, expression, stances, etc.):
	Comments:
	Style of Communication: Passive ____
	Assertive ____ Aggressive ____
	Comments:

(continues)

Table 2-4. (continued)

Time Sense	Observations
Do you wear or use a watch?	Arriving at scheduled appointment
Do you use a schedule or date book?	Early _____ On time _____
Do you usually arrive early, late, or right on time to planned events?	Late _____
Is that pattern typical in your family or community?	Comments:

Social and Spatial Organization	Observations
What are some activities you enjoy? (OR What are your hobbies? OR What do you like to do during your free time?)	Touch (e.g., startles or withdraws when touched, accepts touch/ touches others w/ or w/o difficulty):
What are your roles? (OR What is your role in your family/community?)	Degree of comfort with space/ Distance in conversations:

Health/Locus of Control

What is good health to you?

Is there anything in your heritage/background that affects your approach to being well/healthy?

What do you think is going to make you or keep you well? (OR What is going to keep you from getting well?)

SUMMARY:

Source: Adapted from Giger and Davidhizar's Transcultural Assessment Model.

Summary

Occupational therapy intervention occurs within both environmental and cultural contexts. Occupational therapists must continually broaden their skills in these areas to provide competent services in a client-centered tradition. Furthermore, the unique focus on occupation within these contexts makes the occupational therapist a key member of the treatment team and also opens the possibility for a role as consultant or program developer. Mental health is directly affected by both the environmental and cultural contexts of individual clients. All members of a treatment team, including the occupational therapist, must understand the impact of these contexts on client function.

Review Questions

1. How does environment affect assessment?
2. Why is it important for OTs to be familiar with TM/CAM?
3. How does cultural competence affect OT assessment and intervention?

References

Allen, C. (1985). *Occupational therapy for psychiatric diseases: Measurement and management of cognitive disabilities*. Boston: Little, Brown.

American Psychiatric Association. (2000). *Diagnostic and statistical manual of mental disorders* (4th ed.-text revised). Washington, DC: Author.

Barker, S. B., & Dawson, K. S. (1998). The effects of animal-assisted therapy on anxiety ratings of hospitalized psychiatric patients. *Psychiatric Services, 49*(6), 797–801.

Blais, L. (1997). The issue of mental health in the context of poverty [French]. *Canadian Journal of Community Mental Health, 16*(1), 5–22,

Brown, C. (2001). What is the best environment for me? A sensory processing perspective. *Occupational Therapy in Mental Health, 17*(3/4), 115–125.

Canadian Association of Occupational Therapists. (2003). *Position statement: Universal design and occupational therapy*. CAOT.

Chou, K., Lu, R., Chang, M. (2001). Assaultive behavior by psychiatric in-patients and its related factors. *Journal of Nursing Research, 9*(5), 139–51.

Christiansen, C., & Baum, C. (1997). Person-environment-occupational performance: A conceptual model for practice. In C. Christiansen & C. Baum (Eds.), *Occupational therapy: Enabling function and well being* (pp. 46–70). Thorofare, NJ: Slack.

Christophersen, J. (2002). *Universal design: 17 ways of thinking and teaching*. Oslo, Husbanken.

Cole, K. M., & Gawlinski, A. (2000). Animal-assisted therapy: The human-animal bond. *AACN Clinical Issues, 11*(1), 139–49.

Creek, J. (1997). *Occupational therapy and mental health* (2nd ed.). Edinburgh: Churchill Livingstone.

Dillard, M., Andonian, L., Flores, O., Lai, L., MacRae, A., & Shakir, M. (1992). Culturally competent occupational therapy in a diversely populated mental health setting. *American Journal of Occupational Therapy, 46*, 721–726.

Dunn, W., Brown, C., & McGuigan, A. (1994). The ecology of human performance: A framework for considering the effect of context. *American Journal of Occupational Therapy, 48*(7), 595–607.

Dunn, W., Brown, C., & Youngstrom, M. (2003). Ecological model of occupation. In P. Kramer, J. Hinojosa, & C. B. Royeen (Eds.), *Perspectives in human occupation*. Philadelphia: Lippincott Williams & Wilkins.

Dressler, J., & MacRae, A. (1998). Advocacy, partnerships, and client centered practice. *Occupational Therapy in Mental Health, 14*(1/2), 35–43.

Fick, K. M. (1993). The influence of an animal on social interactions of nursing home residents in a group setting. *American Journal of Occupational Therapy, 47*(6), 529–534.

Giger J. N., & Davidhizar, R. E. (1999). *Transcultural nursing* (3rd ed.). St. Louis, MO: Mosby.

Hagedorn, R. (2000). *Tools for practice in occupational therapy.* Edinburgh: Churchill Livingstone.

Hagedorn, R. (2001). *Foundations for practice* (3rd ed.). Edinburgh: Churchill Livingstone.

Hall, E. T. (1966). *The hidden dimension.* Garden City, NY: Doubleday.

Hall, E. T. (1976). *Beyond culture.* Garden City, NY: Anchor/Doubleday.

Hammon, A., Kellegrew, D., & Jaffe, D. (2000). The experience of pet ownership as meaningful occupation. *Canadian Journal of Occupational Therapy, 6,* 271–278.

Harris, C. H. (2000). Educating toward multiculturalism. *OT Practice, 5*(6), 7–8.

Hartery, T., & Gahagan, T. (1998). Social stratification and social class. In D. Jones et al. (Eds), *Sociology and occupational therapy.* Edinburgh: Churchill Livingstone.

Hoppes, S., Davis, L. A., & Thompson, D. (2003). Environmental effects on the assessment of people with dementia: A pilot study. *American Journal of Occupational Therapy, 57*(4), 396–402.

Jacobshagen, I. (1990). The effect of interruption of activity on affect. *Occupational Therapy in Mental Health, 10*(2).

Kielhofner, G. (1995). *A model of human occupation: Theory and application* (2nd ed). Baltimore: Williams & Wilkins.

Law, M., Cooper, B., Strong, S., Steward, D., Rigby, P., & Letts, L. (1996). The person-environment occupation model: A transactive approach to occupational performance. *Canadian Journal of Occupational Therapy, 63,* 9–23.

Law, M., & Mills, L. (1998). Client centred occupational therapy. In M. Law (Ed.), *Client centered occupational therapy.* Thorofare, NJ: Slack.

MacDonald, R. (1998). What is cultural competency? *British Journal of Occupational Therapy, 6*(7), 325–328.

MacRae, A. (1992). The issue is: Should music be used therapeutically by occupational therapists? *American Journal of Occupational Therapy, 46,* 275–277.

McGruder, J. (2003). Culture, race, ethnicity, and other forms of human diversity. In E. B. Crepeau, E. S. Cohen, & B. A. B. Shell (Eds.), *Willard and Spackman's occupational therapy* (10th ed.). Philadelphia: Lippincott Williams & Wilkins.

Nelson G., Hall, G. B., & Walsh-Bowers, R. (1998). The relationship between housing characteristics, emotional well-being and the personal empowerment of psychiatric consumer/survivors. *Community Mental Health Journal, 34*(1), 57–69.

Occupational Therapy Practice Framework: Domain and Process. (2002). *American Journal of Occupational Therapy, 56*(6), 614–639.

Peloquin, S. (1991). Time as commodity: Reflections and implications. *American Journal of Occupational Therapy, 45*(2), 147–154.

Perrins-Margalis, N., Rugletic, J., Schepis, N., Stepanski, H., & Walsh, M. (2000). The immediate effects of a group-based horticulture experience on the quality of life of persons with chronic mental illness. *Occupational Therapy in Mental Health, 16*(1), 15–32.

Polgar, J. M. (2003). Critiquing assessments. In E. B. Crepeau, E. S. Cohen, & B. A. B. Shell (Eds.), *Willard and Spackman's occupational therapy* (10th ed.). Philadelphia: Lippincott Williams & Wilkins.

Roenke, L., & Mulligan, S. (1998). The therapeutic value of the human-animal connection (1998). *Occupational Therapy in Health Care, 11*(2), 27–43.

Rowles, G. D. (2003). The meaning of place as a component of self. In E. B. Crepeau, E. S. Cohen, & B. A. B. Shell (Eds.), *Willard and Spackman's occupational therapy* (10th ed.). Philadelphia: Lippincott Williams & Wilkins.

Schade, J. K., & Schultz, S. (1992). Occupational adaptation: Towards a holistic approach for contemporary practice: Part I. *American Journal of Occupational Therapy, 46,* 829–838.

Schwarzberg, S. (2002). *Interactive reasoning in the practice of occupational therapy.* Upper Saddle River, NJ: Parson Education.

Spector, R. (2004). *Cultural diversity in health and illness* (6th ed.). London: Prentice-Hall.

Topf, M. (2000). Hospital noise pollution: An environmental stress model to guide research and clinical interventions. *Journal of Advanced Nursing, 31*(31), 520–528.

Wade, B., & Franciscus, M. L. (1954). Occupational therapy for the mentally ill. In H. Willard & C. Spackman (Eds.), *Principles of occupational therapy* (2nd ed.). Philadelphia: Lippincott.

Wells, S. A., & Black, R. M. (2000). *Cultural competency for health professionals*. Bethesda, MD: American Occupational Therapy Association.

Wilcock, A. (1998). *An occupational perspective of health*. Thorofare, NJ: Slack.

Wong, E. (1996). *Feng-Shui: The ancient wisdom of harmonious living for modern times*. Boston: Shambhala.

World Health Organization (WHO). (2001). *International classification of functioning, disability and health (ICF)*. WHO.

World Health Organization Press Release WHO/38 (2002, May 16). *Who launches the first global strategy on traditional and alternative medicine*. WHO.

Suggested Reading

Clitheroe, H., Stokols, D., & Zmuidzinas, M. (1998). Conceptualizing the context of environment and behavior. *Journal of Environmental Psychology, 18*, 103–112.

Cooper Marcus, C., & Barnes, M. (1999). *Healing gardens: Therapeutic benefits and design recommendations*. Indianapolis: Wiley.

Fadiman, A. (1997). *The spirit catches you and you fall down: A Hmong child, her American doctors, and the collision of two cultures*. New York: Noonday.

Fearing, V., & Clark, J. (2000). *Individuals in context: A practical guide to client-centered practice*. Thorofare, NJ: Slack.

Fitzgerald, M. H., Mullavey-O'Byrne, C., & Clemson, L. (1997). Cultural issues from practice. *Australian Occupational Therapy Journal, 44*(1), 1–21.

Friedman, S., and Wachs, T. (1999). *Measuring environment across the life span: Emerging methods and concepts*. Washington, DC: American Psychological Association.

Howarth, A., & Jones, D. (1999). Transcultural occupational therapy in the United Kingdom: Concepts and research. *British Journal of Occupational Therapy, 62*(10), 451–458.

Jones, D., et al. (Eds). (1998). *Sociology and occupational therapy*. Edinburgh: Churchill Livingstone.

Leavitt, R. (Ed.). (1999). *Cross-cultural rehabiliation: An international perspective*. London: Saunders.

Letts, L., Rigby, P., & Stewart, D. (2003). *Using environments to enable occupational performance*. Bethesda, MD: American Occupational Therapy Association.

Linde, P. R. (2002). *Of spirits and madness: An American psychiatrist in Africa*. New York: McGraw Hill.

Pomerinke, K., Crawford, J., & Smith, D. (2003). *Therapy pets: The animal human healing partnership*: Amhurst, NY: Prometheus.

Purnell, L., & Paulanka, B. (1998). *Transcultural health care*. Philadelphia: F. A. Davis.

Sims, E. M., Pernell-Arnold, A., Graham, R., Hughes, R., Jonikas, J., Naranjo, D., Onaga, E., & Sardinas, M. (1998). Principles of multicultural psychiatric rehabilitation services. *Psychiatric Rehabilitation Journal, 21*(3), 219–223.

Well, S. (1997). *Horticulture therapy and the older adult population*. Binghamton, NY: Haworth.

Theoretical Concepts

Part II includes two chapters that focus on the theoretical underpinnings of psychosocial occupational therapy. Chapter 3 traces the thinking of the founders and the societal events of their time to describe the evolution of psychosocial occupational therapy. The strong emphasis on occupation is the historical cornerstone of our profession and has been "rediscovered" in current occupational therapy models of practice.

In the first edition of this text, Chapter 3 was titled, "Psychological Models." In this edition, this material is covered in Chapter 4, whose title has been changed to "Theories of Mental Health and Illness." It is the authors' position that the approaches discussed in this chapter are not discipline specific, but rather guide our understanding of mental illness from an interdisciplinary perspective. This chapter also discusses the unique ways that occupational therapy has been influenced by and incorporates these approaches.

Missing from this second edition is a specific chapter on occupational therapy models. This deletion does not negate their importance. On the contrary, the proliferation of conceptual and practice models in occupational therapy has made it impractical to do justice to them in this text. Instead, the authors of all chapters in this book have emphasized their own use of occupational therapy models as they are applied in practice. Readers are also encouraged to read current primary sources on the many occupational therapy models.

The History and Philosophy of Psychosocial Occupational Therapy

Kathleen Barker Schwartz, EdD, OTR/L, FAOTA

Key Terms

curative occupations
electroconvulsive therapy (ECT)
habit training
moral treatment

neurasthenia
psychoanalysis
psychobiological

Chapter Outline

Introduction
Treatment of the Insane before the Twentieth Century
The Founding of Occupational Therapy
    William Rush Dunton: Moral Treatment, Crafts, and Science
    Adolph Meyer: Psychobiology, Occupation, and Habits
    Eleanor Clarke Slagle: Curative Occupations and Habit Training

Introduction

In order to understand psychosocial occupational therapy fully, it is necessary to know how practice has evolved from its inception to today. The history of psychosocial occupational therapy is rich in ideas, events, and people who have helped to shape its development. The purpose of this chapter is to provide a history of psychosocial occupational therapy with an emphasis on the field's philosophical underpinnings, including the values and ideas upon which the profession was founded, and to describe how these ideas changed over time. Thus, this chapter provides the broader context from which to understand how contemporary practice has been influenced by earlier events, people, and ideas.

TREATMENT OF THE INSANE BEFORE THE TWENTIETH CENTURY

Prior to the twentieth century, care of the insane (the term *mental illness* is modern terminology) took place primarily at home or in asylums. For example, in France in 1860, the situation was described as follows:

> In our rural areas, where people are still imbued with absurd prejudices, public opinion sees having madness in the family as shameful and will not send the person to an asylum. This is the principal reason that motivates our peasants to keep poor afflicted individuals at home. If the insane person is peaceful, people generally let him run loose. But if he becomes raging or troublesome, he's chained down in a corner of the stable or an isolated room, where his food is brought to him daily. (Caradec as quoted in Shorter, 1997, p. 11)

In England if people were not kept at home they might be sent to workhouses or poorhouses, and the situation in the United States was similar to that in Europe. In rural Massachusetts in 1840, social reformer Dorothea Dix noted finding a woman in a cage in Lincoln, a man chained in a stall in Medford, and four women in animal pens in Barnstable (Dix, 1971/1943, pp. 5–7). In addition, she visited almshouses such as the one in Danvers, where she came upon a woman beating on the bars of a cage, "the unwashed frame invested with fragments of unclean garments, the air so extremely offensive, though ventilation was afforded to all sides save one, that it was not possible to remain beyond a few moments" (p. 6).

Before 1800 there were only two hospitals in the United States that admitted the insane: Pennsylvania Hospital, established in 1752 by the Religious Society of Friends, and New York Hospital, which had a separate psychiatric building that was called the Lunatic Asylum.

Asylums, which had existed in Europe since the Middle Ages, were frequently referred to as madhouses, and, for obvious reasons, were regarded as places to be avoided. That began to change with the introduction of a new approach in the nineteenth century that became known as **moral treatment**. Phillipe Pinel of France is commonly recognized as its initiator, although efforts were under way in all of Europe and England to create new-style asylums based on moral treatment philosophy. Moral treatment was humanitarian and therapeutic. Pinel's philosophy was a humanistic one characterized by kindness and respect, in which clients would be treated with dignity and optimism in place of the previous view of persons with mental illness as dangerous and incurable. The asylums for moral treatment were designed around the belief that orderly routines and occupations would have a therapeutic effect on clients. Pinel (1809) advocated a carefully planned treatment approach based on the use of "occupational activities of different kinds according to individual taste; physical exercise, beautiful scenery, and from time to time soft and melodious music" (p. 260).

What began in Europe ultimately came to the United States, where several private institutions were created under the moral treatment philosophy. They included McLean Asylum in Massachusetts, Hartford Retreat in Connecticut, Friends Hospital in Pennsylvania, and Sheppard Enoch Pratt Asylum in Maryland. Public asylums using the moral treatment approach were also established, with one of the most prominent founded in Worcester, Massachusetts. These facilities were impressively equipped with a variety of craft rooms, gardens, and recreational areas designed to provide clients with an active schedule of productive, creative, and recreational occupations. Figures 3-1 and 3-2 show samples of the occupational therapy environment where clients engaged in furniture making and repair as well as textile creation at Sheppard Enoch Pratt Asylum (now Sheppard Pratt Health Systems). Another such program, Gardner State Colony in Massachusetts, also provides a typical example of the rich occupation base of treatment: the clients were largely responsible for the development of 1,500 acres of productive farmlands that yielded 142,526 quarts of milk and 2,000 dozen eggs (Occupational Treatment of Patients in State Hospitals, 1914, p. 302). Inside the facility there was a carpenter shop, furniture factory, machine shop, shoemaking department, and rug weaving department (p. 304). "But it is not all work at Gardner. The patients have a good time . . . [with] tennis, golf . . . reading and entertainment. They have their orchestra and have musicals frequently. They have an excellent library, bowling and billiard rooms, and on the whole it is not such a terrible thing to be insane if one can be sure of the happy, even passage of one's life at a place like Gardner" (p. 305).

In a way, the success of the asylums based on moral treatment ultimately led to their demise. Once asylums gained a good reputation, people were willing to be admitted to them. After a while there were more people than could be

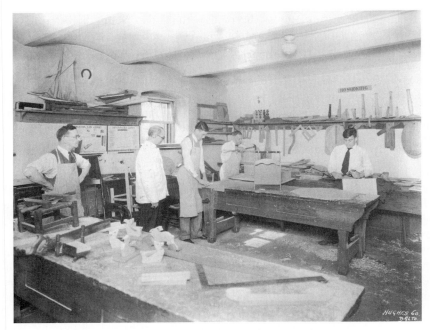

Figure 3-1. Furniture Making at Sheppard Enoch Pratt Asylum

Source: Reprinted with permission from Sheppard Pratt Health System.

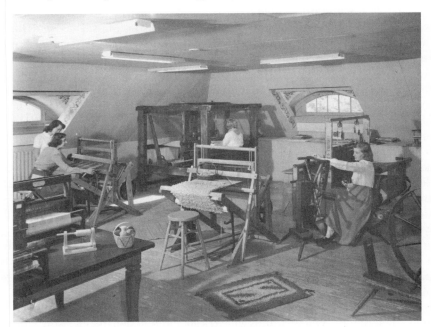

Figure 3-2. Textiles at Sheppard Enoch Pratt Asylum

Source: Reprinted with permission from Sheppard Pratt Health System.

accommodated with the available resources. Ultimately, the asylums did not have the funding to support the increasing numbers of individuals needing care. This resulted in overcrowded conditions and understaffing (Rothman, 1971). Moreover, by the beginning of the twentieth century, there was a shift in the view of mental illness away from the beliefs of moral treatment that centered on the importance of the therapeutic environment to the view that the science of brain pathology would provide the information that would ultimately lead to a cure.

THE FOUNDING OF OCCUPATIONAL THERAPY

The National Society for the Promotion of Occupational Therapy (NSPOT, later to be renamed the American Occupational Therapy Association) was founded in 1917. Although at the time occupational therapy was not divided into specialty areas, there were several people who were particularly instrumental in articulating the ideas that would provide the foundation for psychosocial occupational therapy. They were William Rush Dunton, Jr., Adolph Meyer, Eleanor Clarke Slagle, and Herbert James Hall. We will examine their backgrounds, work, and ideas in order to understand the significance of their contributions. As we do so, we will also introduce any relevant ideas in psychiatry or society at large that may have influenced their thinking.

William Rush Dunton: Moral Treatment, Crafts, and Science

At the founding meeting of NSPOT, Dunton (1917) presented a paper in which he traced the philosophical roots of occupational therapy to the moral treatment movement of the 1800s. At the time Dunton was a psychiatrist and supervisor of occupation classes at the prestigious Sheppard-Pratt Hospital in Towson, Maryland. He had received his medical training at the University of Pennsylvania, and began his career as an assistant physician at Sheppard Asylum (as it was then called) in 1895. Although Dunton initially worked in the laboratory, he became frustrated by the lack of progress and began to work directly with clients on the clinical wards. Dunton was introduced to the concept of therapeutic occupations by Edward Brush, MD, the superintendent of Sheppard. In 1902 a separate building for occupation classes was created, and Dunton took responsibility for overseeing client occupations, which included leatherwork, weaving, art, metalwork, bookbinding, electrical repair work, and printing (Fields, 1911). Dunton's ideas about occupational therapy can be found in a published outline of lectures (AOTA, 1925), of which he was primary author. These guidelines exemplified the principles of moral treatment in their focus on productive employment in occupation based on each client's capabilities and interests, and "carried on by encouragement, not criticism" (p. 279).

Dunton was a craftsman himself, and firmly believed in the therapeutic value of crafts. His interest in crafts was supported by the proliferation of arts and crafts societies in the United States in the early 1900s. The arts and crafts movement originally began in England in the late 1800s with John Ruskin and William Morris, who were disturbed by the negative effects that industrialization and bureaucracy were having on British society. They proposed a return to a simpler way of life in which objects were handcrafted. They argued that handcrafted goods were natural, honest, and pleasing whereas manufactured goods were neither aesthetic nor moral because the worker who produced them was treated like an extension of the machine (Levine, 1987). In the United States craftsmanship offered to the middle class the promise of a return to a life that was slower-paced and grounded in familiar values, and was therefore very attractive (Boris, 1984). Crafts were also taught at settlement houses such as Hull House as a way to help immigrants assimilate into their new culture and to offer them an opportunity to learn a potential skill (Addams, 1911).

Dunton and his colleagues took the arts and crafts movement one step further: they applied the concept of engagement in crafts to the treatment of children and adults with emotional disabilities. "Handcrafts have a special therapeutic value as they afford occupation which combines the elements of play and recreation with work and accomplishment. They give a concrete return and provide a stimulus to mental activity and muscular exercise at the same time, and afford an opportunity for creation and self-expression" (Johnson, 1920, p. 69). Particularly in the treatment of the mentally ill, crafts became the chief occupation of choice.

One approach to using crafts in occupational therapy was to divide the clients and the crafts by levels of function and complexity. Haas (1924) proposed three "classes" of clients and three levels of crafts. The first group could not be entrusted to work with tools, so it was recommended that they engage in "preliminary" crafts that required modest tool use, such as basketry, weaving, brush making, and chair caning. The second group were those who could be trusted with tools but were at times confused as to their use. Crafts that were more structured and required less technical skill were recommended for these individuals, such as cement work, bookbinding, and printing. The third group was the highest-functioning and consisted of individuals who could use tools and were interested in the crafts. For them, the more complex and artistic crafts were recommended, including metal work, jewelry, carpentry, and pottery.

The challenge to occupational therapists using crafts was to plan the treatment so that it combined a therapeutic process with a satisfying outcome. It was commonly acknowledged that craft work must be of value and interest to the client. "With adults one thing above all is essential, that the work be important . . . Therefore all products should be useful, at least, as well made as is possible, and in some instances should be artistically beautiful" (Haas, 1924, p. 416). At the same time, "therapeutic value should not be lost sight of. Care should be taken not to discourage one who, after an effort, produces a very poor piece of work. The important thing is the therapeutic satisfaction it has given him. For him it is and should be an achievement" (Haas, 1924, p. 416). Most therapists tried to solve the process versus product issue by creating a balance so that clients engaged in crafts that were of interest to them and matched their abilities.

Dunton (1928) was a proponent of making the use of crafts "scientific" in order to justify occupational therapy practice within the medical community. In this case, the science consisted of elaborate activity analyses in which the mental processes (i.e., interest, concentration, initiative) were described, along with the physical requirements (i.e., ankle flexion, controllable posture, good eye-hand coordination); gradation of the activity was determined (from simple to complex, and slow to rapid); and a description was provided of those clients who would be best served by this particular craft (Analysis of Crafts, 1928). There was debate, however, about whether such a classification system was wise or feasible. "There seems to be a feeling that before it can be admitted to the rank of a therapeutic science the kinds of work to be used in occupational therapy must be labeled and arranged like the bottles on the pharmacist's shelves to be administered each for its specific disease. How far is such a definite classification possible or desirable?" (Humphrey, 1922, p. 554). In particular, there was concern about the use of a classification system when it came to the treatment of those with mental illness.

> Along physical lines the classification is comparatively simple . . . and work can be selected according to the required movements. Knotting gives finger movements, weaving gives arm and body development . . . jig-saws furnish foot and leg exercises . . . But where the mental effect upon the patient is the primary end, our whole problem takes on a different aspect. As soon as we get away from the physical standpoint, we at once realize that there is not firm basis for a rigid classification. The demand is not for the exercise of a group of muscles, but the reorganization of a per-sonality (p. 554).

This debate highlights the conflicting ideals underlying the use of arts and crafts in occupational therapy. A rigid ("scientific") classification of crafts and matching diseases goes against the humanistic, individualistic approach of moral treatment. Humphrey (1922) argued that in the treatment of mental illness, the occupational therapist should be free to choose any craft that might be helpful, regardless of its classification, as long at it was suited to the client's interest, intel-lectual capability, and disability. On the other hand, as a physician, Dunton (1928) was well aware of the need for occupational therapy to establish itself within the medical community as a health profession with a basis in science. The best way for occupational therapists to have their work recognized as a legitimate therapeutic endeavor was to be able to document its efficacy scientifically.

Adolph Meyer: Psychobiology, Occupation, and Habits

As one of the leading psychiatrists of the early twentieth century, Meyer was well aware of science and its importance in the treatment of people with mental ill-ness. However, Meyer was concerned that scientific thinking could be reduc-tionistic and mechanistic: "The great mistake of an overambitious science has been the desire to study [human beings] altogether as a mere sum of the parts, if possible of atoms . . . and as a machine, detached, by itself" (Meyer, 1948/1921, p. 3). In contrast, Meyer argued that nurture and nature were both important. He proposed **psychobiological** as an approach, which considered an individual's performance and occupational history, in addition to biological and neurological data. "We take up a survey of functions of the person beginning with the full-fledged performances and achievements and attempt to give an idea of the individual; the personal care, the jobs and hobbies . . . family, sociability, public life, education, religious activity, etc . . . . [all] interests and ambitions, one's perceptive life (sensual and esthetic gratification) dreaming, thinking, acting" (1948/1934, p. 319).

Meyer earned his MD in Zurich in 1892 and immigrated to the United States to study neurology. At the time there was no recognized specialty examination in psychiatry, so practitioners called themselves by various titles: alienist, psychiatrist, psychologist, neurologist, pathologist, or internist. Meyer's first appointments were as a researcher. Ultimately, he tired of pathology and decided that the study of psychiatry was best done at the bedside. He was appointed professor of psychiatry at Johns Hopkins in 1910, where he came to know both Dunton and Slagle.

Meyer was a supporter of occupational therapy, and in response to Dunton's request, he published his thoughts in a paper entitled "The Philosophy of Occupation Therapy" in 1922. In this paper he conceptualized mental illness as "problems of living, and not merely diseases of a structural and toxic nature on the one hand or of a final lasting constitutional disorder on the other" (Meyer, 1922a, p. 4). He emphasized the importance of viewing each individual from a holistic and temporal perspective, and of balancing work and rest: "Our body is not merely so many pounds of flesh and bone figuring as a machine, with an abstract mind or soul added to it. It is throughout a living organism pulsating with its rhythm of rest and activity . . . Our conception of man is that of an organism that maintains and balances itself in the world of reality and actuality by . . . acting its time in harmony with its own nature and the nature about it" (p. 5).

Meyer proposed engagement in occupation as a way to address the problems of living. "Our role consists in giving opportunities rather than prescriptions. There must be opportunities to work, opportunities to do and plan and create, and to learn to use material" (p. 7). One important aspect of occupation was habits. "It will be our duty to define in actual cases what sets of habits we find interwoven and with what effect. This directs the attention to the investigation of matters which are open to influence in education, and to a more rational management of dementia praecox [an early term for schizophrenia], as well as many other mental disorders" (1948/1905, p. 181). Meyer proposed that "habit disorder is to be treated by habit training" (p. 180). As the director of the Phipps Clinic at Johns Hopkins Hospital, Meyer was in an excellent position to see that his ideas on **habit training** were implemented. He recruited Eleanor Clarke Slagle to direct the first Occupational Therapy Program.

Eleanor Clarke Slagle: Curative Occupations and Habit Training

At a retirement dinner in Slagle's honor, Harriet Robeson (1937) characterized Slagle as a "pioneer by nature, with a searching mind and a keen interest in social problems and their psychological aspects" (p. 3). Slagle brought to the new profession of occupational therapy her dedication to social reform in mental hygiene. She first became acquainted with the concept of therapeutic occupations when she took a course in **curative occupations** conducted at Hull House in 1911. The course was designed to educate "institution attendants in occupations for the insane" (Taylor, 1909, quoted in Quiroga, 1995, p. 42). Later, in 1912, Slagle was recruited by Meyer and came to Phipps clinic to oversee the new Department of Occupational Therapy.

One of her contributions was the creation and implementation of a habit training program, based on Meyer's focus on habits. According to Meyer (1948/1922b, p. 486), "the first point is development of habits which can be thoroughly satisfied in harmony with the environment and with ample opportunity for satisfaction . . . There must be habits of work for which there is a market and call, habits of care of oneself in keeping with the probable opportunities, habits of recreation easily enough dovetailed with life, habits of melioristic self-culture—social, educational, civil and religious habits and contacts."

Habit training required the health practitioner to "make distinctions of various types of habit disorganization, to study the working of the various sets of activities and habits in the patient, determine their relative value by accurate observation . . . and shape our therapeutic measures in accord with these principles" (Meyer, 1948/1905, p. 181).

Slagle designed a habit training program for a group of the most profoundly ill clients, who were diagnosed as having dementia praecox. "To visualize the picture more clearly, let us consider a group of sixteen untidy, destructive, assaultive, abusive and rapidly deteriorating young women" (Slagle, 1924, p. 100). Slagle structured the program so that the clients followed a strict schedule of self-care, physical activities, occupation classes, and meals. At the end of a year, she judged their progress as quite successful. "This group are entirely retrained in decent habits of living and are now being trained in carefully graded tasks" (p. 100).

Stimulated by Meyer and Slagle's example, habit training programs were introduced at other mental health facilities. Wilson (1929), chief occupational therapist at Brooklyn State Hospital, New York, described the program she supervised as a "progressive schedule through which the patient is carried to the highest level of adjustment possible to that particular individual" (p. 189). She vividly portrays the extent of the mental disorders they attempted to address through habit training.

> The regressed mental patient has been unable to adjust at an adult level of existence, but has slipped back to a lower level at which he feels comfortable, content and safe. This level may be so low that he leads a practically vegetative existence. He may not feed, dress or undress himself and frequently wets and soils bed and clothing; in fact he does nothing for himself, and is a great economic burden to those charged with his care. He is often mute, stuperous, and resistive. (p. 190)

The habit training program was the most successful treatment approach for these severely involved clients, Wilson argued, because it provided "intensive care and re-education." However, she noted that this intensive care made it possible to treat only a small, select group of individuals. (She recommended that the ratio of clients to employees be no more than 10:1.) Thus, similar to moral treatment, the habit training programs could be overwhelmed by the large number of clients requiring services alongside the inadequate staffing and resources.

Herbert James Hall: Neurasthenia and Work Therapy

At the turn of the twentieth century it was much more comforting for clients to suffer from "nerves" than insanity. For this reason many more people identified themselves as needing relief from nervous disorders than from mental illness. In Europe, people went to spas and sanitariums, which employed psychiatrists to oversee the therapeutic regimen that commonly included rest, diet, and water therapy. Psychiatrists in the United States coined the term **neurasthenia** to refer to nervous conditions such as hysteria, hypochondria, depression, compulsive behavior, and anxiety. The typical treatment was the same as in Europe—the rest cure—and was equally expensive.

Herbert Hall did not believe that rest was the answer; instead, he advocated work as the remedy. "Probably every practitioner of medicine has felt that if he could get his weary and irritable neurasthenic to care for something outside his own little circle of troubles, to work perhaps at some absorbing occupation, a cure would be accomplished. It is, no doubt, normal and right for a man to be busy; or unoccupied for any length of time, his nervous energies turn in upon themselves and are likely to create mental confusion and depression" (1913, p. 5). Hall designed a treatment regimen that began with a few days of rest, followed by a program in which the hours of rest were gradually decreased and the hours of work increased "until the day is full of interest and self-forgetfulness . . . The progression leads to the shop and depends upon the work there, to fix and render permanent the improvement" (pp. 9–10).

His pioneering work brought him to the attention of Dunton and Slagle, and Hall became an early spokesperson and leader within occupational therapy. Hall graduated from Harvard University Medical School in 1895, where he did an internship at Massachusetts General Hospital. Like all doctors at the time, he had no special training in psychiatry, and therefore gained his knowledge in his practice treating individuals with neurasthenia. In an article on what he called the "high-grade neurasthenic," Hall (1921) described his clients as people "who go from one physician to another, who are sometimes cured by Christian Science or Chiropracty, by a tonic or a few weeks at a sanatorium and unfortunately also, they are the patients who often do not get well or reach a level of efficiency and comfort which they or we may fairly call health" (p. 232).

Hall founded the Devereux Workshops in order to implement his ideas about the value of work as a remedy. He ran an announcement that read: "Through the generosity and understanding of a friend of Occupational Therapy, it has become possible to establish at Marblehead, Massachusetts, a small experimental station for the study of problems of invalid occupations" (Research in Occupational Therapy). He went on to say that the workshop would be staffed by designers and craftsmen who would help "in the development of new occupations which will be elastic enough to meet the varied requirements of invalids and which will, at the same time result in really valuable products." Ultimately, one of the popular occupations that evolved was toy making. Hall describes how "this shop or laboratory, as it may be called, has supplied its toys to more than seventy-five different hospitals scattered all over the country . . . The wooden toy stands very high among the crafts available for the handicapped" (Hall, 1922, p. 63).

Hall's workshop emphasized engagement in craftwork that was not only intrinsically valuable but also commercially viable.

> Surely here is a brave and practical way of looking at the problem of occupations for the handicapped. Every man who can be made fit must be reinstated in his old trade. Those who cannot compete with able-bodied labor may nevertheless resume their own trades under special and favored conditions. Those who cannot go back to their original work may find remunerative employment in their own homes or in especially devised handicapped workshops. Why is this not a sensible model for all handicapped industries in our own country? If the little shops, the hospital industries can be made self-supporting, well and good; if not, they have served a larger purpose. (Hall, 1917, p. 384)

Besides his clients with neurasthenia, Hall was concerned with the many wounded soldiers who were returning after World War I. Hall likened the "shell shock" that the soldiers suffered to the neurasthenia of his clients. Hall, along with his colleagues, justified the creation of the new profession of occupational therapy by emphasizing its potential to enable clients to return to useful, productive lives. It was this aspect of the new profession that most captured the imagination of the public (Ambrosi & Schwartz, 1995). This was in part due to society's preoccupation with what would happen to the soldiers who had suffered psychological or physical injury as a result of World War I. This concern is reflected in the platforms of both major political parties in the 1924 elections, in which they cite as one of their goals the restoration of the veteran with disability to a position of social usefulness (Full text, 1924; Text of platform, 1924). It was also in keeping with the values of American society during the Progressive era, which emphasized economic self-sufficiency, social contribution, and the Protestant work ethic (Wiebe, 1967).

Thus, occupational therapy promoted itself as the profession that would restore persons with mental and physical disabilities to full economic and social usefulness. Slagle (1923) described occupational therapy as an evolutionary process in which individuals make "a complete change in their whole relationship to life . . . from the position of a liability to that of an asset" (p. 57). Dunton asserted that occupation teachers could play an important role in the instruction of veterans in crafts that could help them earn a living (Seek Occupations for War Cripples, 1917). Thomas Kidner and George Barton, two of the profession's founders, created environments that would foster the abilities of clients to return to satisfying, remunerative work. Kidner (1925), former vocational secretary of the Canadian Military Hospitals Commission, developed the "pre-industrial shop" to promote "re-adjustment to normal living by affording opportunity for the development of habits of industry that have been impaired by disease or injury" (p. 188). Barton created Consolation House in an effort to "get away from institutional life" to one where the individual "could be happy, get well, and become self-supporting" (Newton, 1917).

The Arequipa Sanatorium in Marin, California, addressed the problem of "remunerative permanent occupation" by teaching the women clients to make pottery. "As originally planned, it was not intended to do more than provide an interesting occupation during the tedious convalescence from depression and disease and possibly [make] enough profit to contribute to the support of the patient. But the unexpected development of latent talent, as well as the impossibility in many cases of returning to the old employment, led to a consideration of possible connection with the working world and permanent remunerative occupation in the future" (Brown, 1917, p. 394). Brown, who was the medical director, noted that of the 66 clients who learned pottery making, "twenty-four have made good" (p. 395), meaning that they were able to be discharged and to live on their earnings independently. Arequipa pottery came to be highly valued, and some of the craftswomen, with the support of wealthy patrons, went on to become acclaimed artists.

It was not uncommon for state mental hospitals and private asylums to have clients perform work around the institutions as part of their "occupational" therapy. Thus, clients were given the opportunity to "earn something toward the support of their families" (Hospital Will Restore the Industrial Wounded, 1923, p. 3). The reason the New York State Hospital Commission recommended the hiring of occupational therapists was so that they could train clients with mental illness for a useful activity (Hard Times Cause Record in Insane, 1922). Hall (1917) wholeheartedly agreed with this approach. He wrote that his experience with therapeutic occupations led him to conclude that "the more useful the work, the better its therapeutic effect; and conversely, the more trivial and valueless the product of the work, the less effective" (p. 383).

The work of these four individuals reflect the ideas that laid the foundation for psychosocial occupational therapy practice. The roots of psychosocial occupational therapy are founded in the humanistic philosophy of moral treatment, which provided engagement in occupations and a regularity of schedule as the focus of the treatment for the mentally ill. Engagement in occupation is at the center of the therapeutic process. Occupations provide a way to address the holistic needs of the individual and to help create a balance of work, play, and rest. Habit training is proposed as a way to decrease negative habits by instilling a healthy regimen of daily activities. Arts and crafts are advocated to arouse interest, promote good work habits, and increase skills. Engagement in work is promoted as a way to motivate and reinvigorate individuals, and to develop new skills that will ultimately enable people to return to socially productive lives.

TREATMENT OF MENTAL ILLNESS IN THE TWENTIETH CENTURY

The twentieth century was a time of great experimentation in the treatment of mental illness. Since no one thus far had discovered a cure for mental illness, any and all theories, modalities, and approaches that might work were tried. The century began under the influence of Emil Kraepelin (1883), a German psychiatrist, who revolutionized the psychiatric world by proposing the classification of symptoms into major psychiatric disease entities, such as manic-depressive illness and dementia praecox. He based his findings on the careful, systematic study of a large number of his clients over time. These studies revealed that the diagnoses presented with different symptoms and the courses of the diseases were different as well. Although his classifications were a precursor to the *Diagnostic and Statistical Manual of Mental Disorders (DSM)*, Kraepelin's motivation was not to pigeon-hole people into a diagnosis. Rather, as a clinician, he wanted to understand and be able to help families understand the probable course over time of their loved one's disease. In the United States his constructs were adopted by psychiatrists such as Meyer. Indeed, Meyer's ideas about habit training were specifically directed at the treatment of clients with dementia praecox.

However, even with a better understanding of the various disease entities and knowledge of their probable clinical course, practitioners were still uncertain as to what treatments would be most effective. **Psychoanalysis** offered a new theory and a new hope for an effective treatment. (See Chapter 4 for further discussion.) Sigmund Freud, the founder of psychoanalysis, proposed that psychological problems arose as a result of unconscious conflicts over past events, especially of a sexual nature (Gay, 1989). Treatment consisted of the client spending considerable time with the therapist, examining past events and possible feelings that they evoked. Thus, the psychoanalytic process emphasized the importance of the doctor-client relationship. Freud's approach spread from Vienna to the rest of Europe, and ultimately to the United States, where it became a pervasive force in psychiatry from 1930 through the 1970s. Although psychoanalysis was originally directed toward individuals with neurosis, American psychiatrists such as Meyer and Harry Stack Sullivan proposed it could be used with clients with serious mental illness. Thus, many of the private hospitals that had originally been founded under the moral treatment model, including Phipps Clinic and Sheppard and Enoch Pratt Hospital, added psychoanalysis to their treatment approach.

At the same time that psychoanalysis was spreading, alternative approaches were being tried in an attempt to address the many clients who were stagnating in the state mental institutions, as asylums had come to be called. "Walking through the wards, one would see the schizophrenics who spent their entire day in assumed statuesque postures . . . or in rocking rhythmically and tirelessly backwards and forwards" (Rollin, 1990, p. 191). Drugs, including morphine, phenobarbital, and chloral hydrate, were used to try to diminish symptoms. **Electroconvulsive therapy**, or ECT, was first introduced in the United States at the New York Psychiatric Institute in 1940. Although some clients developed fractures as a result of their movements during the convulsions, as well as a myriad of other side effects, for many clients it made a profound change in their condition. By 1959 ECT had become the treatment of choice for major depression (Shorter, 1997). Psychosurgery was practiced in the United States from 1936 to 1954 in the form of the lobotomy. In the lobotomy, part of the brain's frontal lobe was excised, making clients much calmer and less threatening but also depriving them of judgment and social skills. By 1951 no fewer than 18,608 individuals had undergone psychosurgery (Grob, 1991).

At the same time in England, the concept of the therapeutic community was introduced as an alternative to psychoanalysis, drugs, physical modalities, and surgery. It built upon the ideas from moral treatment about respect for the client and the belief that the environment was a significant influence in the therapeutic process. It added a new dimension in advocating that the client should have autonomy and a voice in determining how the therapeutic community would be run. Joshua Bierer introduced the concept of milieu or therapeutic community therapy in London in the late 1930s. Bierer (1980), a psychotherapist who fled Vienna for London during World War II, proposed that psychotherapy groups be run by the clients. In order to provide a suitable environment for the groups to meet, Bierer also established one of the first psychiatric day hospitals. Thus, a therapeutic community was created where clients could run their group sessions, and where they could also receive counseling, occupational therapy, and other supportive services. The idea of the therapeutic community became so popular in the United States that by 1960 almost all mental health facilities claimed to use this approach. Shorter (1997) argues that the American version of the therapeutic community was significantly different from the English, in that the necessary resources to make it successful were never provided and it was not fully embraced by psychiatrists who remained enamored with psychoanalysis.

By mid-century, despite all these therapeutic innovations, mental hospitals still contained many seriously ill people who could not benefit from any of the therapeutic approaches or modalities. That situation began to change in 1954 when chlorpromazine was introduced in the United States. Clinical trials revealed that this drug calmed agitated clients and ameliorated the severe behaviors associated with psychosis (Rollin, 1990). Thus began the era of psychopharmacology, which has since seen the development of many sophisticated antipsychotics, antimanics, and antidepressants. There is little doubt that the introduction of these drugs represented a significant step forward for the many people who would have been lifelong inmates in institutions. Many of them could now lead relatively normal lives in the community. The drugs, however, did come at a price. One problem was the side effects, particularly of the early drugs. The most tragic consequence was an unintended one: as the numbers of clients in the state and county institutions decreased substantially, these institutions were closed. In theory, discharged clients were to be supported by resources in the community, thus linking the deinstitutionalization movement to the community mental health movement. In practice, the funding was paltry or nonexistent and many clients were left to fend for themselves on the streets (Torrey, 1988).

THE EVOLUTION OF PSYCHOSOCIAL OCCUPATIONAL THERAPY

The history of mental health treatment in the twentieth century provides a backdrop from which to view the evolution of psychosocial occupational therapy. It is important to remember that the profession did not develop in a vacuum, and in fact responded to changes in mental health treatment by coming up with its own innovative version of treatment, which blended work in occupations and activities with new ideas about treatment of the mentally ill. This portion of the chapter examines the ideas, approaches, and treatments that most influenced psychosocial practice during the decades that followed the profession's founding.

The 1920s and 1930s

From the founding years through the 1930s, psychosocial occupational therapy practice remained focused on improving clients through their engagement in occupations. "The therapist, through stimulating the patient to engage in certain activities, aims to awaken interest, develop concentration, restore coordination, revive hope, inspire confidence, and give satisfaction through personal achievement" (Haas, 1931, p. 244). Practice took place primarily in the state hospitals, where occupational therapy was responsible for overseeing the environment in which the occupations occurred. Clients worked throughout the hospital, including the laundry, the shops, the sewing room, and the farm (Patterson, 1931). On the ward clients were engaged in habit training and crafts (Fagley, 1931). Physical activities were also deemed important, such as walks, dances, baseball, and fishing trips. At the time therapy was still very much influenced by a humanistic philosophy: "Our patients are people, like you and me, to whom something has happened, and as a result [they] are unable to make satisfactory adjustments to life . . . and must be treated accordingly" (Stevenson, 1931, p. 85).

The 1940s and 1950s

During these decades psychosocial practice shifted in response to the establishment of the psychoanalytic perspective as a part of occupational therapy's treatment rationale. This does not mean that occupational therapy abandoned its belief in the importance of adaptation and the environment. "Persons suffering from mental disease are generally ill as a result of an accumulation of unsuccessful efforts on the part of the individual to adjust to the environment" (Wade, 1947, p. 83). The psychoanalytic perspective was simply added to the occupational therapy treatment rationale. In the first edition of the Willard and Spackman text, Wade (1947) describes occupational therapy as a "supplement" to psychoanalysis. "In the type of treatment, consisting primarily of psychotherapy using the psychoanalytic approach, occupational therapy functions as indirect therapy. It provides a socially acceptable means of sublimation for the conscious expression of the instinctual urges of the patient" (p. 104).

By the late 1950s the psychoanalytic object relations approach had become a recognized rationale to treat persons with schizophrenia (AOTA, 1959). Its major proponents were Fidler (1958) and the Azimas (1959). Gail Fidler (1958) argued that the primary goal of treatment was ego integration and maturation: "The development of a realistic self concept and ego strength can occur for the schizophrenic only to the extent that his primitive narcissistic needs are gratified" (p. 10). Fidler (1957) recommended that occupational therapy activities use objects and object relations as the primary treatment method. "Activities used as treatment provide an almost unique situation in which the patient as an active participant can deal with his actions as well as his feelings and thoughts" (p. 8). Crafts were advocated as an excellent medium in that they offered the opportunity for creative expression and affective display (Smith, Barrow, & Whitney, 1959). For example, clay was commonly used with "regressed patients, on the assumption that unstructured manipulation . . . is at once an easy and satisfying anal activity" (p. 21). Occupational therapists were also urged to use art (Friedman, 1952) and music (Reese, 1952) as occupations that would encourage expression of feelings.

However, Fidler (1957) envisioned a much larger significance for occupational therapy than simply enabling the client to experience certain feelings as she or he hammered a copper tray. "Occupational therapy provides the patient with a laboratory for living, a situation in which he can learn and practice new skills in living, experiment in a give and take relationship with others, utilize insights gained in psychotherapy, and learn and test more effective means of communication" (p. 8). Hand in hand with providing a "laboratory for living" was the therapist's own ability to influence the interaction. This came to be termed "the therapeutic use of self" and was formally recognized as an important therapeutic tool by the profession (AOTA, 1959). Indeed, Huntting (1953) argued that the occupational therapist should put as much thought into how she or he related to the client as to the choice of activity.

Near the end of the 1950s, occupational therapists began to document the effects of thorazine and serpasil on clients with major psychoses (Elkins & Van Vlack, 1957). The changes seen in clients were quite substantial: they became much more relaxed and organized, and were able to participate more fully in occupational therapy activities (Clauer & Wise, 1958). However, it was also noted that at high doses of thorazine clients showed signs of incoordination and Parkinson-like symptoms. Occupational therapists also treated clients who underwent ECT or lobotomies. "Occupational therapists must be alert to the anxiety and dread of shock therapy by the patients and try to alleviate it through their interest in activity" (Elkins & Van Vlack, 1957, p. 269). The focus of treatment after the ECT was to prevent relapse (Clauer & Wise, 1958). Occupational therapists who treated clients with lobotomies were urged to use graded activities to decrease their confusion and regression (Shalik, 1955).

The 1960s and 1970s

These decades were a time of great concern with the role of psychosocial occupational therapy. One way to view this crisis was to see it within the larger context of the field of mental health. Shimota (1965), a psychologist, suggested in an address to occupational therapists that their questions were similar to those raised by other mental health professionals who were questioning the effectiveness of current approaches to treatment. Many of these questions concerned the effectiveness and appropriateness of psychoanalysis, particularly in the treatment of schizophrenia. Questions were also raised by psychiatrists such as Szasz (1960), who proposed that mental illness was a myth—a social construct. At the root of these questions, he believed, was a concern for "the ineffectiveness of current forms of treatment. If one method does not work, we have to find a new one but, had it worked, we'd be quite satisfied with it" (p. 80).

Woodside (1971), in a paper ostensibly about the history of occupational therapy, situated the problem within the profession itself. "Psychiatric occupational therapy could cease to exist because other professions are rapidly absorbing our body of knowledge, they appear to the public to be offering the same services that we offer, and they are selling their programs to other professionals and the public more effectively than we are" (p. 229). As an occupational therapist Woodside was discouraged when she saw nurses, psychologists, social workers, vocational counselors, and recreation, music, art, dance, and activity therapists doing aspects of occupational therapy. "*Their* 'therapy' looks very similar to ours and I wonder if we can adequately explain our uniqueness to those concerned with the rising costs of medical care and the overlapping of professional services" (pp. 229–230). Psychosocial occupational therapy was floundering, Woodside argued, because it was unable to articulate its uniqueness and to fight for its services. "I suggest that occupational therapy is gradually losing its professional role in psychiatric care because we have always been unsure of our unique professional responsibilities . . . and have not fought to maintain the boundaries of our services to patients, but have repeatedly capitulated to more established and more verbal professions" (p. 230). Woodside ended her address with a warning and a challenge to all psychosocial occupational therapists: "Society may lose a profession with a vibrant history and the potential for a healthy future. What are you doing to prevent this?" (p. 230).

In answer to Woodside's question, innovative ideas were being offered within psychosocial occupational therapy. Howe and Dippy (1968) proposed that the next site for practice should be the new comprehensive community mental health centers funded by the federal government as well as the psychiatric day hospitals that were becoming increasingly popular. This idea built on the growing recognition within the profession that the best environment for psychosocial occupational therapy was the community. "If the fundamental principles of occupational therapy are carefully examined, the idea emerges that the most meaningful place to carry out such treatment would be in the home and in the community. The most natural social context in which to treat a patient would be with the family or people with whom he lives" (Watanabe, 1967, p. 353).

Sandra Watanabe (1967) argued that community treatment enabled the occupational therapist to focus on the "life tasks of the patient—his education and work, avocational and social interests, and all activities of daily living, including self care, housekeeping and child-rearing" (p. 354). In particular, she emphasized the importance of treatment based on a knowledge of the habits and patterns the individual had adopted. She proposed that the primary treatment modalities were to be found in the client's home: making a cup of tea, doing financial planning, developing child care techniques, practicing vocational skills, or initiating a hobby. She deemphasized crafts except where they were contextually appropriate: "the most realistic tasks and objects would be the life tasks and personal objects of the individual" (p. 353). The ultimate advantage of treatment in the community, she argued, was that it promoted occupational therapy treatment that was client-centered. "When the consultation is patient-centered, we direct our attention to general case management, with a life task focus [on] the activities of daily living, motivational techniques and enriching activities" (p. 355).

Another important idea was the activity or task-oriented group led by the occupational therapist, as a complement to the psychotherapy group. Shannon and Snortum (1965) argued that the occupational therapist was in a perfect position to initiate activity groups where clients could have an opportunity to learn and practice new skills. "While intensive group psychotherapy is useful as a point of origin for verbal insights, patients require assistance in converting verbal insights into new behavior. By working in a group of limited size, the patient could be provided with a more closely supervised opportunity for practicing rudimentary social skills and could receive needed feedback from actual experience" (p. 345). They urged therapists to think beyond their traditional beliefs about their work: "Traditionally the responsibility for group psychotherapy in psychiatric hospitals has rested with the psychiatrist, psychologist or the social worker. The failure of the occupational therapist to become actively involved in this area may be attributed to the belief that group work is not the occupational therapist's responsibility" (p. 344).

Fidler (1969) envisioned the task-oriented group as one context in which her "laboratory for living" could take place. "The nature of the occupational therapy setting which expects active involvement in doing, provides a microcosm for life-work situations which can be seen and explored as they occur rather than in retrospect" (p. 69). She proposed that the intent of the task-oriented group was to provide a shared work experience where the relationship between "feeling, thinking and behavior, their impact on others and on task accomplishment, and productivity can be viewed and explored" (p. 45). She defined a task as any activity or process directed toward creating a service or end product. Examples included publishing a newspaper, cooking, gardening, and planning an outing. A primary goal of the groups was to promote problem solving: "Responsibility for selecting and accomplishing a task provides opportunity for the group to explore problem-solving and decision-making skills, [and] to have concrete evidence of their ability to function" (p. 45). Even though the group might take place in an institution, the task-oriented group, as Fidler defined it, more closely resembled living in the community, and thereby provided practice in learning those skills needed for community adjustment.

In response to questions raised at the University of Southern California as to whether psychosocial occupational therapy practice should remain a legitimate part of the university curriculum, Mary Reilly (1966) set up a model occupational therapy program. Reilly observed that there was little theory or research to substantiate its effectiveness. The model program had several key components. One was that clients would graduate from classes in the Department of Occupational Therapy to employment in various departments of the hospital and then to work in the community. Thus, the program was set up on a developmental model that assumed that old behaviors could be reconstituted and new behaviors could be learned. It also emphasized the importance of work in an individual's life. A second principle was that the program was focused on developing the individual's capacity for self-direction and decision making. This was based on the belief that therapy needed to go beyond simply guiding and directing, by giving the client sufficient autonomy to take responsibility for his or her own decisions. Otherwise, Reilly felt that treatment just perpetuated social disability. The third principle focused on the importance of providing normal living experiences that were performed at natural times. Thus, each client had a structured schedule that more or less corresponded to the "natural social order of daily living" (p. 63). This principle drew on Meyer's ideas regarding habits, routine, temporal adaptation, and balance of work and play. For these ideas Reilly credits Meyer and urges a recommitment to his principles. We can see in this program the foundation for a theoretical model that Reilly and her colleagues would call Occupational Behavior and ultimately would become the Model of Human Occupation (Kielhofner, 2002).

Summary

One way to see the psychosocial occupational therapy of today is to view it as an amalgam of past best practices. In looking at the past 80 years we can identify many ideas that have been retained, albeit in a somewhat different form, whereas other approaches have been dropped. In part this is due to the fact that mental health practice has changed, and so occupational therapy treatment has changed along with it. For example, psychoanalysis no longer provides the predominant framework for treatment that it did in the 1940s and 1950s. But occupational therapists still retain the notion of the importance of meaning in occupation, which one could argue was derived from the focus on the symbolic nature of the projective activities.

At times the founding concepts of occupational therapy were deemphasized, as new approaches and techniques were introduced. However, by the end of the twentieth century there was a reemphasis on the founding ideas, as psychosocial occupational therapy practice appears to have returned to its roots. Today we see practice that is still grounded in the humanistic philosophy of moral treatment, "the conception that occupational therapy is based first and foremost upon respect for human individuality and on a fundamental perception of the individual's needs to engage in creative activity" (Bockoven, 1971, p. 223).

The central concept of occupational therapy is the same as that articulated by the founders: engagement in valued occupations (Law, 2002). Occupations continue to provide a way to help create a balance of work, play, and rest (Kielhofner, 2002). Habits are seen as integral to optimal performance in both personal and instrumental activities of daily living (Occupational Therapy Practice Framework, 2002). Arts and crafts remain a viable medium for motivating, promoting good work habits, and increasing skills. Vocational occupations help to develop new skills and productive habits that can sustain independent living in the community.

In addition to the founding concepts, innovations from the 1960s have also been incorporated into today's practice. Much psychosocial treatment today is done in groups and conducted in the community. Treatment is client-centered and focused on providing functional living skills (Melville, Baltic, Bettcher, & Nelson, 2002). Drug management has become a critical aspect of treatment for most clients, and this has allowed many to live in the community with the support of occupational therapy services. Thus, contemporary psychosocial practice consists of some of the best ideas of the past reformulated into models and treatments that also reflect today's beliefs regarding mental illness.

As this book demonstrates, psychosocial occupational therapy has come through its professional crisis, and therapists today are actively engaged in many aspects of practice. However, although Woodside's warnings about the demise of psychosocial occupational therapy were premature, there is still a need for vigilance and innovation. Conflicts remain over which mental health professional should provide which service, and the need to justify services to third-party payers has become of critical importance. Psychosocial occupational therapists must continue to clearly articulate what occupational therapy can do and to fight for its services in the treatment of individuals with mental illness. It is hoped that this history will help psychosocial occupational therapists understand their rich past as well as future promise.

Review Questions

1. How are the contributions of the founders exemplified in current psychosocial occupational therapy practice?
2. What values have endured from the founding of occupational therapy to the present?
3. Describe six innovations introduced by occupational therapy leaders in the 1950s and 1960s that contribute to practice today?

References

Addams, J. (1911). *Twenty years at Hull House*. New York: Macmillan.

Ambrosi, E., and Schwartz, K. B. (1995). The profession's image, 1917–1925: Occupational therapy as represented in the media. *American Journal of Occupational Therapy, 49*, 715–719.

American Occupational Therapy Association. (1925). An outline of lectures on occupational therapy to medical students and physicians. *Occupational Therapy and Rehabilitation, 4*(4), 277–292.

American Occupational Therapy Association (1959). The schizophrenic patient. In AOTA (Ed.), *The objectives and functions of occupational therapy* (pp. 130–136). Dubuque, IA: Wm. C. Brown.

Analysis of Crafts. (1928). Continuation of the Report of the Committee on Installations and Advice. *Occupational Therapy and Rehabilitation, 7*, 417–420.

Azima, H., & Azima, F. (1959). Outline of a dynamic theory of occupational therapy. *American Journal of Occupational Therapy, 13*, 215–221.

Bierer, J. (1980). From psychiatry to social and community psychiatry. *International Journal of Social Psychiatry, 26*, 77–79.

Bockoven, J. S. (1971). Legacy of moral treatment: 1800's to 1910. *American Journal of Occupational Therapy, 25*(5), 223–225.

Boris, E. (1984). *Art and labor: John Ruskin, William Morris, and the craftsman ideal in America 1876–1915.* Philadelphia: Temple University Press.

Brown, P. K. (1917). The potteries of Arequipa Sanatorium. *Modern Hospital, 8*(6), 394–396.

Caradec, L. (1860). Topographie medico-hygienique du departement du Finiestere. In E. Shorter (1997), *A history of psychiatry.* New York: Wiley.

Clauer, C., & Wise, K. (1958). Tranquilizing drug effects on the schizophrenic patient in occupational therapy. *American Journal of Occupational Therapy, 12*, 69–73.

Dix, D. (1971/1943). *Report to the legislature of Massachusetts.* New York: Arno, pp. 5–7.

Dunton, W. R. (1917). History of occupational therapy. *Modern Hospital, 8*(6), 380–382.

Dunton, W. R. (1928). The three "r's" of occupational therapy. *Occupational Therapy and Rehabilitation, 7*, 345–348.

Elkins, H., & Van Vlack, N. (1957). Changes in occupational therapy due to the tranquilizing drugs. *American Journal of Occupational Therapy, 111*, 269–272.

Fagley, R. C. (1931). The value of occupational therapy in treatment of mental cases. *Occupational Therapy and Rehabilitation, 10*, 291–298.

Fidler, G. S. (1957). The role of occupational therapy in a multi-discipline approach to psychiatric illness. *American Journal of Occupational Therapy, 11*, 8–35.

Fidler, G. S. (1958). Some unique contributions of occupational therapy in treatment of the schizophrenic. *American Journal of Occupational Therapy, 12*, 9–12.

Fidler, G. S. (1969). The task-oriented group as a context for treatment. *American Journal of Occupational Therapy, 23*, 43–48.

Fields, G. E. (1911). The effect of occupation upon the individual. *American Journal of Insanity, 8*, 103–109.

Friedman, I. (1952). Art therapy, an aid to reintegrative processes. *American Journal of Occupational Therapy, 6*, 64–65.

Full text of the Republican platform as reported to the convention last night. (1924, June 12). *New York Times*, 4.

Gay, P. (1989). *The Freud Reader.* New York: Norton.

Grob, G. (1991). *From asylum to community: Mental health policy in modern America.* Princeton, NJ: Princeton University Press.

Haas, L. J. (1924). The men's occupational therapy work at Bloomingdale Hospital. *Modern Hospital, 22*(4), 410, 420.

Haas, L. J. (1931). Precision in presenting occupational therapy to the mentally and nervously ill. *Occupational Therapy and Rehabilitation, 10*, 241–249.

Hall, H. (1913). *The systematic use of work as a remedy in neurasthenia and allied conditions.* Boston: W. M. Leonard.

Hall, H. (1917). Remunerative occupations for the handicapped. *Modern Hospital, 8*(6), 383–386.

Hall, H. (1921). The high-grade neurasthenic. *Boston Medical and Surgical Journal, 185*(8), 232–235.

Hall, H. (1922). Occupational therapy in 1921. *Modern Hospital, 18*(1), 61–63.

Hard Times Cause Record in Insane. (1922, January 2). *New York Times*, 12.

Hospital Will Restore the Industrial Wounded. (1923, July 8). *New York Times*, 3.

Howe, M., & Dippy, K. (1968). The role of occupational therapy in community mental health. *American Journal of Occupational Therapy, 22*, 521–524.

Humphrey, E. F. (1922). Classifying therapeutic occupations from the standpoint of mental patients. *Modern Hospital, 18*(6), 554–556.

Huntting, I. (1953). The importance of interaction between patient and occupational therapist. *American Journal of Occupational Therapy, 7*, 107–109.

Johnson, S. C. (1920). Instruction in handicrafts and design for hospital patients. *Modern Hospital, 15*, 69–75.

Kidner, T. B. (1925). The hospital pre-industrial shop. *Occupational Therapy and Rehabilitation, 4*(3), 187–194.

Kielhofner, G. (2002). *Model of human occupation* (3rd ed.). Philadelphia: Lippincott Williams & Wilkins.

Kraepelin, E. (1883). *Compendium der psychiatrie.* Leipzig: Abel.

Law, M. (2002). Participation in the occupations of everyday life. *American Journal of Occupational Therapy, 56,* 640–649.

Levine, R. E. (1987). The influence of the arts-and-crafts movement on the professional status of occupational therapy. *American Journal of Occupational Therapy, 41*(4), 248–254.

Melville, L., Baltic, T., Bettcher, T., & Nelson, D. (2002). Patients' perspectives on the self-identified goals assessment. *American Journal of Occupational Therapy, 56,* 650–659.

Meyer, A. (1948/1905). The role of habit-disorganizations: Paper for the New York Psychiatrical Society. In A. Lief (Ed.), *The commonsense psychiatry of Dr. Adolph Meyer: Fifty-two selected papers* (pp. 178–183). New York: McGraw Hill.

Meyer, A. (1948/1921). The contributions of psychiatry to the understanding of life problems: An address at the celebration of the 100th anniversary of Bloomingdale Hospital. In A. Lief (Ed.), *The commonsense psychiatry of Dr. Adolph Meyer: Fifty-two selected papers* (pp. 1–15). New York: McGraw Hill.

Meyer, A. (1922a). The philosophy of occupation therapy. *Archives of Occupational Therapy, 1,* 1–10.

Meyer, A. (1948/1922b). Normal and abnormal repression: Address to the Progressive Education Association. In A. Lief (Ed.), *The commonsense psychiatry of Dr. Adolph Meyer: Fifty-two selected papers* (pp. 479–490). New York: McGraw Hill.

Meyer, A. (1948/1934). The birth and development of the mental hygiene movement. In A. Lief (Ed.), *The commonsense psychiatry of Dr. Adolph Meyer: Fifty-two selected papers* (pp. 312–319). New York: McGraw Hill.

Newton, I. (1917). Consolation House. Archives of the Wilma L. West Library, American Occupational Therapy Association, Bethesda, MD.

Occupational Treatment of Patients in State Hospitals. (1914). *Modern Hospital, 2*(4), 302–305.

Occupational Therapy Practice Framework: Domain and Process. (2002). *American Journal of Occupational Therapy, 56,* 609–639.

Patterson, W. L. (1931). Occupational therapy in a state hospital for the insane. *Occupational Therapy and Rehabilitation, 10,* 281–289.

Pinel, P. (1809). *Traite medico-philosophique sur l'alientation mentale* (2nd ed.). Paris: J. A. Brosson.

Reilly, M. (1966). A psychiatric occupational therapy program as a teaching model. *American Journal of Occupational Therapy, 20,* 61–67.

Research in Occupational Therapy: An Announcement. Archives of the Wilma L. West Library, American Occupational Therapy Association, Bethesda, MD.

Reese, M. R. (1952). Music as occupational therapy for psychiatric patients. *American Journal of Occupational Therapy, 6,* 14–49.

Robeson, H. (1937). A testimonial to Eleanor Clarke Slagle. Twenty-first Annual Meeting of the American Occupational Therapy Association, September 14. Archives of the Wilma L. West Library, American Occupational Therapy Association, Bethesda, MD.

Rollin, H. R. (1990). The dark before the dawn. *Journal of Psychopharmacology, 4,* 109–114.

Rothman, D. J. (1971). *The discovery of the asylum.* Boston: Little, Brown.

Seek Occupations for War Cripples. (1917, September 4). *New York Times,* 20.

Shalik, H. (1955). Refining the use of occupational therapy with the lobotomized patient. *American Journal of Occupational Therapy, 9,* 118–120.

Shannon, P., & Snortum, J. (1965). An activity group's role in intensive psychotherapy. *American Journal of Occupational Therapy, 19,* 344–347.

Shimota, H. (1965). Psychiatric occupational therapy. *American Journal of Occupational Therapy, 19,* 79–82.

Shorter, E. (1997). *A history of psychiatry.* New York: Wiley.

Slagle, E. C. (1923). Report of the secretary-treasurer. *Archives of Occupational Therapy, 1,* 49–59.

Slagle, E. C. (1924). A year's development of occupational therapy in New York state hospitals. *Modern Hospital, 22*, 98–104.

Smith, P., Barrow, H., & Whitney, J. (1959). Psychological attributes of occupational therapy crafts. *American Journal of Occupational Therapy, 12*, 16–26.

Stevenson, G. H. (1931). The healing influence of work and play in a mental hospital. *Occupational Therapy and Rehabilitation, 11*, 85–89.

Szasz, T. S. (1960). *The myth of mental illness.* New York: Harper & Row.

Taylor, G. (1909, June). Letter from Graham Taylor to Governor Charles Deneen. In V. Quiroga (1995), *Occupational therapy: The first 30 years.* Bethesda, MD: American Occupational Therapy Association.

Text of platform as presented to the Democratic National Convention. (1924, June 29). *New York Times*, 4.

Torrey, E. F. (1988). *Nowhere to go: The tragic odyssey of the homeless mentally ill.* New York: Harper & Row.

Wade, B. (1947). Occupational therapy for patients with mental disease. In H. Willard & C. Spackman (Eds.), *Principles of occupational therapy* (pp. 81–111). Philadelphia: Lippincott.

Watanabe, S. G. (1967). The developing role of occupational therapy in a psychiatric home service. *American Journal of Occupational Therapy, 21*, 353–356.

Wiebe, R. H. (1967). *The search for order, 1877–1920.* New York: Hill & Wang.

Wilson, S. C. (1929). Habit training for mental cases. *Occupational Therapy and Rehabilitation, 8*(3), 189–197.

Woodside, H. (1971). The development of occupational therapy 1910–1929. *American Journal of Occupational Therapy*, 226–230.

Suggested Reading

Hasselkus, B. R. (2002). *The meaning of everyday occupation.* Thorofare, NJ: Slack.

Fidler, G., & Fidler, J. (1954). *Introduction to psychiatric occupational therapy.* New York: Macmillan.

Fidler, G., & Fidler, J. (1963). *Occupational therapy, a communication process in psychiatry.* New York: Macmillan.

Lief, A. (Ed.). (1947). *The commonsense psychiatry of Dr. Adolph Meyer: Fifty-two selected papers.* New York: McGraw Hill.

CHAPTER 4

Theories of Mental Health and Illness

Michael Alessandri, PhD

Elizabeth Cara, PhD, OTR/L, MFT

Anne MacRae, PhD, OTR/L

Key Terms

biopsychosocial focus
eclectic
psychopharmacology

synthetic eclecticism
technical eclecticism

Chapter Outline

Introduction

It is generally understood that a comprehensive understanding of a client, including relevant biological, psychological, and sociocultural factors, creates more effective and meaningful treatments. This greater understanding, including what is meaningful and motivating to her or him, is likely to enhance treatment compliance, thereby facilitating more positive outcomes. It is in this process of developing an understanding of the individual clients and their needs that an appreciation for multiple theories of mental illness becomes critical. Among the more prominent theoretical perspectives are the humanistic, biological, psychodynamic, behavioral, and cognitive. Each perspective represents a unique set of basic assumptions about psychological disorder, including relevant etiological factors and appropriate treatment strategies. In order to familiarize the reader with these theoretical perspectives, the major concepts of each will be presented independently. Although presented separately, it is not our intention to convey that these perspectives are necessarily incompatible. In order to gain a comprehensive understanding of the client, an integration of concepts from the varied perspectives is most useful. After all, no single one exists that is capable of explaining all psychopathology. An appreciation for all mediating influences on one's behaviors, thoughts, and emotions is essential. Attending to the complex array of biological, intrapsychic, and interpersonal factors that may be creating and/or maintaining mental dysfunction allows for a comprehensive **biopsychosocial focus** understanding of the individual client. This, in turn, will foster the development of more individualized and effective treatment protocols.

Most contemporary therapists use an **eclectic** approach, employing ideas and techniques from a variety of perspectives in order to understand and treat effectively a client's presenting problems (Davis & Adams, 1995). **Synthetic eclecticism** describes the integration of distinct theoretical principles, while **technical eclecticism** refers to the adoption of a variety of therapy strategies and techniques from multiple schools of thought. While eclectic approaches and attempts at theoretical integration have become quite popular, they have not always proven very successful (Patterson, 1989). Nonetheless, it seems reasonable to expect that practitioners who are eclectic in their orientation will have more tools available to them to treat the complex mental health disturbances they encounter.

HUMANISTIC PERSPECTIVE

The humanistic perspective emphasizes the value, worth, and potential of the individual, with a focus on the integrity of the client-therapist relationship. This model of psychological functioning offers a philosophy and an approach to dealing with clients in psychological distress to which all practitioners, regardless of theoretical orientation, should attend. With its primary focus on broad dimensions of an individual's life experience, the humanistic view is generally more encompassing than the other perspectives, which attend to rather specific aspects of human functioning such as physiological processes, unconscious conflicts, learned behaviors, and cognitive processes. For example, humanism pays careful attention to the individual's concept of self as well as personal values. Because of their global perspective, humanistic theories are often seen as more than simply explanations of psychological adjustment and personality development. In fact, they are often viewed as philosophies of life (Davis & Adams, 1995).

Development of the Perspective

The basic tenets of humanistic psychology arose in the early twentieth century as an alternative to the two prominent theoretical models of the time: the psychodynamic and behavioral paradigms. Humanistic principles, however, were evident prior to the development of the formal field of humanistic psychology. For example, early humanistic philosophies are evident in the work of G. Stanley Hall and William James, both of whom stressed the unique characteristics of human beings. In addition, the bridge between theoretical humanism and clinical practice was first seen in the early 1800s by Samuel Tuke, an English Quaker. Tuke developed a program, known appropriately as "moral treatment," stressing the humane treatment of the mentally ill. Prior to this time, clients with psychiatric illnesses were locked up in asylums, where they were provided with basic necessities (i.e., food, water, and shelter), but essentially removed from the community at large. Moral treatment encouraged active involvement in the care and upkeep of the asylum, as well as participation in selected self-care and leisure activities, which included woodworking, gardening, and sewing. Tuke found that engagement in daily tasks had a positive, reality-orienting effect on the psychiatric clients with whom he worked. Moral treatment, it seems, was quite consistent with the principles and practice of occupational therapy (Fidler & Fidler, 1963; Schwartz, 2003). Underlying Tuke's treatment principles is the basis of a humanistic treatment approach: the ability to look beyond the psychiatric disease, unconscious conflicts, and environmental precursors of behavior and toward the inherent worth of each individual.

The popularity of humanistic approaches in clinical practice waxed and waned, but the theoretical principles continued to be expounded, especially in Europe, where humanistic principles were closely tied to existential philosophy (also see Chapter 3). The sociocultural trends of the 1950s and 1960s contributed to the reemergence of humanistic principles and practices in psychology. In particular, the theories of Abraham Maslow and Carl Rogers helped humanism become the "third force" in psychology (Association of Humanistic Psychology, 2001), along with behaviorism and psychodynamic theory. Humanists stressed that behaviorism and psychodynamic theory were too reductionist, with the former focusing on environmental stimuli and resulting observable behavior and the latter focusing on human behavior as being primarily sexually driven (Reilly, 1962). Both Maslow (1968) and Rogers (1951) proposed more global and healthy perspectives of human functioning than these other paradigms, and both held as basic the belief that individuals were innately good and driven to achieve self-actualization (i.e., realize their potential as whole and self-contained beings).

Maslow defined a pyramidal hierarchy (shown in Figure 4-1) representing five levels of needs. The lower levels of the pyramid comprise "deficiency," or survival-based, needs (i.e., physiological needs, safety needs, the need to be loved, and the need to belong to a social group). As one moves up the hierarchy, needs become less survival driven and more focused on the components of happiness and personal success. Among these higher-level needs, or "meta-needs," is the need for esteem. Self-actualization, the point at which a person has realized fully his or her potential, lies at the peak of the pyramid. According to Maslow (1968),

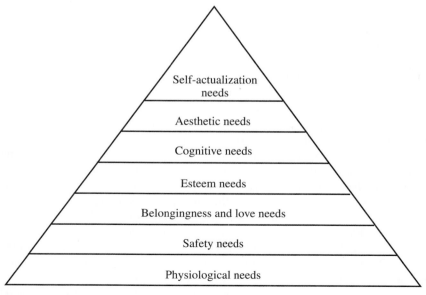

Figure 4-1.   Maslow's Hierarchy of Needs

a person is only able to concentrate on and meet higher-level needs after lower-level needs have been met.

Carl Rogers was heavily influenced by Maslow's hierarchy of needs. He, too, felt the motivating drive of humans was to achieve a state of self-actualization. He believed that it is only through the process of trying to achieve self-actualization that an individual develops an increasingly differentiated self-concept. Reflecting on Maslow's need hierarchy, Rogers proposed that human beings have a basic need for positive regard, especially from parents and significant others in their lives. Rogers conceptualized positive regard as a freely provided and unconditional liking for another person as an individual, without demands or expectations on that person's behavior. When this regard is provided unconditionally to developing children, they will grow up in a better position to realize self-actualization. More often than not, however, children are not raised with unconditional positive regard. Instead, they are taught that positive regard is, in fact, conditional; that is, certain behaviors, thoughts, and emotions valued by the caregiver (typically the parent) are required in order to receive positive regard. What results is a set of conditions of worth, which impacts the child's subsequent behaviors. That is, in an effort to receive positive regard, the child begins to behave in a manner consistent with the conditions and expectations set forth by the caregiver rather than his or her own desires and needs. As a result, the child's need to self-actualize may be in direct competition with his or her need to receive positive regard from the caregiver. The adoption of the standards and values of others may inhibit self-actualization, especially if the standards are very restrictive. It is the discrepancy between one's experience (shaped by conditions of worth) and one's self-concept that creates psychological abnormality. In order to maintain the integrity of the self-concept, discrepant experiences are distorted and denied. The self-concept itself becomes distorted over time as it begins to internalize the conditions of worth set forth by others.

Rogers (1942; 1951; 1961) applied humanistic principles to create client-centered therapy, a nondirective therapeutic approach focused on helping individuals realize their potential by creating a safe, supportive environment to promote self-enhancement. Characteristics present in this nonjudgmental environment include empathy, unconditional positive genuineness, and regard (Davis & Adams, 1995). *Empathy* refers to experiencing the world from the client's perspective. This is accomplished through the use of active listening and reflecting techniques in which the therapist communicates an understanding and acceptance of the client. *Genuineness* involves responding to the client as a human and not just as a therapist. It also requires that therapists stay in touch with their own feelings and be able to communicate them to the client in an effective, appropriate manner. Finally, an environment of *unconditional positive regard* should be created so that clients feel comfortable and secure when engaging in the change process. That is, clients should not feel judged in this environment; they should feel valued and accepted regardless of their thoughts, behaviors, and emotions.

Although notably more existential than humanistic, the beliefs of Victor Frankl (1967; 1972), a survivor of the Nazi concentration camps, represent another strong influence in this phenomenological domain. Frankl disagreed with Rogers and Maslow that the motivating drive toward fulfillment in life is self-actualization. Instead, he postulated that there was a basic drive toward meaning in life and, therefore, that psychiatric disturbances arose from an inability to find meaning in life. This parallels the thinking in occupational therapy, as the significance of the personal meaning of occupation has been well documented in the literature. The founders of occupational therapy certainly recognized the need for meaning in activity (see Chapter 3) and today the search for meaning is a pivotal principle of occupational science (Larson, Wood, & Clark, 2003). Also, the emphasis on client-centered practice (Law, 1998) and on the acknowledgment of spirituality as a fundamental orientation that provides inspiration, personal meaning, and motivation (Occupational Therapy Practice Framework, 2002) have contributed to the recognition of the essential need for and the driving force of meaning. However, Frankl's interpretation of meaning was not limited to the meaning of doing that is often implicit in the occupational therapy literature.

Frankl, along with other existentialists, asserted that there was an anxiety, shared by all humans, that resulted from the knowledge that death, or "nonbeing," is a known outcome of being. It was Frankl's belief that some people resolve this anxiety by finding meaning in their lives. *Meaning* represents different things to different people. It does not have to represent actions toward a specific goal, but it may represent the freedom to take responsibility for an attitude or belief, even if unspoken. Frankl argued that meaning could also be found through the ability to believe in one's inherent worthiness. Accordingly, a person could create meaning or purpose in life simply through the act of taking the responsibility to believe a certain way.

It is the humanist perspective in both psychology and occupational therapy that provides the focus on the whole human being and acknowledges the interconnectedness of the mind, body, and spirit. There are other shared philosophical tenets of humanistic psychology and occupational therapy that are quite striking. Early humanistic psychologists, especially Abraham Maslow, recognized the quality of human adaptation (Rowan, 2004), which is also a cornerstone of occupational therapy (Schultz & Schade, 2003).

Applications in Occupational Therapy

Applications of the theories of Rogers, Maslow, and Frankl have been extended into the arena of occupational therapy practice through the integration of humanistic and existential principles into prominent occupational therapy models. Moreover, as noted by Mosey (1980), the philosophical basis of occupational therapy appears to be grounded in humanistic and existential principles. As previously stated, inherent in the occupational therapy theory base is the belief that individuals find meaning through occupation (Fidler & Fidler, 1978). Occupational therapists are taught to see each client as an individual with unique qualities. This is reflected in the development of goals and treatment objectives, all of which are defined by the client. In today's managed care environment, insurance companies define which services are covered, thus dictating a structure within which goals must be chosen. However, occupational therapists can, and should, define treatment priorities within this structure according to client needs.

Humanistic principles reinforce the notion that no matter how well conceived the therapeutic protocol, the treatment outcome depends on both the client's capacities and his or her choice to utilize them (Yerxa, 1967; Law, 1998). This basic concept highlights perhaps the most salient contribution of humanistic theory—the importance of the individual client in determining his or her own outcomes. Humanistic theories remind therapists that "man, through the use of his hands . . . can influence the state of his own health" (Reilly, 1962, p. 6). Approaching therapy with this dictum in mind encourages therapists to assume a more nondirective approach with the clients they treat. Taking such an approach with a client who has become disabled allows him or her to gain a better understanding of his or her own areas of interest and determine the extent to which his or her own cultural and spiritual identity will impact treatment priorities. Empowering a client to take an active role in the healing process may be the first step toward helping him or her to reestablish meaning in life and therefore the will to live. As Yerxa eloquently states, "I believe our broad purpose is to produce a reality-orienting influence upon the client's perceptions of his physical environment and self" (1967, p. 5).

In summary, the client-centered principles of the humanistic model are very useful in establishing rapport and trust between client and therapist. This is a significant predictor of treatment outcome in all disciplines, including occupational therapy. The practicing occupational therapist, therefore, would be well served by employing humanistic principles as part of the therapeutic process. Being nonjudgmental and genuine toward clients and understanding their perspective or frame of reference (i.e., providing empathy) may be critical to the change process (see Chapter 18 on approaches and techniques). In general, therapists should make every effort to create a nonjudgmental environment in which the vulnerable client feels safe in expressing himself or herself and in learning new, and relearning old, skills.

BIOLOGICAL PERSPECTIVE

The biological perspective has sought to understand the physiological mechanisms underlying behavior. This knowledge allows us to understand the behavior of clients from a biological or medical perspective. According to this model, symptoms of psychological disorder are caused by underlying biological factors. Included among these causal factors may be viral infections, neuroanatomical defects, biochemical (i.e., neurotransmitter and hormonal) imbalances, and genetic predispositions. While other perspectives propose theories regarding the nature of thinking, learning, feeling, and perceiving, this branch attempts to reduce these processes to their simplest components in order to study the mechanisms that produce them.

Although biological factors were long considered as possible determinants of abnormal behavior, it was not convincingly demonstrated that mental illness had an organic basis until syphilis was identified as the cause of a constellation of psychological symptoms, including delusions of grandeur as well as paralysis. From this key discovery, scientists began to speculate about the causal factors of other mental disorders, stimulating revived interest in biological explanations of psychopathology. This perspective views abnormal behavior as an illness caused by malfunctioning parts of the organism, primarily the brain (Gershon & Rieder, 1992; Rosenzweig, Leiman, & Breedlove, 2001). Therefore, a brief overview of brain structure and function is presented next.

The Brain

The brain is made up of billions of neurons and many more support cells, called glia. Groups of neurons form brain regions, such as the hindbrain, midbrain, and forebrain; further differentiation is noted within each region and is shown in Figure 4-2. For example, the hindbrain is comprised of the medulla, pons, cerebellum, and reticular activating system; it is connected to the spinal cord. The forebrain consists of the cerebrum (i.e., the two cerebral hemispheres), thalamus, and hypothalamus. The midbrain coordinates communication between the forebrain and hindbrain regions.

Within the forebrain, the cerebrum is further differentiated into the cerebral cortex, corpus callosum (which connects the two brain hemispheres), basal ganglia, and amygdala. The cerebral cortex has four distinct regions: the frontal, parietal, temporal, and occipital lobes, as is shown in Figure 4-3. The frontal lobe is located near the front of the brain and contains the motor cortex. The parietal lobe contains the somatosensory cortex. The temporal lobes are located on the

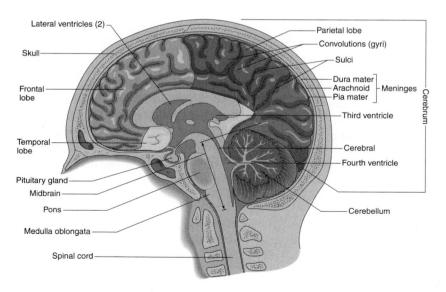

Figure 4-2. Structures of the Brain

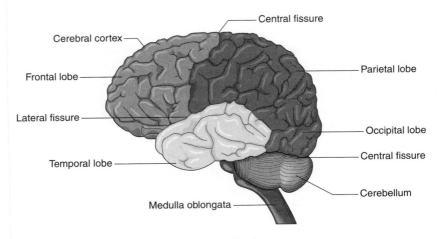

Figure 4-3. The Four Lobes of the Cerebral Cortex

sides of the brain and contain the auditory cortex, and the occipital lobe, at the back of the brain, contains the visual cortex. Finally, the limbic system is located at the base of the forebrain and includes portions of the thalamus, hypothalamus, and amygdala.

Each of these brain regions and subregions is comprised of neurons responsible for specific brain functions. The medulla controls heart rate, respiration, and gastrointestinal function. The pons is involved in sleeping, waking, and dreaming; it is also a pathway for motor information traveling from the cerebral hemispheres to the cerebellum. The cerebellum receives and processes information from peripheral sensory structures (i.e., hair cells of the inner ear, joint receptors, and muscle spindles). It also is responsible for processing feedback from the motor centers of the cortex (e.g., the coordination of head/eye movements; force and timing when reaching for an object, etc.). The reticular activating system screens incoming information and stimulates other brain regions whose pathways pass through the pons and medulla; it is thought to be primarily responsible for the mediation of states of arousal.

In the forebrain, the thalamus is important in processing and relaying information between other regions of the central nervous system and the cerebral cortex. Specifically, it directs incoming sensory information from the visual, auditory, and somatosensory systems to the correct locations within the cerebral cortex. The cerebral cortex is primarily responsible for sensory processing, motor control, and higher mental functions, such as learning, memory, planning, and judgment. The hypothalamus helps regulate body temperature, hunger/satiety, thirst, and the sex drive. It also controls the release of hormones by the pituitary and modulates feelings of pleasure and aggression. The amygdala is involved in the coordination of the autonomic nervous system and the endocrine system, as well as emotional states.

Similar to other brain regions, each of the lobes of the cerebral cortex has specific brain functions. The frontal lobe is involved in higher mental functions such as thinking and planning, as well as in the control of the body muscles. The parietal lobe processes information about pain, pressure, and body temperature. The temporal lobes are involved in memory, perception, and language processing, and the occipital lobe is responsible for visual processing.

Causal Factors of Psychopathology

Psychopathology can be caused by any number of physiological dysfunctions. Included among the possible physiological causes of psychopathology are infections, such as syphilis. Anatomical aberrations may also be present. That is, the size or shape of certain brain regions may be abnormal, thereby creating abnormal behavior. For example, Huntington's disease, which presents with violent emotional outbursts, memory and other cognitive difficulties, delusions, suicidal thinking, and involuntary body movements, has been traced to a loss of neurons in the brain area called the basal ganglia.

However, infections and brain structure defects are not the only determinants of abnormal behavior. It may also be that neurons are not communicating effectively with one another due to improperly functioning neurotransmitter substances and systems. It is via the neurotransmitter substances that neurons transmit electrical impulses to other neurons; thus, these substances are critical in the transmission of information in the brain. Hormonal imbalances may also contribute to aberrant behavior. Neurotransmitter dysfunction and hormonal imbalances represent biochemical causal factors of psychopathology. In addition, genetic factors may also be operating in the manifestation of a psychological disorder.

Biochemical Factors.   Biochemical factors, including neurotransmitter dysfunction and hormonal imbalances, have been implicated as possible causal factors in many psychological disorders. Several of the neurotransmitter substances receiving particular attention in psychopathology research are serotonin, dopamine, gamma-aminobutyric acid (GABA), and norepinephrine. Each of these neurotransmitters has been found to be related to the symptom presentations of specific psychological disorders. To understand how neurotransmitter dysfunction can impact behavior first requires a good understanding of the structure of nerve cells and the mechanism of communication among these cells.

Neurons are comprised of several parts: the cell body, or soma; dendrites; and an axon (shown in Figure 4-4). Most neurons have one axon and numerous dendrites attached to the cell body. The cell body houses the basic cellular components (i.e., ribosomes, endoplasmic reticulum, mitochondria, and Golgi apparatus), which manufacture vital nutrients for the cell's survival. The cell body is also the manufacturing plant of neurotransmitters, the chemical messengers whose transport between cells forms the basis for cellular communication. The axon transports these chemical messengers to its distal end, where they are stored in vesicles until needed. The axon also serves to conduct an electrical signal from its proximal end (by the cell body) to its distal end (where the vesicles are stored).

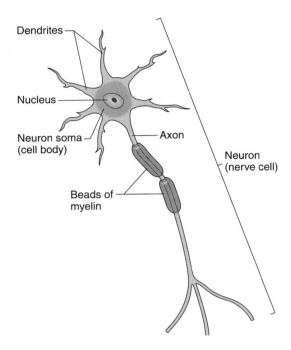

Figure 4-4.   The Neuron

The dendrites are comparable to the antennae of a radio; they receive chemical messages from the axons of other cells. A neuron's axon does not form a direct connection with another neuron's dendrites. Rather, a small gap (approximately 20 billionths of a meter wide) separates them (Thompson, 1993). This space between two neurons is referred to as the synapse.

An electrical impulse is received by a neuron's dendrites (located at one end of a neuron) and then travels down its axon (a long fiber) to the axon's terminus, where it stimulates the release across the synapse of tiny packets of neurotransmitter substances in chemical form. These substances cross the synapse and bind to receptors (actually proteins) on the dendrites of the next neuron. Depending on the nature of the neurotransmitter substance, this binding either stimulates or inhibits the firing of the next neuron. In either case, neurotransmitter substances are essential to effective communication between the neurons.

Normally, the electrical current generated by the bonding of one neurotransmitter on a dendrite is not enough to excite a cell. However, if enough excitatory neurotransmitters bind to the dendrites of a cell in either a short time (temporal summation) or a small space (spatial summation), the cell will build a large electrical charge at the area where the cell body connects with its axon, called the axon hillock. If the axon hillock builds a large enough charge (normally −70 millivolts), gates on the membrane of the axon will open up and allow the charge to propagate down the axon.

A synapse has both a presynaptic and a postsynaptic terminal. The presynaptic terminal lies at the distal end of an axon and contains the vesicles that house the neurotransmitters. The postsynaptic terminal lies on the distal end of a dendrite and contains "locks" with shapes specific for the entry of certain neurotransmitter "keys." The electrical signal, upon reaching the distal end of the axon, causes a chain of reactions to take place as follows. Calcium ions are released, causing the vesicles (housing the neurotransmitters) to bind with the distal end of the axon and, in effect, opening a door through which the neurotransmitters escape from the vesicle within the axon and move into the open space of the synapse beyond. Once in the synapse, the neurotransmitter key is drawn toward the lock on the postsynaptic membrane (on the dendrites of the second cell). If the key fits the lock (in a chemical sense), the neurotransmitter will bind to the membrane and either excite or inhibit the next cell, depending on its function. At this point, the process begins again. This chain of events serves as the basis for communication between neurons.

Many different types of neurotransmitter substances have been discovered in the brain. It has also been discovered that different types of neurotransmitters serve different brain regions; that is, each neuron uses only certain kinds of neurotransmitters (Barondes, 1993). Neurotransmitter problems may include:

a. excessive or insufficient amounts of neurotransmitter substances in the synapse
b. too few receptor sites on the postsynaptic membrane
c. the presence or absence of other chemicals that interfere with neural transmission
d. the interrelationships between different neurotransmitter systems (environmental factors such as stress can also inhibit neural transmission)

Neurological studies have indicated that abnormalities in the activity of different neurotransmitters can cause different mental disorders. Dopamine regulation is the leading neurological hypothesis for the etiology of schizophrenia and norepinephrine is thought to play a major role in the development of depression. However, recent studies suggest that the role of serotonin is also significant in both schizophrenia and mood disorders (Sadock & Sadock, 2003).

Increased knowledge of biochemistry, specifically the role of neurotransmitters, have led the way to the development of the most widely used form of intervention, which is **psychopharmacology.** However, dependence on biological theory alone is insufficient for successful pharmacological treatment. "Many variables affect the practice of psychopharmacology, including drug selection and administration, the psychodynamic meaning to the patient, and family and environmental influences" (Sadock & Sadock, 2003, p. 974). Medication is not the panacea once hoped for. Nevertheless, it is an important component of many treatment plans and often stabilizes the client sufficiently for other forms of therapy to be effective. Knowledge of brain function continues to grow and, as a result, a plethora of new drugs have been developed that not only are more effective in reducing symptoms but often do so with fewer side effects. (See Appendix A for further discussion of psychopharmacology.)

Increased understanding of the special regions of the brain, the mechanisms surrounding neural connectivity, and the functions of the neurotransmitters has certainly furthered our understanding of the biological basis of behavior. However, our knowledge of the physiological factors present in psychopathology is by no means complete. In an effort to develop a more comprehensive biological understanding of abnormal behavior, another biochemical system, the endocrine system, has become the subject of investigation. Unlike the neural connections, this system communicates by means of the circulatory system. The hypothalamus regulates endocrine system functioning in one of two ways: (1) by releasing hormones directly into the bloodstream, and (2) by emitting hormone release factors, which stimulate the anterior pituitary gland to release the appropriate hormone into the bloodstream. In both cases, hormones circulate throughout the body until they bind to target receptors. Similar to the lock-and-key mechanisms of neurotransmitters, the target receptors are selective for the particular hormones with which they bind.

One frequently studied hormone is adrenocorticotropin (ACTH). The target receptor site of ACTH is the adrenal gland. When ACTH binds to the adrenal gland, it causes steroid hormones to be released. One of these is cortisol, which serves to elevate blood sugar and increase metabolism. When a person is under significant stress, the hypothalamus stimulates the pituitary gland to secrete large amounts of cortisol. The increases in blood sugar, and thus in metabolism, are necessary for cells to sustain themselves in the midst of excessive activity. The energy expended in increasing metabolism and blood sugar levels lessens the energy available for other bodily functions (specifically, self-defense). Thus, the link between high levels of stress and a weakened immune system may lie in the excessive secretion of ACTH from the pituitary gland (Kalat, 1988).

Genetic Factors in Psychopathology.   Many theorists who follow the biological perspective believe that inherited vulnerabilities mediate psychological disorders. Certain personality traits, temperamental styles, and specific disorders may have a genetic component (Bouchard, Lykken, McGue, Segal, & Tellegen, 1990). In fact, researchers and clinicians have long noted that certain disorders tend to run in families. In an effort to study the genetic influence on psychopathology, researchers have utilized studies of twins, family pedigrees, adoptions, and risk. These research methodologies attempt to tease out the unique genetic contributions to psychopathology from the vast array of influential biological and environmental factors present. In many cases, a unique genetic contribution proves elusive to the investigator. In such cases, it appears likely that a combination of factors is essential to the manifestation of psychopathology. Thus, multiple genes—or, more likely, a genetic predisposition—coupled with psychological risk factors may be required for psychological disorders to manifest themselves. The theoretical model outlining this possibility is the diathesis-stress model. According to this model, diatheses (i.e., genetic or other biological predisposing factors) must be present along with psychological stressors in order for abnormal behavior to develop. This model has been used to explain the etiology of psychological disorders such as schizophrenia (Meehl, 1962), as well as the development of personality characteristics such as temperament (Plomin, DeFries, & McClearn, 1990).

Twins are frequently studied in the effort to learn more about the genetic influences on psychopathology. There are two types of twins, monozygotic (identical) and dizygotic (fraternal). While identical twins share all the same genes, fraternal twins have an average of only half their genes in common. Twin studies often help to tease out genetic contributions to psychology because twins are typically raised in the same environment, thus controlling external influences to a large degree. Research on several disorders, such as schizophrenia, autism, and bipolar disorder, has demonstrated that identical twins are more likely to share the same disorder than dizygotic twins. When both twins have a disorder, they are referred to as *concordant twins*. When only one twin has a disorder, they are *discordant*.

Family pedigree studies are designed to assess how many members of a given family have a specific disorder. The notion here is that if more members of a given family have a disorder than would be expected in the general population, there may be a genetic predisposition to the disorder that is being transmitted across the generations. For example, evidence from such studies has demonstrated that depression occurs at greater frequencies within families than in the general population (Bloom, Lazerson, & Hofstadter, 1985).

Adoption studies help to further delineate the roles of nature and nurture in the development of psychopathology. One type of adoption study is to compare adopted children to their adoptive and biological parents. Another, perhaps stronger, methodology is to study twins who have been adopted by different families and therefore reared apart. Studies such as these have demonstrated that numerous personality traits, such as IQ, alcohol and drug use, crime and conduct problems, depressiveness, danger seeking, and neuroticism are strongly related in identical twins and related, but to a much lesser degree, in fraternal twins (Bouchard et al., 1990; Bouchard & McGue, 1990; Waller, Kojetin, Bouchard, Lykken, & Tellegen, 1990).

Risk studies target the family members of identified clients to determine the frequency of an identical psychological disorder among them. Studies such as these help to clarify the relative risk of developing that psychological disorder. For example, it has been found that the risk of developing depression is greater for those family members whose biological relationship is closest to the identified client (Gottesman, 1991).

Applications in Occupational Therapy

The biological perspective provides much useful information to the occupational therapist working with clients who have mental illness. An understanding of the biological basis of the disorder can guide clinicians in the formulation of appropriate treatment plans. For example, understanding the biological basis of schizophrenia allows a clinician to appreciate the importance of medication management in the treatment of symptoms. Thus, working with a client to develop a medication routine or schedule may be a treatment priority. (See Appendix A for further information.) Furthermore, family members and caretakers may find some relief in understanding the biological basis of the disorder. Additionally, understanding that a disorder reflects overactivity in the limbic system and frontal lobe area of the brain may lead a clinician to develop theories of treatment focusing on the remediation of skills in the affected areas. For example, teaching appropriate social interaction skills and how to dress for a work environment may assist an individual with schizophrenia in acquiring a job.

Understanding the biological basis of disorders such as attention deficit hyperactivity disorder (ADHD) or autism may allow the clinician to develop a teaching style that is appropriate for the particular child. For example, understanding that a child with ADHD may have an uninhibited reticular formation would allow a clinician to predict that this child will have difficulty focusing attention. When setting up to evaluate or treat this client, the clinician should prepare by modifying the environment. Modifications may include dimming bright fluorescent lights, choosing a confined work area with minimal distractions, selecting well-organized activities, and using a timer to allow the child to self-monitor the time left on a task. Knowing that attention requires a lot of energy for this child, periods of attentiveness should be handsomely rewarded.

In summary, the biological perspective may very well be the fastest growing perspective. Due to recent scientific advances such as magnetic resonance imaging (MRI), positron emission tomography (PET) scanning, and computerized axial tomography (CAT) scanning, scientists are now able to study the brain and its processes more closely. These technological breakthroughs, along with the tremendous advances in the use of pharmacological treatments to ameliorate psychological disorders, have enabled clinicians to develop a better understanding of the physiological mechanisms underlying aberrant behavior. Scientific advances have also triggered a renewed interest in researching the appropriate and focused use of electroconvulsive therapy (ECT) and psychosurgery (Sadock & Sadock, 2003).

The enhanced appreciation for the role of biology facilitates the work of all service providers, including occupational therapists, who work directly with clients with psychological disorders. Biological factors, however, are not the only determinants of psychological disturbance; psychological factors, such as unconscious conflicts, learning histories, and cognitive processes, may also be etiologically significant. The perspectives described in the remainder of this chapter attempt to explain psychopathology in terms of these psychological factors.

PSYCHODYNAMIC PERSPECTIVE

The psychodynamic perspective primarily focuses on the emotional and personality development of the individual and emphasizes early childhood experiences as formative. According to psychodynamic theorists, both normal and abnormal behaviors are largely determined by unconscious psychological forces and internal processes. It is the interaction among these forces that creates behavior, thoughts, and emotions. Abnormal behavior results when these dynamic forces come in conflict (intrapsychic conflict). Psychodynamic theorists assume a deterministic view of behavior. That is, all behavior can be seen as the product of forces beyond the immediate awareness and control of the individual. Although patterns of behavior are viewed as having their origins in early childhood, they may not emerge until adulthood.

The most prominent of the psychodynamic theories was developed by the Viennese neurologist Sigmund Freud in the early twentieth century. His interest in hypnosis as a form of treatment for hysterical illnesses (i.e., physical ailments with no apparent medical explanation) and his early work with the neurologist Jean Charcot and the physician Josef Breuer ultimately led to the formulation of his theory of psychoanalysis, which was the first truly psychological theory of normal and abnormal behavior. This theory postulates that unconscious factors are responsible, not only for hysterical illnesses, but for all psychological functioning, both normal and abnormal. Treatment involves the use of free association, hypnosis, dream analysis, and the interpretation of resistances and transference (i.e., the process by which the client comes to attribute characteristics of important figures from childhood to the therapist) in order to help unconscious conflicts become conscious. Once available to consciousness, psychological conflicts can be worked through and resolved.

Psychoanalytic Concepts

Psychoanalytic theory represents a set of elaborate assumptions about human behavior that are quite complex and, due to their abstractness, often difficult to comprehend. Moreover, the theory evolved throughout the twentieth century. Various therapists have expanded on the original theory, and it has been influenced by different cultural beliefs. Indeed, Freud expanded and changed his own ideas through his lifetime. In order to familiarize the reader with psychoanalytic theory, the following discussion is meant to be a cursory review of some of the key Freudian concepts, including structures of the mind, ego defense mechanisms, levels of consciousness, and psychosexual developmental stages (Comer, 1995; Freud, 1923/1976; Sadock & Sadock, 2003). However, the intricacies and depth of Freud's theoretical notions cannot possibly be captured in such a review.

Structure of the Mind. Freud believed that personality was comprised of three dynamic and interactive forces operating at the unconscious level. The terms used to describe these three forces are *id, ego,* and *superego;* they refer respectively to instinctual needs, rational thinking, and moral standards. It is the interaction among these three forces that shapes human behavior, thoughts, and emotions. In fact, psychoanalysts assert that what distinguishes abnormal and normal behavior is the manner in which psychic energy is distributed among these three "structures." If the id or the superego is too overpowering, it will render the ego ineffective and abnormal behavior will result.

The id, which is innate, represents an individual's instinctual needs, drives, and impulses. Freud believed that these instincts were primarily sexual in nature. The id, which was viewed by Freud to be the primary motivating force in personality, is most prominent in psychoanalytic theory. The id strives for immediate and constant gratification, thereby operating in accordance with the pleasure principle. The id operates without consideration of realistic constraints or regard for consequences. Two sources of id gratification have been described in psycho-analytic writings: direct or reflex activity and primary process thinking. An example of reflex activity is an infant seeking and receiving milk from the mother to satisfy hunger. A description of primary process thinking involves activating a memory or image of the desired object. For example, when a hungry child's mother is unavailable, the child may imagine her breast. As Comer (1995) notes in this example, such images are at least partially satisfying because the id is unable to distinguish between objective and subjective realities. *Wish fulfillment* is the Freudian term used to describe the gratification of id instincts by primary process thinking.

As we come to recognize that our environment will not meet every instinctual need, a separate force develops out of the id. This force, the ego, strives for gratification unconsciously but does so in accordance with the reality principle. The ego engages in secondary process thinking, which involves planning, reasoning, remembering, evaluating, and decision-making processes. That is, the ego determines whether it is safe or dangerous to express an impulse by considering the factors present in reality. The ego experiences anxiety and/or guilt when the id presses to make its desires conscious or get them gratified.

In an effort to control unacceptable id impulses and reduce the anxiety and/or guilt they arouse, the ego develops unconscious coping responses, called ego defense mechanisms, to protect the self. Defense mechanisms are unconscious methods generated by the ego to protect itself from anxiety and guilt related to unacceptable id impulses. Examples of these mechanisms are repression, denial, fantasy, projection, displacement, rationalization, reaction formation, intellectualization (isolation), undoing, regression, identification, overcompensation, and sublimation (several of these are described in Table 4-1). The principal function of the ego, then, is to mediate the impulses of the id and also the moral and ethical value constraints posed by the superego (comprised of the conscience and the "ego ideal"). Psychological abnormality is thought to result when the ego is not mediating effectively, whereas psychological adjustment results when the ego is able to regulate internal conflicts effectively.

The superego develops from the ego during the phallic stage of psychosexual development. In interaction with our caregivers (typically parents), we learn that many of our id impulses are not acceptable and should not be expressed. Thus, parental values and judgments come to be unconsciously introjected (incorporated), thereby becoming the standards against which we come to judge our own behaviors. The superego is comprised of two components, according to Freud: the conscience and the ego ideal. It is the conscience that reminds us that certain behaviors, thoughts, and emotions are acceptable or unacceptable. The ego ideal represents the person we are striving to become; it incorporates all the values and standards of our caregivers. It is important to remember that the superego is just as irrational as the id. It has no concern for reality and can be overly critical and controlling, generating feelings of guilt and worthlessness when standards are violated.

Table 4-1.	Ego Defense Mechanisms
Mechanism	*Description*
Repression	Preventing unacceptable impulses or desires from becoming conscious
Denial	A primitive or early defense mechanism by which a person disavows or refuses to acknowledge the external source of anxiety
Projection	Attributing personally unacceptable impulses or desires to the external world
Displacement	Shifting repressed desires and impulses from a dangerous object to one that is more safe and acceptable
Reaction Formation	Adopting behavior that is in direct opposition to one's unacceptable impulses or desires
Intellectualization	Repressing of the emotional components of one's experience, but not the informational components
Regression	Retreating to an earlier, more immature developmental stage in response to anxiety
Identification	Adopting the values and feelings of a person who causes anxiety in an attempt to increase self-worth
Sublimation	Expressing sexual and aggressive impulses in a socially acceptable manner

According to Freud, these personality forces are fueled by psychic energy. One critical component of this (finite supply of) psychic energy is sexual energy, which is present in the child long before adult sexuality develops. Prior to the development of mature sexual interests and expression, this sexual energy exists as libido according to Freudian theory. Early in life, libido is associated with pleasurable activities related to the gratification of biological needs; later in life, social and psychological needs become prominent. (This will be discussed further when the psychosexual developmental stages are presented in the next section.)

Levels of Consciousness.   Freud (1923/1976) initially conceptualized that the human mind was comprised of three levels of consciousness: the unconscious, the preconscious, and the conscious. The intrapsychic conflicts he noted to be central to his theory of personality could occur at any of these varying levels of awareness. Relating these concepts to the structural model, the id is unconscious, while the ego and superego function at various levels of consciousness (shown in Figure 4-5). The unconscious contains elements, such as instincts or drives, that actively seek to become conscious but are typically prevented from doing so by psychic forces. That is, they may be viewed as unacceptable for expression by the ego (creating anxiety) or by the superego (creating guilt) and, therefore, prevented from being expressed consciously. A large portion of mental activity is unconscious, meaning that it occurs outside a person's normal awareness and is not readily accessible, according to this theory. In fact, psychoanalysts assert that most behaviors, thoughts, and emotions are unconsciously motivated. On the

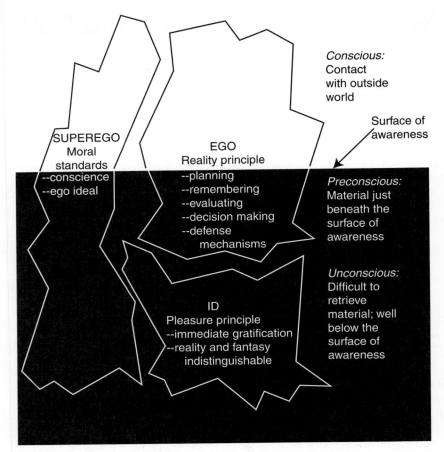

Figure 4-5. Levels of Consciousness and Related Structures of the Mind

other hand, the preconscious level of the mind contains elements that can
become conscious; this, however, requires efforts at retrieval on the part of the
individual. Conscious material is that of which we are aware of at any given
moment; thus, the contents change constantly. According to psychoanalysts, consciousness represents only a small part of actual mental life.

Developmental Stages.   Freud believed that individuals pass through a
series of psychosexual stages, each identified by a specific body region most sensitive to sexual stimulation and therefore most capable of gratifying id instincts
(as described in Table 4-2). The satisfactory gratification of the impulses at one
stage allows the individual to move to the next stage. Adjustment problems are
related to impulses that were ungratified or improperly gratified at earlier stages.
Sometimes fixation—excessive attachment to someone or something that is
appropriate to an earlier developmental level—may result. At other times,

Table 4-2. Psychosexual Developmental Stages		
Psychosexual Stage	*Age Range*	*Source of Gratification*
Oral	Birth–1½ years	Oral region (mouth, tongue)
Anal	1½–3 years	Anal region
Phallic	3–6 years	Genitalia
Latency	6–12 years	Sexual desires repressed
Genital	> 12 years	Mature sexual relationships

regression—a reversion to an earlier, more immature form of behavior, which is typically due to stress or internal conflict—may occur. The psychosexual stages are as follows: oral, anal, phallic, and genital. A fifth stage of development, the latency stage, occurs between the phallic and genital stages and represents a period when sexuality is repressed.

During the first psychosexual stage, called the oral stage, the maximum gratification of id impulses comes from sucking, feeding, biting, and other behaviors that center around the mouth or oral region, which represents an erogenous zone, or pleasure center. During the second year of life, pleasure shifts to the anal region as the primary source of gratification. The elimination and retention of feces become primary sources of libidinal satisfaction during this period of development.

Between the ages of three and five, children pass through the phallic stage, during which sexual gratification comes from manipulation of the genitalia. It is during the phallic stage that the superego develops in response to the Oedipus complex in boys and the Electra complex in girls. It is theorized that during these psychic conflicts, incestuous desire for opposite-gender parents is repressed and identification with same-gender parents occurs. Thus, boys begin to adopt aspects of their fathers' personalities, while girls adopt those of their mothers. It is through the process of internalizing parental standards, moral beliefs, and values that the superego begins to develop.

Following the phallic stage, there is a much needed repression of sexual desires (referred to as the latency stage of psychosexual development) so that children can be primarily engaged in nonsexual learning and socialization experiences. This stage lasts roughly until the children are 12 years of age, the time when puberty generally has its onset. The genital stage is the final psychosexual stage. During this developmental period, Freud believed that sexual drives reappear and sexual gratification is achieved through mature sexual relationships. While earlier forms of sexual desire and expression are notably narcissistic (i.e., focused distinctly on self-gratification), this stage of development relates to an emerging and maturing interest in other people, who are no longer seen solely as objects of self-gratification but rather as unique and valuable in their own right. The defense mechanism of sublimation is likely to be evident during this stage of psychosexual development.

Neo-Freudian Theories

Freudian theory has been altered over the years by many theorists who believe strongly in the power of the unconscious and intrapsychic conflict but who disagree with other aspects of Freud's theory. The neo-Freudians, as they have come to be called, placed less emphasis on the role of sexuality than did their predecessor. For example, Carl Jung developed analytical psychology, which combined Freudian and humanistic theories. Compared to Freud, he believed the unconscious to be more positive, creative, and spiritual, and he deemphasized the role of sexuality as a motivator of behavior. He also believed that in addition to the personal unconscious, there also exists a collective unconscious, which represents all the experiences of all people over the centuries.

Other theorists took exception to Freud's focus on psychosexual development and instead attended to psychosocial aspects of personality development. Alfred Adler, for example, believed that human beings were motivated more by social needs than sexual drives. According to Adler's theoretical notions, children's goals evolve from selfish to more social over the course of development. Harry Stack Sullivan similarly emphasized the importance of interpersonal relationships in personality development on the grounds that one's developing personality cannot be separated from one's social context. He also stressed that human beings have a basic need for security, as we live in a potentially hostile world. The concept of security and the importance of social relationships in achieving security were also addressed by Karen Horney, who believed that childhood relationships were most critical in determining security and adjustment later in life. The experience of anxiety, according to her theoretical notions, was due primarily to social (i.e., interpersonal) factors rather than factors that were biological or sexual. Finally, Erik Erikson conceptualized a life span theory of psychosocial development in which he emphasized the relationship between individuals and the social context in which they live their lives. Erikson also stressed the impact of this changing relationship on personality development from infancy through old age. Each of these stages is characterized by a specific developmental challenge, or crisis, whose resolution affects how the individual deals with subsequent stages.

Although the neo-Freudian's ideas developed separately and apart from original Freudian concepts, these newer ideas about the creative and collective unconscious, the need for security, the influence of the social environment, life-span development, and interpersonal relationships in turn later influenced and enriched psychoanalytic ideas.

Contemporary Psychodynamic Theories

Contemporary psychodynamic theories currently stress the importance of one's social environment in individual development. Psychoanalytic theory is now considered a two-person theory instead of the one-person theory it previously was. That is, psychoanalytic theories now recognize that change takes place in the presence of another person, and we can no longer think that change takes place in an individual alone. Presence does not imply only physical presence but also includes mental representations that are derived from concrete interactions and that are formed in an individual's mind. These two-person concepts have given rise to two theoretical developments in psychotherapy and research. In both theoretical developments, the primary relationship, usually with a mother, but also with whoever is the significant caregiver, is considered the basis for later personality development. The primary relationship particularly shapes how people represent their self or others in their minds (Bretherton, 1990a; 1990b; Zeanah & Anders, 1987). These self- or other representations then guide people's interactions throughout their lives. These later ideas about relationship and primary caregiver evolved from the British school of psychoanalysis called object relations and from the British psychiatrist John Bowlby's ideas about attachment (Bowlby, 1988a; Bretherton, 1992; Cassidy & Shaver, 1999). Currently, object relations and attachment theory ideas influence a wide range of psychotherapy practice (Stern et al., 1998), child development (Sroufe, 1998; Stern, 1985), and theories of research and practice. In another development, psychotherapeutic approaches recognize the importance of early relationships in organizing psychic structure, or one's psychological self (Sroufe & Waters, 1977). These approaches focus on how intersubjectivity influences relationships (Beebe, 2003) and therapy (Stern, 2003; Stolorow, 1994; Stolorow, Atwood, & Branchaft, 1994) and on how early relationships may affect one's later actions, primarily through forms of guilt (Weiss, 1993).

In addition, specific research and programs of psychotherapy have borrowed from Freudian and neo-Freudian ideas. For example, programs for people with borderline personality disorder follow Freud's (Gabbard, 2001) and Harry Stack Sullivan's (Benjamin & Pugh, 2001) theories with modifications and additions. (See Chapters 9 and 18 for more information about these programs and theories of psychotherapy practice.)

Applications in Occupational Therapy

Gail S. Fidler has been credited as being the first occupational therapist to use a psychodynamic approach in treatment (Hopkins, 1988). She encouraged the study and use of projective techniques to guide the interpretation of nonverbal communication displayed by the clients within her activity groups (Fidler & Fidler, 1954). Fidler believed a person's relationships with objects in the environment to be integral to the development of the ego. Because occupational therapy used activities requiring clients to interact with both human and nonhuman objects, she felt it was a rich medium through which clients could reveal both feelings and needs and through which the therapist could ascertain unconscious conflicts and the strength of clients' ego defense mechanisms (Miller, Seig, Ludwig, Shortridge, & Van Deusen, 1988).

Fidler has continued her explorations into the meaning of activities (Fidler & Velde, 1999) and their associated action processes and objects. Her recent work "examines the potential of activities in their own right to represent, reflect, and infer social, cultural, and personal meanings and to communicate and call into play certain physical, affective, and cognitive responses" (p. xi). She continues to promote a psychoanalytic or introspective approach, though not necessarily from an ego psychology perspective. Her current perspective acknowledges the importance of an unconscious inner life to "open the door to a fuller understanding of how one level influences processes at another" (p. 13).

Anne Cronin Mosey was heavily influenced by Gail Fidler and also described psychiatric function from a psychodynamic frame of reference. She believed that "occupational therapy attempted to bring . . . unconscious content to consciousness and integrate it with conscious content" (Hopkins, 1988, p. 29). Since that time, other occupational therapists have written about the use of projective tests within the realm of occupational therapy but generally have cautioned that the interpretation of an activity in this way requires additional education and collaboration with psychologists and/or psychiatrists. Generally, such authors suggest that a therapist can learn about a client's self-esteem, the presence of underlying conflicts (i.e., control or expression of anger), the ability to relate to the therapist, and the use of ego defense mechanisms through such activities as making tile mosaics, drawings, clay sculpture, and magazine collages (Sheffer & Harlock, 1980).

In summary, psychodynamic theory has had a profound impact on Western culture. Its influence can be seen in our educational system, literature, the arts, and, of course, all the mental health professions. Although the theoretical concepts of Freud and his followers may be regarded as outdated and lacking in empirical validity, they are still in use today by many clinicians. In addition, even though psychodynamic principles may have had less impact on the practice of occupational therapy than the other perspectives, this does not negate the potential value they may have in practice. In particular, a knowledge of psychodynamic concepts can assist the occupational therapist in becoming sensitive to intrapsychic factors (e.g., psychological factors not immediately accessible to consciousness) and early childhood experiences impacting an individual client's functioning. An awareness of defense mechanisms and maladaptive coping mechanisms may also prove to be clinically useful for the occupational therapist. Moreover, a self-reflective, "analytical" way of thinking about the self as therapist stems from the psychoanalytical model. Assessing such factors may facilitate the therapy process as well as the development of more effective treatment plans for clients.

BEHAVIORAL PERSPECTIVE

Behaviorism is the branch of psychology that studies the interaction of a person and her or his environment. The behavioral perspective emphasizes the study of objective behavior and generally rejects all schools of thought based on subjective reports of thoughts and feelings. Behaviorism is based on a mechanistic model of behavior that is reflective of the early thinking of René Descartes. Descartes described the difference between involuntary and voluntary behavior as a function of what initiated it: a stimulus from the external environment (involuntary) or a higher mental process (voluntary) (Nevin, 1973). Sir Charles Sherrington (1906) expanded this concept by describing the stimulus-and-response mechanisms of reflexes within the human nervous system. A classic example of a stimulus-response paradigm is the stretch reflex elicited by a tendon tap. A tap to the tendon of the quadriceps causes the quadriceps to shorten, resulting in knee extension (i.e., straightening of the knee). In this example, a tendon tap (the stimulus) elicits knee extension (the response).

According to behaviorists, all behavior, whether normal or abnormal, is learned. Furthermore, the learning of such behavior can occur in three distinct ways: through classical or respondent conditioning; operant or instrumental conditioning; or modeling.

Classical Conditioning

Psychologists became interested in the application of reflex properties to behavior through the work of Ivan Pavlov, a physiologist who separated and studied the difference between "inborn" behavior, such as the act of pulling one's hand away from a hot stove, and learned behavior, such as engaging in a withdrawal response after hearing someone scream "Fire!" (Schwartz & Reisberg, 1991). In studying the digestive process in dogs, Pavlov observed that salivation was always elicited by placement of food in the dog's mouth. He termed the food an unconditioned stimulus (UCS), in that it always caused the same reaction (salivation). A UCS must be shown to produce reliably a desired response without prior training (Gormezano, Prokasy, & Thompson, 1987). He termed the salivation an unconditioned response (UCR), as it was always triggered by the taste of the food. Subsequently, Pavlov noticed that dogs salivated upon the sight of a person bringing the food to them. Pavlov then observed that ringing a bell on successive trials (a conditioned stimulus, or CS), in conjunction with presenting the animal with food (an unconditioned stimulus, or UCS) caused salivation (the UCR) to occur. After repeated pairings of the UCS with the CS, Pavlov found that he was able to elicit salivation using the CS in isolation. He now termed the appearance of salivation a conditioned response (CR) because the response was now elicited by the conditioned stimulus (bell) alone (i.e., without the presentation of the unconditioned stimulus). Over time, the conditioned stimulus fails to elicit the conditioned response if it continues to be presented without the unconditioned stimulus. This is referred to as extinction. This process of learning by temporal association is what behaviorists refer to as classical or respondent conditioning.

John B. Watson was strongly influenced by Pavlov's theories and rejected other psychological theories of his day as being too subjective. He felt that unobservable events (i.e., thought processes, perceptions of stimuli, and feelings and emotions) should not be a part of any scientific theory. Instead, Watson felt that stimuli and responses elicited by those stimuli should form the basis of scientific analysis. Watson is best known for applying Pavlov's theories of classical conditioning to human learning. In one study, Watson and Rayner (1920) "trained" a young boy to be frightened of a furry, white rabbit by presenting it in conjunction with a loud noise. Not only did the boy learn to associate the harmless rabbit with the fear response, he also generalized the response to other white, furry objects.

This study formed the basis for a technique developed by Joseph Wolpe (1958) to treat phobias, which is known as systematic desensitization. This technique

focuses on the use of progressive muscle relaxation procedures and gradual exposure to feared stimuli at increasing levels of intensity in order to eliminate phobias. The basic premise is built on the concept of reciprocal inhibition, which
simply states that one cannot feel anxious and relaxed at the same time. Thus, if
you can create a state of relaxation and pair it with the presentation of a feared
stimulus, the anxiety will ultimately be extinguished. This technique is often successful when used with clients who have specific phobias or who are afraid to
engage in certain types of activities.

Operant Conditioning

Edward L. Thorndike studied the goal-directed behavior of cats attempting to
escape from a box to obtain food (1898). The box was equipped with a lever that
opened the door and allowed the cat to escape. Thorndike described the cat's initial attempts at escape as purely random movements that accidentally tripped the
lever, allowing the cat to escape and obtain food. However, with increasing numbers of learning trials, the amount of time between placement in and escape from
the box decreased. Thorndike also observed that the cat's behavior came closer
and closer to the target behavior with each learning trial in that the cat used less
random, unnecessary movements and more efficient, goal-directed ones. Thorndike concluded that when a response (i.e., pushing the lever) is followed by a positive event (i.e., escape and food), it is more likely to be repeated; conversely, if a
response (i.e., random movement) is followed by a negative event (i.e., inability
to escape and lack of food), it is likely to cease. This principle is known as the law
of effect and serves as the basis for a type of learning known as operant or instrumental conditioning.

B. F. Skinner expanded Thorndike's theory by studying the behavior of hungry
rats in a device known as the Skinner box, which contains both a lever and an
empty food plate (1938). In his studies, lever pushing initially did not cause anything to happen. In this situation, the rats rarely pressed the lever. Subsequently,
the lever was connected to a food container such that depression of the lever
resulted in a few food pellets being delivered into the food plate. Skinner then
observed that the incidence of lever pressing increased dramatically. He concluded that behavior followed by a positive consequence will result in an increase
in that behavior. Skinner then hooked up a device that hit the rat's paw each time
it attempted to press the lever. As predicted, the incidence of lever pressing
decreased dramatically compared to the condition in which the rats were given
food for reinforcement. Skinner thus concluded that behavior followed by a negative consequence (i.e., punishment) will result in a decrease in that behavior.

Skinner cited these and other studies to support his theory of operant conditioning, which states that behavior can be modified by its consequences. Operant
and classical conditioning differ in that the behaviors elicited by operant conditioning are voluntary, while those elicited by classical conditioning are involuntary. Skinner then renamed the law of effect, now referring to the concept as the
principle of reinforcement. He also asserted that reinforcement is the primary
mechanism for learning and for explaining human behavior.

Skinner (1938; 1953) described the different types of reinforcement and punishment contingencies he used in operant conditioning trials. Positive and negative reinforcement both serve to increase the occurrence of target behaviors, while positive and negative punishment serve to decrease behaviors. Positive reinforcement can best be explained as rewarding a person or animal for a behavior after its occurrence. Rewards can be given in such forms as food, praise, hugs, or new clothes—anything qualifies as long as the person receiving the reward perceives it positively. Negative reinforcement also increases the likelihood of a behavior reoccurring, but it does so through the removal of an aversive stimulus. Positive punishment refers to the delivery of an aversive stimulus in response to a behavior. Spanking or yelling are examples of positive punishment. Negative punishment refers to the removal of a positive stimulus in response to a behavior. An example of negative punishment is taking food away from a brain-injured client who is purposefully spitting it out on the table. Taking away privileges (e.g., going for a walk, watching TV, earning an allowance or tokens) from a child for inappropriate behavior may be an effective negative punishment.

Edwin Guthrie (1935) conducted studies providing valuable insight into the importance of the time interval between the presentation of a stimulus and the subsequent presentation of a reward. He found that if the reward is delayed following a correct response to a stimulus, the learner may attribute another response (made during the time delay) to reward acquisition. This principle is especially important when treating children or clients with cognitive deficits, for whom immediacy in delivering reinforcements is critical to promoting behavior change.

Reinforcement schedules describe differences in the elapsed time interval and rate with which behaviors are reinforced. Differences in schedules of reinforcement lead to different response sets. There are two general types of reinforcement schedules: continuous and intermittent. In continuous reinforcement, every occurrence of a target behavior is reinforced, while in intermittent reinforcement, some, but not all, instances of a behavior are reinforced. Intermittent reinforcement can be based on either the number of behaviors required for reinforcement (ratio schedules) or the amount of time that must elapse before a behavior is reinforced (interval schedules). Ratio and interval schedules can be either fixed (i.e., a set number of responses or elapsed time is required prior to the delivery of reinforcement) or variable (i.e., the number of responses and elapsed time required for reinforcement constantly changes). Response rates vary according to the reinforcement schedules used. The use of continuous reinforcement schedules is advised when teaching new behaviors, while intermittent reinforcement schedules are recommended for the maintenance of acquired skills (S. M. Deitz, 1985).

Skinner described different methods of teaching behaviors using principles of reinforcement. Shaping and chaining represent two such methods. Both can be used in clinical settings to teach more complex behaviors. Shaping involves reinforcing a person for closer and closer approximations of a target behavior. Initially, only a simple response is required. The criteria for reinforcement are then gradually made more stringent in an attempt to elicit more complex or refined target behaviors (Becker, 1985). This technique is widely used to teach verbal behavior (i.e., language), whereby closer and closer approximations of the required sound, word, or phrase are needed to obtain reinforcement. Clients with head injury, mental retardation, or autism often benefit from this form of teaching.

Chaining refers to a method of reinforcement involving the linking of component skills to teach a more complex behavior. This procedure involves reinforcing in a particular sequence simple behaviors that are already in the individual's repertoire in an effort to teach more complex skills (D. E. D. Deitz, 1985a). Chaining can be accomplished in either a forward or backward format. Forward chaining refers to the teaching of a task's subcomponents in the order in which they are to be performed so as to complete the task (D. E. D. Deitz, 1985b), while backward chaining teaches the subcomponent skills in reverse order. In this case, the final response is taught first, then the preceding response, and so on, until the first response in the sequence has been taught (Schreibman, 1985). A benefit of backward chaining is that the client produces the final product each time, which makes tasks more meaningful and less frustrating. Backward chaining generally appears to be the more effective of the two methods, although both are widely used clinically.

A final concept studied by Skinner was the extinction of behaviors. *Extinction* refers to the decline in rate of a target behavior and ultimate elimination of that behavior. Skinner found that he could eliminate (or extinguish) a response by removing the reinforcement that followed it; this is referred to as operant extinction (Poling, 1985). In laboratory studies, it has been demonstrated that animals initially continue to elicit behaviors following the removal of reinforcement, sometimes even at an increased rate, but that response rates decline and eventually fade with time. Skinner did note that some behaviors were more resistant to extinction than others, which had to do with the schedule of reinforcement used during the skill acquisition phase of learning. Specifically, behaviors that are reinforced more variably prove more resistant to extinction procedures, while those on a fixed schedule are extinguished more easily. Behaviors can also be eliminated using respondent extinction, in which unconditioned stimuli consistently fail to follow conditioned stimuli, thereby weakening the likelihood of the conditioned response reoccurring (Poling, 1985).

Modeling

In addition to the classical and operant conditioning explanations for the acquisition of behavior, Albert Bandura (1977; 1997) recognized that learning also occurred through observation and imitation of the behaviors of others. Bandura expanded Skinner's theory of operant conditioning by stating that persons can learn by observing the consequences that people receive for their behaviors. For example, if a child observes her sibling receive a piece of candy for making her bed, she may learn vicariously that making one's bed results in receiving treats. Consequently, she may be more likely to make her bed in the future. Bandura differs from Skinner in that he differentiates learning from the performance of learned behaviors. Bandura claims that although the child in this example may have learned that making one's bed results in reinforcement, she may neverthe-less choose to not perform the task. This may be due, in part, to appraisals she makes about the relative value of the reinforcement to the task requirements. Thus, Bandura integrates cognitive components into his understanding of mod-eling and observational learning.

Bandura (1986) has cited four critical factors necessary for a behavior to be learned observationally and subsequently performed. First, in order for observa-tional learning to occur, the learner must attend to the modeled behavior. Sec-ond, the learner must form and retain a mental image of the modeled behavior for later use. Third, the learner must reproduce the modeled behavior from the stored image. That is, he or she must take the stored mental image and con-vert it into overt behavior. Fourth, the observational learning process requires that the learner be sufficiently motivated to reproduce the modeled behavior. Bandura's understanding of behavior acquisition clearly reflects his appreciation for the mediating influence of cognitive processes in learning. Proponents of the cognitive model, in fact, assert that cognitive processes are primary in determin-ing psychopathology.

Applications in Occupational Therapy

Behavioral principles are widely used in contemporary society (e.g., in the edu-cational, legal, and employment systems) in an effort to promote productive and prosocial behaviors of individuals. Related procedures are also commonly used in health professions, such as occupational therapy. Behavioral systems are particu-larly used in programs for adolescents and milieu treatment. Additionally, some behavioral principles, such as reinforcement and reward, are commonly incorpo-rated into day treatment models and long-term care facilities for people with mental illness.

Because behavioral strategies are relatively concrete and do not require complex verbal, cognitive, or psychosocial abilities, they can be used effectively with a variety of clinical populations (e.g., individuals with mental retardation, autism, or schizophrenia). Attending to a client's learning history, including rein-forcement contingencies that influence behavior, can be very useful to the prac-ticing occupational therapist when designing treatment protocols. In addition, using conditioning and modeling procedures in therapy certainly will facilitate more positive outcomes for clients (especially individuals with cognitive deficits, young children, and clients lacking sufficient internal motivation to comply with treatment).

Cognitive-behavioral therapy (CBT), which merges elements of both behav-ioral and cognitive perspectives, is now widely used in occupational therapy as well as in other mental health disciplines. For example, Strong (1998) showed positive results using this approach in occupational therapy for pain manage-ment. Giles also advocates using a behavioral perspective as well as CBT within an occupational therapy framework. This approach has shown to be successful with various populations, including those with eating disorders such as anorexia nervosa and bulimia (Giles, 1985), as well as with people with traumatic brain injury (Giles, Ridley, Dill, & Frye, 1997).

COGNITIVE PERSPECTIVE

Although interest in cognitive processes has a long history, a clinical model of their etiological significance in psychopathology only began to emerge in response to traditional behavioral notions that rejected the mediating influence of mental processes on abnormal behavior. Proponents of the cognitive perspective, therefore, believe that behavior is influenced by factors other than observable environmental stimuli and the responses they elicit. These theorists argue strongly that what people think, believe, expect, remember, and attend to influences how they behave (O'Leary & Wilson, 1987). Specifically, dysfunctional cognitive processes are thought to produce psychological disorder. Furthermore, altering a person's cognitions (i.e., making him or her more functional and adaptive) can ameliorate psychological difficulties. Although the behaviorists, such as Skinner (1971), acknowledged that mental life existed, they denied the causal role of cognitions in behavior. Cognitive psychologists, on the other hand, view cognitions as primary causal agents in psychopathology, and therefore, as first-order treatment targets.

Cognitive psychologists take issue with the basic stimulus-response conditioning theories of behaviorists, which they find far too passive and simplistic. These theorists believe that the learner actively interprets novel information relative to previously acquired information, which they refer to as a schema (Neisser, 1976). Rescorla (1988) even conceptualizes classical conditioning as an active process by which individuals learn about relationships among events.

The application of cognitive psychology concepts and principles to the understanding and treatment of psychopathology is a relatively recent phenomenon and is becoming increasingly popular, especially when combined with behavioral approaches in cognitive-behavior therapy. The focus of related treatments generally is to alter cognitions and cognitive processes in order to facilitate behavioral and emotional changes. The general term for this treatment approach is *cognitive restructuring*. Several prominent professionals in the field have proposed cognitive theories of psychopathology that bear mentioning. Notable figures include Albert Bandura, Aaron Beck, and Albert Ellis. For the purposes of therapy, cognitive processes can be divided into those that are short term and those that are long term. Short-term processes, including expectations, appraisals, and attributions, are processes of which we either are or can become aware through practice. On the other hand, long-term processes, including beliefs, are generally not readily available to consciousness.

Expectations

Expectations refer to cognitions that anticipate future events. In his seminal work on modeling and observational learning, Albert Bandura assessed the impact of expectations on the performance of learned behaviors. Bandura demonstrated that individuals learn behavior, not only by receiving reinforcement directly for the expression of that behavior, but also by observing others receiving reinforcement for the same behavior. As a result of this evidence for vicarious learning, Bandura hypothesized that learning must involve expectations in addition to operant conditioning principles (Bandura, 1977; 1978; Bandura & Walters, 1959). According to Bandura's theory, two types of expectations are relevant to behavior change: an outcome expectation and an efficacy expectation. An outcome expectation is a person's belief that a given behavior will lead to a desired outcome, while an efficacy expectation is the person's belief that he or she can, in fact, perform the behavior necessary to produce the desired outcome. Both are critical to understanding the mechanisms underlying the acquisition and application of learned behavior. In fact, it has been shown that individuals may learn that a specific behavior will result in a desired outcome but, because they do not believe they have the capacity to perform the target behavior, it nonetheless fails to be produced. As a result, some desired outcomes do not occur (Bandura, 1977; 1978; Bandura & Adams, 1977).

Appraisals

Human beings are constantly evaluating events occurring in their everyday lives. Sometimes these appraisals are evident. Other times, these evaluative processes are not conscious, but rather automatic, most likely due to a lifetime of practice. In his cognitive explanations for psychopathology, Aaron Beck (1976) emphasizes automatic thoughts as causal agents of psychological disorder; in fact, he argues that emotion states are always preceded by related thought processes. In therapy, the individual is taught to slow down and become aware of relevant negative automatic thoughts so that they may then be restructured (Goldfried, Decenteceo, & Weinburg, 1974).

Beck is primarily interested in cognitive processes related to depression (Beck, 1967; 1976; Beck, Rush, Shaw, & Emery, 1979), but his theoretical concepts have also been successfully applied to other psychological conditions, including personality and anxiety disorders. Specifically, Beck noted that depressed individuals tend to distort their realities by engaging in dysfunctional thought processes. Beck's cognitive therapy of depression is primarily concerned with altering negative thoughts about one's self, the world, and the future and with correcting general misinterpretations of life events that individuals with depression typically possess. The pattern of negative thinking described by Beck is called the "cognitive triad," which refers to negative self-evaluation, a pessimistic view of the world, and a sense of hopelessness regarding future outcomes. These thoughts reflect the drawing of false conclusions by selectively attending to isolated aspects of a situation (selective abstraction), the exaggerating of the importance of negative events (magnification), and the generalizing of the significance of isolated events for one's life (overgeneralization). These pervasive negative thoughts represent primary treatment targets in Beck's cognitive therapy for depression. The goal of therapy, therefore, is to help the client monitor and systematically refute illogical and negative self-statements.

Attributions

Attributions are an individual's beliefs about cause-and-effect relationships. For example, an individual might make internal or external attributions (Rotter, 1966), stable or unstable attributions (Weiner, 1974), or global or specific attributions (Abramson, Seligman, & Teasdale, 1978; Seligman, 1991); the specific array of attributions made determines differential behavioral outcomes. Internal attributions emphasize the causal role of intrapersonal variables, while external attributions focus on the role of the environment or other factors out of the individual's personal control. Stable attributions are those that are persistent over time, whereas unstable attributions are considered transient. Finally, global attributions emphasize the persistence of behavior across tasks, while specific attributions relate to one's understanding that a certain behavior is specific to a certain task. The goal of cognitive therapists is to alter the attributions that individuals make so that they become more rational and adaptive.

Beliefs

Albert Ellis (1962) argues that irrational beliefs, instilled in us over the course of our lives by parents and society, are at the root of psychological disorder. In addition to being maladaptive in and of themselves, these beliefs are also presumed to shape short-term, dysfunctional expectations, appraisals, and attributions. Specifically, maladaptive behaviors and emotions are due to false assumptions (e.g., illogical "shoulds" and "musts") that individuals make about their behavior and the world. As defined by Ellis, six such assumptions are as follows:

1. Adult human beings must be loved and approved by all significant others.
2. In order to be worthy, one should be competent, adequate, and successful in all possible respects.
3. It is catastrophic when things are not the way one would like them to be.
4. Unhappiness is externally caused, and one has little or no control over negative events.
5. Past history is the critical determinant of present behavior, and events that strongly affect one's life will continue to do so.
6. There is always a perfect solution to one's problems, and it is catastrophic if that ideal solution is not found (Ellis, 1962).

Ellis's rational emotive therapy (RET) actively confronts and challenges these assumptions or false beliefs and attempts to replace them with those that are more rational and, hence, more adaptive to an individual's functioning.

Applications in Occupational Therapy

The cognitive perspective is clearly among the more prominent in contemporary thinking. Its focus on cognitive processes that mediate behavior has proven to be a very rich area for empirical study. In addition, the inclusion of cognitive components in psychological assessment and intervention has resulted in more comprehensive and effective treatment outcomes for many clients. By attending to dysfunctional appraisals, expectancies, attributions, and beliefs, therapists may be better able to facilitate and maintain behavioral and emotional changes in their clients. Research in the area of cognitive function has also enhanced our understanding of the importance of providing clients with meaningful tasks and therapeutic activities that are consistent with their level of cognitive functioning.

Many of the life skills workbook activities used by occupational therapists are examples of how occupational therapists apply cognitive therapy. (See Suggested Readings.) Also, one aspect of activity gradation uses a cognitive perspective to simplify and structure a task, and the cognitive disabilities model (Allen, 1985) uses a cognitive perspective to analyze and treat the needs of individuals to "support participation in contexts" (Occupational Therapy Practice Framework, 2002).

Summary

The broad perspectives discussed in this chapter contribute to occupational therapy's underlying philosophy and also contribute to the tools and strategies used in OT treatment. These theoretical concepts (as well as the philosophical tenets described in Chapter 3) provide the basis of psychosocial occupational therapy. This is essential knowledge not only for use in mental health settings, but also for all occupational therapy practice in order to address the psychosocial needs of clients. Kielhofner (1997) describes an emerging paradigm of occupational therapy, in which the major themes "affirm the value of occupation and emphasize a client-centered practice and respect for the subjective perspectives of clients and patients. These themes also affirm that therapy is a process of active engagement and empowerment that must be guided by a balance of art and science" (p. 88). The Occupational Therapy Practice Framework (2002) reaffirms this paradigm by stating that "engagement in occupation to support participation in context is the focus and targeted end objective of occupational therapy intervention" (p. 611).

Since every client is unique, treatment plans must be personalized in order to assure that the goals of treatment are those that are most meaningful to the particular client. To understand clients' behavior, it is imperative that occupational therapists have a comprehensive understanding of the biological, intrapsychic, and interpersonal factors mediating that behavior. For example, it is essential to have an understanding of the clients' level of cognitive and perceptual functioning, their ability to process sensory input and produce motor output, their cultural belief system, personality factors that were present prior to injury or disease onset, and valued life roles. Only then can a therapist establish and carry out a treatment plan that is meaningful to the particular client. Psychological theory and research provides many of the tools necessary to develop effective treatment plans. Although the theoretical concepts presented here from the biological, psychodynamic, behavioral, cognitive, and humanistic perspectives are distinct in their understanding and treatment of psychological disorders, they are not necessarily incompatible. In fact, the integration of concepts should provide the practicing clinician with a better understanding of the biopsychosocial factors influencing behaviors, thoughts, and emotions. Theoretical integration should also allow for the development of individualized treatment plans that are both more comprehensive and more effective.

Review Questions

1. Describe the benefits and disadvantages to using an eclectic approach to therapy.
2. Explain Maslow's hierarchy of needs and its relevance to occupational therapy.
3. What are the differences between classical psychoanalytic concepts (Freudian) and neo-Freudian concepts?
4. Which client groups are most likely to benefit from behavioral interventions?

References

Abramson, L. Y., Seligman, M. E. P., & Teasdale, J. (1978). Learned helplessness in humans: Critique and reformulation. *Journal of Abnormal Psychology, 87,* 49–74.

Allen, C. (1985). *Occupational therapy for psychiatric diseases: Measurement and management of cognitive disabilities.* Boston: Little, Brown.

Association of Humanistic Psychology (AHP). (2001). A brief history of the humanistic psychology movement. www.ahpweb.org.

Bandura, A. (1977). *Social learning theory.* Englewood Cliffs, NJ: Prentice-Hall.

Bandura, A. (1978). The self system in reciprocal determinism. *American Psychologist, 37,* 122–147.

Bandura, A. (1986). *Social foundations of thought and action: A social cognitive theory.* Englewood Cliffs, NJ: Prentice-Hall.

Bandura, A. (1997). *Self efficacy: The exercise of control.* New York: Freeman.

Bandura, A., & Adams, N. E. (1977). Analysis of self-efficacy theory of behavioral changes. *Cognitive Theory and Research, 1,* 287–310.

Bandura, A., & Walters, R. H. (1959). *Adolescent aggression.* New York: Ronald.

Barondes, S. H. (1993). *Molecules and mental illness.* New York: Scientific American.

Beck, A. T. (1967). *Depression: Clinical, experimental, and theoretical aspects.* New York: Harper & Row.

Beck, A. T. (1976). *Cognitive therapy and the emotional disorders.* New York: International Universities Press.

Beck, A. T., Rush, A. J., Shaw, B. F., & Emery, G. (1979). *Cognitive therapy of depression.* New York: Guilford.

Becker, R. E. (1985). Shaping. In A. S. Bellack & M. Hersen (Eds.), *Dictionary of behavior therapy techniques* (p. 205). New York: Pergamon.

Beebe, B. (2003). *Forms of intersubjectivity in infant research and their implications for adult treatment.* Paper presented at the New Developments in Attachment Theory: Applications to Clinical Practice, Los Angeles, CA.

Benjamin, L. S., & C. Pugh. (2001). Using interpersonal theory to select effective treatment interventions. In W. J. Livesley (Ed.), *Handbook of personality disorders: Theory, research and treatment* (pp. 414–436). New York: Guilford.

Bloom, F. E., Lazerson, A., & Hofstadter, L. (1985). *Brain, mind, and behavior.* New York: Freeman.

Bouchard, T. J., Lykken, D. T., McGue, M., Segal, N. L., & Tellegen, A. (1990). Sources of human psychological differences: The Minnesota study of twins reared apart. *Science, 250,* 223–228.

Bouchard, T. J., & McGue, M. (1990). Genetic and rearing environmental influences on adult personality: An analysis of adopted twins reared apart. *Journal of Personality, 58,* 263–292.

Bowlby, J. (1988a). Developmental psychiatry comes of age. *American Journal of Psychiatry, 145*(1), 1–10.

Bretherton, I. (1990a). Communication patterns, internal working models, and the intergenerational transmission of attachment relationships. *Infant Mental Health Journal, 11*(3), 237–252.

Bretherton, I. (1990b). *Open communication and internal working models: Their role in the development of attachment relations.* Paper presented at the Nebraska symposium on motivation.

Bretherton, I. (1992). The origins of attachment theory: John Bowlby and Mary Ainsworth. *Developmental Psychology, 28*(5), 759–775.

Cassidy, J., & Shaver, P. R. (1999). *Handbook of attachment: Theory, research and clinical applications.* New York: Guilfod.

Comer, R. (1995). *Abnormal psychology* (2nd ed.). New York: Freeman.

Davis, J. M., & Adams, H. E. (1995). Models. In L. A. Heiden & M. Hersen (Eds.), *Introduction to clinical psychology* (pp. 21–46). New York: Plenum.

Deitz, D. E. D. (1985a). Chaining. In A. S. Bellack & M. Hersen (Eds.), *Dictionary of behavior therapy techniques* (p. 53). New York: Pergamon.

Deitz, D. E. D. (1985b). Forward chaining. In A. S. Bellack & M. Hersen (Eds.), *Dictionary of behavior therapy techniques* (p. 131). New York: Pergamon.

Deitz, S. M. (1985). Schedules of reinforcement. In A. S. Bellack & M. Hersen (Eds.), *Dictionary of behavior therapy techniques* (p. 189). New York: Pergamon.

Ellis, A. (1962). *Reason and emotion in psychotherapy.* New York: Lyle Stuart.

Fidler, G. S., & Fidler, J. W. (1954). *Introduction to psychiatric occupational therapy.* New York: Macmillan.

Fidler, G. S., & Fidler, J. W. (1963). *Occupational therapy: A communication process in psychiatry.* New York: Macmillan.

Fidler, G. S., & Fidler, J. W. (1978). Doing and becoming: Purposeful action and self-actualization. *American Journal of Occupational Therapy, 32,* 305.

Fidler, G., & Velde, B. P. (1999). *Activities: Reality and symbol.* Thorofare, NJ: Slack.

Frankl, V. E. (1967). *Psychotherapy and existential papers on logotherapy.* New York: Square.

Frankl, V. E. (1972). *The doctor and the soul.* New York: Knopf.

Freud, S. (1976). *The ego and the id.* In J. Strachey (Ed. & Trans.), *The complete psychological works* (Vol. 19). New York: Norton. (Original work published 1923)

Gabbard, G. O. (2001). Psychoanalysis and psychoanalytic psychotherapy. In W. J. Livesley (Ed.), *Handbook of personality disorders: Theory, research and treatment* (pp. 359–376). New York: Guilford.

Gershon, E. S., & Rieder, R. O. (1992). Major disorders of the brain. *Scientific American, 267,* 127–133.

Giles, G. M. (1985). Anorexia and bulimia: An activity oriented approach. *American Journal of Occupational Therapy, 39,* 510–517.

Giles, G. M., Ridley, J. E., Dill, A., & Frye, S. (1997). A consecutive series of adults with brain injury treated with a dressing retraining program. *American Journal of Occupational Therapy, 51,* 256–266.

Goldfried, M. R., Decenteceo, E. T., & Weinberg, L. (1974). Systematic rational restructuring as a self-control technique. *Behavior Therapy, 5,* 247–254.

Gormezano, I., Prokasy, W., & Thompson, R. (1987). *Classical conditioning* (3rd ed.). Hillsdale, NJ: Erlbaum.

Gottesman, I. I. (1991). *Schizoprenia genesis: The origins of madness.* New York: Freeman.

Guthrie, E. R. (1935). *The psychology of learning.* New York: Harper.

Hopkins, H. L. (1988). A historical perspective on occupational therapy. In H. L. Hopkins & D. H. Smith (Eds.), *Willard and Spackman's occupational therapy* (7th ed., pp. 16–37). Philadelphia: Lippincott.

Kalat, J. (1988). *Biological psychology* (3rd ed.). Belmont, CA: Wadsworth.

Kielhofner, G. (1997). *Conceptual foundations of occupational therapy.* Philadelphia: F. A. Davis.

Larson, E., Wood, W., & Clark, F. (2003). Occupational science: Building the science and practice of occupation through an academic discipline. In W. Blesedell Crepeau, E. Cohn, & B. Schell (Eds.), *Willard and Spackman's occupational therapy* (10th ed.). Philadelphia: Lippincott Williams & Wilkins.

Law, M. (Ed.). (1998). *Client centered occupational therapy.* Thorofare, NJ: Slack.

Maslow, A. H. (1968). *Toward a psychology of being.* New York: Van Nostrand-Reinhold.

Meehl, P. E. (1962). Schizotaxia, schizotypy, schizophrenia. *American Psychologist, 17,* 827–838.

Miller, R., Seig, K., Ludwig, F., Shortridge, S., & Van Deusen, J. (1988). *Six perspectives on theory for the practice of occupational therapy.* Rockville, MD: Aspen.

Mosey, A. C. (1980). A model for occupational therapy. *Occupational Therapy in Mental Health, 1,* 11–31.

Neisser, U. (1976). *Cognition and reality.* San Francisco: Freeman.

Nevin, J. (1973). *The study of behavior: Learning, motivation, emotion, and instinct.* Reading, MA: Addison-Wesley.

Occupational Therapy Practice Framework: Domain and Process. (2002). *American Journal of Occupational Therapy, 56*(6), 614–639.

O'Leary, K. D., & Wilson, G. T. (1987). *Behavior therapy: Application and outcome.* Englewood Cliffs, NJ: Prentice-Hall.

Patterson, C. H. (1989). Eclecticism in psychotherapy: Is integration possible? *Psychotherapy, 26,* 157–161.

Plomin, R., DeFries, J. C., & McClearn, G. E. (1990). *Behavioral genetics* (2nd ed.). New York: Freeman.

Poling, A. (1985). Extinction. In A. S. Bellack & M. Hersen (Eds.), *Dictionary of behavior therapy techniques* (p. 124). New York: Pergamon.

Reilly, M. (1962). Occupational therapy can be one of the greatest ideas of twentieth century medicine. *American Journal of Occupational Therapy, 16,* 1–16.

Rescorla, R. A. (1988). Pavlovian conditioning: It's not what you think it is. *American Psychologist, 43,* 151–160.

Rogers, C. R. (1942). *Counseling and psychotherapy: Newer concepts in practice.* Boston: Houghton Mifflin.

Rogers, C. R. (1951). *Client-centered therapy: Its current practice, implications, and theory.* Boston: Houghton Mifflin.

Rogers, C. R. (1961). *On becoming a person: A therapist's view of psychotherapy.* Boston: Houghton Mifflin.

Rosenzweig, M. R., Leiman, A. L., & Breedlove, S. M. (2001). *Biological psychology: An introduction to behavioral, cognitive, & clinical neuroscience* (3rd ed.). Sunderland, MA: Sinauer.

Rotter, J. B. (1966). Generalized expectancies for internal versus external control of reinforcement. *Psychological Monographs, 80*(1).

Rowan, J. (2004). *A guide to humanistic psychology.* Alameda, CA: Association for Humanistic Psychology.

Sadock, B., & Sadock, V. (2003). *Kaplan and Sadock's synopsis of psychiatry* (9th ed.). Philadelphia: Lippincott Williams & Wilkins.

Schreibman, L. (1985). Backward chaining. In A. S. Bellack & M. Hersen (Eds.), *Dictionary of behavior therapy techniques* (p. 22). New York: Pergamon.

Schultz, S., & Schade, J. (2003). Occupational adaptation. In W. Blesedell Crepeau, E. Cohn, & B. Boyt Schell (Eds.), *Willard and Spackman's occupational therapy* (10th ed.). Philadelphia: Lippincott Williams & Wilkins.

Schwartz, B., & Reisberg, D. (1991). *Learning and memory.* New York: Norton.

Schwartz, K. (2003). The history of occupational therapy. In W. Blesedell Crepeau, E. Cohn, & B. Boyt Schell (Eds.), *Willard and Spackman's occupational therapy* (10th ed.). Philadelphia: Lippincott Williams & Wilkins.

Seligman, M. E. P. (1991). *Learned optimism: The skill to conquer life's obstacles, large and small.* New York: Random House.

Sheffer, M., & Harlock, S. (1980). Tell us what your drawings say. *Occupational Therapy in Mental Health, 1,* 21–38.

Sherrington, C. S. (1906). *The integrative action of the nervous system.* New Haven, CT: Yale University Press.

Skinner, B. F. (1938). *The behavior of organisms: An experimental analysis.* New York: Appleton-Century-Crofts.

Skinner, B. F. (1953). *Science and human behavior.* New York: Macmillan.

Skinner, B. F. (1971). *Beyond freedom and dignity.* New York: Knopf.

Sroufe, L. A. (1998). The role of infant-caregiver attachment in development. In T. Nezworski (Ed.), *Clinical implications of attachment* (pp. 18–38). New York: Erlbaum.

Sroufe, L. A., and Waters, E. (1977). Attachment as an organizational construct. *Child Development, 48,* 1184–1199.

Stern, D. (1985). *The interpersonal world of the infant.* New York: Basic.

Stern, D. N. (2003). *Attachment and intersubjectivity.* Paper presented at the New Developments in Attachment Theory: Applications to Clinical Practice, Los Angeles, CA.

Stern, D. N., Sander, L. W., Nahum, J. P., Harrison, A. M., Lyons-Ruth, K., Morgan, A. C., et al. (1998). Non-interpretive mechanisms in psychoanalytic therapy: The "something more" than interpretation. *International Journal of Psycho-Analysis, 79,* 903–921.

Stolorow, R. (1994). The intersubjective context of intrapsychic experience. In R. Stolorow, G. Atwood, & B. Brandchaft (Eds.), *The intersubjective perspective.* Northvale, NJ: Jason Aronson.

Stolorow, R., Atwood, G., & Brandchaft, B. (Eds.). (1994). *The intersubjective perspective.* Northvale, NJ: Jason Aronson.

Strong, J. (1998). Incorporating cognitive-behavioral therapy with occupational therapy: A comparative study with patients with low back pain. *Journal of Occupational Rehabilitation, 8*(1), 61–71.

Thompson, R. (1993). *The brain: A neuroscience primer.* New York: Freeman.

Thorndike, E. L. (1898). Animal intelligence: An experimental study of the associative processes in animals. *Psychological Review Monograph Supplement, 2*(8).

Waller, N., Kojetin, B., Bouchard, T., Lykken, D., & Tellegen, A. (1990). Genetic and environmental influences on religious interests, attitudes, and values. *Psychological Science, 1,* 138–142.

Watson, J. B., & Rayner, R. (1920). Conditioned emotional reactions. *Journal of Experimental Psychology, 3,* 1–4.

Weiner, B. (Ed.). (1974). *Achievement motivation and attribution theory.* Morristown, NJ: General Learning.

Weiss, J. (1993). *How psychotherapy works.* New York: Guilford.

Wolpe, J. (1958). *Psychotherapy by reciprocal inhibition.* Stanford: Stanford University Press.

Yerxa, E. J. (1967). Authentic occupational therapy. *American Journal of Occupational Therapy, 21,* 1–9.

Zeanah, C. H., & Anders, T. F. (1987). Subjectivity in parent-infant relationships: A discussion of internal working models. *Infant Mental Health Journal, 8*(3), 237–249.

Suggested Reading

Barris, R., Kielhofner, G., & Watts, J. (1988). *Occupational therapy in psychosocial practice.* Thorofare, NJ: Slack.

Bruce, M., & Borg, B. (1993). *Psychosocial occupational therapy: Frames of reference for interventions.* Thorofare, NJ: Slack.

Canadian Association of Occupational Therapists. (1993). *Occupational therapy guidelines for client-centered mental health practice.* Toronto: Minister of Supply and Services.

Cole, M. (1998). *Group dynamics in occupational therapy.* Thorofare, NJ: Slack.

Creek, J. (Ed.). (1997). *Occuapational therapy and mental health* (2nd ed.). New York: Churchill Livingstone.

Ellis, A. (1973). *Humanistic psychotherapy: The rational-emotive approach.* New York: McGraw-Hill.

Fearing, V., & Clark, J. (2000). *Individuals in context: A practical guide to client centered practice.* Thorofare, NJ: Slack.

Frankl, V. (1978). *The unheard cry for meaning: Psychotherapy and humanism.* New York: Simon & Schuster.

Hagedorn, R. (2001). *Foundations for practice in occupational therapy* (3rd ed.). New York: Churchill Livingstone.

Korb-Khalsa, K., Leutenberg, E., & Leutenberg Brodsky, A. (2001). *Life management skills V: Reproducible activity handouts created for facilitators.* Beachwood, OH: Wellness Reproductions.

Morihisa, J. M. (Ed.). (2001). *Advances in brain imaging.* Washington, DC: American Psychiatric Publishing.

Mosey, A. C. (1986). *Psychosocial components of occupational therapy,* New York: Raven.

Rogers, C. (1965). *Client-centered therapy: Its current practice, implications and theory.* Boston: Houghton Mifflin.

Schwartzberg, S. (2002). *Interactive reasoning in the practice of occupational therapy.* Upper Saddle River, NJ: Prentice-Hall.

Shannon, P. (1977). The derailment of occupational therapy. *American Journal of Occupational Therapy, 31*(4), 229–234.

Diagnosis and Dysfunction

The first chapter in Part III on psychopathology and the diagnostic process (Chapter 5) reviews the major symptoms seen with mental illness and the diagnostic process used in mental health practice. However, in this edition, further emphasis has been placed on an international understanding of these concepts and addresses not only the *DSM-IV-TR* categories but also the World Health Organization's *International Classification of Functioning*. It is the authors' beliefs that a thorough understanding of both psychopathology and diagnosis are critical in providing competent mental health care. However, this background alone is not sufficient. Therefore, each chapter in this section addresses symptoms and diagnosis and places this information in context while discussing environments, assessment, and interventions in a client-centered, occupation-based approach.

C H A P T E R 5

Psychopathology and the Diagnostic Process

Anne MacRae, PhD, OTR/L

Key Terms

diagnosis
DSM-IV-TR
dysfunction

ICF
psychopathology
symptom

Chapter Outline

Introduction

The purpose of this chapter is to provide a brief overview of psychopathology and diagnosis. It is not intended to replace or represent the more extensive knowledge found in abnormal psychology and psychiatric courses or textbooks. Indeed, several of the authoritative psychiatric and psychological texts are sources for this chapter (American Psychiatric Association, 2000; Andreasen & Black, 2001: Bernstein, Milich, & Nietzel, 2002; Maxmen & Ward, 1995; Rosenzweig, Leiman, & Breedlove, 2001; Sadock & Sadock, 2003). In addition, the categories presented in this chapter are implicitly consistent with body function descriptions of the **ICF**, or *International Classification of Function* (WHO, 2001) and the Occupational Therapy Practice Framework (2002). However, rather than simply restating the information from these sources, there is an emphasis in this chapter on the most commonly seen problems in mental health settings as well as OT clinical application, and the functional implications of psychopathology and diagnosis.

   The terminology used in mental health settings can often be confusing, especially since the terms are often misused by the general public. It is important to be as specific as possible and to be clear as to whether a phenomenon is a **symptom, dysfunction,** or **diagnosis,** even though there is often much overlap. In other words, an individual may experience a particular symptom that is typical of a specific disorder but still not meet the criteria for that diagnosis. Moreover, neither the symptom nor the diagnosis will give the clinician a true indication about the level or type of dysfunction. It is a common error to assume that some diagnoses automatically imply a greater level of dysfunction, when actually, "psychiatric diagnosis does not always predict functional performance" (Bonder, 1991/1995, p. xxi). The following case illustrations compare brief psychiatric histories of three people in order to show the differences between symptoms, diagnosis, and dysfunction.

CASE ILLUSTRATIONS: Symptoms, Diagnosis and Dysfunction

Ms. Jones complains of feeling bored and depressed (symptoms). She has alienated all of her friends and is now isolated from social contact (dysfunction). Ms. Jones also meets the criteria for borderline personality disorder (diagnosis).

   Mr. Nguyen has recently been fired from his job for reportedly "slipshod" work (dysfunction). His doctor has been treating him for dysthymia (diagnosis) for several years, but lately Mr. Nguyen has been feeling more lethargic and melancholic (symptoms).

Mrs. Garcia is hospitalized for an episode of major depression (diagnosis). She expresses feelings of hopelessness and suicidal ideation (symptoms) and is disinterested in performing basic self-care tasks such as caring for personal hygiene (dysfunction).

PSYCHOPATHOLOGY

Symptoms of mental illness may present in a wide variety of combinations, and there are various schemas for organizing the information. The following is one example of a categorical organization of **psychopathology** and descriptions of common symptoms within each category.

Thought

Thought includes what are considered to be the higher intellectual functions of abstraction, reasoning, judgment, and analysis. The most common deficits seen in this area are concrete thinking and an inability to recognize or correct errors (which may be due to increased impulsivity). Concrete thinking includes thought processes focused on immediate experiences and specific objects or events as well as an inability to think metaphorically or abstractly.

A specific form of psychopathology involving the content of thought is delusions, which are deep-seated beliefs not based in reality. The presentation of factual proof will not typically change such beliefs. There are many types of delusions, including delusions of grandeur as well as self-deprecating and paranoid delusions. These are typically not an exaggeration of real experiences, but rather an essentially inaccurate, though powerful, belief. For example, an individual with a delusion of grandeur may believe he or she has supernatural powers, is a famous historical figure, or has an important secret mission to accomplish. Some delusions are relatively harmless with little associated dysfunction, while others leave an individual extremely incapacitated in daily living activities, or, as sometimes is the case with paranoid delusions, make him or her a danger to herself or himself or to others.

Another form of disordered thought is obsession, which is a specific and repetitive thought that is typically unwanted and cannot be eliminated by reason. Obsessions are often found in conjunction with compulsions, whereby a person attempts to extinguish the obsession by acting upon it. Although obsessive-compulsive disorder (OCD) is a diagnosis, it is possible to have either or both symptoms without meeting the criteria for OCD or any other diagnosis. Again, the level of associated dysfunction is quite variable.

Language

Speech disturbances are often considered to be part of thought disorder, but they are so common in severe mental illness that it is easier to study them as a separate category. Some people who experience these symptoms seem oblivious to the oddity of their speech, but other people find it exhausting to engage in casual conversation and may avoid it whenever possible. Occupational therapists must be knowledgeable of these symptoms in order to appreciate the effort clients may be expending in conversation and also to understand the meaning of their communication. Table 5-1 provides examples of some of the abnormal speech patterns that can occur with severe mental illness.

Although language is usually considered a cognitive ability, speech or language production is motoric in nature. A decreased intelligibility of speech (dysarthria) may be due to long- and short-term side effects of psychotropic medication. Also, in general, illnesses that affect the nervous system have the potential for causing a variety of problems that can interfere with the production of speech and language.

Perception and Sensation

Perception is the ability to attain information via the senses and then process and interpret the stimuli. Another closely related term is *sensory processing*. Although problems in both areas can exist independently, they often overlap and it is sometimes difficult to clearly identify the resulting dysfunction as attributable to one or the other. Perception is usually considered a cognitive process with the emphasis on interpretation, whereas the term *sensory-processing deficits* implies that the dysfunction is in the delivery or integration of the sensory message. It is well documented that people with persistent mental illness (particularly schizophrenia) commonly experience hallucinations, but it is also true that there is a higher than average incidence of other perceptual disturbances, as well as problems with sensory processing and integration, which are found in this population (Brown et al., 2001; Doniger et al., 2001; Blakeney, Stickland, & Wilkinson, 1983). These deficits include distorted time sense and spatial awareness, poor visual perception, poor body scheme, hyper- or hyposensitivity to stimuli, and astereognosis, which is the inability to identify common objects by touch. Also, people with serious mental illness may display a variety of sensorimotor symptoms either as a direct result of the illness or as side effects of psychotropic medication. These include abnormal muscle tone, abnormal gait, and apraxia, which is an inability to plan and coordinate complex motor actions. In addition, a decreased pain and temperature response as well as an increased sensitivity to sunlight may also be found in people with severe mental illness. These deficits are often subtle and may go unrecognized. However, a careful evaluation of these possible conditions is essential, as they pose potential safety threats to the individual.

Hallucinations. Hallucinations are perceptual images experienced as sensations but not based on actual stimulation from the external environment. Hallucinations can involve any of the senses: visual (seeing images), auditory (hearing voices or sounds), tactile (feeling sensations on the skin surface), gustatory (taste), olfactory (smell), and somatic (feeling sensations within the body). There have been many attempts to correlate kinds of hallucination with an actual diagnosis, but care must be taken not to oversimplify the relationship between symptom and diagnosis. For example, there are many theories regarding damage to the brain and the presence of visual and tactile hallucinations, yet there are also many exceptions. Nevertheless, there are some significant patterns regarding kinds of

Table 5-1. Abnormal Speech Patterns Associated with Mental Illness

Term	Description	Example
Concreteness	Extremely literal verbal responses due to concrete thinking patterns. The speaker does not recognize the nuances of language, including abstractions or metaphors.	"Reading can open a whole new world." *Response:* "And then the lava flows out of the cracks."
Loosening of Associations	Ideas shift from one subject to another that is completely unrelated. The speaker does not show any awareness that the topics are unconnected.	"What is your name?" *Response:* "A rose by any other name . . . I wish I could get out of here . . . Jigsaw puzzles are fun."
Perseveration	Repetition of the same word, phrase, or idea. Also, an inability to shift from one task to another.	"What do you want to do today?" *Response:* "Today is Tuesday, I always do wash on Tuesday, always on Tuesday it's wash."
Circumstantiality and Tangentiality	The person digresses, giving unnecessary, irrelevant information. When speech is circumstantial there is difficulty getting to the point of the conversation, yet in the person's mind, the answers are related. In tangential speech the person starts answering a question but then rapidly digresses.	"When were you in the hospital?" *Circumstantial response:* "I went to this great concert last summer after I visited my aunt." *Tangential response:* "In the fall . . . the leaves were so beautiful . . . They were like my paintings . . . My art is my soul."
Echolalia	Repetition (echo) of the words and phrases of others. This speech is repetitive and persistent.	"What is your name?" *Response:* "What is your name? Your name, your name."
Clanging	The sound or rhyme of the words takes precedence over the meaning or content of the replies.	"What is your occupation?" *Response:* "I used to be a lawyer, now a liar, lollipops, licenses, and licorice."
Neologism	An invented word that may closely resemble an existing word or may be known only to the individual.	"Why were you admitted to the hospital?" *Response:* "It come from too much normiation, a sort of infesteration of some sort. I was being institized."

hallucinations and diagnosis. For example, visual or olfactory hallucinations may precede grand mal seizures. Tactile hallucinations are often experienced during alcohol or drug withdrawal, and gustatory hallucinations may indicate brain trauma.

Hallucinations seem very real to the person experiencing them and can cause dysfunction in several ways. The relationship between the manifestation of hallucinations and specific dysfunctions is described in the model of functional deficits (MacRae, 1997) and shown in Table 5-2.

The model of functional deficits is a framework for examining the phenomenon of hallucinations from an occupational therapy perspective. In this model, various types of dysfunction are correlated to specific manifestations of hallucinations.

Table 5-2. Model of Functional Deficits Associated with Hallucinations

Classification		*Observable Behavior*
Class 0	Insufficient information	None identifiable.
Class I	No hallucinations	None.
Class II	Intermittent hallucinations with minimal or no functional deficits	Phenomena reported upon questioning or in appropriate settings. Individual may appear withdrawn.
Class III	Intermittent or persistent hallucinations with functional deficits related to the content of the phenomena	Evidence of poor self-esteem, such as frequent self-deprecating remarks, poor posture, lack of social interaction, and poor motivation.
Class IV	Intermittent or persistent hallucinations with functional deficits directly related to the intrusiveness of the phenomena	Inappropriate behavior while apparently responding to internal stimuli. Inappropriate affect such as giggling not related to the outside environment. Conversations with the self. Poor attention to the task on hand but can be redirected to task and surroundings.
Class V	Intermittent or persistent hallucinations with functional deficits related to *both* content and intrusiveness of the phenomena	See classes III and IV.
Class VI	Persistent hallucinations with profound functional deficits. Generally acute	Inability to appropriately respond to the external environment.

Source: Adapted from MacRae (1991, 1997).

For example, when the dominant feature of the hallucinations is the *content* (such as what the voices are saying), typically there is evidence of poor self-esteem and observations may include frequent self-deprecating remarks, poor posture, lack of social interaction, and poor motivation. However, when the dominant feature of the hallucinations is the *intrusiveness* of the phenomenon, dysfunctions will more likely include inappropriate behavior while apparently responding to internal stimuli. Observations might include behaviors such as giggling for no apparent reason, conversations with the self, and poor attention to tasks.

Illusions.   A milder form of perceptual distortion is an illusion, in which the outside object causing the stimuli is real but the person misinterprets the object (for example, a lamppost may be mistaken for a robot). Like hallucinations, illusions may involve any of the senses, but auditory and visual illusions are most common.

Affect

Affect refers to the observable behavior representing one's emotions, but (as shown in Figure 5-1, which depicts classical drama masks) it is not always possible to know what someone is feeling. It is also sometimes difficult to determine a pathological affect because there are normal fluctuations in everyone's emotional state. The demonstration of emotions is partially dictated by culture, so awareness of and sensitivity to a person's background are essential. Disturbances of affect can be a direct result of a mental illness or a neurological disorder such as cerebrovascular accident (CVA). Changes in affect can also be drug induced. *Flat*

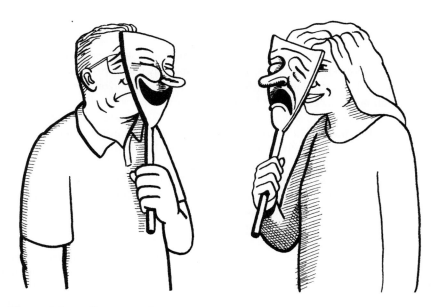

Figure 5-1.   Affect Is an Observable Behavior Representing Emotion

affect refers to a lack of observable emotion. Other emotional states, such as anxiety or hostility, may be considered pathologic if the emotional state is either inappropriate or out of proportion to the environmental stimuli.

Depression.   Depression is one of the most common affective symptoms. It may be seen with many psychiatric diagnoses, including not only major depression and dysthymia but also schizophrenia, the dementias, and personality disorders. Mania is a condition in which the individual responds in an eager, exuberant, and even joyful manner, regardless of the environmental reality. Although mania is considered a disordered affect, the dysfunction resulting from the manic state is usually caused by the associated features of poor judgment and impulsivity. Therefore, mania might best be described as a syndrome consisting of affect, thought, and motor dysfunctions.

Lability.   Lability is a state of unstable emotions, which may present in many different ways. For example, one individual may swing rapidly between laughter and tears, while another person may cry uncontrollably yet be unable to identify a reason for the tears. Paying particular attention to the individual's previous level of emotional display and cultural background is necessary to identify a true lability accurately.

Because *affect* refers only to the observable behavior associated with feelings, it is difficult to categorize or even identify some altered or impaired feelings. For example, a person with a mental illness may experience intense feelings of rage and yet have no visible signs of such intense feelings. Another altered emotional state common in mental illness is anhedonia, which is an inability to experience pleasure. Some individuals experience a milder form of this symptom known as hypohedonia, which is defined as a decreased ability to experience pleasure.

Orientation

Orientation refers to a person's awareness of time, place, and person. Typically, the first orientation to be lost is time. The individual may know where and who he or she is, yet not know the date, month, or even year. The second orientation to be lost is orientation to place, and the last is orientation to person, which includes the recognition of both the self and significant others. This pattern is so predictable that a standard method of charting has been developed to represent orientation. O (orientation) × 3 means that the individual is oriented to time, place, and person; O × 2 means orientation is to place and person only; and O × 1 means that the person is oriented only to person. If orientation was lost in a different order than that of time, place, and person, this must be explicitly stated. Table 5-3 provides examples of this form of documentation.

Memory

The most common categorization of memory is the simple division into short-term and long-term. However, memory is quite complex and further categorization is helpful to determine specific functional deficits associated with its loss. Table 5-4 describes one classification system of types of memory and their clinical significance. A knowledge of these specific types of memory will help the clinician iden-

Table 5-3. Orientation to Time, Place, and Person

Description	Clinical Interpretation	Charting
Mrs. Wong states that she is in Hong Kong in 1948 when she is actually in present-day San Francisco. She recognizes her children and can report her own name.	Mrs. Wong is not oriented to place or time; she is oriented to person.	O x 1
Mr. Geary recognizes all of his family members, as well as his doctor. He is aware that he is presently hospitalized in his hometown but frequently is unclear about the day and month and occasionally does not know the year.	Mr. Geary is clearly oriented to person and place; however, his time disorientation fluctuates in severity.	O x 2
Ms. Tenaka was administered a mental status exam during which she was able to accurately report her name, her presence in the psychiatric emergency room, and the correct date.	Ms. Tenaka is fully oriented to time, place, and person.	O x 3

tify an individual's assets as well as deficits and plan treatment accordingly. For example, procedural memory is often retained when declarative memory is not. By designing a treatment plan that allows desired responses to become automatic, the therapist can help clients become more functional.

Another example of clinical significance is the identification of prospective memory, which is important for independent living. Examples of prospective memory include remembering to pay bills, go to the doctor, and turn off the stove.

People who have severe memory deficits, as is found with dementia of the Alzheimer's type or substance-induced persisting amnestic disorder, often engage in confabulation. Confabulation is the unknowing fabrication of events to fill in the gaps of true memory. It is not intentional lying, as the person is not aware that he or she is doing so. It is also not delusional, as the person will not be particularly invested in, or attached to, the confabulated statements.

Energy and Motoric Response

Observable changes in the energy or activity level of a person with a mental illness are sometimes assumed to be a consequence of psychotropic medications. The *Diagnostic and Statistical Manual,* 4th Edition, Text Revised (***DSM-IV-TR***) includes classifications of drug-induced movement disorders to assist the clinician in identifying specific neurological patterns associated with high levels of psychotropic medication (APA, 2000). While drugs can have such effects, it is also common to experience increased or decreased energy levels due directly to a

Table 5-4. Types of Memory

Type	Description	Example
Procedural memory	An automatic sequence of behavior such as conditioned responses	Despite significant deterioration of her mental status, Mrs. Makiba remembers to retrieve the newspaper from the porch and make a pot of coffee by 8 A.M. as she has done every day for years.
Declarative memory	Memory specific to consciously learned facts such as school subjects	Mr. Alvarado is diagnosed with schizophrenia. He has a history of failure in jobs and has been unable to pass classes at the community college due to poor attendance. Nevertheless, he is able to recall much of the material from the lectures he was able to attend and he is quite knowledgeable about current events.
Semantic memory	The knowledge of the meaning of words and the ability to classify information or ideas	Mr. Hackett lives in a supervised residential care home, where he is considered to be quite proficient at solitary crossword puzzles.
Episodic memory	The knowledge of personal experiences	Mrs. Yen spends three mornings a week meeting at the cultural center, where she enjoys sharing stories and reminiscing with her friends.
Prospective memory	The capacity to remember to carry out actions in the future. In essence, "to remember to remember"	After a home evaluation, the occupational therapist concluded that Ms. Cohen can live independently. She has been able to keep all her appointments and safely operates a stove in the kitchen.

mental illness. It is not always possible to predict when, or if, this fluctuation will accompany a mental illness or what form it will take. For example, one person with depression may appear lethargic while another person is quite agitated and yet a third person with depression shows little or no change in energy level.

Many people with serious mental illness experience disruption of the sleep-wake cycle. For example, either excessive or insufficient sleep patterns are often found in people experiencing major depression. Too little or too much sleep can contribute to poor overall functioning and to worsening of other symptoms.

Changes in sleep patterns can also be the result of psychotropic medication. Medication-induced sleep problems may be resolved by changes in dose, frequency, or time of administration of medication. (See Appendix A for further discussion of medication.)

Specific motor symptoms may be related to the severity of the mental disorder. For example, catatonia, which is rigidity or immobility, would most likely be observed during an acute and severe psychotic episode rather than as a persistent state. Other possible symptoms involving motor function are stereotypy, the repetition of apparently senseless actions; tics, involving muscular spasms or twitching; and compulsions, which are repetitive, irrational behaviors acted out in response to an overwhelming urge.

DIAGNOSIS

The determination of a clinical diagnosis in psychiatry is, at best, an inexact process based on both deductive and inductive reasoning. One view of this process is that it is a constructive way of ordering knowledge about a person's dysfunction in order to better understand the mental illness. However, diagnoses are also viewed by some as a destructive force that serves only to inappropriately label and dehumanize individuals. There are inherent dangers in labeling, and it is the clinician's responsibility not to make assumptions about an individual's behavior or abilities based on diagnosis alone. On the other hand, a structured diagnostic process attempts to make psychiatric terminology more uniform, which is important because of the stigma attached to mental illness. The implications of these disorders at a societal level are great, which means that the careless use of volatile terms must be avoided, regardless of the purpose of diagnosis. Indeed, the occupational therapist can play an important role in educating the public about the myths of mental illness and the misuse of clinical terminology. For example, calling someone "a schizophrenic" implies that the individual's main identifying feature is an illness, which is simplistic and dehumanizing. It is both more appropriate and more accurate to identify the individual as a "person with schizophrenia." Figure 5-2 suggests other ways to use labels intelligently and sensitively.

Another criticism of the diagnostic process is the lack of precise data on psychiatric illness. It is rare that measurable or visible objective data such as X-rays and blood tests, as are used in physical diagnosis, can be used in psychiatry. "Much of the controversy stems from a lack of accurate measurements to validate the diagnosis, thereby allowing for differences of opinion of a highly subjective nature" (Mathis, 1992, p. 253).

Still another significant concern about diagnosis is cultural bias. "In a world in which ethnic and cultural pluralism is daily becoming more politically salient, it is striking that North American professional constructs of personality and psychopathology are mostly culture bound" (Lewis-Fernandez & Kleinman, 1994, p. 67), with, specifically, a white, male, Judeo-Christian orientation. The awareness of this limitation is increasing, but it remains essential that clinicians be aware of the inherent ethnocentrism found in the current diagnostic system. "A clinician who is

LANGUAGE

Mental illnesses are frequently the subject of news stories, or of dramatic films or television programs. NAMI, the Nation's Voice on Mental Illness, offers the following guidelines for use of medical and slang terms about mental illnesses:

- words like "crazy," "nuts," "wacko," "sicko," "psycho," "lunatic," "demented" and "loony" are offensive

- terms like "insane" are inappropriate except when used in a specific medical or legal context (e.g., the term "criminally insane" in a courtroom scene)

- referring to a "person with a severe mental illness" is preferable to "the mentally ill," which depersonalizes—highlighting the illness, not the person

- terms like "schiizophrenia" and "manic depressive illness" have very specific meanings and apply only to certain groups of people; such scientific labels not to be checked carefully for accuracy; they should not be used to refer to "schizophrenic weather" or other uses unrelated to the illnesses themselves

■ ■ ■ ■ ■ ■ ■

For more information, contact the NAMI, a self-help organization providing mutual support, public education, research and advocacy for people with serious mental illnesses:

Public Relations Director
National Alliance for the Mentally Ill
2107 Wilson Boulevard,
Suite Colonial Place Three
Arlington, VA 22201
www/nami.org

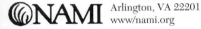

ABOUT MENTAL ILLNESS

Figure 5-2.   Language about Mental Illness

Source: Reprinted with permission from NAMI.

unfamiliar with the nuances of an individual's cultural frame of reference may incorrectly judge as psychopathology those normal variations in behavior, belief, or experience that are particular to the individual's culture" (APA, 2000, p. xxxiv).

Given these limitations, why are diagnoses used at all? Despite legitimate controversy, the diagnostic process helps facilitate interdisciplinary communication and fosters research, both of which are essential for high-quality mental health care. It is hoped that as research continues, the process of diagnosing will become increasingly objective, culturally sensitive, and accurate.

The most commonly used instrument to record diagnoses, disorders, and symptoms is the World Health Organization's (WHO) *International Classification of Diseases,* currently in its 10th edition (*ICD-10*). However, the *ICD* is not limited to mental illness and does not contain the diagnostic specificity found in the American Psychiatric Association's *Diagnostic and Statistical Manual* (*DSM*). For the purposes of this chapter, discussion is primarily limited to the *DSM*; however, with each revision of these documents, there is increased agreement and mutual influence (APA, 2000).

WHO also publishes a companion document known as the *International Classification of Function* (*ICF*), which not only covers the diagnostic concerns of body structure and functions but also includes ratings of activities and participation, and contextual factors such as the influence of personal causation and environment (WHO, 2001). This is very consistent with an occupational therapy approach and indeed was used to develop the language of the Occupational Therapy Practice Framework (2002), which is discussed throughout this book. Table 5-5 is an overview of the *ICF* and its structures.

Table 5-5. An overview of ICF

	Part 1: Functioning and Disability		Part 2: Contextual Factors	
Components	Body Functions and Structures	Activities and Participation	Environmental Factors	Personal Factors
Domains	Body functions Body structures	Life areas (tasks, actions)	External influences on functioning and disability	Internal influences on functioning and disability
Constructs	Change in body functions (physiological) Change in body structures (anatomical)	Capacity Executing tasks in a standard environment Performance Executing tasks in the current environment	Facilitating or hindering impact of features of the physical, social, and attitudinal world	Impact of attributes of the person
Positive aspect	Functional and structural integrity	Activities Participation	Facilitators	Not applicable
	Functioning			
Negative aspect	Impairment	Activity limitation Participation restriction	Barriers/ hindrances	Not applicable
	Disability			

From *International Classification of Functioning, Disability and Health (ICF)* (WHO, 2001). Reprinted with permission of the World Health Organization (WHO), and all rights are reserved by the organization.

Overview of the *Diagnostic and Statistical Manual* of *Mental Disorders* (*DSM*)

The concept of multiaxial diagnosis had been discussed in the European psychiatric literature since the 1940s. Nevertheless, American psychiatry has only had practical application since the publication in 1980 of the third edition of the American Psychiatric Association's *Diagnostic and Statistical Manual of Mental Disorders* (*DSM-III*). This multiaxial system provides a comprehensive view of an individual's mental health, with each axis addressing a different domain. This system minimizes the likelihood that pertinent information will be overlooked in interdisciplinary treatment planning. An overview of the multiaxial assessment process according to *DSM-IV* is provided in Table 5-6.

Study of the *DSM* is a significant part of the academic curricula of mental health professionals. Unfortunately, it is sometimes difficult for students to keep in mind that the information being presented is not clear-cut, concrete, or complete. It is important to analyze the data critically and be aware of its limitations. As stated in the *DSM-IV*, "The specific diagnostic criteria included in DSM-IV are meant to serve as guidelines to be informed by clinical judgment and are not meant to be used in a cookbook fashion" (APA, 2000, p. xxxii). Furthermore, the process of evaluation and treatment planning is far more comprehensive than can be covered in a manual such as the *DSM*, and each particular discipline has some-

Table 5-6. An Overview of the DSM-IV-TR Axes

Axes	*Description*	*Comments*
Axis I	Clinical Disorders; Other conditions that may be a focus of clinical attention	Reason for referral or principal diagnosis is listed first if multiple diagnoses are present
Axis II	Personality Disorders, Mental Retardation	May also be used to record maladaptive personality features and defense mechanisms
Axis III	General Medical Conditions	Condition is related to the mental disorder and is consistent with the *International Classification of Diseases* (*ICD*)
Axis IV	Psychosocial and Environmental Problems	If the problem is the primary focus of treatment it is also recorded on Axis I under "Other conditions that may be a focus of clinical attention"
Axis V	Global Assessment of Functioning	Impairment in functioning due to physical or environmental limitations is not considered

Source: Reprinted with permission from the *Diagnostic and Statistical Manual of Mental Disorders*. Fourth Edition-Text Revised (APA, 2000). Copyright 2000, American Psychiatric Association.

thing unique and specific to offer. It is important to be familiar with the information in the *DSM*; however, it should not be assumed that this knowledge is all that is required for practice, as it barely constitutes a beginning.

Theory and the *DSM*

Although the APA states that the *DSM* is atheoretical, theories pervade both our conscious and unconscious thought, so it may not be possible to eliminate theoretical bias. However, the association did make a serious attempt to avoid defining disorders based on the beliefs of a particular school of thought. This is a valuable unifying concept for all the professions involved in mental health because of the diversity of beliefs that are found in practice, particularly regarding the etiology of mental illness. Rather than defining disorders based on an individual theory, such as behaviorism or psychoanalytic thought, the multiaxial system uses what is known as a biopsychosocial approach to assessment. This model is an attempt to be holistic by providing a wide range of information without necessarily referring to the etiology of the disorder or defining it according to one theoretical belief. Figure 5-3 illustrates the communication difficulties encountered when theoretic beliefs are the sole basis of diagnosis. While various theories have significance for treatment, diagnosis becomes problematic when clinicians base their diagnosis solely on theoretical premises.

The Role of Occupational Therapy

> Occupational therapists work within a system in which diagnosis is important, but their view of disorder differs from that of other mental health professionals. The difference revolves around the importance of function in everyday activities, the causes of dysfunction, goals of treatment, and methods for intervening. (Bonder, 1991/1995, p. 17)

As previously mentioned, the occupational therapy approach is very consistent with the language and intent of the *ICF* and the profession can play a pivotal role in advocating for its expanded use in mental health settings. Nevertheless, the *DSM* will likely continue to be the primary source used for the diagnosis of mental illness, at least in the United States.

Occupational therapists are not responsible for determining diagnosis; however, in settings where an interdisciplinary approach is utilized, they often contribute to the diagnostic process by providing the team with specific information from evaluations. A knowledge of the first three *DSM* axes is essential for effective communication with the team, but from an occupational therapists' perspective, a more valuable focus is on axes IV and V. Occupational therapy intervention is based on the assessment of an individual's unique assets and deficits, and diagnosis on Axis I and Axis II alone cannot provide this information. An attempt is made in the *DSM* to denote the severity of some disorders; however, this is not always indicative of the individuals' functional level.

Axis IV is used to report the psychosocial and environmental problems in an individual's life. The problem groups used with this axis include problems with the

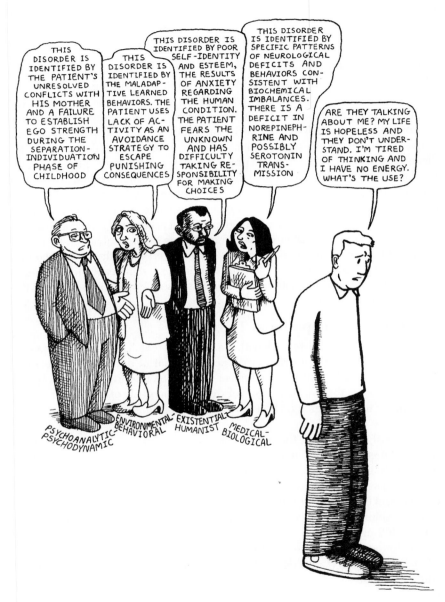

Figure 5-3. Problems with Theoretically Based Communication

primary support group and those related to the social environment; educational, occupational, housing, and economic problems; problems with access to health care services and those related to interaction with the legal system and crime; and other psychosocial and environmental problems (APA, 2000). Occupational therapists often uncover relevant information for this axis during an initial assessment and use the data in the development of the treatment plan. Axis IV is used to specify all problems that are deemed relevant to the individual's diagnosis and treatment. This is a significant improvement from the Axis IV rating scale in the *DSM III* because it documents specific, concrete problems, whereas the former scale rated a problem's severity based on an assessment of an "average" person's response to the same stressor without consideration of the role of multiple stressors.

Axis V is the Global Assessment of Functioning (GAF) scale. The purpose of the GAF (reproduced in Figure 5-4) is to assess a person's overall levels of psychological, social, and occupational functioning. Clearly, this is very much in line with the evaluation process of occupational therapy, where assessment is based on performance in areas of occupation such as activities of daily living, education, work, play, leisure, and social participation (Occupational Therapy Practice Framework, 2002). Axis V measures are somewhat reliable and valid; however, they are not widely used (Goldman, Skodol, & Lave, 1992). The *DSM-IV-TR* provides greatly expanded instructions for the GAF, which includes "a four-step method to ensure that no elements of the GAF scale are overlooked when making a GAF rating" (APA, 2002, p. 829). Hopefully, this addition will increase the use of this valuable tool by all mental health clinicians, including occupational therapists.

The *DSM-IV-TR* has proposed several additional scales for more specific tracking of an individual's functioning. These include the Social and Occupational Functioning Assessment Scale (SOFAS), the Global Assessment of Relational Functioning (GARF), and the Defensive Functioning Scale. As these are newly introduced scales in the DSM, their usefulness in clinical practice is yet to be shown. However, in some settings they would be ideal data collection tools for research conducted by many disciplines, including occupational therapists. The case illustrations of Cathy and David illustrate the use of the axis system in diagnosis. As you are reading, look for the pertinent information that led to the information on the axes.

CASE ILLUSTRATION: Cathy—Application of the *DSM*

Cathy is a 33-year-old woman who was referred to the day treatment center with the goals of increasing structure in her life, improving her social skills, and enhancing her poor self-image. Despite having a master's degree, she has never held a job for more than a couple of months and has been unemployed for the last three years. She presently receives disability payments and lives alone in an apartment. However, she is angry at her landlord so she stopped paying the rent. He, in turn, is threatening to evict her. Cathy freely admits that it is hard

Global Assessment of Functioning (GAF) Scale

Consider psychological, social, and occupational functioning on a hypothetical continuum of mental health or illness. Do not include impairment in functioning due to physical (or environmental) limitations.

Code *(Note: Use intermediate codes when appropriate, e.g., 45, 68, 2.)*

100 | 91	Superior functioning in a wide range of activities, life's problems never seem to get out of hand, is sought out by others because of his or her many positive qualities. No symptoms.
90 | | 81	Absent or minimal symptoms (e.g., mild anxiety before an exam), good functioning in all areas, interested and involved in a wide range of activities, socially effective, generally satisfied with life, no more than everyday problems or concerns (e.g., an occasional argument with family members).
80 | | 71	If symptoms are present, they are transient and expectable reactions to psychosocial stressors (e.g., difficulty concentrating after family argument); no more than slight impairment in social, occupational, or school functioning (e.g., temporarily falling behind in schoolwork)
70 | | 61	Some mild symptoms (e.g., depressed mood and mild insomnia) OR some difficulty in social, occupational, or school functioning (e.g., occasional truancy, or theft within the household), but generally functioning pretty well, has some meaningful interpersonal relationships.
60 | 51	Moderate symptoms (e.g., flat affect and circumstantial speech, occasional panic attacks) OR moderate difficulty in social, occupational, or school functioning (e.g., few friends, conflicts with peers or co-workers).
50 | 41	Serious symptoms (e.g., suicidal ideation, severe obsessional rituals, frequent shoplifting) OR any serious impairment in social, occupational, or school functioning (e.g., no friends, unable to keep a job).
40 | | | 31	Some impairment in reality testing or communication (e.g., speech is at times illogical, obscure, or irrelevant) OR major impairment in several areas, such as work or school, family relations, judgment, thinking or mood (e.g., depressed man avoids friends, neglects family, and is unable to work; child frequently beats up younger children, is defiant at home, and is failing at school).
30 | | 21	Behavior is considerably influenced by delusions or hallucinations OR serious impairment in communication or judgment (e.g., sometimes incoherent, acts grossly inappropriately, suicidal preoccupation) OR inability to function in almost all areas (e.g., stays in bed all day; no job, home or friends).
20 | 11	Some danger of hurting self or others (e.g., suicide attempts without clear expectation of death; frequently violent; manic excitement) OR gross impairment in communication (e.g., largely incoherent or mute).
10 | 1	Persistent danger of severely hurting self or others (e.g., recurrent violence) OR persistent inability to maintain minimal personal hygiene OR serious suicidal act with clear expectation of death.
0	Inadequate information.

Figure 5-4. The Global Assessment of Functioning (GAF) Scale

for her to "pay bills and stuff," stating, "I'm just not that organized a person." She frequently spends her entire monthly check on the day it is cashed and then resorts to "borrowing" money from her sister and neighbors.

Cathy has a history of getting quite enthusiastic about a particular therapist for a short while and then "firing" him or her. She has dropped out of several mental health programs in the past. Cathy has had several hospitalizations for attempted suicide. Her suicidal threats and attempts are usually very dramatic (i.e., slashing her wrists or threatening to jump out of a building) and often coincide with the perceived "failure" of the most recently fired therapist. Recently, she has become quite attached to the occupational therapist at the day treatment center and states, "She is the only one who really understands me."

AXIS I	V71.09—No diagnosis or condition on Axis I
AXIS II	301.83 Borderline Personality Disorder
AXIS III	None
AXIS IV	Occupational problems—unemployment; housing problems—discord with landlord
AXIS V	60 (current)

CASE ILLUSTRATION: David—Application of the *DSM*

David is a 14-year-old boy who was brought to the emergency psychiatric service after it took three police officers to subdue his vicious physical attack, in which he used a baseball bat on another youth. It was originally thought that David might be on the street drug PCP, but his blood levels proved negative and he became quite calm and somewhat aloof during the hospital admission process. Formal charges against David are pending.

David is presently undergoing evaluation on the adolescent psychiatric unit. Reports from the school and family reveal a history of aggressive behaviors at school since third grade, but with a recent increase in frequency. David has been involved in several physical fights with classmates over the past two semesters and was reported for two incidents of vandalism. He also is frequently truant from school. David says he has no "real friends," and he shows no remorse for his acts of violence. His academic record shows substantially below-average reading ability, although he maintains a passing grade in math and workshop classes. His mother reports that she cannot control him and that, in order to provide basic care for David and his four sisters, she must work two jobs, one as a housekeeper and the other on a night shift at a local factory. Six months ago, David's father was convicted of assault and robbery and is presently serving a five-year sentence in the state penitentiary.

AXIS I	312.8—Conduct Disorder, Childhood-Onset Type, Severe; 315.00 Reading Disorder (Provisional)
AXIS II	V71.09—No diagnosis on Axis II
AXIS III	None

| AXIS IV | Problems with primary support—father incarcerated, mother unable to provide discipline; educational problems—below-average academic performance, discord with teachers and classmates; problems related to interaction with legal system/crime—recent arrest |
| AXIS V | 50 (current) |

Summary

This chapter provides a brief overview of the terminology commonly used in mental health settings. Much of the terminology related to mental health care is misunderstood or misused. Consequently, clinicians practicing in the field need to be as specific and clear as possible in professional discussions and documentation. Furthermore, clinicians can be role models for the sensitive use of terminology and advocates for educating the public about mental health.

Occupational therapists primarily focus their practice on the alleviation of dysfunction for engagement in occupation, but a thorough understanding of symptoms and diagnoses is essential for all clinicians working in mental health. People with mental illness present with a range of symptoms and dysfunctions of varying frequency and severity, and it is not possible in this chapter to do justice to all presentations. However, forthcoming chapters on specific disorders provide more in-depth discussions of commonly seen diagnoses, dysfunctions, and symptoms.

Review Questions

1. How are symptoms related to diagnosis?
2. What is the relationship between thought and language in relation to psychopathology?
3. How would you justify the use of the *DSM* for diagnosis?
4. What argument would you offer against use of the *DSM*?

References

American Psychiatric Association (APA). (2000). *Diagnostic and statistical manual of mental disorders,* Fourth Edition, Text Revision. Washington, DC: Author.

Andreasen, N., & Black, D. (2001). *Introductory textbook of psychiatry* (3rd ed.). Washington, DC: American Psychiatric Press.

Bernstein, D. A., Milich, R., & Nietzel, M. T. (2002). *Introduction to clinical psychology.* (6th ed.). Prentice-Hall.

Blakeney, A., Strickland, L. R., & Wilkinson, J. (1983). Exploring sensory integrative dysfunction in process schizophrenia. *American Journal of Occupational Therapy, 37*(6), 399–407.

Bonder, B. (1995/1991). *Psychopathology and function* (2nd ed.). Thorofare, NJ: Slack.

Brown, C., Tollefson, N., Dunn, W., Cromwell, R., & Filion, D. (2001). The Adult Sensory Profile: Measuring patterns of sensory processing. *American Journal of Occupational Therapy, 55*(1), 75–82.

Doniger, G., Silipo, G., Rabinowicz, E., Snodgrass, J., & Javitt, D. (2001). Impaired sensory processing as a basis for object-recognition deficits in schizophrenia. *American Journal of Psychiatry, 158*(11), 1818–1826.

Goldman, H., Skodol, A., & Lave, T. (1992). Revising Axis V for DSM-IV: A review of measures of social functioning. *American Journal of Psychiatry, 149*(9), 1148–1156.

Lewis-Fernandez, R., & Kleinman, A. (1994). Culture, personality, and psychopathology. *Journal of Abnormal Psychology, 1,* 67–71.

MacRae, A. (1997). The model of functional deficits associated with hallucinations. *American Journal of Occupational Therapy, 51,* 57–63.

Mathis, J. (1992). Psychiatric diagnosis: A continuing controversy. *Journal of Medicine and Philosophy, 17,* 253–261.

Maxmen, J., & Ward, N. (1995). *Essential psychopathology and its treatment* (2nd ed.). New York: Norton.

Occupational Therapy Practice Framework: Domain and Process. (2002). *American Journal of Occupational Therapy, 56*(6), 614–639.

Rosenzweig, M. R., Leiman, A. L., & Breedlove, S. M. (2001). *Biological psychology: An introduction to behavioral, cognitive, & clinical neuroscience.* Sunderland, MA: Sinauer.

Sadock, B. J., & Sadock, V. A. (2003). *Kaplan and Sadock's synopsis of psychiatry: Behavioral sciences, clinical psychiatry* (9th ed.). Philadelphia: Lippincott Williams & Wilkins.

World Health Organization (WHO). (2001). *International classification of functioning, disability and health (ICF).* Geneva: WHO.

Suggested Reading

Sadock, B. J., & Kaplan, H. I. (2003). *Study guide and self-examination review for Kaplan and Sadock's synopsis of psychiatry.* Philadelphia: Lippincott Williams & Wilkins.

Spitzer, R. L., Gibbon, M., Skodol, A. E., Williams, J. B., & First, M. B. (Eds.). (2002). *DSM-IV-TR casebook: A learning companion to the Diagnostic and Statistical Manual of Mental Disorders. Fourth Edition, Text Revision.* Washington, DC: American Psychiatric Press.

In addition, many new terms have been introduced in this chapter that will also be used in other chapters. Therefore, it is strongly recommended that students have at least one medical dictionary to study clinical terminology. Suggested sources include the most recent editions of the following:

Dorland's medical dictionary. Philadelphia: Saunders.

Miller, B., & Keane, C. *Encyclopedia and dictionary of medicine, nursing, and allied health.* Philadelphia: Saunders.

Taber's cyclopedic medical dictionary. Philadelphia: F. A. Davis.

CHAPTER 6

Schizophrenia

Anne MacRae, PhD, OTR/L

Key Terms

cognitive deficits
negative symptoms
positive symptoms

psychosis
psychotropic

Chapter Outline

Introduction

Schizophrenia is a common disorder affecting approximately one in every 100 people. According to the National Institute of Mental Health (NIMH), approximately two million people will develop schizophrenia in their lifetime.

The disorder of schizophrenia has probably existed as long as humankind, but it has been interpreted in various physical, emotional, and spiritual ways by different generations and cultures. Even after the condition was recognized as a specific disease entity, diagnostic criteria have varied historically as well as geographically. In other words, depending on when and where diagnosticians were trained, they may or may not agree on the diagnosis of schizophrenia. Kraepelin (1919/1971) was one of the first European clinicians to recognize schizophrenia as a specific disease process. He called the condition dementia praecox because of its relatively early onset (usually in young adulthood) and its tendency to produce cognitive and behavioral changes in the individual. Bleuler (1911/1950) concluded that the term *dementia praecox* was essentially inadequate because there was not always cognitive deterioration and the disorder was not necessarily degenerative, as had been thought by Kraeplin. It was Bleuler who first suggested that schizophrenia was really one of several possible diseases that present in similar fashion. Therefore, he suggested that the term *dementia praecox* be replaced with *the group of schizophrenias*. Current diagnostic criteria have been strongly influenced by Kurt Schneider's (1959) identification of "first rank" symptoms of schizophrenia. These symptoms primarily consist of hallucinations (auditory especially), delusions, and bizarre behavior. This emphasis on the psychotic, or "positive," symptomatology of the disorder may not give an accurate representation of the functional level of people with schizophrenia.

Schizophrenia is referred to as a thought disorder, but not all forms of the disorder include long-term **cognitive deficits**. It is also referred to as a psychotic disorder, yet **psychosis** may be present only for some period during the course of the disease, not as a chronic condition. Both the terms *psychotic* and *thought disorder* could be applied to other conditions and lack the specificity needed to identify schizophrenia accurately.

MYTHS AND MISCONCEPTIONS

To this day, the term *schizophrenia* is often misused and the concept is frequently misunderstood. The misconceptions regarding this condition are rampant and must be dispelled before any meaningful understanding can be reached.

Eight Common Myths

Myth #1: "Split personality."   A person suffering from schizophrenia does not have a split personality. This is an unfortunate, and essentially inaccurate, description. Schizoprenia is not a personality disorder. The concept of split personality more accurately describes multiple personality disorder, which is now called, in the *DSM-IV-TR*, dissociative identity disorder (American Psychiatric Association, 2000).

Myth #2: Bad parenting.   People with schizophrenia are not a product of bad parenting. No one can cause another person to have schizophrenia. It is caused by a combination of factors, including hereditary predisposition. If someone who inherits the predisposition to schizophrenia is in a particularly stressful environment, the illness may manifest itself earlier, have greater severity and frequency, and lead to a poorer outcome, but environment alone is not believed to cause the disorder. The vast majority of people who experience even catastrophic levels of stress do not develop schizophrenia. Although the popularity of this myth is waning, it still persists and is particularly damaging and painful to families—the very people who might best support people with schizophrenia.

Myth #3: Drug experimentation.   Schizophrenia is not caused by taking drugs. It is a complicated disease, not the result of drug experimentation. People who have schizophrenia may have an acute exacerbation if they use certain drugs because of the disinhibiting effect of many substances. Moreover, a prime time for drug experimentation is adolescence and young adulthood, which happens to coincide with the usual onset of schizophrenia. It is not uncommon for people with schizophrenia to have a coexisting diagnosis of substance abuse. In many cases, people with schizophrenia use drugs and alcohol in an maladaptive attempt to control their symptoms and the related distress.

Myth #4: Lack of motivation. People with schizophrenia do indeed try to get better. No one wants to have a disorder such as schizophrenia. People who take their prescribed medication and maintain psychosocial support usually fare better, but dysfunction may persist regardless of the level of treatment. **Psychotropic** medications typically dampen or reduce the severity of the more obvious symptoms, but they often fail to eliminate them. In the 1990s the atypical antipsychotic agents, such as clozapine, risperidone, and olanzapine, were introduced and hailed as a major breakthrough in the treatment of schizophrenia. Indeed, some people switching from one of the earlier medications, such as haloperidol, experienced a significant reduction in both symptoms and side effects (Csernansky, Mahmoud, & Brenner, 2002). However, current research suggests that these medications may have only small added value in the overall treatment of psychotic disorders (Lewis, 2002). Maxmen and Ward (1995) state that clozapine and risperidone are effective in about one-third of people with schizophrenia who exhibit resistance to other antipsychotic medication. In other words, there remains a significant minority of people with schizophrenia who continue to display symptoms even while taking medication.

There are a variety of reasons why someone may not be compliant with treatment. In some cases, appropriate treatment is simply unavailable. People with schizophrenia benefit the most from consistent and maintained intervention, yet community and outreach programs are scarce. The consequence is a "revolving door" syndrome whereby people decompensate and are recurrently hospitalized. (Further discussion of this dilemma can be found in Chapter 21, "Case Management.")

Myth #5: Rising incidence.   The incidence of schizophrenia is not on the rise, and there is no evidence to support the myth that it is increasing. However, modern Western society is stressful, particularly in the urban areas, so there may be a trend for people with schizophrenia to be more seriously disabled by the condition. Moreover, the deinstitutionalization movement created a situation in which people with schizophrenia are more visible in the community. This has had some positive effects but also many negative ones. The National Mental Health Association estimates that 25% to 35% of homeless people in the United States have schizophrenia.

Myth #6: Institutionalization and disability.   People with schizophrenia do not always live in institutions and are not always profoundly disabled. While it is true that in the past there were greater numbers of people who were institutionalized, they never constituted the majority of people who have schizophrenia. Most people with the disorder live with families, in residential care facilities in the community, or independently. The disorder has the potential for being gravely disabling and it is a serious mental illness. However, the actual functional deficits are highly variable, and it is possible for some people to work, go to school, and raise a family.

Myth #7: Low intelligence.   People with schizophrenia do not have below-average intelligence. Instead, the actual range of IQs of people with schizophrenia is highly variable. It is possible to have schizophrenia and be quite brilliant; it is also possible to have a coexisting developmental disability. Many, but not all, people with schizophrenia have a variety of cognitive deficits, but these do not necessarily include decreased intelligence. Rather, the cognitive deficits may include poor abstraction, judgment, and processing time, which can be misinterpreted as low intelligence.

Myth #8: Danger and violence.   People with schizophrenia are generally not dangerous and violent. This is a persistent and highly damaging myth largely fostered by the media. The sensationalization of stories such as accounts of the "Son of Sam" murders in New York and assassinations of prominent figures have distorted the facts. People who are actively psychotic, particularly if they are paranoid, sometimes do become very violent, and this can be understandably frightening. "The major predictors of violent behavior are male gender, younger age, past history of violence, noncompliance with antipsychotic medication, and excessive substance use" (APA, 2000, p. 304). Statistically, however, people who have schizophrenia, who live in the community, are no more likely to commit a serious crime than people in the general population.

People with psychotic symptoms are more likely to hurt themselves than someone else (MacRae, 1993). Self-inflicted violence includes a wide variety of injuries, including mutilation and starvation. It also unfortunately includes successful suicide attempts. The APA estimates that 10% of people with schizophrenia commit suicide (2000). Sadock and Sadock (2003) state that 10% to 15% of people with schizophrenia die by suicide and as many as 50% attempt suicide. It is also true that family members or significant others may sometimes be the target of violent outbursts (discussed in Chapter 1).

Several recent reports have indicated that violent crimes committed by people with serious mental illness are on the rise. One explanation for this is the increased number of people with dual diagnoses. Clearly, violence related to drug and alcohol use is a significant problem, regardless of whether there is concurrent schizophrenia (see also Chapter 9).

Another explanation for this increase in violence is the shortage of appropriate treatment. As cutbacks in mental health and social services continue, people are forced to do without necessary treatment, become more disenfranchised, and experience both acute exacerbations and gradual decompensations of their illness. It could well be true that if the present trends continue, what started out as a myth about violence may become a self-fulfilling prophecy.

ETIOLOGY OF SCHIZOPHRENIA

Ideas regarding the cause of schizophrenia are constantly changing, but it is now generally accepted that there is some level of organic involvement, and many believe that at least a predisposition to the disease is hereditary. Stress may play a role in the onset of episodes and the severity of the disorder, but it is not the single causative factor.

Much of the neurological information about people with schizophrenia is due to the development of technology, including computerized tomography (CT) and magnetic resonance imaging (MRI) (Sadock & Sadock, 2003). Unfortunately, however, understanding of the findings lags behind the information explosion created by these new technologies. The list of hypothesized causes of schizophrenia is somewhat daunting and may, on the surface, seem contradictory, but it highlights the need for much further research. Currently in the United States, research dollars available to study schizophrenia are only a small fraction of the money spent to research other diseases. Also complicating the research efforts is the awareness that schizophrenia, like many other diseases, is probably caused by a combination of many factors. One of the criticisms of neurologic, and particularly structural, theories of etiology is that they cannot account for the episodic nature of the disease in some people or for its highly variable clinical outcome. Future research will most likely focus on the interaction of many variables rather than a single entity.

Many different structural anomalies have been discovered in the brains of people with schizophrenia. These include lesions in the brain stem, enlargement of the ventricles, brain atrophy, and abnormalities in the limbic structures, cerebellum, and corpus callosum. There is a growing body of evidence that frontal lobe dysfunction, possibly related to the basal ganglia, plays a role in the development of negative symptoms. Structural abnormalities in the brain are clearly more common in people with schizophrenia than in the general population. However, the clinical significance of these findings is far from understood. The National Institute for Mental Health (NIMH) is currently conducting research exploring the human genome and the possibility that schizophrenia is a developmental disability that manifests itself after puberty (Spearing, 1999).

One of the most prevalent theories of etiology concerns the role of the neurotransmitter dopamine. It is hypothesized that people with schizophrenia have either an excess of dopamine or an excessive quantity of dopamine receptors, making the neurotransmitter more effective. No reliable measure presently exists to determine specific amounts of neurotransmitters in the brain, but it is known that antipsychotic medication, which often decreases overtly psychotic symptoms, affects dopamine levels. Therefore, it might be assumed that excessive dopamine is particularly related to positive symptoms. Although there has been a tremendous amount of emphasis placed on the role of dopamine, other neurotransmitters, specifically norepinephrine, serotonin, and glutamate, as well as certain neuropeptides, are also being studied (Sadock & Sadock, 2003).

Another promising area of research is the role of a virus or viruses in the development of schizophrenia. There are viruses that stay inactive for many years and then start to grow slowly. Thus, it is hypothesized that a possible cause of schizophrenia is exposure to certain viruses prenatally while involved areas of the brain are being developed (Coleman & Gillberg, 1996). The person's subsequent deterioration in adolescence or young adulthood may be the direct result of a virus or an autoimmune reaction triggered by a virus. Evidence to support this theory is limited, but certain demographic data on people with schizophrenia is suggestive. For example, there is a higher than average incidence of people with schizophrenia who are born in the winter or spring months, which coincides with the epidemiological patterns of many viruses. Moreover, low birth weight is more common than average in people with schizophrenia, possibly suggesting a viral infection in utero. Recent research suggests that advanced paternal age at the time of birth of the offspring may also be a risk factor for adult schizophrenia (Brown, et al., 2002).

There are many theories about the role of food substances in both the cause and treatment of schizophrenia. One promising area of research is in the use of fish oil or other fatty acids. A research literature review conducted by the Cochrane Collaboration Project concluded that polyunsaturated fatty acid supplementation to standard treatment or as primary intervention for schizophrenia may be acceptable to people with schizophrenia and have a moderately positive effect (Joy, Mumby-Croft, & Joy, 2002).

The School of Occupational Therapy and Physiotherapy in Aarhus, Denmark, currently includes the subject of nutrition and psychiatry in their occupational therapy curricula and encourages occupational therapists to incorporate meal planning that reduces caffeine intake and increases fatty acid intake (Cold, 2002).

Other deficiencies in diet and vitamins have been examined as possible causes of schizophrenia, but so far the results have been largely discounted or considered to be anecdotal. Nevertheless, considering what is still unknown about neurochemistry, these avenues of study may still hold promise.

DIAGNOSIS OF SCHIZOPHRENIA

There is criticism that schizophrenia tends to be overdiagnosed, particularly with people demonstrating bizarre or flagrant behaviors. Some societies more than others appear to tolerate "eccentric" behavior without necessarily considering it pathological. For a person to act "odd" or "different" does not necessarily mean that he or she has a disease. Even with the presence of obvious psychosis, it cannot be assumed that a pathological condition exists. For example, it has been well documented that hallucinations can occur as part of specific religious and cultural rituals, drug-induced behavior, or even within the realm of "normal" experience (MacRae, 1991).

For the purposes of this chapter, schizophrenia is considered a group of disorders that meet the minimum criteria as described in the *DSM-IV-TR* (APA, 2000). These criteria are as follows:

A. Characteristic symptoms: two or more of the following, each present for a significant portion of time during a one-month period (or less if successfully treated):

1. delusions
2. hallucinations
3. disorganized speech (i.e., frequent derailment or incoherence)
4. grossly disorganized or catatonic behavior
5. negative symptoms (e.g., affective flattening, alogia, or avolition)

B. Social/occupational dysfunction: for a significant portion of the time since the onset of the disturbance

C. Some signs of the disorder must be continuously present for at least six months.

Clinicians should be aware, however, of the limitations of the *DSM*. As Andreason and Carpenter state: "Somehow, the existence of such criteria gives the sense that we know what schizophrenia is when in fact we do not. Schizophrenia remains a clinical syndrome comprising an unknown number of disease entities or pathologic domains" (1993, p. 203).

Another way of classifying schizophrenia is to differentiate distinct syndromes based on the predominance of either **positive symptoms** or **negative symptoms**. Two syndromes of schizophrenia have been identified by Crow (1985). Type 1 is characterized by positive symptoms, and Type 2 is characterized by negative symptoms. Table 6-1 further describes the differences between these two syndromes. It remains controversial as to whether these syndromes are distinct entities. A third category has been recently added that describes a mix of positive and negative symptoms, including thought disorder and disorganized behavior as well as cognitive and attention deficits (Sadock & Sadock, 2003). In some cases there may be interplay between positive and negative symptoms. For example, deficits in perception (usually considered a positive symptom) "may contribute to the muted world experience of patients with persistent negative symptoms of schizophrenia" (Doniger, Silipo, Rabinowicz, Snodgrass, & Javitt, 2001, p. 1818).

Not all conditions presenting with psychosis are schizophrenia. There are many disorders that may present where psychosis is transient but is not a defining feature of the disorder. The *DSM-IV-TR* also recognizes several disorders as being primarily a type of psychotic disturbance, including the following:

Table 6-1. Syndromes of Schizophrenia: A Comparison of Types 1 and 2

Type	Symptomatology	Prognosis	Response to Treatment
1	Predominance of positive symptoms with minimal or no cognitive deficits	Characterized by a fluctuating course of exacerbations and remissions. Usual onset involves a full-blown psychotic episode	Generally responds well to antipsychotic medication. May need little or no other therapeutic intervention between psychotic episodes providing there is a stable environment
2	Predominance of negative symptoms, typically with some degree of cognitive deficits	Usually a chronic course. Onset may be insidious but is generally identified by early adulthood	Responds poorly to typical antipsychotic medication but may experience a reduction of negative symptoms with an atypical agent. Usually needs ongoing supportive therapy for both rehabilitation and maintenance of living skills

- Schizophreniform disorder
- Schizoaffective disorder
- Delusional disorder
- Brief psychotic disorder
- Shared psychotic disorder
- Psychotic disorder due to a general medical condition
- Substance-induced psychotic disorder
- Psychotic disorder not otherwise specified

POSITIVE SYMPTOMATOLOGY

The most common positive symptoms associated with schizophrenia are delusions and perceptual distortions, especially hallucinations. However, various other perceptual and behavioral disturbances may also present as positive symptoms. Abnormal affect, such as uncontrolled laughing or silliness, is particularly common with the disorganized type of schizophrenia. Language disturbances may include bizarre speech, echolalia, and, more frequently, circumstantiality, tangentiality, loosening of associations, incoherency, and pressured speech. Changes are possible in motoric responses, including pacing, rocking, restlessness, and lethargy, as well as disturbances of sleep patterns. It is important to recognize that the range and severity of symptoms varies with the individual.

Delusions

Delusions vary in content. Typical delusions found with schizophrenia are considered bizarre in that they are implausible within the context of the individual's environment and culture. William Bowden, a man diagnosed with schizophrenia, paranoid type, described the intractable nature of delusional thinking in this first-person account: "My belief has withstood attack from anyone I've shared it with. It is also something that I truly wish would stop. I also wish, even if this phenomenon is true, that I did not believe it" (1993, p. 165).

Paranoid delusions are certainly not limited to schizophrenia, but they do partially account for the suspicious and guarded behavior sometimes seen with the disorder. The delusions of schizophrenia also take various forms of presentation. For example, a delusion may be in the form of thought broadcasting, which occurs when the individual believes that his or her thoughts can be transmitted. Thought insertion and thought withdrawal are the beliefs that someone or something is responsible for either putting thoughts into one's brain or removing one's thoughts (and ability to think). Thought control is also attributed to someone other than the person having the delusion and usually also implies action control (for example, someone who commits a crime and attributes the action to the force of a spirit or devil).

Presentations of thought broadcasting, insertion, withdrawal, and control are relatively consistent throughout different cultures and in historical reports of suspected delusions. What does change is the individual's rationale for what is happening. Thus, descriptions of these phenomena are remarkably similar throughout the world except for the individual's explanation for the phenomena. For example, a person who experienced a delusion of thought control in the European Middle Ages would have typically explained the control as coming from a demonic force, while in the decade of the 1950s in the United States, when the Cold War was raging, it was common for "the communists" to be blamed for thought control delusions. It is understandable that people would attempt to explain something happening to them that is out of the realm of the ordinary; therefore, these rationales are usually common themes found in the culture. The forms of the rationale may be political, religious, supernatural, scientific, or pseudo-scientific.

Perceptual Distortion

People with schizophrenia may experience many different kinds of perceptual disturbances, which also vary in severity. Hallucinations are probably the most common, particularly in acute phases of the disorder. However, illusions are also possible, as well as other perceptual disturbances indicative of sensory-integrative or sensory-processing dysfunction (Blakeney, Strickland, & Wilkinson, 1983; King, 1974; APA, 2000; Doniger et al. 2001). These deficits may also include poor body schema and personal boundaries, tactile defensiveness, and distorted figure-ground (Eimon, Eimon, & Cermak, 1983), spatial, and time relations.

Distemporality does not fit neatly into a description of positive or negative symptoms, as it includes perceptual distortion and disorientation but also behaviorally presents as avolition. People with schizophrenia often report a sense of being stuck in present time, living only in the moment and unable to process the events of the past or determine a future course. Moneim El-Meligi stated that change in subjective time is "by far the most neglected area in both psychiatric evaluation and psychodiagnostic testing" (1972, p. 226).

Hallucinations are considered one of the hallmark symptoms of schizophrenia, but it has often been inaccurately considered that only auditory hallucinations are found in this disorder. Auditory hallucinations are probably the most common presentation, and they may lead to the greatest personal distress, possibly causing them to be reported with greater frequency. However, it is the phenomenon of multiple presentations of hallucinations that probably causes the greatest level of dysfunction. In other words, the more senses are involved with hallucinatory experiences, the more difficult it is for an individual to stay oriented to reality (MacRae, 1993).

Interestingly, the vividness or frequency of the hallucinations is not necessarily indicative of the severity of the disorder. Some people with quite pronounced perceptual distortion manage to develop adequate coping skills, while others with only a minimal disturbance remain severely impaired. In schizophrenia, the presence of negative symptoms, cognitive deficits, and a poor ability to manage environmental stimuli decreases the ability to cope with hallucinations, therefore creating a greater level of dysfunction.

CASE ILLUSTRATION: Maureen—Positive Symptoms

Maureen is a 23-year-old college student who was accompanied by her roommate to the Emergency Psychiatric Services at the county hospital. She arrived in a wildly agitated state, claiming, "They are all trying to kill me." During an initial interview, Maureen admitted that she had been hearing voices commanding her to kill herself. The voices had apparently worsened over the last several days to the point where she was unable to sleep or concentrate on any activities. It was decided that Maureen was a danger to herself, and she was admitted to the acute inpatient locked unit. Further interviews revealed that Maureen had a history of repeated psychotic episodes starting in high school. Six years ago she had been diagnosed with schizophrenia, paranoid type. When she took her medication, her symptoms remained under control and she was able to function relatively well. However, her attempts to finish college had been hampered by acute exacerbations of her illness at times when she stopped taking her medication.

Discussion

Maureen's behavior is characteristic of someone with predominantly positive symptoms, minimal cognitive deficits, a fluctuating course of exacerbations and remissions, and good response to antipsychotic medication, which aids her functioning.

NEGATIVE SYMPTOMATOLOGY

Many researchers and theorists have recently concentrated on negative symptomatology in schizophrenia. This effort has been strongly influenced by the work of Nancy Andreason, who developed the Scale for the Assessment of Negative Symptoms (1984). The scale includes the following broad categories:

- Affective flattening or blunting—a limited ability to express emotions and feelings
- Alogia—impoverished thought process that is manifested in speech patterns
- Avolition—a lack of interest or energy unaccompanied by depressed affect
- Anhedonia—an inability to experience pleasure or sustain interest in activities
- Inattention—an inability, of which the person may be unaware, to sustain concentration or attention

From an occupational therapy perspective, the term *hypohedonia* (decreased enjoyment) rather than *anhedonia* probably more accurately reflects the emotions, affect, and potential of the person with Type 2 schizophrenia. A study conducted by Emerson, Cook, Polatajko, and Segal (1998) suggests that people with schizophrenia, even with negative symptoms, are able to experience joy given occupations or activities that are challenging but not overwhelming. Research conducted by Ivarsson, Soderback, and Ternestedt (2002) concurred with these findings, stating that occupational therapy "alleviated their symptoms, gave them belief in the future, strengthened their self esteem and feeling of capability, and all this appeared to give them satisfaction" (p. 108).

Because negative symptoms are most often observed during sustained and social activity, the occupational therapist has a critical role in the accurate assessment of function. Moreover, the occupational therapy emphasis on activities of self-care, work, and leisure makes it essential that the therapist understand the nature of negative symptoms. A meaningful treatment plan reflects an awareness of these symptoms and efforts to be made to help the individual cope with, and compensate for, existing deficits.

CASE ILLUSTRATION: James—Negative Symptoms

James has lived in a residential care facility for the past seven years. He has not been hospitalized since living in this home but had several hospitalizations in the five years prior to this move. James takes antipsychotic medication, which seems to completely control the hallucinations he experienced in the past. Nevertheless, even in the absence of psychosis, James remains unable to function independently. He reports that he does nothing all day but has no plans for changing his lifestyle. He has been enrolled in several rehabilitative programs, including sheltered workshops, but was unable to follow through with their recommendations. James also attempted to complete an associate's degree at the local community college but dropped out during his first semester. Poor attendance and difficulty attending to tasks were the primary reasons for this cycle of failure. James also has great difficulty in social situations. He tends to be passive, avoiding conversation and relationships even though he states he is lonely.

Discussion

James's functioning is severely influenced by his negative symptoms of avolition, anhedonia, and inattention.

PROGNOSIS

Schizophrenia is a serious and persistent mental illness, but data on its prognosis is unreliable. "Because of the variability in definition and ascertainment, an accurate summary of the long-term outcome of schizophrenia is not possible" (APA, 2000, p. 309).

The severity and prognosis of schizophrenia may be affected by cultural and environmental influences. For example, the World Health Organization (WHO) concluded that schizophrenia has a more benign course in the Third World. This may be explained by different family structures and types of treatment, a less urban environment, or the possibility that the disorder found in the Third World may have a different biological basis. Severity and clinical presentation are also partially determined by gender. Women generally have a later onset of the disorder than men with the potential for a more benign course. However, it is not known if these differences are due to different sociocultural conditions or biologically separate disease processes (Castle, 2000). The presence or absence of cognitive deficits is currently thought to be the strongest indicator of long-term functional deficits (Green, 1996).

The long-held belief that schizophrenia is always a chronic and possibly deteriorating condition is currently being challenged (Kruger, 2000; McGuire, 2000). It has been suggested that some people with schizophrenia may have a natural remission after two to three decades. In other words, recovery rates may actually be much higher than previously estimated, but only after a prolonged course of illness (possibly 20 to 30 years). According to Liberman and Kopelowicz:

> Long-term follow-up studies of persons who had experienced severe forms of schizophrenia earlier in their lives have discovered that over 50 percent of these individuals are living what may be considered "normal" lives—working, socializing, playing, living without close supervision and with little or no psychotic symptoms—20 to 30 years after their illness began. These "recoveries" have been documented in Japan, Germany, Switzerland, Scotland, France, and the USA. (1994, p. 67)

These studies have many ramifications for treatment. Hypothetically, if a young man developed schizophrenia at the age of 17, by the time he was 40 years old the disease might have run its course, but by that time his identity will also be firmly entrenched as a "disabled person." Many functional deficits would continue because of lifestyle, habits, and societal expectations and, most important, because of the missed developmental milestones of adolescence and young adulthood. Role dysfunction, which is considered an integral part of schizophrenia, may be minimized if aggressive rehabilitation is provided early in the course of illness. "The onset of psychotic disorder often disrupts a person's ability to perform competently in occupational and social roles, thus adolescents with psychotic disorders are appropriate candidates for occupational therapy intervention" (Henry & Coster, 1996, p. 171).

It also must be acknowledged that poor prognosis may be linked to inadequate treatment. It has been repeatedly documented that outcome is improved when people with schizophrenia are given comprehensive and consistent long-term treatment. It is possible that if such treatment were universally available, there would be a higher incidence of full recovery. It is certain that, given comprehensive and consistent treatment, functional outcome and quality of life would be improved even if the course of the disease remains chronic.

INTERDISCIPLINARY TREATMENT

In the acute phase of illness, hospital treatment may be necessary and beneficial, but typical hospitalization stays have shortened considerably over the last decade, and in the United States they are often only three to seven days in length. The hospitalization of people with schizophrenia usually only occurs when the individual has a severe psychotic episode, has grossly decompensated in function, and is considered either a danger to the self, a danger to others, or gravely disabled. The primary goal of acute hospitalization is to provide a thorough evaluation and stabilize the person on medication. Acute care hospitalizations also help stabilize clients by providing a safe environment with adequate rest and nutrition. This is becoming especially pertinent as the incidence of homelessness among people with schizophrenia increases. Depending on the length of stay, the beginnings of a rehabilitation program may be commenced, but it is unrealistic to assume that brief hospitalizations will serve as sufficient intervention. People with schizophrenia require consistent treatment, typically of long duration, with a combined interdisciplinary approach. "Psychopharmacologic and psychosocial treatments appear to be additive in their efficacy. Combining social skills training with maintenance of antipsychotic medication yields better social functioning while minimizing relapse" (Liberman & Kopelowicz, 1994, p. 69). Treatment should include psychotropic medication, supportive services, and rehabilitation that includes both verbal and activity-based therapies.

Goal Setting

A key component of an interdisciplinary treatment plan is setting the goals of treatment. Ideally, these goals are determined by the individual in conjunction with the team. This cornerstone of client-centered practice "does not negate the importance of professional expertise, but is guided by a commitment to listen and respond to each client. The clients' personal knowledge and experience of living with a mental illness enable them to explain their lives, goals, and plans and allows them to seek personal meaning in their lives" (Dressler & MacRae, 1998, p. 37). It is highly desirable to also include the family and significant others, provided the person in treatment consents. Unfortunately, there are many constraints to this ideal situation. The trend toward managed care has placed great limits on the amount of services that can be provided, and too often, services are predetermined by agency mandate. Moreover, Western society has a long history of an authoritarian approach to health care, whereby professionals are viewed as "experts" who know what is best for the client. Although the "expert" model is changing to a more collaborative one, vestiges of the authoritarian health care system remain in practice.

Cooperative goal setting can also be hampered by the individual's pathology. People with delusions, poor insight, concrete thinking, or avolition may be incapable of healthy and realistic goal setting. Nevertheless, within the person's capabilities, every effort should be made to seek out and honor his or her expressed interests and desires, even if they sometimes conflict with the team's opinion.

CASE ILLUSTRATION: Diamond—Goal-Setting Conflict

Diamond, 38, has been diagnosed with schizophrenia, undifferentiated type. She has a long history of repetitive decompensations while living in the community. During her most recent hospitalization, the team recommended that she be placed in a residential care facility to help monitor her symptoms and medication. Diamond strongly objected, stating that she likes living alone in an apartment and that her goal is to return to independent living. After repeated discussions with the team, Diamond reluctantly agreed to the placement. Two weeks later, Diamond walked out of the facility and has not gotten in touch with her therapist in the ensuing month.

Discussion

This scenario might have been avoided if more effort had been made to comprehend Diamond's goals. While a residential care facility may be a safer alternative than independent living, it cannot be a feasible alternative without the individual's cooperation. Negotiation about follow-up care in the community, including day treatment and case management options, might have addressed the team's legitimate concerns while allowing Diamond to remain in an independent living situation.

Agreement as to what are "realistic" goals is not an easy task. The goals of the treatment team members may be quite different from those of the person with schizophrenia, whose ideas may also differ from the goals and expectations of the family. Professionals have been accused of contributing to chronicity by fostering dependency on the system and discouraging individuals from pursuing goals of independence in housing, employment, or school. On the other hand, for some people the demands of independent living exacerbate their symptoms, leading to a cycle of failure. "The patient with schizophrenia . . . is often walking a tightrope between exposure to understimulating or overstimulating environments" (Lukoff, Liberman, & Nuechterlein, 1986, p. 579). Either overestimating or underestimating a person's potential can have adverse effects, so it is essential that goal setting not be based on diagnosis or preconceived ideas of outcome but rather be founded on an assessment of the particular individual's strengths, deficits, interests, needs, and level of support. In client-centered occupational therapy, "the targeted outcome is a vision of the future shared by the client and therapist and driven by the dream and desire of the individual. Dreams are unique to each individual, thus, targeted outcomes will also be" (Clark & Bell, 2000, p. 80).

Psychotropic Medication

A significant part of the treatment of schizophrenia involves antipsychotic medication prescribed by a physician. However, the role of drug therapy has often been misunderstood. Antipsychotic medication does not cure schizophrenia. It typically decreases symptoms, but treatment that involves only drug therapy is inadequate. The primary benefit of **psychotropic** drugs is to stabilize the individual sufficiently that he or she may benefit from other treatment.

Side effects do occur with antipsychotic medication, including extrapyramidal symptoms (EPS), autonomic nervous system signs, endocrine side effects, and skin changes. Therefore, it is important that drug trials be closely monitored to determine the best choice of drug and optimum dosage. In the medical model, there is often an overemphasis on decreasing symptoms, even at the expense of overall function. For example, a person on relatively high dosages of medication may experience a complete elimination of hallucinations but be too sedated to engage in meaningful activity, while a lower dose may cause some of the positive symptoms to persist but allow the individual to continue functioning while coping with the symptoms.

It is theorized that the typical antipsychotic agents primarily act as antagonists of typical dopamine. Their therapeutic effect is believed to come from blockage of dopamine in the frontal cortex and limbic system, which is responsible for behavior and affect. However, these traditional antipsychotic drugs also block dopamine in the basal ganglia, causing unwanted extrapyramidal symptoms. Antipsychotic medication tends to readily cross the blood-brain barrier and eventually attain a higher concentration in the brain. Because of this process, systemic side effects of antipsychotic medications will usually appear before the therapeutic effects. (See Appendix A for further information.)

A major concern in drug therapy for people with schizophrenia is a relatively high incidence of noncompliance. Given the extent of side effects experienced with these medications, it should not be a surprise that people may not want to take their medication, but there are many additional reasons for noncompliance. People with schizophrenia find themselves in a paradoxical situation in that the very symptoms that need treatment may prevent them from taking their medication. These symptoms may include delusional thinking regarding the harm of the drugs or lack of insight regarding their illness. Moreover, people with schizophrenia often have cognitive deficits such as forgetfulness, confusion, and poor time orientation, making it difficult for them to manage medication independently.

Noncompliance can be minimized by providing education and supportive interventions to help the individual manage both symptoms and side effects. Moreover, people with cognitive deficits can benefit from simplified drug regimes, and time and memory management techniques. However, the most important predictor of compliance is the therapeutic relationship and level of trust the individual feels with the prescribing physician and treatment team as a whole. Unfortunately, the current state of mental health care makes it difficult for a consistent treatment team to follow people, who frequently become "lost in the system."

OCCUPATIONAL THERAPY INTERVENTION

Team treatment of people with schizophrenia is common and, depending on the model of treatment used, various disciplines may be involved. For the purposes of this chapter, discussion is limited to the role of the occupational therapist. It must be acknowledged, however, that in some team approaches, several disciplines may overlap with occupational therapy or conduct evaluation and treatments typically viewed as occupational therapy. In some cases, occupational therapists may also take on roles outside their traditional domain. Regardless of the model of intervention, the needs of the client should dictate the services provided.

Evaluation

The choice of assessment tools is influenced by the therapist's theoretical frame of reference. One such theory-bound evaluation is Allen's Cognitive Levels test, which is based on Claudia Allen's model of cognitive disability (Allen, 1985). The information derived from this evaluation is helpful in structuring the environment and interactions to best compensate for the person's cognitive limitations.

Another commonly used formal evaluation for people with schizophrenia is the Kohlman Evaluation of Living Skills (KELS) (Kohlman Thomson, 1992). This is an easily administered evaluation, which provides information on an individual's ability to perform a variety of tasks necessary for independent living. The KELS is not intended as a diagnostic tool, as it does not give specific information on the causes of dysfunction. For this reason, it is not a sufficiently sensitive tool for treatment planning. However, it is very valuable for discharge planning, especially if placement of the individual is in question. For example, when a client is being prepared for discharge from an acute care hospital, it is crucial that the treatment team have a clear understanding of the level of assistance needed. Based on the information provided by the KELS, recommendations may be made for independent living or a range of assisted living environments.

Another functional evaluation is the Assessment of Motor and Process Skills (AMPS) developed by Anne Fisher. "The AMPS is an observational assessment that permits the simultaneous evaluation of motor and process skills as a person performs two or three complex or instrumental activity of daily living (IADL) tasks (e.g., meal preparation, home maintenance, laundry) of his or her choice" (Fisher et al., 1992, p. 878). The AMPS is not specific to any diagnosis, but considering that people with schizophrenia often have both cognitive and sensorimotor deficits that result in dysfunction, it is very useful for this population. As stated by Pan and Fisher,

> Limitations in function of clients with psychiatric disorders are a major factor affecting their independence and need for service . . . [and] therefore, occupational therapists need to use valid, reliable, and sensitive functional assessment instruments that can guide the intervention process and measure change. (1994, p. 775)

One of the most recent additions to occupational therapy assessments is the Adult Sensory Profile (Brown, Tollefson, Dunn, Cromwell, & Filion, 2001). Considering the well-documented sensory-processing deficits and perceptual distortions found in schizophrenia, this assessment may be valuable in developing successful interventions, especially in the areas of coping strategies and environmental modifications.

Occupational therapists also use an interview to build a therapeutic relationship, determine interests and skills, and develop goals. A particularly useful interview format is the Canadian Occupational Performance Measure (COPM), which measures the client's self-perception of occupational performance by using a semistructured interview. The structure of the COPM helps the client and therapist develop goals that are both realistic and applicable for occupational therapy intervention. It can also be used as an outcome measure of the client's perception of performance and satisfaction, if it is administered at the beginning of treatment and then readministered at the time of discharge (Law et al., 1998). An interview also discloses much information regarding symptoms related to thought processes, but it is not the most effective method of determining function. A more useful tool for evaluating the functional skills of people with schizophrenia is task analysis. The observation of an individual engaged in routine activities provides a wealth of information about functioning that could not be uncovered through an interview.

Treatment

Group work is the most common approach used by occupational therapists in mental health. (For discussion of groups, see Chapter 19.) Groups are especially effective for building social skills, but the importance of one-to-one personal contact should not be underestimated, especially in the early stages of treatment, when it aids in developing a relationship and performing evaluation. Unfortunately, occupational therapists working with budget and time constraints often must forgo individual treatments. One-to-one contact is vital for individuals who are withdrawn or are too psychotic to benefit from a group approach. The stimulation of an activity group may place undue demands on some people and exacerbate their symptoms. In addition, individual contact is often a prelude to group involvement. It is helpful if the occupational therapist in a one-to-one interaction explains the purpose of the available groups, and personally invites the individual to join. Attendance and participation in group activities is much more likely if the person already has a relationship with the group leader and knows what to expect.

Individual intervention is often thought to be too expensive, but in fact it is possible to meet specific objectives in a time- and cost-effective manner. For example, an occupational therapist may visit individual rooms on an inpatient unit with a cart stocked with grooming supplies. In this way, the OTR engages in one-to-one contact with clients while providing evaluation and treatment. This activity gives the therapist an opportunity to check in with clients at the beginning of the day. Introductions and orientation to occupational therapy occur simultaneously with activity of daily living (ADL) evaluation and treatment. The actual contact may be quite brief, yet this form of individual treatment paves the way for more sustained one-to-one and group activities.

Although occupational therapists structure their interventions on the individual's strengths, understanding the pathology of the illness is also essential. People who display positive symptoms, especially hallucinations, benefit from activities that divert attention from their symptoms. In the process, the individual can learn self-help coping strategies to minimize the intrusiveness of positive symptomology. However, it is only when people can clearly identify activities with *personal meaning or purpose* that they are able to see them as a viable method of symptom management. While random applications of activities sometimes provides a temporary distraction from hallucinations, it is the use of activities that bolsters the sense of personal achievement and mastery that are consistently deemed as most successful in coping with hallucinations and other positive symptoms (MacRae, 1993; Ivarsson, Soderback, & Ternestedt, 2002).

Negative symptoms have a more profound effect than positive symptoms on an individual's overall ability to function. Understanding that negative symptoms are part of the disease process and not necessarily a learned maladaptive behavior can help the clinician structure interventions to compensate for these deficits. Individuals who display negative symptoms often need highly structured activities with concrete expectations and goals. Specific skill training and psychoeducation are very beneficial to people with negative symptoms, but many individuals need ongoing support to utilize their skills.

Improving overall quality of life for people with schizophrenia is one of the main objectives of treatment. In research conducted by Laliberte-Rodman, Yu, Scott, and Pajouhandeh (2000), three major themes regarding quality of life were identified through the use of focus groups consisting of subjects with schizophrenia, a consumer facilitator, and a nonconsumer facilitator. These themes are managing time, connecting and belonging, and making choices and maintaining control. Occupational therapy techniques and interventions are ideal for mastering and fulfilling these quality-of-life-concerns.

Table 6-2. Occupational Therapy Treatment Formats for People with Schizophrenia	
Types	*Comments*
Structured tasks	Provide habit training, diversion, coping skills, and time management training. Potential for leisure skill development. May also build self-esteem through successful completion
Expressive activities	Nonverbal communication, emotional and creative outlets. Potential for leisure skill development. May also build self-esteem through successful completion
Functional living skills	May include basic self-care, including hygiene, grooming, and dressing. Also includes independent living skills such as meal preparation and money management
Psychoeducation	Can be used to teach living skills but is also used for teaching symptom management, health and safety awareness, and assertiveness training
Social skills training	Especially effective in groups; includes verbal and nonverbal communication. Role playing is one technique used
Vocational training	Includes basic skill preparation as well as time management and social skills. Vocational pursuits must be carefully graded and may require ongoing support

Considering the global dysfunction associated with schizophrenia, there is a wide range of possible interventions, which address the occupational performance areas of self-care, work, and leisure as well as the performance components of motor, sensory-integrative, cognitive, psychological, and social functioning. Most activities can address more than one component or area, and the therapist must adapt and grade the activities to best meet the needs of the individual patient or group. Treatment goals may be accomplished in many different ways using a variety of individual and group techniques. Table 6-2 describes some of the specific treatment formats used with this population by occupational therapists.

Summary

Schizophrenia is a complicated disorder affecting over a million people throughout the world. Its effects can be devastating on a person's ability to function but, moreover, individuals with schizophrenia additionally experience dysfunction from society's reaction to them for being ill. Schizophrenia is largely misunderstood by the general public, and clinicians have a responsibility to combat the myths and misconceptions about this disorder. Many people with schizophrenia can lead productive, meaningful lives, but only with consistent and comprehensive treatment. A knowledge of the underlying pathology of the illness, an ability to work with a team approach, and a willingness to relate to the person with schizophrenia are essential for successful intervention.

Review Questions

1. Why is schizophrenia commonly misunderstood?
2. What is believed to be the cause of schizophrenia?
3. How does the presence of positive symptoms affect occupational therapy intervention?
4. How does the presence of negative symptoms affect occupational therapy intervention?
5. How does occupational therapy intervention for people with schizophrenia differ from other mental health professions?

References

Allen, C. (1985). *Measurement and management of cognitive disabilities*. Boston: Little, Brown.

American Psychiatric Association (APA). (2000). *Diagnostic and statistical manual of mental disorders* (4th ed., Text Revision). Washington, DC: APA.

Andreason, N. (1984). *Scale for the Assessment of Negative Symptoms (SANS)*. Iowa City: University of Iowa Press.

Andreason, N., & Carpenter, W. (1993). Diagnosis and classification of schizophrenia. *Schizophrenia Bulletin, 19*(2), 199–213.

Blakeney, A., Strickland, L. R., & Wilkinson, J. (1983). Exploring sensory integrative dysfunction in process schizophrenia. *American Journal of Occupational Therapy, 37*(6), 399–407.

Bleuler, E. (1950/1911). *Dementia praecox, or the group of schizophrenias* (J. Zinkin, Trans.). New York: International Universities Press.

Bowden, W. (1993). First person account: The onset of paranoia. *Schizophrenia Bulletin, 19*(1), 165–167.

Brown, A., Schaefer, C., Wyatt, R., Begg, M., Goetz, R., Bresnahan, M., Harkavy-Friedman, J., Gorman, J., Malaspina, D., & Susser, E. (2002). Paternal age and the risk of schizophrenia in adult offspring. *American Journal of Psychiatry, 159*, 1528–1533.

Brown, C., Tollefson, N., Dunn, W., Cromwell, R., & Filion, D. (2001). The Adult Sensory Profile: Measuring patterns of sensory processing. *American Journal of Occupational Therapy, 55*(1), 75–82.

Castle, D. (2000). Women and schizophrenia: An epidemiological perspective. In D. Castle, J. McGrath, & J. Kulkarni (Eds.), *Women and schizophrenia*. Cambridge: Cambridge University Press.

Clark, J., & Bell, B. (2000). Collaborating on targeted outcomes and making action plans. In V. Fearing & J. Clark (Eds.), *Individuals in context: A practical guide to client-centered practice*. Thorofare, NJ: Slack.

Cold, J. (2002). *Occupational therapists' use of nutrition in psychiatry with focus on schizophrenia and depression*. The School of Occupational Therapy and Physiotherapy in Aarhus. Web retrieval: www.efaa.dk/webpublications.

Coleman, M., & Gillberg, C. (1996). *The schizophrenias: A biological approach to the schizophrenia spectrum disorders*. New York: Singer.

Crow, T. J. (1985). The two-syndrome concept: Origins and current status. *Schizophrenia Bulletin, 11*, 471–486.

Csernansky, J., Mahmoud, R., & Brenner, R. (2002). A comparison of risperidone and haloperidol for the prevention of relapse in patients with schizophrenia. *New England Journal of Medicine, 346*(1), 16–22.

Doniger, G., Silipo, G., Rabinowicz, E., Snodgrass, J., & Javitt, D. (2001). Impaired sensory processing as a basis for object-recognition deficits in schizophrenia. *American Journal of Psychiatry, 158*(11), 1818–1826.

Dressler, J., & MacRae, A. (1998). Advocacy, partnerships, and client centered practice. *Occupational Therapy in Mental Health, 14*(1/2), 35–43.

Eimon, M., Eimon, P., & Cermak, S. (1983). Performance of schizophrenic patients on a motor-free visual perception test. *American Journal of Occupational Therapy, 37*(5), 327–332.

Emerson, H., Cook, J., Polatajko, H., & Segal, R. (1998). Enjoyment experiences as described by persons with schizophrenia. *Canadian Journal of Occupational Therapy, 65*(4), 183–192.

Fisher, A., Liu, Y., Velozo, C., & Pan, A. W. (1992). Cross-cultural assessment of process skills. *American Journal of Occupational Therapy, 46*(10), 876–885.

Green, M. F. (1996). What are the functional consequences of neurocognitive deficits in schizophrenia? *American Journal of Psychiatry, 153*, 321–330.

Henry, A., & Coster, W. (1996). Predictors of functional outcome among adolescents with psychotic disorders. *American Journal of Occupational Therapy, 50*(3), 171–183.

Ivarsson, A., Soderback, I., & Ternestedt, B. (2002). The meaning and form of occupational therapy as experienced by women with psychosis. *Scandinavian Journal of Caring Science, 16*, 103–110.

Joy, C. B., Mumby-Croft, R., & Joy, L. A. (2002). Polyunsaturated fatty acid (fish or evening primrose oil) for schizophrenia (Cochrane Review). *The Cochrane Library,* Issue 3. Oxford: Update Software.

King, L. J. (1974). A sensory-integrative approach to schizophrenia. *American Journal of Occupational Therapy, 28*(9), 529–536.

Kohlman Thomson, L. (1992). *The Kohlman Evaluation of Living Skills.* (3rd ed.). Bethesda, MD: American Occupational Therapy Association.

Kraepelin, E. (1971/1919). *Dementia praecox and paraphrenia* (R. M. Barclay & G. M. Robertson, Trans. & Eds.). Edinburgh: E. & S. Livingstone.

Kruger, A. (2000). Schizophrenia: Recovery and hope. *Psychiatric Rehabilitation Journal, 24*(1), 29–37.

Laliberte-Radman, D., Yu, B., Scott, D., & Pajouhandeh, P. (2000). Exploring the perspective of persons with schizophrenia regarding quality of life. *American Journal of Occupational Therapy, 54*(2), 137–147.

Law, M., Baptiste, S., Carswell, A., McColl, M., Polatajko, H., & Pollock, N. (1998). *Canadian Occupational Performance Measure (COPM)* (3rd ed.). Thorofare, NJ: Slack.

Lewis, D. (2002). Atypical antipsychotic medications and the treatment of schizophrenia. *American Journal of Psychiatry, 159*(2), 177–179.

Liberman, R. P., & Kopelowicz, A. (1994). Recovery from schizophrenia: Is the time right? *Journal of the California Alliance for the Mentally Ill, 5*(3), 67–69.

Lukoff, D., Liberman, R. P., & Nuechterlein, K. H. (1986). Symptom monitoring in the rehabilitation of schizophrenic patients. *Schizophrenia Bulletin, 12*, 578–597.

MacRae, A. (1991). An overview of theory and research on hallucinations: Implications for occupational therapy intervention. *Occupational Therapy in Mental Health, 11*(4), 41–60.

MacRae, A. (1993). *Coping with hallucinations: A phenomenological study of the everyday lived experience of people with hallucinatory psychosis.* Ann Arbor, MI: University Microfilms.

Maxmen, J., & Ward, N. (1995). *Essential psychopathology and its treatment* (2nd ed.). New York: Norton.

McGuire, P. (2000). New hope for people with schizophrenia. *Monitor on Psychology, 32*(2), 24–28.

Moneim El-Meligi, A. (1972). A technique for exploring time experiences in mental disorder. In H. Yaker, H. Osmond, & F. Cheek (Eds.), *The future of time* (pp. 220–271). Garden City, NY: Anchor.

Pan, A. W., & Fisher, A. (1994). The assessment of motor and process skills of persons with psychiatric disorders. *American Journal of Occupational Therapy, 48*(9), 775–782.

Sadock, B. J., & Sadock, V. A. (2003). *Kaplan and Sadock's synopsis of psychiatry: Behavioral sciences, clinical psychiatry.* Philadelphia: Lippincott Williams & Wilkins.

Schneider, K. (1959). *Clinical psychopathology* (M. W. Hamilton, Trans.). London & New York: Grune & Stratton.

Spearing, M. (1999). *Schizophrenia.* National Institute of Mental Health. NIH Publication No. 99-3517.

Suggested Reading

Andreasen, N. (1984). *The broken brain: The biological revolution in psychiatry*. New York: Harper & Row.

Backlar, P., & Andreasen, N. (1994). *The family face of schizophrenia: Practical counsel from America's leading experts*. New York: Putnam.

Burrows, G., Norman, T., & Rubenstein. G. (Eds.). (1986). *Handbook of studies on schizophrenia*. New York: Elsevier.

Fuller-Torrey, E. (2001). *Surviving schizophrenia: A manual for families, consumers & providers*. New York: Harper Trade.

Keefe, R., & McEvoy, J. (2000). *Negative symptom and cognitive deficit treatment response in schizophrenia*. Washington, DC: APA.

Marneros, A., Andreasen, N., & Tsuang, M. (Eds.). (1991). *Negative versus positive schizophrenia*. Berlin: Springer–Verlag.

Miller, R. (Ed.). (2002). *Diagnosis: schizophrenia: A comprehensive resource for patients, families, and helping professionals*. Columbia University Press.

Sullivan, E., Shear, P., Zipursky, R., Sagar, H., & Pfefferbaum, A. (1994). A deficit profile of executive, memory, and motor functions in schizophrenia. *Biological Psychiatry, 36*, 641–653.

Weidenbeck, P. (1999). *Breakthroughs in antipsychotic medications*. New York: W. W. Norton.

Mood Disorders

Elizabeth Cara, PhD, OTR, MFT

Key Terms

cyclothymia
depression
dysthymia
mania

melancholia
mood
referential thinking

Chapter Outline

Introduction

Mood disorders have been described throughout history. Descriptions of depressive episodes are found in the Old Testament and in classical Greek literature. Originally, in ancient times, they were thought to be a curse of the gods, and therefore, sufferers were treated by priests. In the sixth century B.C., Hippocrates, "the father of physicians," introduced the terms **melancholia** and **mania** in clinical descriptions that are still accurate today. He also placed mental functioning, or malfunctioning, in the brain rather than in the spirit. Therefore, mania and melancholia became the domain of the medical doctor rather than the priest. Although the disorders continued to be recognized throughout different periods of history, it was not until recently, in the nineteenth century, that the current diagnostic properties of manic and depressive illness were formally categorized (Sadock & Sadock, 2000).

Many people living in the twenty-first century can identify with the term **depression** because they have some idea of what it feels like to be sad, blue, "under the weather," or to temporarily lose a sense of meaning in their lives. Many people can also identify with the term *mania*, because, due to today's fast-moving society, they have some idea of what it is like to feel "pressured," "pressed," "speedy," or "hyper." Perhaps because of our general ability to experience a range of emotions, depression and mania (to a lesser extent) have become household words.

Perhaps because these terms have become familiar and because, generally, people can identify the emotions associated with each term, beginning clinicians are often not prepared for the depth of the symptoms or for how extremely and strongly mood and behavior are affected. Although recognizing that there is a range of severity of symptoms accompanying depression and mania, this chapter will refer mostly to the extreme syndromes or symptoms of mania and major depression.

DIAGNOSTIC CRITERIA

The *DSM-IV-TR* (APA, 2000) describes a group of disorders with the essential feature of a disturbance in **mood** that is not due to any other mental or physical disorder, medication, substance use, or other psychiatric condition. These disorders are classified as *mood disorders*. Former classifications described the same disorders as *affective disorders*, so this term may be used interchangeably (Sadock & Sadock, 2000).

The *DSM-IV-TR* uses three groups of criteria to diagnose problems regarding mood: episodes, disorders, and specifiers that describe a most recent episode and a recurrent course (Morrison, 1995). *DSM-IV-TR* divides mood disorders into bipolar disorders and depressive disorders. The essential feature of a bipolar disorder is the presence of one or more manic episodes (often with a history of at least one major depressive episode). The essential feature of depressive disorders is one or more periods of depression, but not necessarily with a manic episodic history. **Dysthymia** is a milder form of major depressive episode, but it lasts for a longer period of time. **Cyclothymia** is a milder form of bipolar disorder, and it also has a longer duration. Bipolar and depressive disorders range from mild to severe and may include psychotic features. They usually cause considerable distress and/or impairment in all occupational areas of functioning.

Episodes

A mood episode refers to any time at which a client feels abnormally happy or sad. The mood disorders are constructed from these episodes, that is, the episodes are the foundation from which the disorders are arranged (Morrison, 1995).

   Major depressive.   At least five of the following symptoms must be present for two weeks and represent a change from previous level of functioning. At least one of the symptoms is either depressed mood or loss of interest and pleasure.

1. daily depressed mood, indicated by subjective report or the observation of others. In children or adolescents, the mood can be irritable.
2. very marked decrease of interest or pleasure in most daily activities
3. significant weight loss (when not dieting) or weight gain or significant increase or decrease in appetite. For children this could be represented by failure to gain expected weight through normal growth.
4. inability to sleep or sleeping most of the day
5. psychomotor agitation or its opposite, psychomotor retardation
6. extreme fatigue or loss of energy
7. feelings of extreme worthlessness or inappropriate guilt nearly every day
8. indecisiveness or lack of concentration
9. recurring thoughts of death, suicidal ideas, or a suicidal plan or attempt

   Manic.   There is a distinct period of abnormal, elevated, expansive, or irritable mood lasting at least one week. During this period at least three or more of the following symptoms are significantly present. There may be psychotic features or hospitalization may be necessary to prevent harm to the self or others.

1. grandiosity or overinflated self-esteem
2. decreased need for sleep
3. talking more than usual or pressured talking
4. the experience that thoughts are racing
5. extreme distractibility
6. increase in goal-directed activity (this can take form in different areas, e.g., socially, at work or school, or sexually) or psychomotor agitation
7. excessive involvement in pleasurable activities that have the potential for later painful consequences (such as buying sprees, imprudent investments, or indiscreet sexual activity)

   Hypomanic.   The elevated mood must last at least four days, be observably different from the usual nondepressed mood, and include three of the symptoms of mania. The episode does not cause marked impairment in occupational or social functioning, call for hospitalization, or include psychotic features.

Mixed. The criteria for both manic and major depressive episodes are met nearly every day for at least one week. The impairment in functioning is identical to that of the manic and major depressive episodes.

Disorders

A disorder is a pattern of illness due to an abnormal mood. Most people who have a mood disorder experience depression at some times, and some also have high moods. Most mood disorders are diagnosed on the basis of a mood episode (Morrison, 1995).

Major depressive disorder. A major depressive disorder, single episode, is diagnosed if there is a single major depressive episode and there has never been a manic, mixed, or hypomanic episode. A major depressive disorder, recurrent episode, is diagnosed if there have been two or more major depressive episodes at least two months apart and there has never been a manic, mixed, or hypomanic episode. A dysthymic disorder is a depressed mood that lasts most of the day for a majority of days over at least two years. In children and adolescents the mood can be irritable, and symptoms must be present for at least one year. To qualify for diagnosis, during the period of symptoms, the person should not have been symptom free for more than two months at a time and he or she should have experienced no major depressive, manic, mixed, or hypomanic episode or cyclothymic disorder. There also must be at least two of the following symptoms:

1. poor appetite or overeating
2. insomnia or too much sleeping
3. fatigue
4. low self-esteem
5. poor concentration or difficulty with decisions
6. hopelessness

Bipolar Disorders. The various bipolar disorders are distinguished by the presence of either a manic episode or a major depressive episode. They are classified as either bipolar I or bipolar II, depending on which is the dominant mood. Bipolar I features a dominant manic mood, and bipolar II features a dominant depressed mood. As with the other disorders, the symptoms cause significant distress or impairment in important daily areas of functioning; they are not the result of use of a substance, medication, or medical condition; and they cannot be better accounted for by positing the existence of other disorders.

In bipolar I, single manic episode, there is the presence of a manic episode and there have been no major depressive episodes in the past. In bipolar I, most recent episode hypomanic, there is currently a hypomanic episode and there has been at least one manic, or mixed episode in the past. In bipolar I, most recent episode manic, there is a manic episode and there has been at least one major depressive, manic, or mixed episode in the past. In bipolar I, most recent episode mixed, there is a mixed episode and there has been at least one major depressive, manic, or mixed episode in the past. Finally, in bipolar I, most recent episode depressed, there is currently a major depressive episode and there has been in the past at least one manic or mixed episode.

In bipolar II, there is one or more major depressive episodes and at least one hypomanic episode in the past, but there has never been a manic or mixed episode. In cyclothymic disorder there have been periods of hypomanic symptoms with periods of depressive symptoms for at least two years and the person has not been symptom free for more than two months. Moreover, there has been no major depressive, manic, or mixed episode during that time (APA, 2000).

Specifiers

Specifiers are descriptors that help qualify disorders or episodes. One set describes the most recent major depressive episode and manic episode. "Atypical features" describes individuals who eat and sleep a lot, feel weighted down and almost immobile, and are extremely sensitive to rejection. "Melancholic features" describes what can be considered the classic features of depression: early morning awakening with a mood that improves later in the day, loss of appetite, guilt, and feeling slowed down or agitated, with loss of interest and pleasure in those events and experiences that usually bring pleasure. "Catatonia" describes features of either extreme motor hyperactivity or extreme inactivity. "Postpartum onset" describes either a manic or a depressed episode experienced by a woman within a month of giving birth.

The other set of descriptors describes the overall course of a disorder. "With or without full interepisode recovery" describes the presence or absence of symptoms between episodes. "Rapid cycling" describes a person who has had at least four episodes within a year. "Seasonal pattern" describes those who become ill with regularity at the same time each year.

CAUSES, OCCURRENCE, AND THEORIES OF MOOD DISORDERS

In all industrialized countries, major depression is twice as common in females as in males (Sadock & Sadock, 2000). Resaons for this difference include hormonal and endocrine system involvement and other gender-related stresses, such as childbirth and social conditions related to women's sex roles (see also Bracegirdle, 1991; Feder, 1990; 1991). Bipolar disorder is reported to be almost equally common among males and females. Major depression is 1.5 to 3 times more common among relatives of people with the disorder than in the general population. Bipolar disorder clearly occurs at a much higher rate in first-degree relatives. Up to 1.2% of the adult population is estimated to have bipolar disorder. Pelissolo and Lepine (2001) cite the average age of onset of bipolar disorder in the United States as 18 years, while Marneros and Angst (2000b) state that the peak onset for a bipolar episode is between ages 25 and 30, and for a unipolar episode, the late 30s. The lifetime prevalence of major depressive disorder ranges from 4.4% to

5.8% for those 18 and older. Though some (APA, 2000) estimate the prevalence of major depression as high as 26% for women and 12% for men. The age of onset for major depression varies from children to adults. An interesting statistic is that the incidence of depression has increased among individuals who matured after World War II, and the age of onset for a major depressive episode has decreased (Pelissolo & Lepine, 2001).

Causes and Occurrence

The causes of mood disorders are unknown; however, most agree that there are multiple factors involved in mood disorders, such as genetic/biochemical, psychosocial, and socio-environmental, which interact in very complex ways. Table 7-1 discusses the factors implicated in both mood disorders.

Physical diseases such as Addison's and Cushing's disease, thyroid disorders, diabetes, syphilis, multiple sclerosis, and chronic brain syndromes related to arteriosclerosis may induce depression. Thyroid disorders may also be implicated in bipolar illness, although thyroid disorders are generally ruled out prior to making the bipolar diagnosis. Other physical disorders are associated with depression, including mononucleosis, anemia, malignancies, hypoglycemia, colitis, congestive heart failure, rheumatoid arthritis, and asthma. Some medications are also associated with depression, including antiparkinsonian agents, hormones, steroids, and antihypertensives (Sadock & Sadock, 2000).

Other Theories

Various authors present interesting theoretical ideas regarding major depressive and bipolar illnesses. There was an explosion of information in the 1990s, particularly regarding bipolar illness. When discussing the centrality of cycling to the bipolar disorder, Koukopoulos et al. (2000) believe that there is not a unipolar disorder but more likely recurrent depressions preceded or followed by mild hypomanias, and that cyclothymic or hyperthymic clients belong to the bipolar group. They think of bipolar disorder in terms of energy. There is an increased level of energy in mania and a decreased need for sleep. Periods of excitement, like a fire, consume much energy and may exhaust the biological processes that create it. As a result of this exhaustion, depression occurs and a genetic flaw may then prevent recovery of the energy, leading to long-lasting depression.

Temperament is also related to both major depression and bipolar illness and "affective disorders predominantly arise in persons with great emotional reactivity" (Koukopoulos et al., 2000, p. 330). Temperaments may be dysthymic (depressive), hyperthymic (manic), irritable, or cyclothymic (cycling) (Akiskal cited in Koukopoulos et al., 2000). Although the concept of bipolar I and bipolar II was used in the *DSM-IV-TR*, there is much support (Marneros & Angst, 2000; Marneros, 2000) for a spectrum of disorders on a continuum of affectivity (see Table 7-1) that distinguishes between hypomania, cyclothymia, mania, mania and mild depression, mania and major depression, and major depression and hypomania. Usually there is a normal level of human behavior and activity that moves between the two poles of depression and mania. However, with some people

	Table 7-1. Major Etiologic Theories of Depression and Bipolar Illnesses	
	Depression	*Bipolar*
Biochemical	The neuronal response may be influenced by multiple signals from serotonin and other neurotransmitters such as acetylcholine or melatonin, hormones, or neuropeptides that modulate mood (Loosen et al., 2000).	As in depression, the neuronal response may be influenced by multiple signals from serotonin and other neurotransmitters such as acetylcholine or melatonin, hormones, or neuropeptides that modulate mood (Loosen et al., 2000).
	The hypothalamic-pituitary-adrenal (HPA) and hypothalamic-pituitary-thyroid (HPT) systems are believed to be involved in major depression.	
Neuroendocrine	Almost half of those with major depression show a higher secretion of cortisol than those who are not depressed. The level returns to normal when depression abates. A small dose of thyroid hormone accelerates the effects of antidepressants in women and for both sexes the hormone is responsible for making those who do not respond to antidepressants more responsive than usual (Loosen et al., 2000).	Stress affects the hypothalamic-pituitary-adrenal (HPA) axis; the HPA then disrupts social and circadian rhythms, leading to mood instability (Hlastala & Frank, 2000).
Genetic	Family studies, twin studies, and adoption studies support the role of genes in transmission of major depressive disorder (Tsuang & Faraone, 2000).	Family studies, twin studies, and adoption studies support the role of genes in transmission of bipolar disorder (Tsuang & Faraone, 2000).
Socioenvironmental	Life events, particularly the death or loss of a loved one. (Support for other predisposing factors in combination with life events is the fact that fewer than 20% of those who report a loss become depressed.	Life events, such as a change in social roles (becoming a parent or getting a divorce), changes in routines (travel across time zones), or loss (death of a loved one) and birth of a child (Hlastala & Frank, 2000).
Psychosocial	Behavioral theories concerning control and reinforcement predominated in the late twentieth century; however, currently a popular behavioral theory is that depression develops when a person cognitively misinterprets life events and develops a cognitive triad of a negative view of	People with bipolar illness may be affected by family members and relatives who often explicitly express (often critical) emotions. These high emotion expression (HEE) families may promote relapses in the early stages of the illness, depending on the bipolar person's style,

continues

Table 7-1. (continued)		
	Depression	*Bipolar*
	self, of the experience, and of the future. The views one keeps in the mind are called schemas or schemata and all events become interpreted through the negative schemata (Loosen et al., 2000).	self-concept, age, psychological status, rehabilitation planning, and social environment (Mundt, Kronmuller & Backenstraf, 2000).
Psychophysiological	Affective disturbance is associated with lack of daylight (called seasonal affective disorder, or SADD). People tend to be depressed in fall and winter, but not so in spring and summer.	Physiological cycles are influenced by the seasons and the environment, so in bipolar illness the individual is not able to mediate adaptation to changes in the physical environment (Koukopoulos et al., 2000).

there is a disruption of the normal homeostasis, with resulting restriction as in depressive disorders or expansion as in bipolar disorders. More recently, the spectrum has expanded to encompass diagnostic subgroups called *soft bipolar spectrum* (described by Akiskal, as cited in Marneros & Angst, 2000c, p. 26).

This soft spectrum of affectivity (Marneros, 2000; Marneros & Angst, 2000c) would include a bipolar III classification of recurrent depression that changes to hypomania with antidepressant treatment and the speculation that people with hyperthymic temperaments belong to the bipolar spectrum and that certain personality disorders, such as histrionic-sociopathic or borderline-narcissistic, may belong to cyclothymic temperaments. Support for this soft spectrum could be found in the fact that 84% of those who have a bipolar disorder also have another disorder. Of those who have a comorbid condition, over 50% have an axis I or axis III disorder and up to 30% have a coexisting axis II personality disorder. However, these subgroups need to be researched further to move beyond speculation.

The kindling and sensitization model of recurrent affective disorders (Hlastala & Frank, 2000) proposes that people with bipolar illness become so sensitized to stress because of so many episodes that they eventually only require the slightest stimulus to precipitate an episode. Also, the episodes will be increasingly severe and time between episodes will shorten. So far, research has been equivocal, with about an equal number of studies supporting or not supporting the hypothesis. Age, symptom severity, type of bipolar illness, and other factors, such as self-esteem, relationships, social support, and personality, may be important mediating factors in the role of sensitization.

Another interesting speculation (Crow, 2000) is an evolutionary theory connecting the division of the spheres of the brain and language acquisition with bipolar disorders as well as psychotic disorders. This theory proposes that the same gene responsible for the evolution of language in humans was also responsible for the psychoses. Furthermore, the psychoses and affective disorders can be viewed on a continuum, with the schizophrenic disorders developing first in a person followed later by the affective disorders. Crow puts forth evidence for his hypothesis by correlating the psychotic symptoms of thought insertion, withdrawal, and broadcast and auditory hallucinations with a language disorder (indeed, they are classified as disorders of language in *DSM-IV-TR*). Additionally, some affective symptoms, such as pressured speech or mutism, are also disorders of speech production. Further evidence that the disorders relate to brain lateralization are that affective disorders are often associated with spatial orientation and face recognition difficulty generally attributed to the nondominant hemisphere. Also many who have psychotic or affective disorders are ambidextrous, and thus lateralization is not specialized.

Another evolutionary theory (Sloman & Gilbert, 2000) focuses on depression. The authors propose that an evolutionary-biological model, the social competition model, is involved in mood disorders, primarily depression. According to this model, humans, like nonhuman primates, developed strategies for dominance and control or submission in conflicts that are related ultimately to survival. In every conflict a person has to decide if she or he can be victorious (dominate and control) or not. Just as in other evolutionary mechanisms like attachment, if one assesses a situation to be such that she or he cannot win, then she or he will involuntarily trigger submission strategies. These dominant or submission strategies involve actual behavior to fight or flee and internal mechanisms to read the situation and activate or deactivate physiological mechanisms, such as arousal or inhibition of the HPT axis.

Sloman and Gilbert (2000) propose that depressed people find themselves in situations or instances that can be actual or imagined that they believe they cannot control. Therefore, "involuntary defeat strategies" (IDS) are activated. Thus the individual avoids defeat and accommodates to control. However, the depression results when the IDS are not deactivated and areas for fight are suppressed and flight are blocked. The IDS continue and result in physiological and intrapsychic signals that both lead to depression and continue the maladaptive strategies. Some situations typical of arrested fight and resulting anger of suppression are dependence on the object of one's own anger as in a boss who could fire an employee, or a spouse who could leave the partner, or fear of making a fool of oneself, or shame for one's anger. Some typical situations of arrested flight leading to feelings of entrapment are external, such as loss of resources or lack of alternatives, or internal, such as fear of asking for help due to worry about what the other may think, fear that one cannot cope alone, or moral concerns about hurting others and resulting guilt. Ironically, the same cortical advantages that humans evolved that enable self-awareness, self-evaluation, anticipation, and planning are also responsible for the maladaptive internalization of signals that activate the subordinate psychobiological response patterns.

CLINICAL PICTURE

Most people experience varying moods at different times in their lives. Generally, moods can be described as ranging from happiness, elation, and joy to sadness, despair, and hopelessness. The usual feelings that one experiences in daily life should not be confused with the syndromes of mania and depression. Most happy, energetic people do not have a manic disorder, and unhappiness or sadness does not signal a depressive disorder. Both the manic and depressive disorders can be viewed according to the degree and duration of symptoms. Like other disorders they have to be viewed in the context of how an individual usually functions and to what degree and how long a change in function occurs.

Individuals experiencing a manic episode present themselves with a very elevated mood and their behavior is generally very expansive and irritable. There is heightened psychomotor activity, and they speak, think, and move very rapidly. Usually they have seemingly boundless energy. Often they feel very creative, and indeed, they are usually flooded with some ideas that are imaginative. Popular lore would have us envy those who are manic for their creative qualities. However, although there may be heightened motor activity, there is usually little productivity. An individual who is manic rarely completes projects; attention is fragmented and activity has a purposeless quality to it. Increased activity often takes the form of sexual provocativeness and promiscuity, exaggerated political and religious concern, or purchasing many expensive items regardless of their affordability. Essentially, all activities are carried out with a gross lack of judgment.

An individual who is manic may be euphoric and have an infectious quality, but there is also an accompanying quality of being "driven." He or she may be humorous but, due to a low frustration tolerance, may also easily become irritable and angry. The grandiose behavior and sense of importance may give way to psychotic delusions. It is not unusual to think that one is God, and an individual may show considerable contempt for other people. Due to this grandiosity; frequent, loud speech; and an interruptive manner accompanied by poor social judgment, those with manic behavior are often socially rejected (Kaplan & Sadock, 1989, 1991). Often, beginning professionals find it difficult to simply "be with" someone who is manic, and therefore should seek out clinical supervision for assistance in tolerating this behavior and working effectively.

In my clinical experience, in the realm of occupational therapy, their heightened activity, difficulty concentrating and attending to tasks, distractibility, and intrusiveness often make individuals experiencing a manic episode candidates for individual treatment with engagement in simple concrete tasks or movement. Working with those who are manic often calls on one's best idea of the therapeutic use of self and the use of a full repertoire of interpersonal skills. At the same time, it also calls for the use of concrete and simple tasks or activities. The seeming contradiction involving requirements of simplicity, on one hand, and the use of complex interpersonal skills, on the other, is often confusing and difficult for new clinicians. Again, this is a time to seek out clinical supervision. Table 7-2 lists major symptoms of mania and depression.

Individuals with major depression present themselves as hopeless with a very despairing mood and their behavior is usually passive and withdrawn. There is usually a marked lack of energy, and they speak, think, and move very slowly. However, this psychomotor retardation (slow movements) can also be accompa-

Table 7-2. Clinical Picture: Major Symptoms of Depression and Mania

Symptoms	Depression	Mania
Emotional	Depleted mood Hopelessness Decreased sense of humor Lack of pleasure	Euphoric mood Grandiosity
Cognitive	Negative thinking Decreased concentration and attention Indecision	Grandiose, expansive thinking Decreased concentration and attention
Motivational	Decreased energy Paralysis of will and initiation Avoidance or escapist wishes	Increased energy Agitation Distraction Low frustration tolerance
Self-Concept	Worthlessness Guilt	Inflated sense of worth and power
Vegetative	Loss of appetite Sleep disturbance Loss of sexual desire	Loss of appetite Sleep disturbance Increased sexual preoccupation

nied by anxiety and agitation, called *psychomotor agitation*. Often, the person complains of not experiencing pleasure, and indeed, is often unable to accept or experience humor in naturally humorous situations. The person with major depression will experience most activity as overwhelming and burdensome. Often, the person will be unable to initiate activity or may vacillate and be unable to make a decision, even the simplest of ones.

Often individuals have trouble concentrating or organizing thinking, usually feel worthless, and make many negative statements about themselves. Often they feel an overwhelming sense of guilt for some imaginary crimes and they often imagine that they are the cause of someone else's misfortune (called *referential thinking*).

Because of their negativity, hopelessness, ambivalence, and lack of humor, they may repel people. The palpable depressed mood or agitated behavior can be difficult to be around. Also, their indecision and ambivalence may make them appear overly dependent. Just as with a person who is manic, it may be difficult for new clinicians to empathize with a person who is depressed, or to tolerate dependency. There may be a tendency to push persons with depression to do things that they are unable to do, or to reject their dependent behavior. If this is the case, then seeking clinical supervision for assistance is indicated just as it is in working with people who are manic.

Suicidal thoughts are experienced by some people who suffer from depression (Beck, 1973; see also Hemphill, 1992). The most dangerous periods often are in the beginning, usually when the person is most anxious and help is not present, and in the later remission period, when the person begins to feel better and then may become frightened of a relapse. At this time, he or she will have regained energy and be able to think clearly enough to commit suicide. It is important to take suicidal statements seriously and inquire if an individual has the means (usually a gun or pills) and a formulated plan. All statements and other information should be immediately reported to the primary therapist and the treatment team.

In the occupational therapy clinic, people who are depressed may have difficulty initiating any task or may protest often that they can do nothing. They may require much prompting and activities that are concrete and simple. They may take a very long time to complete a task or obsess over a perceived error. An individual who is manic may display the opposite behavior, initiating too many tasks, stating that he or she can do everything and anything, flitting from task to task, denying any errors, and requiring much attention and prompting to contain or stop behavior.

COMMON EVALUATION AND MANAGEMENT

There are some common strategies of evaluation and management for depressive and manic disorders that are recognized by most disciplines working in psychiatric settings.

Evaluation

The intensity, severity, and duration of symptoms are obtained by observation, interview, and history taking. Since life events such as loss or psychosocial stressors (e.g., divorce or abusive relationships) are implicated in the timing of both depressive and manic episodes (APA, 2000; Hlastala & Frank, 2000), a life events inventory may be used to supplement a careful history. Some scales are used by other professionals, most notably, the Hamilton Rating Scale for Depression (HRSD) and the Beck Depression Inventory (BDI) (Beck, 1978) and later, similar versions (Burns, 1989), which are easily answered questions referring to symptoms. Due to biological research there are also tests that measure the disorders by various biological means (Kaplan & Sadock, 1991). However, they are expensive and their use and diagnostic efficiency are still questionable.

Usually, symptoms of mania, such as pressured speech, psychomotor agitation, and grandiosity, are easily observable. An interview and a recent history usually suppleement the evaluation. Often, family members may aid in the history. The task is to differentiate the types of bipolar illness from major depressive disorder and other psychotic disorders.

People with major depression and bipolar illness will often have other disorders concurrently with the manic or depressive ones. Having more than one condition at the same time is called comorbidity. Alcohol abuse is frequently comorbid with major depression and bipolar disorders (APA, 2000). Panic and obsessive compulsive disorders are common with depression (APA) and over 50% of those with bipolar disorder are said to have a comorbid axis I or axis III condition, while over 30% have a comorbid axis II disorder (Marneros, 2000).

Management

Psychotherapy amd medications are common methods of managing depression and bipolar disorders (APA, 2000; Belmaker & Yaroslavsky, 2000; Maj, Totorella, & Bartoli, 2000; Moller & Grunze, 2000; Thase, 2000). The kindling and desensitization hypothesis has resulted in more aggressive treatment for the first episodes, primarily for bipolar disorders, less so for major depression, with the belief that later episodes will be prevented or that they will be less severe and shorter in duration.

Medicines that are mood stabilizers for bipolar disorder are lithium and anticonvulsants such as carbamazepine and valproate. Sometimes antipsychotic medicines, including the newer ones, such as clozapine, are used for acute manic episodes. Some (Belmaker & Yaroslavsky, 2000) advocate "rational polypharmacy," a combination of anticonvulsants, lithium, and neuroleptics, and believe that since mania is a symptom of both bipolar I and II that it should be the target of treatment (Koukopoulos et al., 2000).

Optimal medicines for major depression are selective serotonin reuptake inhibitors (SSRIs) and tricyclic medicines such as nortriptyline or desimpramine. Monoamine oxidase inhibitors (MAOIs) are recommended for those who do not respond to other medicine. A combination of medicine and psychotherapy is more effective than medicine alone for those with dysthymia. Those who have comorbid obsessive compulsive, avoidant, dependent, borderline, or narcissistic personality disorders respond to SSRIs and MAOIs rather than tricyclics (APA, 2000).

Evidence-based practice (APA, 2000) indicates that cognitive-behavioral therapy (CBT) and interpersonal therapy (IPT) are the most effective psychotherapy treatments for depression, particularly for acute episodes (Roth & Fonagy, 1996). These therapies work for short-term episodes and when given from four to 20 sessions. However, their efficacy becomes weaker after 20 sessions. Also, the two therapies have not proven as effective for severe depression, though IPT was more effective than CBT for more severe depression. Behavior therapy may be as effective as CBT and IRT, but there have not been enough randomly controlled studies to verify its efficacy (APA, 2000). Marriage and family therapy may be effective for decreasing major depressive symptoms and prevent relapse but if there is not marital distress it may delay recovery and increase vulnerability to major depression (APA, 2000). Short-term psychodynamic therapy has not proven as effective as CBT and IPT and it is unclear how effective long-term psychoanalytic therapy is for depression. IPT (Klerman cited in Markowitz, 1998) focuses on social and interpersonal relationship functioning. It deals with disturbances between the depressed person and others in the environment. In a very structured way the therapist together with the client determines interpersonal problems in the here and now and then the therapist links the problems to the interpersonal problem area. Usually problem areas are classified as ones of grief (complicated bereavement), role disputes (conflicts with significant others), role transitions (moving, changing jobs), or interpersonal deficits (lack of social skills). The therapist very directively works with the client on two problems that the client determines are most emotionally charged using various techniques such as psychoeducation, prescribing activity and socialization, using contracts, and capitalizing on a therapeutic alliance. Family therapy aids in maintaining support for the individual in the environment. Behavioral therapy for depressive disorders is designed to alter behaviors that may be keeping a person isolated or defeatist. It also deals with changing life patterns or situations in the environment that may be negative reinforcers. It may involve skills training, such as assertiveness, self-monitoring, and activity scheduling (APA, 2000). Cognitive therapy (Persons, Davidson, & Tompkins, 2001) is designed to change negative thinking processes that contribute to depression. Distorted thinking is targeted, and the here-and-now therapy interactions and current life situations are the focus for changing thinking.

Psychoanalytic theories attempt to change personality structure. This means targeting for change an individual's experience of trust, intimacy, dealing with loss, coping mechanisms, and recognition of a range of emotions. Usually problems are thought to stem from relationships in early childhood. The therapy process utilizes *transference*; that is, the client transfers perceptions and feelings about important childhood figures and events to the therapist and the therapy situation. Typically these are then interpreted by the therapist and discussed and explored together. In the short-term versions, the therapist quickly points out transference reactions and immediately uses the present session to explore and correct behavior carried over from the past.

Psychotherapy has been emphasized more recently for bipolar disorder. Studies (Marneros & Angst, 2000b; Roth & Fonagy, 1996) show that psychosocial events contribute to the first manic episode and to the timing of subsequent episodes; there are role disturbances between episodes; and medicines such as lithium may be effective for only half of those who take it. Also, psychotherapy is indicated because those with most severe symptoms may experience low self-esteem and fear of recurrence and have social consequences to repair. They also may have interpersonal, family, and vocational problems (Hackman, Ram, & Dixon, 1999).

The use of electroconvulsive therapy (ECT) has stirred controversy for many years (Kaplan & Sadock, 1989) although 80% to 90% respond to ECT (APA, 2000). Some claim it caused a permanent loss of memory, while others claim that ECT was the only intervention that aided their recovery. Some people claim that the practice should be outlawed, and it is illegal in several states. Others point to recent advances in administration of the treatment that make it less harmful. Typically 6 to twelve and not more than twenty treatments are administered every other day (APA, 2000). The method of delivery includes giving a general anesthetic along with a muscle relaxant and then placing electrodes usually bilaterally, which causes a seizure consisting of muscular contractions in face, jaw, and plantar extensions for about 30 to 60 seconds. ECT can be extremely effective when there are very severe symptoms, such as psychomotor retardation, early morning awakening, agitation, decreased appetite and weight, psychotic symptoms, or little response to other antidepressant medications. It is indicated when there is a high risk of suicide or danger to physical health. The mode of action of ECT is thought to be brought about through physiological and biochemical changes in the brain, caused by the seizure. Neurochemical changes are thought to produce changes in neurotransmitter function. Physiological changes are thought to be affected by the reduction of activity in the brain following the seizure.

Studies show an immediate loss of memory shortly after treatment, though clients are back to their baseline memory six months later. Unwanted effects of ECT include anxiety and headache immediately afterward; confusion, nausea, and vertigo a few hours afterward; and some muscle pain. The contraindications include respiratory infections, heart disease, aneurysms, and certain other drugs, such as reserpine. Obviously, the procedure's benefits and risks should be adequately and clearly explained, and the client must sign a standard consent form. Other forms of medicine, such as the newer neurotransmitter drugs, are less controversial (Sadock & Sadock, 2000) but nevertheless, ECT remains a topic of popular discussion.

OCCUPATIONAL THERAPY TREATMENT

Various occupational therapy evaluations may be used depending on which context or performance area and components are being assessed or which occupational therapy model is followed (see Devereaux & Carlson, 1992). There is not yet an occupational therapy assessment specific to depression or bipolar disorders. Notwithstanding that fact, the therapist should always evaluate a client according to the severity of the mood disorder. A person's behavior and statements will indicate the stage of functioning on a *mood continuum*. Where a person's behavior falls on this continuum will indicate a different treatment and interpersonal approach (see Figure 7-1). The following case illustrations demonstrate the difference in people's symptoms, whether severely depressed or severely manic. However, despite different symptoms, their behavior fits on the far ends of the mood continuum and therefore necessitates a similar approach and treatment.

CASE ILLUSTRATION: Tae—Severely Depressed

On Tuesday, Tae did not show up for the partial hospitalization occupational therapy group, "About Depression." When he was called by his therapist, he reported that he was still in bed, he had been there since Friday, and this was the first time he had answered the phone in three days. He reported that he had been ruminating about his life and obsessively thinking that he had hurt another client because of his remarks in a community meeting at the program. He felt as if he could hardly move from his house. However, after reassurance that he was missed and was expected at the program, he said he would try to make it. With prompting from the therapist that she was counting on him, he agreed to come in the next day. Tae did not come the next day and continued to be homebound and noncommunicative. Because the occupational therapist was able to

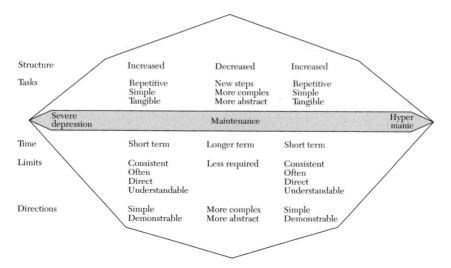

Structure	Increased	Decreased	Increased	
Tasks	Repetitive Simple Tangible	New steps More complex More abstract	Repetitive Simple Tangible	
Severe depression		Maintenance		Hyper manic
Time	Short term	Longer term	Short term	
Limits	Consistent Often Direct Understandable	Less required	Consistent Often Direct Understandable	
Directions	Simple Demonstrable	More complex More abstract	Simple Demonstrable	

Figure 7-1.   The Mood Continuum

provide home visits, she went to his home. He answered the door and was cordial and agreed that he needed motivation to leave the house. The therapist and he designed a concrete, step-by-step list of the exact tasks and times that he would accomplish getting out of bed, dressing, leaving the house, and taking the bus to his group. They included incentives, such as the therapist phoning him the next morning, an agreement to call her on his cell phone from the bus-stop, and rewards, such as a café-latte from the hospital café.

Discussion

Tae had difficulty initiating any task and required much prompting to follow through. He obsessed over self-referential remarks that he perceived as wrong and harmful. He responded to concrete and structured behaviors by the OTR including the therapist going to his house, working on written lists with him, phone contacts, and rewards that were usually pleasurable.

CASE ILLUSTRATION: Maria—Hypermanic

Maria entered the occupational therapy group early, bringing five other clients with her. She proceeded to walk around the room, taking something from every cabinet and announcing how she would lead the group. Before the therapist caught up with her, she commented coquettishly on how sexy the occupational therapist looked and suggested that maybe they could get together since she was available. While thanking her for her willingness to assist and her flattering comments, the OTR assured her that he could aptly lead the group and asked her to take a seat.

Discussion

Maria initiated too many tasks, and did so in a grandiose and expansive manner, in addition to making inappropriate remarks to the therapist. Even though her symptoms were quite the opposite of Tae's, she, too, responded to a direct approach by the OTR.

Occupational therapists' training in analyzing and grading activities means that interventions can, and should, be tailored for anyone at any stage of the mood continuum. Moreover, an occupational therapist's interpersonal approach should also be tailored to stages of the mood continuum (see Figure 7-1).

At the extreme ends of the continuum, represented by severe depression and hypermania, the therapist's focus is on providing structure and meeting demands. Interventions should be concrete and tangible, and activities should be short-term, simple, and success enhancing. The surrounding environment should be carefully arranged so as not to be too distracting. The therapist also should make decisions, provide clear expectations and parameters for activities, and provide limits on expansive behavior and validation for depressed behavior. The therapist's focus is on creating an external structure for the clients. Craft and exercise activities in short segments of 30 to 45 minutes can be most useful at this stage.

As a person improves and moves toward the middle, maintenance stage of the continuum, more abstract activities with more complex steps that require more time can be incorporated. Activities can include more client decision making and fewer limits. Clients can be expected to take more responsibility for functioning and for reflection on their behavior and thoughts. The therapist's focus is to assist the client to realize his or her internal abilities and resources. Useful groups are daily living and vocational, problem solving, and expressive activities; these can be an hour or longer.

The occupational therapy emphasis on independent functioning often leads beginners to insist on independent functioning and decision making from all people at all times. However, occupational therapy also advocates meeting a person at his or her particular level. If an individual clearly is unable to make independent decisions or to engage in daily activities, the occupational therapist should adjust to meet the demands of the person and the environment. Following the concept of the mood continuum helps a therapist know when to focus on the external or internal environments. It allows the OTR to flexibly provide treatment according to whatever the person (internal environment) and stage of the disorder (external environment) require.

Interpersonal Approach

Many occupational therapists may find themselves charmed by an individual who is manic and drawn to take inordinate responsibility for the individual who is depressed. They may be overwhelmed by overactive, expansive behavior or extreme depression. They may become impatient and frustrated. Beginners often make the mistake of expecting too much and therefore frustrating their clients.

When working with someone who is depressed, it is essential to relate with understanding and empathy. The client will not benefit from a "snap out of it" attitude. The depressed individual already feels sad, worthless, humorless, and, often, guilty. Depressed individuals may subject themselves to mental punishment because they are depressed and have been unable to change their condition. They may be stuck in a cycle of negative ruminations. If depressed people could benefit from badgering, they would not be depressed and would certainly help themselves. Often, the tendency is to treat them in an authoritarian manner, and sometimes staff members are unable to tolerate ruminating or negativistic behavior. Some find it difficult to work with people who may not respond immediately or may not be expressive. Although the tendency may be to "encourage independence" and setting limits or to help people see the brighter, often reality-based, alternative, one should provide the opposite: understanding and empathic responses and a validation of the client's feelings or thoughts. Particularly in the early stages of the disorder, one should permit dependence in the form of information about the depressive process and assurance that the person will get better although he or she may not know or feel it now.

CASE ILLUSTRATION: Lizzie—Handling Depressed Behavior

Initially, when Lizzie came to the occupational therapy group she would often sit alone and refuse to work on anything. She felt as if she could hardly move— as if she had a 100-pound pack on her back. To think about making a decision precipitated panic. She worried that she would never get better and would continue to fall into what she described as a "black hole." When approached she would only ruminate about the "black hole," and most interactions were negative statements about herself and her past, present, and future life. People on the unit stayed away from her, and the staff avoided her or attempted to provide reality testing by reviewing how her life "really" was. She became more depressed and hopeless, certain that others hated her, did not understand her, and maybe were unable to help her.

The OTR provided a different approach. She validated Lizzie's statements of how she felt, acknowledged that her state was indeed painful and difficult, and stated that although it seemed there was no light at the end of the tunnel, Lizzie would indeed get better. The therapist shared the information that she had worked with many people who had been severely depressed and had felt similarly hopeless, and that through treatment they did return to former functioning. The OTR was not put off by negative statements and continued to initiate contact. She continued to provide empathic responses and to invite Lizzie to participate in structured groups that included movement and working on very short-term activities. Lizzie's ruminations did not completely stop; however, they decreased. She felt that someone seemed to understand her, did not reject her, and was competent to help. She attempted to participate in groups and began to sense some hope.

Discussion

Lizzie demonstrated symptoms and behaviors of depression, negative rumina-tions, immobility, and hopelessness. These often are responded to with a posi-tive manner that is not perceived as genuine. However, when the therapist responded in an understanding and validating manner and with structure in activities, Lizzie's behavior changed for the better.

When working with an individual who is experiencing a manic episode, it is also essential to relate with understanding and empathy. Empathy means being pres-ent and able to tolerate manic behavior that may be grandiose, obnoxious, intru-sive, and egocentric. Just as with someone who is severely depressed, the person who is severely manic does not deliberately desire to be this way. This client will also not benefit from a heavily authoritarian approach, but he or she will benefit when a therapist consistently demonstrates the ability to be with the client and is not "turned off" by the individual's often-overwhelming behavior. In addition, the client will benefit from direction providing parameters of acceptable behavior, and an honest appraisal of behavior presented in a gentle yet firm, matter-of-fact way. It is not unusual for clients to recognize, acknowledge, and apologize for their behavior when they are less symptomatic.

CASE ILLUSTRATION: Jeremy—Handling Manic Behavior

Jeremy entered the occupational therapy evaluation group with expansive, grandiose behavior, talking about why he did not need the group. He spoke in a nonstop, stream-of-consciousness manner, with pressured speech. He was unable to remain in one place and was distracted by almost everybody and everything in the room. When approached by the OTR, he proceeded to tell her how attractive she was, asked if she was married, and told her how "good" he could be with women. The OTR asked him to begin the assessment. He did not think that he needed to be assessed and stated that, in fact, he could probably "assess" and help her. She stated that she understood that he felt wonderful and probably wanted to make a connection with her, but his behavior was out of line, and, indeed, would distance her, which was probably opposite of what he wanted. Jeremy did begin the assessment but after two minutes, he became dis-tracted in an agitated way and declared to all that this was childish and the OTR "did not have a clue." The OTR gently asked him to return to the activity and continued. Occasionally she validated how agitated and disconnected his behavior made him feel.

When Jeremy's manic behavior subsided, following two weeks of hospital-ization and lithium treatment, he thanked the OTR for giving him directions and reminders to return to his activity at a time when he became distracted every few minutes. He also apologized for any behavior that was offensive or insulting, adding that he actually liked the therapist because she was able to tol-

erate and withstand sexual innuendoes by pointing out what was not acceptable and did so without becoming angry or withdrawing from him.

Discussion

The OTR's approach to Jeremy's manic behavior was also empathic, direct, and consistent, demonstrating her ability to tolerate his behavior and, therefore, conveying that she valued him.

Person-to-person Interventions

Evidence-based practice supports cognitive-behavioral and interpersonal therapies in psychotherapy, primarily for clients with depression, less so for those with bipolar illnesses. As yet there are few research studies that support occupational therapy in general. However, in practice occupational therapists may use techniques or strategies specified by CBT or IPT. In fact, occupational therapists implicitly may have used some of the interventions from both schools, such as focusing on thoughts, activity schedules, and social skills training, for many decades. Occupational therapy also focuses on some of the same areas specified in CBT or IPT manuals, such as role disputes and transitions, explicit rehabilitation planning, or job coaching for employment. Although research should validate the efficacy of occupational therapy's unique contributions (for interesting avenues of research, see Gutman & Biel, 2001), specifying the use of CBT and IPT strategies in practice would provide common ground for dialogues with other professions and eventually might differentiate the uniqueness of occupational therapy strategies and dimensions from these other domains.

Following are practical occupational therapy interventions that can be delivered in a way that makes use of techniques or strategies specified by other schools of therapy. Treatment addresses all symptoms—emotional, cognitive, motivational, self-concept, and vegetative. See Table 7-2 for symptoms of depression and mania.

Particularly when addressing motivational symptoms, occupational therapy provides interventions that directly relate to changing behavior. For an individual who is depressed, it provides evidence of the ability to continue with occupations of everyday life and provides concrete proof, often through working with and mastering crafts, of a continued ability to function. For an individual who is manic, it provides concrete structure through which to focus attention. Concrete evidence of a remaining ability to function combats helplessness and distractibility with hope and defense, which are key motivational symptoms.

Occupational therapy can experientially contract or disprove negative thoughts through its focus on functioning in the everyday occupations and activities of daily life. Occupational therapy can intervene in the depressed person's negative cycle of misconstruing experiences as defeating, regarding oneself as deficient or morally defective, and viewing the future in a negative way. Through its focus on the activities of daily life, occupational therapy can intervene in the manic person's expansive and grandiose cycle by providing a structured environment and activities through which to organize and monitor behavior. Tables 7-3 and 7-4 outline the symptoms, problems, and interventions involved in depression and mania (see also Boswell, 1989; Centoni & Tallant, 1986; Devereaux & Carlson, 1992; Feder, 1991; Meyers, 1991; Stein & Smith, 1989).

Table 7-3 focuses on interventions for depression. Pervasive symptoms of depression lead to problems in all performance areas and all performance components, particularly cognitive and social. Treatment focuses on changing behavior, changing the environment, or changing internal appraisals. The most prevalent emotional symptoms of depression will manifest in a loss of interest in formerly valued activities or the pursuit of only one interest in an exclusive and/or compulsive manner. The individual will tend to withdraw from others and become isolated. Some common interventions are to engage the individual in activities that he or she values or has valued in the past and to provide opportunities to engage in different activities or in activities within a group setting. Sometimes an individual will be reluctant to engage in any activities or group; however, the therapist should maintain an approach that is inviting and confident without being authoritarian and overly demanding. Providing activities that do not require too many choices or steps to complete, and perhaps allowing a person to work while in the presence of others but not necessarily interact will enhance engagement. A more behavioral intervention is to ask the client to monitor the pleasure or value received from working on, and completing, an activity. This can be a self-report, and it often is more effective if a simple, concrete scale is constructed. When a person is less severely depressed (on the mid-stage of the mood continuum), values clarification activities may be introduced.

Cognitive and motivational symptoms will manifest in indecision and ambivalence, difficulty concentrating and attending, difficulty initiating or sustaining activities, and the expression of negative thoughts predominantly rather than positive ones. Activities or occupations that do not require too many choices, can be accomplished successfully in a short time, and are tangible may enhance a person's motivation and self-concept. More behavioral interventions of setting and listing step-by-step, easily achieved goals and crossing them off when accomplished will enhance motivation. Cognitive interventions, such as recognizing and monitoring negative thoughts, changing the internal "tapes" one plays over and over, and questioning unrealistic beliefs can be directed toward cognitive symptoms. Psychoeducational groups concerning symptoms, behavior, recognizing precursors to mood changes, managing medicines, and expanding coping strategies can also address cognitive problems.

Symptoms that relate to one's self-concept are expressed as feelings or thoughts of worthlessness or guilt. Again, short-term concrete activities that can be quickly mastered and completed will add to a person's sense of self. In addition, behavioral interventions that show that goals have been achieved usually also enhance self-esteem. Cognitive interventions that directly challenge self-distortions and expressive interventions that focus on self-awareness, self-expression, and self-exploration will model the power of self-reflection and self-expression. Self-

Table 7-3.	Interventions for Depression	
Symptoms	*Problems*	*Interventions*
Emotional	Loss of interest in formerly valued activities or pursuit of narrow or single interests exclusively and in a compulsive manner	Engage in valued activities Expand opportunities to engage in other than one activity
	Tendency to isolate oneself and withdraw from others	Monitor value and pleasure while doing or completing activities and engage in values clarification activities. Engage in group activities
Cognitive and Motivational	Indecision and ambivalence Inability to concentrate and attend to usual daily activities	Initially provide occupations and do not require too many choices
	Negative attitudes that predominate in all usual activities	Provide opportunities to successfully accomplish short-term, simple, concrete activities
	Inability to initiate or sustain activity Tendency to isolate	Set realistic, step-by-step goals and behavioral "to do" lists, grading activities and environment for successful completion
		Reestablish normal routines: structured planning of daily occupations, simple behavioral lists
		Engage in cognitive therapy, i.e., recognizing, monitoring, and changing thoughts
		Perform reality testing and question unrealistic beliefs
		Engage in psychoeducational groups concerning symptoms and behavior, such as recognizing precursors to mood changes and managing medicines
Self-Concept	Worthlessness Guilt	Provide opportunities to successfully accomplish short-term, simple, concrete activities

(continues)

Table 7-3.	(continued)	
Symptoms	*Problems*	*Interventions*
		Set realistic, step-by-step goals and behavioral "to do" lists, grading activities and environment for successful completion
		Perform cognitive therapy, challenge distorted ideas
		Engage in activities that focus on self-exploration, such as recognizing and dealing with emotions, self-expression, and self-exploration through creative media and expanding coping styles
Vegetative	Failure to sustain basic needs for food, rest, etc.	Provide external structure

exploration can also include exploring and changing styles of coping. Again, it is important to be aware of where a person is located on the mood continuum when introducing interventions that require energy, initiation, imagination, and problem solving.

Table 7-4 focuses on interventions for mania. Emotional symptoms of mania will usually manifest in a person having an overinflated or exaggerated interest in various activities and perhaps attributing excessive meaning to all objects and people in life. Interventions can center around engagement in activities or occupations. The occupational therapist can offer honest, realistic appraisals of an individual's behavior while engaged in activities or can make honest, realistic appraisals of end products. The therapist may elicit the client's appraisal and reflection concerning his or her own behavior and products. Sometimes reality testing (e.g., Socratic questioning) utilizing an appropriate tone may be productively employed, even though this may not bring about an immediate change in behavior. Again, the approach depends on where the behavior is located on the mood continuum.

Cognitive and motivational symptoms may result in distractibility, inability to concentrate and attend, and a desire to initiate too many activities, usually all at once. Once activities have been initiated there may be difficulty following through, and in spite of this inability, there may also be an unrealistic appraisal of the person's abilities. Just as with an individual who is depressed, it is important to provide opportunities to engage in concrete, short-term activities that do not contain many steps. It is also important to provide an environment with few distractions, including noises and visual stimulation. In addition, whenever possible the

Table 7-4.	Interventions for Mania	
Symptoms	*Problems*	*Interventions*
Emotional	Overinflated or exaggerated interest and meaning attributed to all areas of life	Offer an honest, realistic appraisal of behavior and end products while engaging in activities or occupations
		Elicit clients' appraisals and reflection regarding their behavior and end products after engaging in activities
Cognitive and Motivational	Increased energy resulting in distractibility, initiation of too many activities, and inability to sustain activity	Provide opportunities to engage in concrete, short-term activities that include more than two steps
	Inability to concentrate and attend to usual daily activities	Provide clear expectations for behavior and end products
	Inability to follow through on decisions	Arrange a distraction-free environment
	Unrealistically positive attitudes that predominate in all usual daily activities	Assist client to return to goal-directed action whenever distracted
		Eventually assist in goal setting and planning and in anticipating the consequences of actions by monitoring behavior during activities
Self-Concept	Inflated, unrealistic sense of worth and efficacy	Display an accepting, tolerant attitude
	Failure to take responsibility for consequences of behavior	Offer an honest, realistic appraisal of behavior and end products while engaging in occupations
		Engage in activities that focus on self-exploration, such as recognizing and dealing with emotions, self-expression, and self-exploration through creative media and expanding coping styles
Vegetative	Failure to sustain basic needs	Provide external structure

OTR should provide clear expectations for behavior and assist the client to return to the goal whenever he or she becomes distracted.

Symptoms involving one's concept of self will usually result in the expression of inflated, unrealistic ideas about oneself and one's effectiveness, often accompanied by a failure to assume responsibility for any consequences related to one's behavior. An approach that is genuine, authentic, and accepting, even while offering clear limits, is suggested, along with an honest, realistic appraisal of the person's behavior and the end products. It is particularly important to assess where a person with mania is located on the mood continuum. Those on the farther ends may have difficulty being in, and may indeed disrupt, a group setting. Engaging in self-exploration and self-expression can be helpful for symptoms relating to self-concept and for expanding coping styles, but these interventions are usually most helpful when a person has moved to the middle of the mood continuum.

System Interventions

Intervention strategies in different programs (Hackman, Ram, & Dixon, 1999; Linroth et al., 1996) address both depression and bipolar illness. Often the community or outpatient (Yakobina, Yakobina, & Tallant, 1997) programs use CBT and IPT strategies.

People with severe depression and bipolar illness may require continuing care after hospitalization. Typically, they may be referred for maintenance for a period of time in a partial hospitalization or day treatment program. Often the day program consists of various levels of treatment directed to people with illnesses varying from severe to mild. Sometimes treatment will take place in the clients' homes or other places in the community (Hackman, Ram, & Dixon, 1999). Usually, there is an intake period where the clients and staff can observe each other and make decisions about which treatment groups would be most beneficial. Then there is a period of time in which the clients work in groups to achieve goals that they have established themselves. Prior to discharge, clients often will anticipate how to prevent relapses after they have left the program. Sometimes there are visits within a few months or a year for "tuneups" (Linroth et al., 1996).

Groups often address skill development, problem solving, managing symptoms, coping with daily life stressors, simply recognizing pleasure and humor, and self-awareness (including not being so intense) (Linroth et al., 1996). Groups also address employment and vocational issues, managing and coping with stigmatizing behaviors from others, medicine compliance, and family psychoeducation (Hackman, Ram, & Dixon, 1999). These latter groups are particularly important for people with bipolar illness who have more of a community than previously was thought (Hackman, Ram, & Dixon, 1999; Kusznir et al., 1996; Tse & Walsh, 2001).

Following are the treatment processes for Lizzie and Jeremy which illustrate occupational therapy interventions.

CASE ILLUSTRATION: Lizzie—Treatment Process

Observation while performing crafts from the Allen Diagnostic Module (1993) indicated that Lizzie was slow to engage, and many comments indicated a lack of interest in what she was doing. A self-report checklist adapted from the Burns Depression Checklist (Burns, 1989) indicated a high score of 40, indicating particularly that Lizzie felt very sad, discouraged, worthless, inferior, guilty, and unattractive. She was indecisive and irritable, had lost interest in life, and was generally unmotivated. An Occupational Performance History interview (OPHI-II) indicated a history of being newly divorced. She worried about losing her job due to downsizing and feared she would not be able to support her two children. She had become isolated, stopped going to work, and attempted suicide. She felt guilty that she was now hospitalized.

The Occupational Self Assessment (Baron, Kielhofner, Iyenger, Goldhammer, & Wolenski, 2002) indicated that Lizzie liked to cook and bake; she had formerly enjoyed tennis and running and had belonged to a book club. Since her marital separation she had not pursued any of these activities. She reported that she had a few close friends but had withdrawn from them because she felt she was a burden and was generally not presentable to people. She did not see the point in participating in occupational therapy groups since she was feeling hopeless and negative about the present and future. However, she agreed to attend some groups.

Initially she attended a movement/exercise group after being sought out by the leader every day. It was difficult for her to follow the simple exercises, though she eventually did look forward to the group and expressed relief that she could just follow directions and did not have to initiate interactions. At the same time she attended a parallel group where people worked on individual craft projects, and after a few days she finally agreed to start a project after admiring another member's finished work. She found that, although she generally had negative things to say about the project, she actually felt some sense of accomplishment. She also was relieved that she did not have to make decisions or "process her feelings." Within a week she had become an active member and finished projects for both herself and her children.

After a few days, she attended a "Learning about Depression" workshop. She enjoyed receiving a handout about depression, and she was surprised at what she learned from the different theories. She gave the handout to her family and they were able to discuss their concerns about her.

Lizzie was discharged to a partial hospitalization program. She attended a medication management group, a "Learning about Feelings" group, and a group titled, "Preventing Depression/Coping Differently" three times a week in the occupational therapy program. In addition, she participated in a sports group and a community resource group, in which she identified resources in the community, such as Parents without Partners and a 12-step group addressing self-confidence. The OTR worked individually with her to help her learn vocational skills and interests. She completed a vocational assessment (APTICOM®), consisting of aptitude, interest, and skills tests (Vocational Research Institute, cited in Asher, 1996). She began to focus on obtaining a job and to explore alternative careers. She eventually attended the partial program one day a week while she began to work at a new job three times a week. Eventually she began to work full-time and was discharged from the day program. She enjoyed a continuing education group sponsored by the partial program, which focused on self-exploration through creative media.

Discussion

Initially, Lizzie was severely depressed but without cognitive impairment, as indicated on the assessments. Her occupational profile yielded her former interests and present concerns. An analysis of occupational performance identified client factors such as guilt, isolation, and fear that were barriers to engagement in occupation and strengths such as her intellect and intact communication skills. The analysis also identified the contexts, such as work, sports, and community self-help programs in which she desired participation. She responded initially to structured interventions that did not require too much independent decision making and would demonstrate her ability to continue to function. She was able to utilize information regarding her disease, and later, as she improved, to utilize interventions that required more thought and independent decision making. She also responded to a reasoned approach of empathy and validation of her experience.

CASE ILLUSTRATION: Jeremy—The Treatment Process

During his hospitalization, Jeremy was able to attend a directive group (Kaplan, 1986). With structured treatment directed toward his behavior that initially was represented on the extreme ends of the mood continuum (see Figure 7-1) his mood stabilized and he prepared for discharge by attending a "Recovery in the Community" predischarge group. This group essentially engaged members in anticipating problem areas that they might experience after leaving the hospital. After anticipating future difficulties, they worked together to set up ways to handle the potential problems, but they also focused on ways in which they could have a balance to the more intense focus on problems. Initially, Jeremy had a hard time anticipating problems and blithely stated that he could handle anything that came up. With the occupational therapist's Socratic questioning and peer support from the group members, he came to think that maybe he could benefit from continuing treatment, at least two days per week; he was particularly apprehensive about returning to work.

After discharge he attended a partial hospitalization program for two days a week for four weeks. In the program with the facilitation of his occupational therapist and the other members he established goals for repairing family and work relationships and for putting in place ways in which he could deal with distressing situations in his home and work life. He attended a family psychoeducation group offered by social workers and an occupational therapy group that discussed interpersonal skills, particularly how to get along with co-workers. His occupational therapist also worked individually with him to assess his workplace using the Work Environment Impact Scale (Moore-Corner, Kielhofner, & Olson, 1998) to analyze his work situations and develop necessary social and physical accommodations. He was able to recognize which work situations were a hindrance to him, such as having more than one project boss and taking on too many projects at the same time. He was able to recognize how some of his behaviors, particularly when he was manic, caused people at work to stay away from him, thus, causing him to feel isolated and unsupported. He successfully graduated from the partial program after three weeks, but returned each quarter or when needed for maintenance therapy.

Discussion

Initially Jeremy's behavior was very manic and he had difficulty being in a group setting. With structured treatment in addition to valproate, his behavior moved more to the middle of the mood continuum (see Figure 7-1). At first he did not acknowledge that he needed to plan a rehabilitation program that would maintain stability, but his occupational therapist and occupational therapy group facilitated self-awareness. He used a postdischarge partial hospitalization program to tackle work and family issues.

Summary

Mood disorders have been described throughout history. Initially, melancholia and mania were thought to be curses of the gods. Over the centuries, environmental and biological theories have emerged and mood disorders were classified as depressive and bipolar disorders. Research on, and treatment of, mood disorders address biology, personality, behavior, cognition, and life events.

Mania and depression represent opposite ends of what can be considered more than a mood disorder because both include multiple symptoms, which may be emotional, cognitive, motivational, or vegetative. Occupational therapy treatment consists of changing behavior, arranging the environment, and changing internal appraisals. One should tailor the therapy to the severity of the mood disorder. Occupational therapy is particularly important for mood disorders because of its use of tangible concrete activities and its focus on everyday occupations and motivation.

Review Questions

1. What are some reasons for the prevalence of depression in females?
2. Which theories of mood disorders are addressed in occupational therapy treatment?
3. Explain the mood continuum. Why is it important?
4. Name one intervention for cognitive and motivational problems for an individual who is manic.
5. Name one intervention for emotional problems of depression.

References

American Psychiatric Association (APA). (2000). *Diagnostic and statistical manual of mental disorders-Text Revision* (4th ed.). Washington, DC: APA.

American Psychiatric Association. (2000). *Practice guidelines for the treatment of patients with major depressive disorder.* Washington, DC: Author.

Asher, I. E. (1996). *Occupational therapy assessment tools: An annotated index* (2nd ed.). Bethesda, MD: American Occupational Therapy Association.

Baron, K., Kielhofner, G., Iyenger, A., Goldhammer, V., & Wolenski, J. (2002). *The Occupational Self Assessment (OSA) (Version 2.0).* Chicago: Model of Human Occupation Clearinghouse, Department of Occupational Therapy, College of Applied Health Sciences, University of Illinois at Chicago.

Beck, A. (1973). *Depression: Causes and treatment: The diagnosis and management of depression.* Philadelphia: University of Pennsylvania Press.

Beck, A. (1976). *Cognitive therapy and the emotional disorders.* New York: International Universities Press.

Beck, A. (1978). *Beck Depression Inventory.* San Antonio: Psychological Corporation.

Belmaker, R. H., & Yaroslavsky, Y. (2000). Perspectives for new pharmacological interventions. In J. Soares & S. Gershon (Eds.), *Bipolar disorders: Basic mechanisms and therapeutic implications* (pp. 507–528). New York: Marcel Dekker.

Boswell, S. (1989). A social support group for depressed people. *Australian Occupational Therapy Journal, 36*(1), 34–41.

Bracegirdle, H. (1991). The female stereotype and occupational therapy for women with depression. *British Journal of Occupational Therapy, 54*(5), 193–194.

Burns, D. (1989). *The feeling good handbook: The new mood therapy.* New York: Plume/Penguin.

Centoni, M., & Tallant, B. (1986). The projective use of drawings as a treatment technique with the depressed unemployed male. *Canadian Journal of Occupational Therapy, 53*(2), 81–87.

Crow, T. J. (2000). Bipolar shifts as disorders of the bi-hemispheric integration of language: Implications for the genetic origins of the psychotic continuum. In A. Marneros & J. Angst (Eds.), *Bipolar disorders: 100 years after manic-depressive insanity* (pp. 335–348). Boston: Kluwer Academic.

Devereaux, E., & Carlson, M. (1992). Health policy: The role of occupational therapy in the management of depression. *American Occupational Therapy Association, 465*(2), 175–180.

Earhart, C. A., Allen, C. K., & Blue, T. (1993). *Allen Diagnostic Module: The manual.* Colchester, CT: S & S Worldwide.

Feder, J. (1990). Occupational stress and the depressed female client. *Work: A Journal of Prevention, Assessment and Rehabilitation, 1*(2), 55–62.

Feder, J. (1991). Women, depression and work: Treatment strategies for the depressed patient. *Occupational Therapy Practice, 2*(4), 58–67.

Gilbert, P. (2000). Varieties of submissive behavior as forms of social defense: Their evolution and role in depression. In L. Sloman & P. Gilbert (Eds.), *Subordination and defeat: An evolutionary approach to mood disorders and their therapy* (pp. 3–45). London: Erlbaum.

Gutman, S. A., & Biel, L. (2001). Abstract: Promoting the neurologic substrates of well-being through occupation. *Occupational Therapy in Mental Health, 17*(1), 1–22.

Hackman, A. L., Ram, R. N., & Dixon, L. B. (1999). Psychosocial treatment of bipolar disorder in the public sector: Program for assertive community treatment. In J. Goldberg & M. Harrow (Eds.), *Bipolar disorders: Clinical course and outcome* (pp. 259–274). Washington, DC: American Psychiatric Press.

Hemphill, B. (1992). Depression among suicidal elderly: A life-threatening illness. *Occupational Therapy Practice, 4*(1), 61–66.

Hlastala, S. A., & Frank, E. (2000). Biology versus environment: Stressors in the pathophysiology of bipolar disorder. In J. C. Soares & S. Gershon (Eds.), *Bipolar disorders: Basic mechanisms and therapeutic implications* (pp. 353–372). New York: Marcel Dekker.

Kaplan, H., & Sadock, B. (1989). *Comprehensive textbook of psychiatry* (5th ed.). Baltimore: Williams & Wilkins.

Kaplan, H., & Sadock, B. (1991). *Synopsis of psychiatry: Behavioral sciences: Clinical psychology* (6th ed.). Baltimore: Williams & Wilkins.

Kaplan, K. L. (1986). The directive group: Short term treatment for psychiatric patients with a minimal level of functioning. *American Journal of Occupational Therapy, 40,* 474–481.

Koukopoulos, A., Sani, G., Koukopoulos, A. E., & Girardi, P. (2000). In A. Marneros & J. Angst (Eds.), *Bipolar disorders: 100 years after manic-depressive insanity* (pp. 315–334). Boston: Kluwer Academic.

Kusznir, A., Scott, E., Cooke, R. G., & Young, L. T. (1996). Functional consequences of bipolar affective disorder: An occupational therapy perspective [Abstract]. *Canadian Journal of Occupational Therapy, 63*(5), 313–332.

Linroth, R., Zander, S., Forde, S., Hanley, M., & Lins, J. (1996). Ramsey county day treatment services: Day treatment to extended day treatment centers to focus groups. *Occupational Therapy in Health Care, 10*(2), 89–103.

Loosen, P. T., Beyer, J. L., Sells, S. R., Gurtsman, H. E., Shelton, R. C., Baird, R. P., & Nash, J. L. (2000). Mood disorders. In M. H. Evbert, P. T. Loosen, & B. Nurcombe (Eds.), *Current diagnosis and treatment in psychiatry* (pp. 290–327). New York: Lange Medical Books/McGraw Hill.

Maj. M., Tortorella, A., & Bartoli, L. (2000). Mood stabilizers in bipolar disorder. In A. Marneros & J. Angst (Eds.), *Bipolar disorders: 100 years after manic-depressive insanity* (pp. 461–464). Boston: Kluwer Academic.

Markowitz, J. C. (1998). *Interpersonal psychotherapy for dysthymic disorder.* Washington, DC: American Psychiatric Press.

Marneros, A. (2000). On entities and continuities of bipolar disorders. In A. Marneros & J. Angst (Eds.), *Bipolar disorders: 100 years after manic-depressive insanity* (pp. 461–464). Boston: Kluwer Academic.

Marneros, A., & Angst, J. (Eds.). (2000a). *Bipolar disorders: 100 years after manic-depressive insanity.* Boston: Kluwer Academic.

Marneros, A., & Angst, J. (2000b). The prognosis of bipolar disorders: Course and outcome. In A. Marneros & J. Angst (Eds.), *Bipolar disorders: 100 years after manic-depressive insanity* (pp. 406–436). Boston: Kluwer Academic.

Marneros, A., & Angst, J. (2000c). Bipolar disorders: Roots and evaluation. In A. Marneros & J. Angst (Eds.), *Bipolar disorders: 100 years after manic-depressive insanity* (pp. 1–35). Boston: Kluwer Academic.

Meyers, J. (1991). Clinical differentiation between dementia and depression. *Gerontology Special Interest Section Newsletter (American Occupational Therapy Association), 14*(1), 5–6.

Moller, H. J., & Grunze, H. (2000). Antidepressant treatment of bipolar depression. In A. Marneros & J. Angst (Eds.), *Bipolar disorders: 100 years after manic-depressive insanity* (pp. 387–403). Boston: Kluwer Academic.

Morrison, J. (1995). *DSM-IV made easy: The clinician's guide to diagnosis.* New York: Guilford.

Mundt, C., Kronmuller, K., & Backenstraf, S. (2000). Interactional styles in bipolar disorder. In A. Marneros & J. Angst (Eds.), *Bipolar disorders: 100 years after manic-depressive insanity* (pp. 201–213). Boston: Kluwer Academic.

Pelissolo, A., & Lepine, P. (2001). Epidemiology of depression and anxiety disorders. In S. A. Montgomery & J. A. den Doer (Eds.), *SSRI's in depression and anxiety* (pp. 1–23). New York: Wiley.

Persons, J. B., Davidson, J., & Tompkins, M. A. (2001). *Essential components of cognitive-behavior therapy for depression.* Washington, DC: American Psychological Association.

Roth, A., & Fonagy, P. (1996). *What works for whom?* New York: Guilford.

Sadock, H., & Sadock, B. (2000). *Comprehensive textbook of psychiatry* (6th ed.). Baltimore: Williams & Wilkins.

Sloman, L., & Gilbert, P. (Eds.). (2000). *Subordination and defeat: An evolutionary approach to mood disorders and their therapy.* London: Erlbaum.

Soares, J. C., & Gershon, S. (2000). *Bipolar disorders: Basic mechanisms and therapeutic implications.* New York: Marcel Dekker.

Stein, F., & Smith, J. (1989). Short-term stress management programme with acutely depressed inpatients. *Canadian Journal of Occupational Therapy, 56*(4),185–191.

Thase, M. E. (2000). Modulation of biological factors by psychotherapeutic interventions. In J. Soares & S. Gershon (Eds.), *Bipolar disorders: Basic mechanisms and therapeutic implications* (pp. 373–385). New York: Marcel Dekker.

Tse, S. S., & Walsh, A. E. S. (2001). How does work work for people with bipolar affective disorder? [Abstract]. *Occupational Therapy International, 8*(3), 210–225.

Tsuang, M. T., & Faraone, S. (2000). The genetic epidemiology of bipolar disorder. In A. Marneros & J. Angst (Eds.), *Bipolar disorders: 100 years after manic-depressive insanity* (pp. 231–241). Boston: Kluwer Academic.

Yakobina, Y., Yakobina, S., & Tallant, B. K. (1997). I came, I thought, I conquered: Cognitive behavior approach applied in occupational therapy for the treatment of depressed (dysthymic) females [Abstract]. *Occupational Therapy in Mental Health, 13*(4), 59–73.

Suggested Reading

Popular Books about Depression and Mania

Berger, D., & Berger, L. (1991). *We heard the angels of madness: A family guide to coping with manic depression*. New York: William Morrow.

Gold, M. (1995). *The good news about depression: Cures and treatments in the new age of psychiatry*. New York: Bantam.

Ingersoll, B. D. (1995). *Lonely, sad and angry: A parent's guide to depression in children and adolescents*. New York: Doubleday.

Jamison, K. R. (1995). *An unquiet mind: A memoir of moods and madness*. New York: Vintage.

Rosen, L. (1996). *When someone you love is depressed: How to help your loved one without losing yourself*. New York: Free Press.

Salmans, S. (1995). *Depression: Questions you have—Answers you need*. Allentown, PA: People's Medical Society.

Styron, W. (1990). *Darkness visible: A memoir of madness*. New York: Vintage.

Popular Self-Help Books

Colgrove, M., Bloomfield, H., & McWilliams, P. (Eds.). (1991). *How to survive the loss of a love*. Los Angeles: Prelude.

Copeland, M. E. (1994). *Living without depression and manic depression: A workbook for maintaining mood stability*. Oakland, CA: New Harbinger.

Emery, Gary. (1988). *Getting un-depressed: How a woman can change her life through cognitive therapy* (rev. ed.). New York: Touchstone.

Greenberger, D., & Padesky, C. A. (1995). *Mind over mood: Change how you feel by changing the way you think*. New York: Guilford.

Lange, A., & Jakubowski, P. (1976). *Cognitive behavioral procedures for trainers*. New York: Research Press.

Young, J. E., & Klosko, J. S. (1993). *Reinventing your life: How to break free from negative life patterns and feel good again*. New York: Plume/Penguin.

CHAPTER 8

Anxiety Disorders

Vivian Banish Levitt, MA, OTR/L, ATR-BC, MFT

Key Terms

autogenic training
benzodiazapenes
compulsions
depersonalization

derealization
obsessions
psychogenic
vasodilatation

Chapter Outline

Introduction

The occupational therapist invites a client on the psychiatric unit, a 35-year-old man who was found pacing the floors, to attend a stress management group. Wringing his hands, trembling as he talks, and speaking quickly, the client refuses to attend the group and states he is too anxious to concentrate. This man has been diagnosed with generalized anxiety disorder and depression; he is a challenge to the occupational therapist, who wonders how to best intervene and make a therapeutic connection. People experience many kinds and degrees of anxiety, but only when anxiety markedly interferes with daily function is it called clinical anxiety.

The origin of the word *anxiety* lies in the Greek root *angh,* meaning both "to press tight" and "to be heavy with grief" (Taylor & Arnow, 1988), and more recently, in the Latin word *anxietas,* meaning "troubled mind" (Sims & Snaith, 1988). Anxiety disorders are often the most common psychiatric disorders and yet the least treated ones. Approximately 4% to 5% of the population can expect to have an anxiety disorder in his or her lifetime (Weissman, Myers, & Harding, 1978); women outnumber men two to one in this population (Sims & Snaith, 1988).

The number of words in the English vocabulary that describe anxiety highlights its pervasiveness—witness the words *worry, edginess, panic, fright, alarm, terror, jitters, jumpiness,* and *uneasiness.* Anxiety is linked to our primitive flight-or-fight response which, when activated, prepares the body biochemically for meeting possible danger. The heart rate and blood pressure rise, blood goes to the large muscles, adrenaline is secreted, and sensory functions such as sight and hearing become keener.

ENCOUNTERING PEOPLE WITH ANXIETY DISORDERS: SETTINGS

Anxiety is a concern that needs to be addressed in all practice areas, including home and physical rehabilitation settings, due to the related loss of function, uncertainty of prognosis, chronicity of symptoms, and other serious related issues. It is a disorder that is not limited to any age group and is diagnosed in young children as well as older adults. In this chapter, anxiety disorders will be discussed in adult psychiatric populations in psychiatric settings; however, the interventions can be used with almost all ages and in any setting.

Acute Inpatient

The occupational therapist is likely to encounter clients with anxiety disorders on inpatient psychiatric units. Their symptoms are usually so severe that they are unable to function in their daily lives. This incapacitation may sometimes include suicidal thoughts or actual suicide attempts. In both instances, the safe and, perhaps, locked environment of a hospital meets the immediate need for structure and external control.

Outpatient

Clients are often referred to outpatient programs, usually called partial hospitalization programs, if (1) they require further intervention following hospitalization and are unable to immediately return to their former occupations or (2) they need considerable support and structure but are able to manage outside the hospital. In either case, people may be living at home, in halfway houses, or in other, special living arrangements. Clients with anxiety disorders as a primary diagnosis are usually able to function outside the hospital in spite of their distressing symptoms.

Home Care

Occupational therapists work in home care programs for clients with psychiatric as well as physical dysfunction. Isolated at home and too impaired to participate in a structured day program, people with anxiety disorders such as agoraphobia (fear of leaving the house) or obsessive-compulsive behavior (involving intrusive thoughts and ritualized behavior) may benefit from one-on-one programs in time management, activities of daily living, and community reentry.

Changes in health care have dramatically shortened lengths of stay in acute hospital settings. As a consequence of the reduction in client care days, occupational therapists must now focus more on evaluation than on treatment and be ready to make recommendations for discharge early in the hospitalization. Anxiety, especially if it takes a chronic course, will usually not be fully resolved during an inpatient stay. Occupational therapists in these settings must be prepared to help identify problem areas in functioning, begin intervention, and solve problems related to the discharge environment with the client and, often, with family members. The consideration of the entire continuity of client care becomes a crucial piece in treatment so that gains made in one environment may be carried over to the next. Communication with professionals working with the client in a prehospital or posthospital setting helps to both accelerate and consolidate treatment plans and recommendations.

DESCRIPTION OF ANXIETY DISORDERS

The *Diagnostic and Statistical Manual of Mental Disorders,* Fourth Edition (*DSM-IV-TR*) (APA, 2000), describes a number of anxiety disorders, which may occur alone or concomitantly with other *DSM-IV* diagnoses. For example, obsessive-compulsive disorder may overlay another axis I disorder, major depressive disorder. In this case, an individual may have an agitated depression manifested by sleeplessness, excessive motor activity, and extreme feelings of worthlessness (major depressive disorder) compounded by a compelling need to follow rigid behaviors, such as pacing a certain number of times around the halls of the hospital (obsessive-compulsive disorder). However, anxiety is also frequently a component of other psychiatric illnesses without necessarily meeting the definition of a true *DSM-IV* diagnosis of anxiety disorder.

Several different kinds of anxiety are defined in Figure 8-1. For example, people with diagnoses such as eating disorders, personality disorders, and schizophrenia are often highly anxious. Many have trait anxiety, or enduring personality patterns of anxiety. In addition, people without any history of mental disorders commonly experience acute anxiety—time-limited periods of anxiety—when, for example, undergoing uncomfortable and perhaps, life-threatening medical procedures. The mere prospect of dealing with an aversive event such as diagnostic testing, chemotherapy, radiation, or surgery may produce intense levels of anxiety (often called *anticipatory anxiety*). In these examples, the anxiety often diminishes with emotional support and the termination of the stressor. However, there are times when anxiety repeatedly arises around new stressors even after

---

Anxiety: unpleasant emotional, cognitive, behavioral, or physical experiences of stress

Trait Anxiety: enduring personality style that manifests persistent anxiety

Acute Anxiety: time-limited anxiety that diminishes with resolution of the problem

Anticipatory Anxiety: predictive anxiety in response to future actual or imagined situations

Chronic Anxiety: anxiety that persists, developing around new stressors after immediate problems are resolved

Free-floating Anxiety: generalized anxiety, which may be vague in origin

Clinical Anxiety: disruption in function due to anxiety

Figure 8-1.   Definitions of Different Kinds of Anxiety

the resolution of the initial ones. In these circumstances the anxiety is labeled *chronic anxiety*. There are also circumstances when anxiety continues but is generalized and vague without an identifiable stressor. In this case, it is called *free-floating anxiety*.

There are certain medical diseases and conditions that are also likely to produce states or acute experiences of anxiety. However, these symptoms of worry, or even panic, often subside when the medical reason is resolved. Examples include hyperthyroidism, estrogen loss occurring in menopause, congestive heart failure, asthma, hypoglycemia, and temporal lobe epilepsy (Taylor & Arnow, 1988). A number of medications and nonprescription drugs may either cause or worsen acute anxiety symptoms. These include anticholinergic drugs, steroids, aspirin, cocaine, amphetamines, and hallucinogens (Taylor & Arnow, 1988). Caffeine and nicotine, two commonly ingested substances, may also produce symptoms of anxiety. Moreover, withdrawal from alcohol or other addictive substances presents a high risk for acute anxiety states.

The difference between normal anxiety (worry that propels one to act), and clinical anxiety (worry that disrupts function) is not always easily or clearly defined. Anxiety in a limited dose is universal, normal, appropriate, and adaptive as a protection from potential threat. It is almost always associated with the anticipation of future events accompanied by expected loss or pain (Sims & Snaith, 1988). It can be the force that propels people to act, cope, and even perform more efficiently. For example, most college students experience a normal level of anxiety as they prepare for final exams, which usually helps induce studying.

On the other hand, anxiety is often defined as abnormal when it hinders rather than helps the individual. If the person's response to a stimulus is greater than one would expect, if his or her feelings of anxiety persist after the stimulus is removed, or if anxiety is ineffective in dealing with the threat of the stimulus, the anxiety may be called abnormal (Sims & Snaith, 1988). Anxiety of this proportion has been likened to having a faulty burglar alarm that signals nonexistent danger (Agras, 1985). For example, if the college students' anxiety prevents them from taking other exams, then it becomes abnormal.

Clinical anxiety is the name given to abnormal anxiety when it clearly affects and hinders daily function and is no longer serviceable. Anxiety becomes disabling when it persists without stimulating positive action to resolve the stressor or ward off distress. For instance, a woman with intense anxiety was so incapacitated by the feelings of terror associated with an upcoming job layoff that she was unable to develop an alternative survival plan for herself. Such clinical anxiety is seen in many people hospitalized on psychiatric units.

When action is taken to diminish the anticipated threat, there is a great possibility that the anxiety will be reduced. For example, clients who are preparing for discharge from the psychiatric hospital are often very anxious about responding to future inquiries about their hospitalization. They feel vulnerable to the feared onslaught of questions by friends and family and the self-driven expectation to reveal more personal details than they would like. If these concerns are effectively addressed in an assertiveness group led by an occupational therapist, anxiety related to this issue will likely decrease. Clients report feeling more prepared to encounter others after discharge when they have learned and practiced direct forms of communication.

Anxiety can affect a person physiologically, emotionally, behaviorally and cognitively. See Table 8-1 for a list of symptoms of anxiety in each area.

Table 8-1. Symptoms of Anxiety

Emotional	Physiological	Cognitive	Behavioral
Feeling uneasy, off-balance	*Cardiovascular:* increased heart rate (tachycardia), chest pain and pressure	Confusion	Looks preoccupied
Feeling overwhelmed		Poor memory	Immobile, withdrawn
		Distractibility, poor concentration	
Feeling a sense of impending doom	*Gastrointestinal:* diarrhea, constipation, nausea, vomiting, gas, cramps, and loss of appetite	Thought blocking	Overactive, restless, agitated
Feeling helpless and out of control		Loss of perspective, cognitive distortion including catastrophic thinking and negative self-evaluation	Excess or decreased consumption of substances and/or food
Feeling one is going insane	*Respiratory:* dyspnea (shortness of breath) and choking sensations		
Depersonalization (having feelings of unreality, as if in a dream)	*Urinary:* frequency and urgency of urination	Obsessive thoughts	Rituals to Alleviate anxiety
		Fears of loss of control, going crazy, injury, death, and not coping	
Derealization (feeling detached from one's surroundings)	*Genital:* loss of libido, premature ejaculation, and amenorrhea	Poor problem solving	
	Autonomic: sweating, flushing, dry mouth, dizziness, and fainting		
	Muscular: twitching, tremors, spasms, tension, cramping, hypervigilance		

Note: Some of the self-help behavioral methods sought to reduce discomfort may be unintentionally self-destructive and therefore not adaptive. For example, addiction to prescription medications and alcohol, extreme isolation, and regression are common secondary problems that develop from immediate, or nonadaptive, behavioral solutions.

IMPACT ON DAILY FUNCTIONING

The impact of anxiety on a person's life may be dramatic and may affect all aspects of functioning, including work, social life, self-care, parenting, and leisure activities. Performance in all roles may dramatically decline as anxiety symptoms persist.

Employment may suffer because of cognitive impairment. Concentration, problem solving, and memory may all be markedly affected by episodes of acute anxiety, primarily because the individual's primary focus is directed toward combating unpleasant symptoms and not to the task at hand. Tardiness, inaccuracy in completing work, and distractibility are some of the problem behaviors that develop in people who experience persistent anxiety. For example, one client with obsessive-compulsive disorder spent so many hours performing ritualistic hand and clothes washing that he was unable to maintain his required work schedule. Social relationships may decline as the person restricts activities and therefore becomes unavailable to others.

There is also the likelihood that others will be alienated by the rigidity and withdrawal of the anxious person. For example, a woman with panic attacks stopped attending her church and volunteer activities and became reclusive in her small apartment. After some period of time, friends and acquaintances associated with these activities no longer called her because of her continued self-imposed isolation and their experience of personal rejection.

Many persons experience stress with their partners as they curtail previously shared activities or become overreliant on them for assistance. For example, the husband of a client with agoraphobia became resentful of his wife's dependency when she would not leave the house without him, even to complete the smallest task. The decrease in function may affect homemaking, grooming, and parenting activities, as well as leisure occupations. The woman described here sought help from friends to transport her children to school and to her medical appointments when her husband was not available. Another client, an elderly man who was coping poorly with a generalized anxiety disorder, abandoned his avid avocational interest in the stock market because of difficulty in concentrating on the newspaper figures.

Depression commonly develops secondarily to anxiety symptoms. People often feel a sense of desperation as various forms of anxiety immobilize them or cause severe discomfort; therefore, the potential for suicide can be high. From a medical standpoint, clients are prone to certain physical diseases, such as heart problems and gastrointestinal disorders like ulcerative colitis and stomach ulcers. Figure 8-2 highlights the impact of anxiety disorders on daily functioning.

DSM-IV Descriptions of Anxiety

There are ten major diagnostic groups related to anxiety in the *DSM-IV-TR* (APA, 2000). A description of each group, with typical symptoms, follows.

Work: poor habits due to problems in concentration and time management
Social Relationships: diminished due to restriction of activity and isolation
Marital Relationships: decrease in shared activities, dependency on spouse
Activities of Daily Living: homemaking, grooming, and parenting may be
  inadequate secondary to poor concentration, depression, and physical
  symptoms
Leisure Activities: pleasurable activities may be neglected, primarily because
  of an inability to sustain sufficient attention
Depression: feelings of low self-esteem and despair may result, hindering
  involvement in customary activities
Medical Status: susceptibility to numerous diseases such as colitis, ulcers,
  heart disease, stroke, and respiratory disorders, which may decrease the
  ability to work, care for the self, and engage in pleasurable activities alone or
  with family and friends

Figure 8-2.   Impact of Anxiety Disorders on Daily Functioning

Panic Attack

The term *panic attack* defines a limited period of intense fear or distress in which four or more of the following symptoms progress rapidly and peak within 10 minutes: cardiac symptoms (palpitations, pounding, rapid heartbeat), trembling, shortness of breath, feelings of suffocation, chest pain, sensations of choking, nausea or abdominal distress, dizziness or lightheadedness, **derealization**, fear of losing control or going crazy, fear of dying, paresthesias (numbness or tingling), and chills or hot flashes. Panic attacks are most often associated with panic disorder but may also develop in those who have social phobias as well as other anxiety disorders.

Agoraphobia

Usually thought of as a reaction to repeated panic attacks, agoraphobia is often an avoidance of, or suffering through, situations where it might be difficult or embarrassing to leave in the event of a panic attack. Feelings of terror that assistance might not be available in the event of a panic attack is a major feature of this condition and leads to restriction of activity in respect to destination and conditions of travel. People with agoraphobia frequently will not travel without a companion. Although it is in itself not a disorder, this term is included in the description of three of the anxiety disorders.

Panic Disorder without and with Agoraphobia

These distressing conditions usually first appear in teenage or early adult years and may be related to life transitions. Twice as many women as men suffer from panic disorder. An individual has repeated and unexpected panic attacks with at least one attack followed by persistent worry of having additional attacks or dealing with the consequences of an attack. Attacks may occur in clusters or more randomly over longer timeframes. Losing control of one's feelings is a major concern of people with this disorder. To accommodate their anxieties, many people will go to great lengths to avoid those circumstances where fear of panic attacks is strong, such as standing in long lines or crossing bridges. This is called *situational avoidance*. Panic Disorder often is accompanied by depression, alcohol abuse, and/or multiple phobias.

Specific Phobia

This disorder, frequently beginning in childhood or the mid-20s, is characterized by recurrent illogical and excessive fear and anxiety, evoked during either the expectation of, or an actual encounter with, a particular stimulus, object or situation. The stimulus can exist in real life or be imagined, such as what might be seen in a video, book, or dream. The object or situation is fiercely avoided though there is usually insight that the reaction is exaggerated and irrational. The anxiety responses dissipate if the stimulus is weakened or removed. A phobia in one subtype often leads to other phobias in the same subgroup. The degree to which a phobia impairs functioning appears to relate to the ease and success of avoiding the stressor. One is impaired if behaviors interfere considerably with daily life, such as missing work or giving up a social life. Animals are the most common phobias, followed by spiders, bats, and rats.

Social Phobia

This disorder, also called social anxiety disorder, refers to excessive fears of potentially humiliating social or performance situations in which there is the anticipation of examination or judgment by others. Extreme self-consciousness and worry about ridicule are key factors in limiting social contacts. Concerns about one's mind going blank, having a panic attack, or losing bladder control are some of the fears that may plague a person well in advance of an event. In most cases the disruption in the person's life is not debilitating, and may be focused on discreet situations, such as avoiding eating in front of others. In other circumstances, however, there may be a more pronounced interference with work and social activities, such as compromising possible achievement by quitting a job when duties expand to public speaking, or refusing dates with potential lifetime mates.

Obsessive Compulsive Disorder

This serious and somewhat rare disorder, usually beginning in adolescence or young adulthood, is characterized by recurrent **obsessions** and **compulsions** that cause anxiety or great distress to the individual. Obsessions are persistent thoughts and images that are experienced as intrusive and unwanted. The content often concerns an exaggeration of usual fears. Examples of obsessions are aggressive thoughts, fear of acting improperly, and repeated questioning whether appliances were turned off. Compulsions are the behaviors devised to neutralize or reduce unwanted thoughts and may not be related directly to the obsession.

Counting the number of items in a room, hoarding, hair pulling, and persistent handwashing are some of the behaviors devised to reduce obsessions. When attempts are made to curb these disturbing behaviors, the individual experiences surges of anxiety. Although the individual realizes that the compulsive behaviors, which are attempts to reduce tension, are ultimately fruitless and time-consuming, he or she feels unable to stop them and experiences surges of anxiety when attempts are made to do so. These odd behaviors often may lead to the alienation of others. Because they can be extremely time-consuming (more than one hour daily), they often interfere with occupational functioning and work, school, social, self-care, and homemaking routines. Other axis I diagnoses commonly coexist with OCD, especially depression and eating disorders. Believing affected individuals share traits with people with phobias, Liebgold (2000) has labeled this group "phobocs." He offers educational information as well as exercises in a handbook (Liebgold, 2000) designed for both professionals and clients.

Post-Traumatic Stress Disorder

This disorder, more common in women than men, occurs in people who have been exposed to an overwhelming traumatic event that continues to impact their current daily functioning and causes them severe distress. Exposure to the trauma can be either in the form of witnessing it, such as seeing a murder, or by personally experiencing it, such as living through childhood sexual abuse. The occurrence in most cases is either a perceived or actual life-threatening situation in which terror and helplessness are responses. Natural disasters, combat, mass causalities, serious medical conditions, rape, domestic violence, accidents and observing the death of a loved one, are all calamities that might lead to post-traumatic stress disorder (PTSD). People reexperience the trauma in different ways but the overwhelming symptoms are anxiety and hypersensitivity. Reoccurring dreams or nightmares, intrusive images, or thoughts, called flashbacks, are key to keeping the trauma alive. "Triggers" that evoke the memories can be in the form of smells, sounds, or images. Avoidance of situations where symptoms might occur is a common strategy used by those with this disorder. People also may feel emotionally numb and disconnected to others and at the same time hypervigilant to their surroundings.

The symptoms continue for more than one month and most often occur in close proximity to the traumatic event. Following the 9/11 World Trade Center catastrophe, many cases of PTSD were reported and emergency health care workers streamed in to help victims cope. One study cited 67,000 residents living below 110th Street suffering from the condition. The disorder may also develop months or years following the trauma. For example, a Bosnian refugee, hospitalized for PTSD, had suddenly developed the symptoms of this disorder many years after fleeing his homeland while watching a TV documentary about his country.

Sometimes the disorder is resolved fairly quickly, but other times, it may turn into a chronic, debilitating condition with varying ranges of impairment. Substance abuse and violence, especially related to combat stress, may lead to confrontation with the law. Chronic depression may result in suicide attempts and difficulty with interpersonal relationships.

Acute Stress Disorder

Acute stress disorder is similar to post-traumatic stress disorder in respect to the exposure to a traumatic event and the response of horror, terror, and powerlessness. However, the symptoms of this disorder develop within one month of the event and last only from two days to one month following the exposure. In addition to experiencing at least one symptom of each PTSD cluster (e.g., flashbacks, dreams, and avoidance of the stimuli), an individual feels a sense of detachment. She or he must also exhibit several dissociative symptoms such as numbing, derealization, **depersonalization**, and amnesia. The world seems dreamlike and the individual may feel her or his feelings and body are disconnected. During a major California earthquake a woman could not recall how she had sustained cuts and bruises while trying to evacuate a store. After the earthquake others confessed to waking up frequently during the night with cold sweats and a rapid heartbeat. Although it was very helpful at times for them to talk about the trauma, this was balanced by their need to stay distanced from the event and avoid discussing it or viewing the damage.

Generalized Anxiety Disorder

This common disorder describes persistent, uncontrollable, and excessive anxiety or worry. A It appears twice as often in women than men and develops gradually from childhood to middle age. People often present a pessimistic outlook because they are continually anticipating problems in everyday life. The focus of the worry can change, from work, school, friends, and family to finances. There may be little variation in the intensity of the anxiety experienced, whether it be related to the outcome of a school exam or to the deteriorating health of a family member. People with GAD may be aware of the exaggeration of their worry but feel unable to control it.

Symptoms range from sleep disturbances to fatigue and muscle tension. Abundant sweating, gastrointestinal distress, headaches, lightheadedness, and irritability are common as well as an inability to relax. In addition to not being able to manage excessive anxiety, to have the diagnosis of GAD someone must have experienced the anxiety for at least six months. Generalized anxiety disorder rarely occurs as a primary diagnosis but major depressive disorder and other anxiety orders frequently occur simultaneously.

Anxiety Disorder Due to a General Medical Condition

Anxiety in this group is due to the physiological causes of a medical problem. Any of the previously mentioned anxiety symptoms may be present. For example, rapid pulse caused by cardiac disease may lead to clinical symptoms of anxiety.

Substance-Induced Anxiety Disorder

The physiological effect of a drug medication or toxin causes substance-induced anxiety. The anxiety may be manifested in a variety of ways, as described thus far.

GENERAL TREATMENT STRATEGIES

A variety of treatments are used to diminish the symptoms of anxiety and promote more adaptive functioning. Treatments range from medications to self-management techniques. Figure 8-3 lists types of general treatment strategies.

Psychopharmacology

Medications addressing the physiological component of anxiety are prescribed most often for the relief of both acute attacks of anxiety and for chronic conditions (see Figure 8-4). They are used in conjunction with other types of therapy, such as cognitive behavioral therapy (Taylor & Arnow, 1988; Telch, 1982). Their aim is to reduce the level of arousal through regulation of neurotransmitters and activating hormones in the brain. There are several groups of medications that work in this way. Antianxiety drugs, such as **benzodiazapenes**, are effective for acute anxiety such as those present in panic attacks, generalized anxiety, social anxiety, and phobias, and they quickly reduce distressing symptoms of trembling and rapid heart beat. They are used as short-term therapy or as needed secondary to tolerance. They may be beneficial in the short term (2 to twelve months), however, they may lead to drug dependence and drug tolerance and are therefore not suited to long-term use. Examples of benzodiazapenes are Ativan (Lorazepam) and Klonipin (Clonazepam).

Antidepressant medications are the best long-term treatment and are also commonly prescribed for anxiety disorders, especially when an affective disorder coexists. However, the side effects of these drugs, such as lethargy, gastrointestinal symptoms, and sexual dysfunction, may not be tolerated well and therefore may be discontinued prematurely. The newest classification of antidepressants are selective serotonin reuptake inhibitors (SSRIs), which have fewer unpleasant consequences than the earlier drugs. Fluoxetine (Prozac) and Sertraline (Zoloft) are examples of SSRIs, and may be useful for people with symptoms of OCD, PTSD, panic disorder, and social phobia. The older, tricyclic antidepressants, such as Trofanil (Imipramine), may be especially helpful for individuals with panic disorder. Monoamine oxidase inhibitors (MAOIs) are the third and oldest class of antidepressants, which work by blocking enzymes that break up important neurotransmitters. Because of potentially serious side effects if used in conjunction with prohibited foods and medications, MAOIs are commonly prescribed only after other antidepressants have failed. Nardil (Phenelzine) is an MAOI that is an effective treatment for panic attacks as well as PTSD.

Heart medications such as beta-blockers like Proponolol (Inderal) are sometimes used for social phobias. Also, antipsychotic drugs have proven successful in treating anxiety disorders in which symptoms are so debilitating as to prevent functioning or where delusions are present.

Counseling

There are many verbal approaches designed to help decrease anxiety in its maladaptive form. They range from intense, long-term treatment, such as

CLASS OF DRUGS Brand and (Generic)	Panic Disorder	GAD	Specific Phobia	Social Phobia	OCD	PTSD
BENZODIAZEPINES Ativan (Lorazpam) Klonipin (Clonazepam) Librium (Chlordiazepoxide) Centrax (Prazepam) Restoril (Temazepam) Serax (Oxazepam) Valium (Diazepam) Xanax (Alprazolam)	X	X	X	X		
ANTI-DEPRESSANTS **Selective Serotonin** **Reuptake Inhibitors (SSRIS):** Prozac (Fluoxetine) Luvox (Fluvoxamine) Zoloft (Setraline) Paxil (Paroxetine) Celexa (Citalopram)	X			X	X	X
Tricyclics (TCA'S): Trofanil (Imipramine) Anafranil (Clomiprimine) Aventyl (Nortriptyline) Ludiomil (Maprotiline) Norpramin (Desipramine) Sinequan (Doxepin) Elavil (Amitriptyline)	X				X (Anafranil)	X
Monoamine Oxidase **Inhibitors (MAOI'S)** Nardil (Phenelzine) Parnate (Tranylcypromine) Marplan (Isocarboxid) Eldepryl (Selegilene)	X					X
OTHER ANTIDEPRESSANTS Effexor (Venlafaxine) Serzone (Nefaxadone)	X	X		X	X	
BETA-BLOCKERS Proponol (Inderal) Tenormin (Atenolol)				X		
ANTICONVULSANTS Neurontin (Gabentin)				X		
AZASIPIRONES **BuSpar (Busipirone)**		X				

Figure 8-3. Medications Frequently Used with Anxiety Disorders

Adapted from Anxiety Disorders Association of America
http://www.adaa.org/AnxietyDisorderInfor/Medications.cfm 6/03

Psychopharmacology
Psychotherapy
Biofeedback and Meditation
Behavior Approaches
Cognitive Behavioral Approaches
Couples Therapy
EMDR

Note: These common strategies for treatment of anxiety disorders require expertise and training, and some are more likely to be utilized by certain professionals. For example, psychiatrists prescribe medication, psychologists may provide psychotherapy and exposure therapy, and social workers or marriage and family counselors often provide couples therapy.

Figure 8-4. Treatment Strategies for Anxiety Disorders

psychoanalysis, to short-term, supportive treatment, such as cognitive therapy. Psychotherapy addresses the immediate relief of symptoms and has a direct focus on immediate, pressing issues; supportive psychotherapy enhances the ability to cope through education, reassurance, and empathy. Cognitive interventions help clients to identify faulty, irrational thinking regarding perceived dangers and to substitute more realistic thoughts. Treatment is accomplished through various strategies, including challenging negative thinking and global generalizations. Someone who is convinced that the decrease in the number of e-mails received from her best friend signifies rejection, for example, may be helped to see other possible causes for the change in the friend's behavior. Alternative explanations for her friend's decreased communication could be increased workload on the job, illness, more involvement in her outside pursuits, or marital pressure to spend more time with her spouse and less time on the Internet. Furthermore, the client may have made startling negative generalizations about herself from her perhaps erroneous interpretation of this one specific event. Sweeping statements may take this form: I upset my friend, I'm insensitive, I'm unable to sustain friendships, I'm unlikable, I'm a loser. In this case, the psychotherapist would help the client focus on the specific situation in question and challenge notions that possible rejection by one friend does not signify general unworthiness. This method may be accomplished through seeking "proof" to support these notions. Educational sessions and homework assignments may help to support cognitive interventions.

Behavioral Approaches

Once irrational ideas are identified, behavioral strategies may be applied to practice new behaviors. There is a broad range of behavioral interventions and many are combined to be the most effective.

Exposure Therapy. Exposure therapy (also called "programmed practice") (Agras & Berkowitz, 1994), focuses entirely on real encounters with the objects of the individual's anxiety, while helping him or her to use a variety of techniques (i.e., deep breathing and positive self-talk) to master the situation.

Because of its in vivo (real-life) component, exposure therapy appears to be a highly effective and powerful treatment, which helps to weaken fear and the subsequent avoidant responses, especially with persons with phobic, panic, and obsessive-compulsive disorders.

Systematic Desensitization. Systematic desensitization is a type of incremental exposure that attempts to systematically diminish anxiety related to specific fears primarily through the use of imagery and relaxation and then real contact with the image of or actual object. Used most often with phobic disorders, a trained therapist helps the client devise a hierarchical list of, usually, 10 items to break down the fear into steps according to the subjective rating of their intensity (Wolpe, 1973). For example, someone who fears rats would likely rank touching a rat as very challenging, while looking at a picture of a rat might be the least threatening. Starting with the least troubling item on the list and coupling progressive relaxation with visualization, the person advances up the hierarchy once each level is mastered as evidenced by the absence of an anxiety response. A variation of this intervention is participant modeling (Bandura, 1977), whereby the therapist interacts with the feared object or situation and then encourages the client to interact jointly before performing alone.

Interoceptive desensitization refers to evoking fear in a controlled setting to help manage the symptoms before they mushroom into unmanageable anxiety, as in the case with someone with panic attacks (Bourne, 2000). For instance, someone who fears heights could practice spinning on a desk chair, look at videos of people on roller coasters, and then participate in virtual video games where dizziness might be evoked. Eventually, the real situation is tackled.

Exposure and Response Prevention (ERP). Exposure and response prevention (ERP) (Bourne, 2000) is a treatment applied to people with OCD whereby usual behaviors devised by the client to ward off anxiety caused by obsessional thinking are gradually prevented. For example, a client with OCD was perceptually fearful of germs and scrubbed his hands at least 50 times a day for about six minutes each time. The ERP program slowly and systematically first exposed him to the feared stimulus, in this case, touching doorknobs, and prevented him from the ritual handwashing by incremental restrictions of the behavior. This was accomplished both by curtailing the number of handwashing episodes per day and by the length of time of each handwashing occurrence.

Biofeedback

The goal of biofeedback is to decrease arousal by providing the client with objective data about, and then helping him or her gain control over, biological states that are normally involuntary. Biofeedback techniques target and attempt to alter changes in heart rate, blood pressure, sweating, and skin temperature by providing feedback through instrumentation (Davis, Eshelman, & McKay, 1988; Taylor & Arnow, 1988). Electrodes, blood pressure indicators, and finger sensors in contact with the body are examples of devices used to provide data that tracks how the treatments are impacting physical condition. Once information is received, the client learns methods of altering the body functions to reduce anxiety.

Biofeedback may be seen as a type of behavioral therapy in that objective, observable data is the focus. Meditation has been helpful for those with anxiety disorders and includes styles that draw from both Western and Eastern practices. Calm breathing, thought focusing, repetition of sounds, and posture are aspects that are stressed in varying ways. Mindful meditation has been used for chronic conditions, both physiological and psychological, especially PTSD. What makes this practice unique is that the participant is instructed to observe thoughts without judging, instead of ridding himself or herself of them (Freeman & Lawlis, 2001). Studies have shown that during meditation heart rate, respiration, anxiety level, and oxygen consumption are lowered and positive mood states are raised (Freeman & Lawlis, 2001). Other relaxation exercises are discussed in more detail in the Occupational Therapy Self-Management Techniques section in this chapter.

Eye Movement Desensitization and Reprocessing (EMDR)

This approach, developed by Shapiro (2001) is used to treat a range of psychological disorders from PTSD to phobias. Relatively new and controversial, this multifaceted and short-term form of psychotherapy draws from cognitive-behavioral approaches, combining eye movements with evocation of feelings, sensations, thoughts, and memories in order to reprocess them in the brain. Negative feelings such as anxiety associated with memories of traumatic events are induced during directed experiences by a trained therapist, who combines eye exercises with verbal instructions. Clients are instructed to track a light or the therapist's finger as it moves back and forth horizontally. This intervention stimulates both sides of the brain. The expected result is that the client gains insight and assumes more adaptive and integrated behavior.

Research in the field of anxiety disorders has investigated the effectiveness of different types of therapeutic interventions. These results as described by Roth and Fonagy (1996) are summarized as follows. For panic disorder, cognitive and exposure therapy in combination with applied relaxation are most helpful. Systematic desensitization is the treatment of choice for someone with a specific phobia. A combination of social skills training and exposure therapy is most useful for an individual treated for social phobia. In addition to tricyclic medications, someone with OCD would be most helped by mass exposure and response prevention for behavioral aspects of the condition and cognitive therapy for ruminations. Those managing symptoms of PTSD would benefit from anxiety management strategies, especially CBT. CBT has also been most effective with individuals with GAD in conjunction with short-term use of benzodiazapenes.

Couples Therapy

How couples interact may greatly influence both the generation of anxiety and how it is managed. Marriage counselors and other psychotherapists help the client with anxiety and his or her partner to identify the dynamics of their relationship that trigger anxiety and to cope with a range of feelings such as anger, discouragement, and resentment. Improving communication, receiving mutual support, and understanding secondary gains (gains that may occur due to the cessation of usual activities) are other possible benefits of marital counseling.

OCCUPATIONAL THERAPY AND SELF-MANAGEMENT TECHNIQUES

Most of the anxiety disorders have a chronic course with periods of remission. Therefore, the foremost task is learning how to manage anxiety in order to continue functioning and to face, rather than avoid, situations that irrationally generate fear. The avoidance of fear-producing stimuli is an attempt at self-protection, but it is maladaptive if it interferes with the fulfillment of environmental and internal needs (Depoy & Kolodner, 1991). Avoidant behavior also reinforces a sense of helplessness. Occupational therapists can help people develop a range of self-efficacy techniques that help to increase the feeling of influence or mastery over one's circumstances (Bandura, 1995). A problem-focused approach is especially useful with this population, for it helps people to respond rationally, rather than emotionally, to potentially fear-producing situations. Self-efficacy has been said to be a major factor in fear reduction (Taylor & Arnow, 1988). In fact, self-efficacy as a goal is a major tenet of the Model of Human Occupation and so addressing self-efficacy fits seamlessly with an occupational therapy approach (Kielhofner, 2002).

Assessment

Many tools exist for measuring the degree and type of anxiety. Occupational therapists, provided they have the required education, qualifications, and experience in using these general anxiety measurement tools, sometimes administer them in research settings. The Hospital Anxiety and Depression Scale (HAD) (Zigmond & Snaith, 1983) is composed of 14 questions that identify levels of both factors in hospitalized clients. Differentiating between state and trait anxiety, the State/Trait Anxiety Scale (STAI) (Spielberger, 1983) looks at whether anxiety is either a temporary or more permanent condition. A third general anxiety assessment is the IPAT (Krug, Scheier, & Cattell, 1976). This self-assessment of 40 questions investigates factors such as tension and guilt-proneness and measures clinical anxiety. This measure is typically used with a clinical population. Physiological measures of heart rate and body temperature are also used as indicators of changes in heart rate. By using these immediately in conjunction with interventions, clinicians can help clients monitor probable decrease in levels of anxiety. Typically occupational therapists are interested in how anxiety impacts daily functioning. Their target, therefore, is assessing impairment caused by anxiety.

In order to develop strategies for improved functioning, the level of impairment of the person with anxiety must be assessed. The assessments serve to highlight the extent of the disorder's interference in daily life activities.

Interviews, surveys, observation of performance, role checklists, function questionnaires, self-assessment of activities, and activity configurations listed in Figures 8-5 through 8-8 elicit information about how anxiety impacts a person's

ROLE CHECKLIST

NAME _____ AGE_____ DATE_____

SEX: ☐ MALE ☐ FEMALE   ARE YOU RETIRED: ☐ YES   ☐ NO

MARITAL STATUS: ☐ SINGLE ☐ MARRIED ☐ SEPARATED ☐ DIVORCED ☐ WIDOWED

The purpose of this checklist is to identify the major roles in your life. The checklist, which is divided into two parts, presents 10 roles and defines each one.

PART I

Beside each role, indicate, by checking the appropriate column, if you performed the role in the past, if you presently perform the role, and if you plan to perform the role in the future. You may check more than one column for each role. For example, if you volunteered in the past, do not volunteer at present, but plan to in the future, you would check the past and future columns.

ROLE	PAST	PRESENT	FUTURE
STUDENT: Attending school on a part-time or full-time basis.			
WORKER: Part-time or full-time paid employment.			
VOLUNTEER: Donating services, *at least once a week,* to a hospital, school, community, political campaign, and so forth.			
CARE GIVER: Responsibility, *at least once a week,* for the care of someone such as a child, spouse, relative, or friend.			
HOME MAINTAINER: Responsibility, *at least once a week,* for the upkeep of the home such as housecleaning or yardwork.			
FRIEND: Spending time or doing something, *at least once a week,* with a friend.			
FAMILY MEMBER: Spending time or doing something, *at least once a week,* with a family member such as a child, spouse, parent, or other relative.			
RELIGIOUS PARTICIPANT: Involvement, *at least once a week,* in groups or activities affiliated with one's religion (excluding worship).			
HOBBYIST/AMATEUR: Involvement, *at least once a week,* in a hobby or amateur activity such as sewing, playing a musical instrument, woodworking, sports, the theater, or participation in a club or team.			
PARTICIPANT IN ORGANIZATIONS: Involvement, *at least once a week,* in organizations such as the American Legion, National Organization for Women, Parents Without Partners, Weight Watchers, and so forth.			
OTHER:_____ A role not listed which you have performed, are presently performing, and/or plan to perform. Write the role on the line above and check the appropriate column(s).			

Figure 8-5.   Role Checklist

Source: Reprinted with permission from Frances Oakley, MS, OTR, FAOTA.

life. For example, accounting for daily activities by filling out typical schedules (Figure 8-8) reveals significant information in respect to productive activities as well as role functioning. Someone with agoraphobia may stay indoors the majority of each day, during which time expected activities are not performed, with the roles of hobbyist, homemaker, or worker being lost.

Treatment Interventions

The primary occupational therapy interventions utilized with anxiety disorders are listed in Table 8-2. The selection of strategies will depend on the nature of the

PART II

The same roles are listed below. Next to *each* role check the column which best indicates how valuable or important the role is to you. Answer for *each role,* even if you have never performed or do not plan to perform the role.

ROLE	NOT AT ALL VALUABLE	SOMEWHAT VALUABLE	VERY VALUABLE
STUDENT: Attending school on a part-time or full-time basis.			
WORKER: Part-time or full-time paid employment.			
VOLUNTEER: Donating services, **at least once a week,** to a hospital, school, community, political campaign, and so forth.			
CARE GIVER: Responsibility, **at least once a week,** for the care of someone such as a child, spouse, relative, or friend.			
HOME MAINTAINER: Responsibility, **at least once a week,** for the upkeep of the home such as housecleaning or yardwork.			
FRIEND: Spending time or doing something, **at least once a week,** with a friend.			
FAMILY MEMBER: Spending time or doing something, **at least once a week,** with a family member such as a child, spouse, parent, or other relative.			
RELIGIOUS PARTICIPANT: Involvement, **at least once a week,** in groups or activities affiliated with one's religion (excluding worship).			
HOBBYIST/AMATEUR: Involvement, **at least once a week,** in a hobby or amateur activity such as sewing, playing a musical instrument, woodworking, sports, the theater, or participation in a club or team.			
PARTICIPANT IN ORGANIZATIONS: Involvement, **at least once a week,** in organizations such as the American Legion, National Organization for Women, Parents Without Partners, Weight Watchers, and so forth.			
OTHER:_____ A role not listed which you have performed, are presently performing, and/or plan to perform. Write the role on the line above and check the appropriate column(s).			

© Copyright 1981 and Revised 1984 by Frances Oakley, M.S., OTR/L

Occupational Therapy Service, Department of Rehabilitation Medicine, Clinical Center, National Institutes of Health

*U.S. GOVERNMENT PRINTING OFFICE: 1985-526-620:30339

Figure 8-5.   *(continued)*

disorder, the setting in which the client is being treated, and the environment to which the person will return. There is a broad application of principles, including approaches for people suffering more severe impairment (Stein & Nikolic, 1989). Most of the approaches listed in the table have emerged from other disciplines, most notably from psychology and from health and wellness. However, they have become widely used by professionals of all disciplines who practice in mental health. Occupational therapists use the techniques to enhance occupational therapy goals and for engagement in occupation to support participation in context. Naturally, it is assumed that, when employing any strategy, the therapist will become competent through education and training.

Relaxation training.   Relaxation training can be an effective intervention to help people with anxiety disorders diminish arousal states and ultimately cope with stress; the relaxation response and a feeling of well-being are incompatible

WORK

The extent to which my work is impaired because of anxiety

0	1	2	3	4	5	6	7	8	9	10
Never		Slightly		Moderately			Markedly		Very Severely	

SOCIAL ACTIVITIES

The extent to which my social life is impaired because of anxiety
(going out with friends, dating, outings, entertaining)

0	1	2	3	4	5	6	7	8	9	10
Never		Slightly		Moderately			Markedly		Very Severely	

LEISURE ACTIVITIES

The extent to which engagement in leisure activities is impaired because of anxiety
(hobbies, use of free time)

0	1	2	3	4	5	6	7	8	9	10
Never		Slightly		Moderately			Markedly		Very Severely	

HOME, SELF-MAINTENANCE, AND FAMILY RESPONSIBILITIES

The extent to which my ability to care for myself and others is impaired by my anxiety
(cleaning house, meal preparation, carpooling, doing laundry, paying bills, grooming)

0	1	2	3	4	5	6	7	8	9	10
Never		Slightly		Moderately			Markedly		Very Severely	

Figure 8-6. Function Questionnaire

Source: Adapted from the Fear Questionnaire in Taylor & Arnow, 1988.

Table 8-2. Occupational Therapy and Self-Management Techniques

- *Relaxation Training*
  Breathing Exercises
  Progressive Muscle Relaxation
  Visualization
  Autogenic Training
- *Assertiveness Training*
- *Community Mobility/Reentry*
- *Expressive Activities*
  Journal Writing
  Craft and Art Activities
- *Functional Behavior Training*
- *Education/Lifestyle Alterations*
- *Rational/Cognitive Approaches*
- *Time Management*

Self-Assessment of Activities

Name:_____

Date:_____

This checklist will be used to help develop an Occupational Therapy program for you. Mark the appropriate column for each item and add any comments you feel would be helpful.

Activity	Never a problem	Sometimes a problem	Always a problem	N.A.	Comments
Grooming					
Bathing or showering					
Preparing meals					
Food shopping					
Doing errands					
House cleaning					
Doing yardwork					
Caring for others					
Managing money					
Transportation					
Socializing					
Attending school					
Working					
Volunteering					
Exercising					
Concentrating					
Problem solving					
Communicating					
Coping with stress					
Managing time					
Managing impulses					
Doing leisure activities					

Figure 8-7. Self-Assessment of Activities

with anxiety. Initially, clients usually require external direction, but the overall goal is to teach them to recognize and manage their own anxiety while it is "young" (still of short duration) to prevent major anxiety attacks, as well as to avert attacks if they occur. It is important to help people generalize from treatment sessions to the variety of life situations where anxiety is likely to occur. The Function Questionnaire (see Figure 8-7) targets these areas effectively. The client rates the extent to which anxiety interferes with daily activities from a quantitative and qualitative standpoint. The next step is to focus on these areas one at a time and strategize how relaxation techniques could be incorporated into the

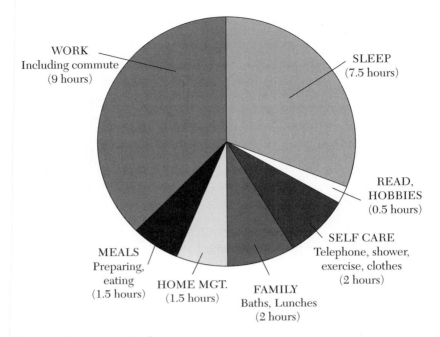

Figure 8-8. Activity Configuration

activities. For example, this method was successful with a construction worker who often became panicky when working on roofs. Utilizing abdominal breathing just before she went on the roof or while she was working on it greatly helped to reduce her symptoms of rapid pulse and queasiness.

Typically, occupational therapists teach a variety of relaxation skills (after they themselves have been sufficiently trained). These skills include deep breathing, progressive muscle relaxation, visualization, and **autogenic training** among others. As described by Benson (1976), who is a pioneer of relaxation training, all relaxation interventions involve the following: (1) the person has a passive attitude, (2) there is a decrease in muscle tone, (3) the environment is quiet, and (4) a mental device is used, such as an image or sound. Anxious people often lack the ability to engage in all steps of the relaxation activity; therefore, it is helpful to teach specific relaxation exercises that have an action component in addition to the distraction of a mental device. Progressive muscle relaxation (discussed in a subsequent section) has this feature. Sessions usually last up to about 30 minutes. Because of the quiet atmosphere generated by the relaxation training, it is wise to include people with the same attention span and to exclude those who are extremely restless or distractible. People should be given the option of keeping their eyes open or closed and the choice of sitting in a chair or sitting or lying on the floor. A protective covering such as a sheet should be available for hygienic reasons. If an individual chooses to use a chair, the therapist should make certain that there is back support by putting the chair against the wall. This will protect the person's neck from possible injury should he or she fall asleep.

Each person will have a preferred technique. Therefore, it is helpful to briefly introduce a variety of methods so as to gain feedback from the client as to which is the most useful. This can be accomplished by having people rate their subjective levels of anxiety on a scale from 1 to 10 before and after the exercises, by taking respiratory and heart rates before and after tasks, by asking which exercise was the most effective, or by observing the person's apparent level of concentration during the exercises. Sampling a variety of relaxation techniques within one session has the advantage of addressing problems of limited attention span and restricted opportunities for treatment due to the increasingly short lengths of stay on inpatient units or treatment in a home setting.

Making personalized audiotapes for relaxation can be extremely helpful, but commercial tapes are also readily available in a variety of forms, from soothing music or nature sounds to directed sessions. When making or selecting tapes, it is essential to consider the concentration level as well as the particular needs of each person. If given a choice, most people will state a preference for either a male or female narrator; therefore, having both available is useful. Some clinicians are finding that having clients make their own tapes facilitates a deeper sense of personal control (H. Stein, personal communication, June 2, 2003, Grand Rounds, Stanford Hospital and Clinics). Once the individual learns and masters the selected techniques, he or she should be helped to apply the skill to everyday barriers. For example, a person with social phobia may learn to practice a few minutes of deep breathing before meeting coworkers for lunch, an individual with agoraphobia may visualize a pleasant spot before leaving the house, and a person with PTSD may engage in relaxation exercises to counteract insomnia.

People should also be encouraged to differentiate, and then apply, other resources they have previously used to enhance the relaxation process, such as music, meditation, lighting, warm baths, and humor.

Breathing exercises. Abdominal breathing can effectively address relaxation, especially when people learn to self-monitor the technique by placing their hands on the abdomen and witnessing them rise on inhalation. This is a logical first task for an individual with an anxiety disorder for it can be short in duration and requires limited direction. However, clients should be introduced to this technique slowly to avoid lightheadedness from the increased oxygen consumption. Breathing exercises have been found to be a useful strategy to use during panic attacks (Clark, Salkovskis & Chalkley, 1985), with the addition of the client counting to 5 between breaths. Under stress, many anxious people hyperventilate, causing blood chemistry changes that lead to unpleasant sensations, such as dizziness. It is this reaction that may actually precipitate the panic and fear. Respiratory control by means of slow, paced breathing counteracts the patterns of hyperventilation thought to contribute to acute anxiety attacks. Sometimes other types of breathing exercises are more effective or can be used in conjunction with abdominal breathing. Imagining the words, "I am," as one inhales, and, "relaxed," as one exhales helps to slow the breath and focus on breathing patterns. Synchronizing breathing with counting slowly or the visualization of color is also effective. Clients seem to respond favorably to imagining the inhalation of clear colors, such as yellow or blue, and the exhalation of gray.

Progressive muscle relaxation. Progressive muscle relaxation, which was first described by Jacobson (1938), teaches clients to tighten and release voluntary muscle groups slowly and methodically in a progressive fashion, thereby contrasting the states of tension and relaxation. This technique offers a discharge of tension as a means to achieve a state of deep relaxation, with the underlying hypothesis that relaxation of the body leads to relaxation of the mind. For clients with limited concentration, the active involvement of tensing and relaxing can be more engaging and therefore more successful than pure mental activity. Daily sessions are recommended for practicing and mastering the technique.

Visualization. Picturing a pleasant scene is another method used to enhance the relaxation response. It is easiest for people to activate images after anxiety has partially subsided; therefore, it is recommended to precede visualization with breathing exercises. Soothing music may also help to evoke images, but some people will still need guidance. If the therapist provides mental pictures for the client such as floating or diving into water, it is important to know beforehand that the images selected are pleasant. Directions can include visualizing a leaf floating in a stream, walking in a meadow or strolling by a pond, returning to a happy childhood place, imagining a fantasy place, or picturing a comfortable place in one's home. By presenting only a general direction and structure, such as saying, "Imagine a beautiful place you've seen," the therapist encourages the client to fill in more of his or her personal experience. The exercise then becomes more interactive and the client may feel a stronger sense of participation and control. If the client is unable to evoke images easily, simply picturing colors may provide a sufficient degree of pleasant sensation. Visualization exercises are contraindicated for patients experiencing perceptual distortions (hallucinations) or thought disorders (delusions) because these exercises can intensify the psychotic experience and become frightening. If visualization exercises stimulate flashbacks of distressing events in people who have PTSD, another form of relaxation should be introduced. Before beginning the task, the occupational therapist should always inform clients to open their eyes if the exercise evokes unpleasant feelings. The therapist should assume this may be happening if he or she observes crying, restlessness, or the eyes suddenly opening. Visualization methods can also be adapted for use with children.

Autogenic training. Autogenic training, which was developed by German neurologist H. H. Shultz, teaches the body and mind to relax through the person's own verbal commands. The intent is to relax the voluntary and involuntary muscles to provide **vasodilatation** and help regulate the circulatory and respiratory systems (Davis, Eshelman, & McKay, 1988). The occupational therapist can introduce several of the exercises, which are learned methodically over several weeks. They consist of imagining the limbs as heavy and warm, the heart as beating regularly and calmly, the lungs as operating regularly, the solar plexus as feeling warm, and the forehead as feeling cool. Since this method of relaxation has a strong effect on body physiology, it is not recommended for people with serious medical problems. In addition, it is contraindicated for children and for people with severe psychiatric disorders.

Assertiveness and general social skills training. Clients with anxiety disorders often manifest passive behavior. This may be due in part to fears related to anticipated embarrassment in social situations in which they may feel they will have no control. This is particularly true of clients with social phobias and generalized anxiety disorder. For example, a young man with generalized anxiety and depression was exceedingly lonely. Terrified to attend social functions, where he could possibly meet a potential mate, he ruminated about rejection and humiliation. He was unsure of how to approach strangers, initiate conversation, or sustain friendships. The cycle continued as he further isolated himself in spite of craving social contact, which he did in part to manage his anxiety. This client attended assertiveness groups while on a psychiatric unit and was referred to a community class at discharge. The OT group included the following stages: (1) understanding the components of assertive behavior, including differentiation between styles; (2) identifying personal styles and blocks to behaving assertively, including irrational beliefs and fears; and (3) practicing assertive communication and the principles and applications of good communication practices through role-play situations. Assertiveness training helped him to reduce anxiety and taught him to confront intimidating social situations in a way that offered more personal control. Assertiveness training can be an effective means of helping people reduce anxiety because it can help people confront intimidating situations in a way that offers more personal control.

Social skills group can be helpful by teaching other appropriate ways of interacting with others. Topics such as eye contact and other nonverbal communication and problem-solving uncomfortable situations are usually explored through discussion, educational materials, and role playing.

Community mobility and reentry. Isolation is a serious problem for people with anxiety disorders, who may completely withdraw from friends, family, leisure activities, and work in order to curb their anxiety. Not only does such constraint lead to loneliness and depression, but the absence of physical and emotional outlets can also contribute to maintaining the anxiety cycle. With restricted activity, people may become even more focused on their thoughts, sensations, and other internal experiences. Clients with anxiety may benefit from locating community resources that draw on former or current interests and simultaneously provide contact with other people. Some feel most supported in activities provided by mental health agencies, such as support groups or social events, because here they can receive direct help with their anxiety while also engaging in the activity at hand. Other clients feel more comfortable in small classes such as private art, music, or bridge classes, which are offered in many communities. Many prefer noncompetitive enrichment classes over junior college courses such as those offered by adult education programs. The occupational therapist can help locate appropriate programs during an individual or group treatment session.

Expressive activities. Clients experiencing anxiety disorders may benefit from engaging in expressive activities, which provide an outlet and release for the physical and emotional turbulence associated with anxiety. Family members and friends may have limited tolerance for discussing the client's repetitive concerns, so self-reliance techniques can help to preserve social relationships as well as promote independence.

Journal and diary writing. A journal can become a focus and receptacle for distressing thoughts. The symbolic act of writing down concerns and feelings may help the individual become better able to dismiss the troublesome emotions once the book is closed. It is been demonstrated that writing about stressful events can reduce physiological symptoms present in some illnesses (Smyth et al, 1999; Booth & Petrie, 2002). When using a diary, a person has control over the expression of content and amount of time devoted to addressing symptoms. For example, a woman in her early 30s with obsessive-compulsive disorder annoyed her mother, who lived next door, by her persistent criticism of her mother's perceived lack of attention to home maintenance and safety. To improve their relationship, the daughter began to write these worries in a notebook rather than discuss them with her mother, who did not perceive that there was a problem.

Sometimes keeping a journal or diary is suggested by a psychologist or psychiatrist as a means for recording specific anxiety disorder symptoms such as those of panic attacks or phobias. The information included may concern the times during the day when the symptoms emerge, the nature and intensity of the symptoms, and events occurring prior to or after the attack. This data helps the person with anxiety achieve some control over the symptoms by recognizing their patterns, precipitants, and consequences.

Craft and art activities. Structured craft and expressive art activities both have a place in the treatment of anxiety disorders. In structured crafts, the limits of a repetitive and predictive project can offer reassurance to the fearful person and help to contain anxiety. Clients with anxiety disorders often prefer projects with true boundaries, such as plastic "stained glass," sophisticated coloring sheets, and mosaics. Simple greeting cards may have the same effect. Completing these tasks successfully also provides a sense of mastery through accomplishment and increases clients' perceived sense of effectiveness.

The more expressive art activities may offer a release of tension through physical activity, such as ripping paper or using a stippling brush for painting designs on paper or cloth, and thus provide an acceptable substitute for an otherwise inappropriate expression of anxiety. For example, a client with multiple diagnoses including borderline personality disorder repeatedly burned herself with lit cigarettes in order to find relief from intolerable levels of anxiety. The occupational therapist provided her with a large body outline on which she was able to draw cigarette burns when she felt overcome by these impulses. Another client, a middle-aged man with schizophrenia and obsessive-compulsive disorder, was encouraged to draw with large felt pens whenever he began to frantically pace, wring his hands, or shake. His subsequent drawings were usually highly controlled, for example, portraying multitiled houses and paved roads, but his obsessive behavior decreased (see Figure 8-9).

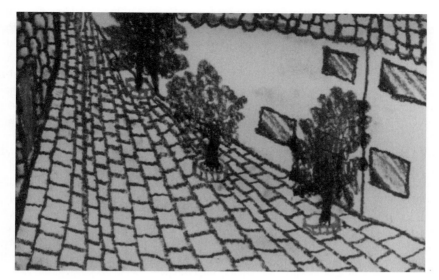

Figure 8-9. Client Drawing in Which Anxiety Is Expressed and Channeled

Expressive art activities may also stimulate self-understanding through the content that emerges. For example, in a group activity, a young mother with tenacious abdominal **psychogenic** pain and anxiety inadvertently drew a representation of her pain similar to the symbol she drew for her husband. When she discussed these similarities with her psychotherapist, she was able to connect the pain in her stomach to anger at her husband for not participating in any of the parenting responsibilities. All the expressive techniques discussed in this section are personally gratifying and increase the internal sense of control and self-mastery.

Functional behavioral training. A psychologist or psychiatrist may ask the occupational therapist to assist in carrying out behavioral programs that directly deal with improving functioning by decreasing symptoms as they relate to daily activities. For example, the plan may take the form of accompanying an agoraphobic client on a community outing to combat anxiety symptoms while riding a bus or going to a store. This intervention (previously referred to as exposure therapy) addresses avoidant behavior and can be an effective approach in treating some of the anxiety disorders, particularly phobias.

The occupational therapist may help the client negotiate difficult tasks through instruction in breathing exercises, refuting irrational thoughts, or suggesting that he or she confront unpleasant sensations as if "riding the wave." More experienced occupational therapists may actually take part in devising the behavioral plan for decreasing symptoms. This might include helping the person identify target behaviors and then breaking them down into smaller, manageable steps. This is traditionally called *grading the activity* by occupational therapists. For example, one client with agoraphobia wanted to be able to go back to his favorite coffeehouse a few times a week. The occupational therapist guided him in making a plan—walking first one block from home with her, walking alone on the same route, buying a newspaper in front of the coffeehouse, and so forth. Another occupational therapist assisted a young woman with obsessive-compulsive disorder who had a fixation on soiled clothes and contamination of the washing machine, which prevented her from performing adequate hygiene routines as she felt impelled to wear the same, unwashed, clothes day after day. The occupational therapist helped her counteract these fears through relaxation training and visualization prior to, and during, the actual laundry activity, resulting in the client being able to carry out the task and thus achieve adequate hygiene.

Education and lifestyle alterations. The relationship between internal (inherent to an individual) and external (outside) factors and anxiety is often not understood by those experiencing anxiety disorders. In particular, reducing caffeine intake, eliminating nonmedically prescribed drugs, exercising regularly, eating a balanced diet, maintaining appropriate weight, sleeping sufficiently, lowering blood pressure, increasing leisure involvement, and managing time effectively are all elements that can positively affect one's ability to cope with anxiety. Sufferers of panic attacks tend to experience fewer attacks when their overall state of arousal is diminished by attending to some of these basic suggestions (Taylor & Arnow, 1988).

Rational-cognitive approaches. The occupational therapist may assist people in coping more effectively by utilizing cognitive interventions (Ellis, 1976) (provided he or she is properly trained in the techniques). Anxious clients are often highly perfectionistic and consequently self-critical of their current or anticipated behavior. They worry in the form of engaging in negative self-talk about their finances, health, job performance, and relationships, expecting failure in every area (Wright & Beck, 1994). The worry becomes even more magnified in obsessive-compulsive disorder. This negative thinking is both time-consuming and self-defeating and usually distorts reality. Cognitive strategies attempt to help replace negative self-talk statements with more favorable ones. One technique is to teach clients to make positive self-statements. For example, when asked to participate in a drawing activity, a good number of clients will disqualify themselves by saying: "I am a terrible artist. I can't do this." The occupational therapist can suggest a reframe of the statement such as, "It makes me nervous to draw but at least I'll give it a try." Another strategy is to help clients relabel internally directed, destructive emotions as more neutral and appropriate ones. For instance, anxiety at failing to meet work deadlines can be changed to "concern," feelings of worthlessness at being criticized can be changed to "annoyance," and guilt at criticizing a child can be changed to "regret" (Davis, Eshelman, & McKay, 1988). These interventions seem to be most effective when they are presented as paper-and-pencil exercises, perhaps because problem solving through writing causes a delay in emotional response. The task can also be applied as a self-management strategy whereby the individual tracks responses over time.

Time management. Anxiety is often manifested by paralysis in goal-directed activity, which arises as a by-product of fears of failure, decreased concentration, or preoccupation with the stressor. Inactivity is further perpetuated by a lack of task mastery, which would likely enhance feelings of self-control and self-esteem. Instead, anxiety is often intensified by the failure to adequately meet personal and environmental demands. Clients may be surprised at the amount of nonproductive time they encounter in a 24-hour day. This is effectively illustrated by an assessment of daily activities whereby clients account for their time hour by hour in either a graphic or a written format.

Learning effective time management techniques is a useful strategy for people with anxiety disorders. For example, the occupational therapist can teach how to prioritize tasks and break them down into manageable and attainable steps. People usually respond favorably to schedules and "to do" lists. Sometimes actually incorporating "worry time" into the daily routine helps to decrease the behavior. For example, one person was horrified that she had written down "worry" as a daily activity that consumed six hours a day. She was helped to plan more productive substitute activities during the vulnerable times of the day. This plan also provided her with access to her former hobbies; for example, she elected to write letters, knit, and practice computer graphics during those times.

Sensory Integration Interventions

There is growing research connecting sensory defensiveness in adults with increased levels of anxiety, depression, and maladjustment (Kinnealey & Fuiek, 1999). Hypersensitivity as well as hyposensitivity to sensory stimuli and difficulty modulating and integrating input are characteristics of sensory defensive individuals. As with clinical anxiety disorders, to outsiders these sources of anxiety, of difficulty in sensory processing, may look harmless when in fact they cause great distress, even leading to panic attacks in the sufferers. Exposure to many sources of sensory input, including certain noises, unexpected movement, tastes, smells, and physical touch, may be interpreted as aversive and anxiety-producing, and therefore are either avoided or approached with great caution (Kinnealey, Oliver, & Wilbarger, 1995). This vulnerability to the environment and decreased coping strategies may lead to significant restrictions in daily activities in order to avoid anxiety and distress, and greatly influences all aspects of life.

It is postulated that since many symptoms of sensory defensiveness may be interchangeable with those of mental disorders, especially GAD, panic disorder, and phobias, poor sensory regulation may actually contribute to the development of anxiety disorders. For instance, someone with tactile defensiveness who avoided going on subways because of the aversive nature of being in physical contact with crowds could also be labeled as having a phobia of subways. On the other hand, because of the pervasive impact on all aspects of one's life, it has been suggested that sensory defensiveness should be viewed as a stand-alone diagnosis, "sensory affective disorder," which encompasses both the physical and emotional aspects of the condition (Wilberger, cited in Heller, 2002).

Current research is exploring sensory integration interventions for decreasing levels of anxiety such as deep pressure, tactile, and proprioceptive activities in both adults and children. Providing a "sensory diet" in order to maintain a balance of arousal and tolerance while incorporating a person's interests and needs is described in the literature (Kinnealey, Oliver, & Wilbarger, 1995). A personal account by a psychologist, survivor, and client advocate, Dr. Pat Deegan, praises the work of an occupational therapist, specializing in treating sensory defensiveness in adults, for her assistance in helping Deegan, as an adult, resolve childhood abuse issues though sensory interventions: joint compression, tactile brushing, and sand blankets (Deegan, 2001). Numerous practical, everyday strategies for managing sensory defensiveness in adults are described in Heller's book *Too Loud, Too Bright, Too Fast, Too Tight* (2002). Recommendations cover a range of topics from doing physical exercises to making the environment more pleasing.

CASE ILLUSTRATION: Sharman—Occupational Therapy Assessment and Treatment

A young, single woman reported problems in job performance following the development of a phobia and subsequent depression. Her usual route to work included driving on a particularly busy street where she had witnessed a catastrophic car accident. Shortly after the accident she developed acute anxiety when driving on this street, so she began to take a more circuitous route to avoid the scene of the accident, which invariably made her late for work. She also became highly distractible, especially during the last hour of the workday as she mentally prepared to go home. In addition, she had difficulty organizing her various work tasks and had been counseled by her employer on several occasions. As her anxiety mounted about losing her job and her performance declined, she took a leave from work in order to attend a partial hospitalization program.

Assessment

Sharman's Role Checklist (see Figure 8-10) indicated difficulty in performing the worker role and the high value Sharman placed on it. The Function Questionnaire (see Figure 8-11) indicated moderate to severe impairment in work because of anxiety. Sharman's Self-Assessment of Activities (see Figure 8-12) reported problems in concentration, job insecurity, excessive worry, poor coping strategies, and problem solving, and Sharman's Activity Configuration (see Figure 8-13) indicated that not enough time was allotted for commuting.

In reviewing the results with Sharman, the occupational therapist confirmed her strong motivation to be able to resume her usual roles, particularly that of employee. Research was shared with Sharman (Prior, 1998) demonstrating that a short-term anxiety management course at a mental health day hospital significantly decreased anxiety in its attendees, as measured by the Hospital Anxiety and Depression Scale (Zigmond & Snaith, 1983). The groups were also rated highly in respect to helpfulness. The content of the course covered the nature of the anxiety and learning techniques for managing it. Homework was included in addition to the class exercises in cognitive and behavioral aspects, breathing and relaxation, and assertiveness. A second study giving credence to a short-

ROLE CHECKLIST

NAME __S. T.__ AGE __26__ DATE __2-24-95__

SEX: ☐ MALE ☑ FEMALE   ARE YOU RETIRED: ☐ YES ☑ NO

MARITAL STATUS: ☑ SINGLE ☐ MARRIED ☐ SEPARATED ☐ DIVORCED ☐ WIDOWED

The purpose of this checklist is to identify the major roles in your life. The checklist, which is divided into two parts, presents 10 roles and defines each one.

PART I

Beside each role, indicate, by checking the appropriate column, if you performed the role in the past, if you presently perform the role, and if you plan to perform the role in the future. You may check more than one column for each role. For example, if you volunteered in the past, do not volunteer at present, but plan to in the future, you would check the past and future columns.

ROLE	PAST	PRESENT	FUTURE
STUDENT: Attending school on a part-time or full-time basis.	✓		
WORKER: Part-time or full-time paid employment.	✓	✓	✓
VOLUNTEER: Donating services, **at least once a week,** to a hospital, school, community, political campaign, and so forth.	✓		
CARE GIVER: Responsibility, **at least once a week,** for the care of someone such as a child, spouse, relative, or friend.			✓
HOME MAINTAINER: Responsibility, **at least once a week,** for the upkeep of the home such as housecleaning or yardwork.	✓	✓	✓
FRIEND: Spending time or doing something, **at least once a week,** with a friend.	✓	✓	✓
FAMILY MEMBER: Spending time or doing something, **at least once a week,** with a family member such as a child, spouse, parent, or other relative.	✓		✓
RELIGIOUS PARTICIPANT: Involvement, **at least once a week,** in groups or activities affiliated with one's religion (excluding worship).	✓		
HOBBYIST/AMATEUR: Involvement, **at least once a week,** in a hobby or amateur activity such as sewing, playing a musical instrument, woodworking, sports, the theater, or participation in a club or team.	✓		✓
PARTICIPANT IN ORGANIZATIONS: Involvement, **at least once a week,** in organizations such as the American Legion, National Organization for Women, Parents Without Partners, Weight Watchers, and so forth.			
OTHER:_____ A role not listed which you have performed, are presently performing, and/or plan to perform. Write the role on the line above and check the appropriate column(s).			

Figure 8-10. Sharman's Role Checklist

Source: Reprinted with permission from Frances Oakley, MS, OTR, FAOTA.

term stress management group for inpatients using a cognitive-behavioral and psychoeducational approach was also described to Sharman (Stein & Smith, 1989). The primary diagnosis of these hospitalized clients was depression, but they too showed significant decrease on the State-Trait Anxiety Scale (Spielberger, 1983) following attendance in the six-session course. As with the other program, they were taught a variety of relaxation techniques and communication skills, but also learned biofeedback and pleasant visualization to reduce anxiety.

PART II

The same roles are listed below. Next to *each* role check the column which best indicates how valuable or important the role is to you. Answer for *each role,* even if you have never performed or do not plan to perform the role.

ROLE	NOT AT ALL VALUABLE	SOMEWHAT VALUABLE	VERY VALUABLE
STUDENT: Attending school on a part-time or full-time basis.		✓	
WORKER: Part-time or full-time paid employment.			✓
VOLUNTEER: Donating services, **at least once a week,** to a hospital, school, community, political campaign, and so forth.		✓	
CARE GIVER: Responsibility, **at least once a week,** for the care of someone such as a child, spouse, relative, or friend.		✓	
HOME MAINTAINER: Responsibility, **at least once a week,** for the upkeep of the home such as housecleaning or yardwork.		✓	
FRIEND: Spending time or doing something, **at least once a week,** with a friend.			✓
FAMILY MEMBER: Spending time or doing something, **at least once a week,** with a family member such as a child, spouse, parent, or other relative.		✓	
RELIGIOUS PARTICIPANT: Involvement, **at least once a week,** in groups or activities affiliated with one's religion (excluding worship).		✓	
HOBBYIST/AMATEUR: Involvement, **at least once a week,** in a hobby or amateur activity such as sewing, playing a musical instrument, woodworking, sports, the theater, or participation in a club or team.			✓
PARTICIPANT IN ORGANIZATIONS: Involvement, **at least once a week,** in organizations such as the American Legion, National Organization for Women, Parents Without Partners, Weight Watchers, and so forth.	✓		
OTHER:_____ A role not listed which you have performed, are presently performing, and/or plan to perform. Write the role on the line above and check the appropriate column(s).			

Occupational Therapy Service, Department of Rehabilitation Medicine, Clinical Center, National institutes of Health

*U.S. GOVERNMENT PRINTING OFFICE: 1985-526-620:30339

Figure 8-10.   *(continued)*

Goals

The overall goal of the occupational therapy program was to assist the client in functioning more effectively in her role as worker, particularly through improved coping strategies. After hearing the evidence about the success of stress management groups in decreasing anxiety, she agreed to attend a similar group three times a week for an hour as well as to work individually with the OTR three times a week for half-hour sessions. In addi-tion, she joined the leisure exploration simulation groups, which each met for one hour weekly. The objectives and interventions to reach this goal were as follows:

Objective	*Intervention*	*Method*
1. Client will have knowledge of alternative forms of transportation	Community mobility through exploration of resources—bus routes, carpool accessibility, and alternative routes for driving	Individual OT Session
2. Client will plan daily schedule to ensure arriving at work on time	Training in time management—prioritization of activities and strategies to follow schedule	Individual OT Session
3. Client will learn and apply one method of relaxation to decrease general anxiety and to facilitate getting to work	Relaxation training—breathing and visualization exercises	Stress Management Group
4. Client will concentrate for 60 minutes on one task while at the program and for 60 minutes on one task at home	Leisure and job simulation activities	Leisure Group and Homework
5. Client will apply one strategy to neutralize fears that impede performance	Cognitive techniques focused on rational thinking	Stress Management Group

Treatment

The occupational therapy program proceeded as follows:

Learning and applying relaxation techniques: Sharman's anxiety was focused primarily on the witnessed accident as she thought about or actually commuted to and from work. However, merely thinking about the accident or about her work problems throughout the day caused rapid heartbeat, nausea, and poor concentration. The occupational therapist initially instructed Sharman in abdominal breathing during a group session. This method taught her to use her lungs more fully through deep breathing, since anxiety symptoms may be exacerbated with shallow breathing. She was trained to be aware of her abdomen rising as she took slow and deep breaths. Her position was supine on the floor on a blanket with her legs bent.

Sharman was told to practice this exercise once a day supine and one or two times a day in a sitting position. Each session was to last two minutes in the

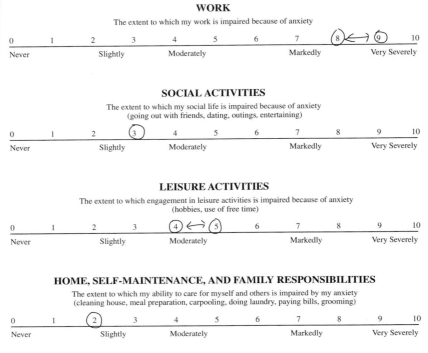

Figure 8-11.   Sharman's Function Questionnaire

beginning and later to be expanded to about five minutes. In addition, she was coached to make use of this technique immediately while sitting in her chair whenever she experienced an initial sign of anxiety. She was also cautioned to return to her normal breathing patterns if she experienced any lightheadedness from increased oxygen flow. Sharman developed skill in using this breathing technique to combat her anxiety symptoms, such as nausea and poor concentration, and subsequently felt less helpless when symptoms appeared during the day.

Visualization and breathing were combined for the second phase. First, the occupational therapist, in an individual session, helped Sharman identify and visualize in her imagination a comfortable, safe place. To help guide the exercise, the OT instructed her to describe places she had been that inspired a sense of well-being. Since Sharman particularly enjoyed the ocean, this was incorporated in the visualization. After first directing her in abdominal breathing, the OT instructed her to imagine being at the beach, while combining sounds, noises, and smells into the picture to strengthen the image. Two 10- to 15-minute sessions a day, to be done at home independently, were prescribed once Sharman had learned to concentrate and attain a state of relaxation with the therapist's assistance. After two weeks, she was able to perform this exercise independently and practiced it before going to the program, work, and bed.

Self-Assessment of Activities

Name: _S T_

Date: _2-2-4-95_

This checklist will be used to help develop an Occupational Therapy program for you. Mark the appropriate column for each item and add any comments you feel would be helpful.

Activity	Never a problem	Sometimes a problem	Always a problem	N.A.	Comments
Grooming	✓				
Bathing or showering		✓			*I tend to stay in too long -- 20 minutes*
Preparing meals	✓				
Food shopping		✓			*I don't like to drive to supermarket*
Doing errands		✓			*If I have to go down a particular street*
House cleaning	✓				
Doing yardwork	✓				
Caring for others				✓	
Managing money	✓				
Transportation			✓		*I am having difficulty driving -- very anxious*
Socializing					
Attending school				✓	
Working			✓		*Not as focused or organized as I used to be*
Volunteering				✓	
Exercising	✓				
Concentrating			✓		*I worry all the time about work, driving.*
Problem solving		✓			*I can't seem to figure out my problems*
Communicating		✓			*Most people O.K. but I avoid my boss*
Coping with stress			✓		*I get overwhelmed by anxiety*
Managing time			✓		*Always a problem regarding getting to work*
Managing impulses		✓			
Doing leisure activities		✓			*Not as motivated as in past*

Figure 8-12. Sharman's Self-Assessment of Activities

The final phase of training focused on the client visualizing, after completing the two previous steps, driving down the dreaded street in her car. When anxiety surfaced during this exercise, she was told to return to the calming image she had learned to picture. She reported difficulty mastering this aspect of treatment although she continued to practice regularly at home as well as deal with the phobia directly with a psychologist using desensitization techniques, by alleviating anxiety through controlled exposure to the scene of the accident.

Overcoming irrational fears: Sharman reported worrying excessively about projected failures; that is, being shunned by her coworkers, being fired by her boss,

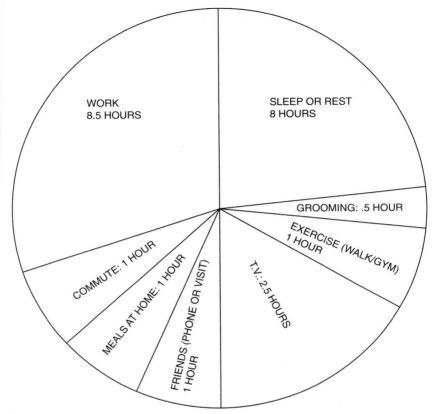

Figure 8-13.   Sharman's Activity Configuration Prior to Treatment

having an anxiety attack while driving, and a host of other events. This response led to a heightened state of arousal and caused her either to avoid important activities or feel distressed while doing them. This negative thinking contributed to her depressive symptoms as well. Sharman responded well to the stress management group session in which cognitive strategies were discussed. The occupational therapist helped her develop more realistic ways to perceive current and future events through changing her self-talk about the expected outcome. This was accomplished by first assisting Sharman in completing worksheets that helped to challenge her irrational thinking and then substitute more realistic thinking. The "Daily Mood Log" (Burns, 1993) was one effective tool for this. Here, using a three-column form, she first documented her negative thoughts, then her distorted thoughts (taken from a preprinted list), and finally positive thoughts she could substitute. Her challenge to her worry that she would be rejected by her co-workers was this was "jumping to conclusions." There was no evidence that others viewed her as defective or weak since she had to take a leave from work. In fact, she had received a few phone calls inquiring about her well-being from people with whom she worked. Her positive thoughts included: (1) people will likely be supportive of my actions to get help; (2) others could feel closer to me since I have exposed my vulnerabilities; (3) even if the people at work reject me, there are many others who like me and it does not mean I am a bad person. Other cognitive strategies included telling herself that her life would not come to an end if she were fired and that searching for a new job would be inconvenient rather than a failure. She further reminded herself that many others had lived through this experience and had even found the subsequent change rewarding.

Improving concentration: Sharman had reported difficulty attending to work tasks. Simulated leisure and work activities were introduced into the treatment program with the goal to work for 60 minutes uninterrupted in occupational therapy and then 60 minutes at home on predefined tasks. If she did work tasks in the program, she did a leisure activity at home, and vice versa.

In the past Sharman had enjoyed ceramics, and in particular, making necklaces. She readily accepted the idea of making jewelry using commercial beads and other materials. Sessions were initially 15 to 30 minutes long and involved uncomplicated techniques such as stringing beads for simple necklaces, but as her concentration improved, they were lengthened to 60 minutes and made to incorporate more complex tasks such as making fashion earrings and constructing beads from a quick-drying substitute clay material. She became so enthusiastic about this activity that she started going to yard sales to buy old, inexpensive jewelry to rework for her new hobby. She also found that engaging in this task helped to dissipate her anxiety at times when it surfaced at home.

Sharman's employment was as office assistant, and her workload consisted of a variety of clerical tasks. The occupational therapist was able to simulate some of these activities by requesting participation in a volunteer project the program had undertaken (assisting with a blood drive). Making up a flyer on the computer, writing letters to local businesses and organizations for support, and compiling blood donation packets were some of the tasks involved. Sharman also made a list of related jobs she needed to accomplish at home; specifically, reorganizing her financial files, working on her tax return, and updating her computer records. She made agreements with the occupational therapist as to the specific tasks and deadlines for jobs to be done at home.

Arriving at work on time: Sharman's late arrival at work was generally the result of not allowing enough time for the task. She was used to her usual half-hour commute prior to the development of the phobia. The OT helped her to adjust other activities by reprioritizing them in order to accommodate the extra one to two hours (round trip) now needed when she drove herself by the longer alternate route. By categorizing her activities away from work from most valued to least valued (Lakein, 1973), she decided to decrease her evening time watching television ("least valued") and to wake up one hour earlier. To make the transition to the earlier wake-up time, she decided to prepare and lay out her clothes the night before, reduce her lengthy shower time, and read only half the newspaper over breakfast. As Sharman advanced in her partial hospitalization treatment program, she discarded television altogether and replaced it with a new hobby and therapy "homework."

In all these activities, the occupational therapist strategized with the client on ways to stay focused on the task at hand. Creating an uncluttered work environment and removing distracting stimuli proved helpful. At home, Sharman turned off her telephone for one hour while she worked, and she agreed to get up from her desk only once during that time. If distracted, she was able to cue herself by saying, "I am able to focus on this task," and doing one minute of deep breathing. Sharman reported increased concentration and was able to meet her goals.

Sharman stayed in the partial hospitalization program for four weeks and then returned to work, commuting by bus. She planned to join a carpool the following month, paying a small fee to members so that she would not be required to drive until her phobia was more resolved through continued work on this issue with her psychologist. She employed relaxation techniques and cognitive strategies to cope with anxiety throughout the day and reported a notable reduction in anxiety and improved concentration. Leisure activities also served as an outlet for her tension as well as a focus through which to override her irrational thoughts. Sharman made the transition into a new daily schedule in order to wake up earlier starting before her actual return to work and consequently was no longer late to her job. She became more self-confident as she showed improved performance in her worker role as well as a newly developed role as a hobbyist.

Summary

Occupational therapists work with people with anxiety disorders in a variety of treatment settings from acute psychiatric hospitals to home care programs. As changes in health care policies reduce the length of hospital stays, treatment is occurring more often in community settings.

Anxiety may be a mental disorder, as outlined in *DSM-IV-TR,* or it may be a component of a physical or other psychiatric illness. The major disorders described in *DSM-IV-TR* include panic disorder without and with agoraphobia, agoraphobia without history of panic attacks, specific phobia, social phobia, obsessive-compulsive disorder, post-traumatic stress disorder, acute stress disorder, and generalized anxiety disorder. When anxiety accompanies a physical illness, it may actually have been induced by a hormonal imbalance or other medical condition. On the other hand, anxiety may be the outcome of coping with a life-threatening illness and thus be likely to dissipate when the medical problem is resolved.

Differentiating between a true anxiety syndrome and normal anxiety is sometimes difficult. Anxiety is universal and often helpful, being related to the fight-or-flight response. However, when anxiety impairs rather than enhances functional performance, it becomes pathological. Anxiety symptoms fall into several categories: emotional, physiological, cognitive, and behavioral. Usually people experience some symptoms in each of these areas.

Treatment strategies aim to reduce symptoms, prevent relapse, and improve functioning. Approaches used by other health professionals include medications, psychotherapy, biofeedback, cognitive interventions, systematic desensitization, and couples therapy.

Occupational therapists work with individuals and families to improve functioning and adaptive behavior in everyday activities as well as the individual's perceived quality of life. Anxiety disorders are always accompanied by great emotional discomfort, which impacts both the client and the family. Anxious people inevitably restrict their lives in order to accommodate the dysfunction. A parent may refuse to take family vacations because of a fear of crossing bridges or flying in an airplane. Another person may give up a satisfying job because of panic attacks. An older adult may drive away everyone in her support system with her excessive, relentless worrying. The challenge for the occupational therapist is to help the client cope and therefore function productively. Improving effectiveness may be accomplished by actually reducing the level of anxiety, or it may be achieved by teaching the client to grapple with life stresses in spite of anxiety. Both strategies involve the development of self-management skills. Empowering the client through instruction in acquiring and developing these skills can be extremely beneficial. Relaxation, assertiveness and general social skills training, community mobility, expressive craft and art activities, the functional behavior approach, education/lifestyle alterations, rational/cognitive approaches, and time management are key strategies. Anxiety often takes a chronic course and requires much adaptation. Many people with anxiety are able to live productively when given the tools to cope more effectively.

Review Questions

1. What occupational therapy goals might a home health clinician establish for a homebound elderly woman who has panic attacks when she attempts to leave the house to visit friends or do daily errands?
2. What types of community programs might assist someone who has not been able to work for several years because of flashbacks that impair concentration?
3. How could an occupational therapist simultaneously address a hospitalized student's stress disorder and depression following the sudden death of a parent?
4. Which types of relaxation training might be most successful with an adult with attention deficit disorder as well as generalized anxiety disorder?
5. What are the first steps you would take to address obsessive compulsive, PTSD, agoraphobia or GAD in a person you treat as part of a home health program?

References

Agras, S. (1985). *Panic: Facing fears, phobias, and anxiety.* Stanford: Stanford Alumni Association.
Agras, S., & Berkowitz, R. (1994). Behavior therapy. In R. E. Hales, S. C. Udofsky, & J. A. Talbott (Eds.), *Textbook of psychiatry* (2nd ed., pp. 1061–1081). Washington, DC: American Psychiatric Press.

American Psychiatric Association (APA). (2000). *Diagnostic and statistical manual of mental disorders*-Text Revision. (4th ed.). Washington, DC: APA.

Anxiety Disorders Association of America. (2002). *Brief overview of anxiety disorders.* Retrieved June 10, 2002, from http://www.adaa.org/AnxietyDisorderInfor/OverviewAnxDis.cfm.

Bandura, A. (1977). Self-efficacy: Towards a unifying theory of behavioral change. *Psychological Review, 84*(2), 191–215.

Bandura, A. (1995). *Self-efficacy in changing societies.* New York: Cambridge University Press.

Benson, H. (1976). *The relaxation response.* Boston: G. K. Hall.

Bonder, B. R. (1991). *Psychopathology and function.* Thorofare, NJ: Slack.

Booth, R. J., & Petrie, K. (2002). Emotional expression and health changes: Can we identify biological pathways? In S. Lepore & J. Smyth (Eds.), *The writing cure* (pp. 157–175). Washington, DC: American Psychological Association.

Bourne, E. (2000). *Anxiety and phobia workbook* (3rd ed.). Oakland, CA: New Harbinger.

Burns, D. D. (1999). *Ten days to self-esteem.* New York: Quill.

Clark, D., Salkovskis, P., & Chalkley, A. (1985). Respiratory control as a treatment for panic attacks. *Behavior Therapy and Experimental Psychiatry, 16*(1), 23–30.

Davis, M., Eshelman, E., & McKay, M. (1988). *The relaxation and stress reduction workbook* (3rd ed.). Oakland, CA: New Harbinger.

Davidson, J. R. (2001). Recognition and treatment of posttraumatic stress disorder. *Journal of the American Medical Association, 286*(5), 584–588.

Deegan, P. E. (2001). *Recovery as a self-directed process of healing and transformation.* Retrieved October 15, 2002, from http://www.intentionalcare.org/art_re.htm

Depoy, E., & Kolodner, E. (1991). Psychological performance factors. In C. Christiansen & C. Baum (Eds.), *Occupational therapy—Overcoming human performance deficits* (pp. 304–332). Thorofare, NJ: Slack.

Ellis, A. (1976). *Growth through reason.* North Hollywood, CA: Wilshire.

Freeman, L. W., & Lawlis, F. G. (Eds.). (2001). *Complementary & alternative medicine.* St. Louis, MO: Mosby.

Hales, R. E., Udofsky, S. C., & Talbott, J. A. (Eds.). (1994). *Textbook of psychiatry* (2nd ed.). Washington, DC: American Psychiatric Press.

Heller, S. (2002). *Too loud, too bright, too fast, too tight: What to do if you are sensory defensive in an overstimulating world.* New York: HarperCollins.

Jacobson, E. (1938). *Progressive relaxation.* Chicago: University of Chicago Press.

Kielhofner, G. (Ed.). (2002). *A model of human occupation: Theory and application* (3rd ed.). Baltimore: Williams & Wilkins.

Kinnealey, M., & Fuiek, M. (1999). The relationship between sensory defensiveness, anxiety, and perception of pain in adults. *Occupational Therapy International, 6*(3), 195–206.

Kinnealey, M., Oliver, B., & Wilbarger, P. (1995). A phenomenological study of sensory defensiveness in adults. *American Journal of Occupational Therapy, 49*(5), 444–451.

Krug, S. I., Scheier, I. H., & Cattell, R. B. (1976). *Handbook for the IPAT anxiety scale.* Champagne, IL: Institute for Personality and Ability Testing.

Lakein, A. (1973). *How to get control of your time and your life.* New York: David McKay.

Liebgold, H. (2000). *Curing anxiety, phobias, shyness, and OCD.* San Rafael, CA: Liebro.

Miller, M. C., & Bakalar, J. (Eds.). (2003). Generalized anxiety disorder: Toxic worry. *Harvard Mental Health Letter, 19*(7), 1–4.

McKay, M., Davis, M., & Fanning, P. (1981). *Thoughts and feelings: The art of cognitive stress intervention.* Richmond, CA: Hew Harbinger.

NIMH. (n.d.). *Anxiety disorders.* Retrieved March 10, 2003, from http:www.nimh.nih.gov/anxiety/anxiety.cfm.

Oakley, F., Kielhofner, G., Barris, R., & Reichler, R. (1986). The role checklist: Development and empirical assessment of reliability. *Occupational Therapy Journal of Research, 6*, 157–170.

Ohio State University. (2003). *Anxiety and stress disorders: Clinic treatment and therapies.* Retrieved June 11, 2003, from http://anxiety.psy.ohio-state.edu/treatment.htm.

Pennebaker, J. (2002). Writing about emotional events: From past to future. In S. Lepore & J. Smyth (Eds.), *The writing cure* (pp. 281–292). Washington, DC: American Psychological Association.

Prior, S. (1998). Determining the effectiveness of a short-term anxiety management course. *British Journal of Occupational Therapy, 61*(5), 207–213.

Roth, A., & Fonagy, P. (1996). *What works for whom: A critical review of psychotherapy research*. New York: Guilford.

Sims, A., & Snaith, P. (1988). *Anxiety in clinical practice*. New York: Wiley.

Smyth, J. M., Stone, A. A., Hurewitz, A., & Kaell, A. (1999). Effects of writing about stressful experiences on symptom reduction in patients with asthma or rheumatoid arthritis. *Journal of American Medical Association, 281*(14), 1304–1309.

Spielberger, C. D. (1983). *State-Trait Anxiety Inventory for Adults*. Redwood City, CA: Mind Garden.

Stein, F., & Nikolic, S. (1989). Teaching stress management techniques to a schizophrenic patient. *American Journal of Occupational Therapy, 43*(3), 162–169.

Stein, F., & Smith, J. (1989). Short-term stress management programme with acutely depressed inpatients. *Canadian Journal of Occupational Therapy, 56*(4) 185–191.

Taylor, B., & Arnow, B. (1988). *The nature and treatment of anxiety disorders*. New York: Free Press.

Telch, M. J. (1982). *A comparison of behavioral and pharmacological approaches to the treatment of agoraphobia*. Unpublished doctoral dissertation, Stanford University, Stanford, CA.

Tickle-Degnen, L. (1998). Using research evidence in planning treatment for the individual client. *Canadian Journal of Occupational Therapy, 65* (31), 152–159.

Weissman, M., Myers, J., & Harding, P. (1978). Psychiatric disorders in a U.S. urban community: 1975–1976. *American Journal of Psychiatry, 135*(4) 459–462.

Wolpe, J. (1973). *The practice of behavior therapy*. Elmsford, NY: Pergamon.

Wright, J. H., & Beck, A. T. (1994). Cognitive therapy. In R. E. Hales, S. C. Udofsky, & J. A. Talbott (Eds.), *Textbook of psychiatry* (2nd ed., pp. 1083–1114). Washington, DC: American Psychiatric Press.

Zigmond, A., & Snaith, R. (1983). *The Hospital Anxiety and Depression Scale*. Windsor, UK: NFER Nelson.

Suggested Reading and Other Resources

Assertiveness Training and Life Management

McKay, M., Davis, M., & Fanning, P. (1983). *Messages: The communication skills book*. Oakland, CA: New Harbinger.

Korb, K., Azok, S., & Leutenberg, E. (1989). *Life management skills I*. Beachwood, OH: Wellness Reproductions.

Korb, K., Azok, S., & Leutenberg, E. (1991). *Life management skills II*. Beachwood, OH: Wellness Reproductions.

Korb-Khalsa, K., Azok, S., & Leutenberg, E. (1994). *Life management skills III*. Beachwood, OH: Wellness Reproductions.

Relaxation

Bourne, E. (2000). *Anxiety and phobia workbook* (3rd ed.). Oakland, CA: New Harbinger.

Burns, D. D. (1999). *The feeling good handbook* (rev. ed.). New York: Penguin/Plume.

Davis, M., Eshelman, E., & McKay, M. (1988). *The relaxation and stress reduction workbook* (3rd ed.). Oakland, CA: New Harbinger.

Ellis, A. (1978). *A new guide to rational living*. North Hollywood, CA: Wilshire.

Gawain, S. (1978). *Creative visualization*. San Rafael, CA: New World Library.

Liebgold, H. (2000). *Curing anxiety, phobias, shyness, and OCD*. San Rafael, CA: Liebro.

McKay, M., Davis, M., & Fanning, P. (1981). *Thoughts and feelings: the art of cognitive stress intervention*. Richmond, CA: New Harbinger.

Wolpe, J. (1973). *The practice of behavior therapy*. Elmsford, NJ: Pergamon.

Expressive Art Activities

Capacchione, L. (1989). *The creative journal*. North Hollywood, CA: Newcastle.
Capacchione, L. (1990). *The picture of health: Healing your life with art*. Carson, CA: Hay House.
Progoff, I. (1992). *At a journal workshop*. New York: G. P. Putnam's Sons. (Originally published 1975).

Relaxation Tapes

East West Book Shop
324 Castro Avenue
Mountain View, CA 94041-1297
(415) 988-9800
http://www.eastwest.comSource (Tapes by Emmet Miller)

P.O. Box 803
Nevada City, CA 95959
(800) 52-TAPES
www.drmiller.com

Time Management

Lakein, A. (1973). *How to get control of your time and your life*. New York: David McKay.

Personality Disorders

Elizabeth Cara, PhD, OTR, MFT

Key Terms

affective instability
dimensions
ego syntonic
"hardwired"

personality
splitting
traits

Chapter Outline

Introduction

There has been a change in the perception of personality disorders over the last two decades based on research, diverse approaches, and contributions from different disciplines (Livesley, 2001). The first edition of this book focused on the difficulties of understanding and working with personality disorders. However, current treatments based on explicit directions and manuals for working with those with personality disorders, primarily borderline personality disorders, have demonstrated empirical efficacy. (See Table 9-1 for a description of various theories of personality disorders that guide treatment.) Also, long-term research studies (Paris, 2002) and a better understanding of biological and genetic origins and developmental mechanisms are changing approaches to treatment and are increasing understanding of personality disorders (Livesley, 2001). Research shows that distress caused by personality disorders can be ameliorated to some extent and there is cause for optimism (Gunderson & Gabbard, 2001).

Individuals with personality disorders can indeed be treated, and occupational therapy, with its focus on adaptive functioning and behavior in everyday life, can be helpful. In fact, individuals with personality disorders often are bright, charming, and creative. Because of the challenges and opportunities for self-learning that may occur in treatment, they can be rewarding and gratifying clients.

Because personality disorders are axis II diagnoses, there will usually be another axis I condition, such as depression, post-traumatic stress, generalized anxiety, or substance addiction that brings an individual with a personality disorder into mental health treatment settings. In addition, people with personality disorders may be seen in other than mental health settings, for example, in a treatment setting for traumatic brain injury subsequent to a failed suicide attempt, in physical rehabilitation subsequent to impulsive behavior that resulted in a diving or driving accident, or in pediatric settings where a child's behavior may in part be a response to poor parenting skills or dysfunctional family relationships. Because occupational therapy focuses on adaptive function and behavior in everyday life, it is a very important aspect of treatment. The methods and strategies grounded in occupations provide opportunities to modify behavior. Because problems manifest in both the social and interpersonal realms, it is necessary for the therapist to be competent not only in occupational treatment methods, but also in the use of self and interpersonal communication. Therefore, a willingness to reflect and understand oneself, including one's conscious and unconscious motivations, values, thoughts, feelings, and responses, is vitally important for the occupational therapist (see Chapter 18, Approaches and Techniques, for a discussion of the self and interpersonal skills).

THE PERSONALITY CONTINUUM AND ETIOLOGY OF PERSONALITY DISORDERS

A brief review of what is entailed in the concept of personality will help to clarify what is meant by a "disorder" or "dysfunction" of personality. Personality could

Table 9-1. Theories of Personality Disorders

Biophysical   Anticipate that chemical deficiencies or other defects will be found that account for symptoms. Just as physical disease represents a disease of the organ system that manifests in the realm of the physical body, psychological disease reflects central nervous system disruptions that will manifest in the realm of behavior, emotions, and thought (Sadock & Sadock, 2000).

Neuropsychiatric   Recognize the influence of the neurobiological system on mood and behavioral symptoms. Neuroanatomical (functional) and neurochemical (operational) aspects are assessed to determine how they are causing or amplifying symptoms. It holds that intrinsic dispositions are modifiable by medicine, environments can be changed, and biological factors underlie some dimensions of personality disorders (Ratey, 1995).

Psychodynamic   Emphasize the impact of early experiences and past events. Early theories were based on the model of the ego, id, and superego that defined the disorder depending on which structure predominated—the id with predominant erotic behavior, the ego with narcissistic behavior, and the superego with compulsive behavior. Traits were later associated with frustrations or indulgences during the psychosexual stages. Character formations were thought to have a defensive function. Currently, Kernberg posits three levels of structural organization: psychotic, borderline, or neurotic. Those with normal personalities have a cohesive sense of self and ego-strength to remain integrated in spite of pressure from internal or external forces and have a mature internalization of social values (Millon, Meagher, & Grossman, 2001) while those with personality disorders experience disintegration of sense of self under pressure and do not fully internalize values. Contemporary theories focus on the infant-caregiver environment.

Behavioral   Emphasize environmental influences and learning from the social environment (Sadock & Sadock, 2000). Currently assess three response systems: verbal-cognitive mode, affective-physiological mode, and overt-motor response system (Millon, Meagher, & Grossman, 2001).

Cognitive   Individuals react to the world depending on their perception of it. A person's way of construing the world determines behavior. Dysfunctional feelings and behaviors reflect biased schemas and result in repetitive interpersonal errors (Millon, 1996).

Interpersonal   Personality is understood in terms of recurrent interpersonal tendencies that are the social product of interactions with significant others (Millon, Meagher, & Grossman, 2001) and shape and perpetuate styles of behavior, thought, and feeling. An individual always transacts with real others or with her or his expectations about them. All important events in life are interpersonal. There are maladaptive causal sequences between interpersonal perceptions, behavior, and others' reactions. Sequences are often activated in inappropriate situations.

Biopsychosocial/Evolutionary   An interaction of biology and environment determines whether traits become disorders. In the presence of psychological risk factors such as trauma, loss, or inadequate parenting, personality traits tend to be amplified. Also called *predisposition stress theory* (Paris, 1994). Newer theory looks at how disorders represent maladaptive functions due to inability to relate in the environment (Millon, 1996).

Neurobiological/Temperaments   Biological constitutional dispositions are central to understanding personality disorders. Attempt to break down constituents of temperament that underlie personality traits, for example, neurotransmitter types may relate to certain dimensions of personality. Traits or dispositions may be associated with a particular neurotransmitter system (Millon, Meagher, & Grossman, 2001).

be considered to comprise a person's lifelong style of relating, coping, behaving, thinking, and feeling. The concept represents a network of traits that emerge from a matrix of biological dispositions and experiential learning, persist over extended periods of time, and characterize the individual's distinctive manner of relating in the environment (Millon, 1996). There are regularities and consistencies in behavior and forms of experience. There is a consistency and coherence to a person's experiences. Personality is not just a collection of traits but an organization that is cohesive and coherent (Livesley, 2001).

Every individual possesses a small and distinct group of primary traits that persist and endure and that exhibit a high degree of consistency across situations. These enduring (stable) and pervasive (consistent) characteristics make up a person's personality. The personality pattern, that is, the repertoire of coping skills and adaptive flexibilities, will determine whether a person will master his or her psychosocial environments. Millon (1996) views personality as composed of three polarities: positive versus negative, self versus other, and active versus passive. These polarities represent an individual's survival mode. That is, people will be motivated by the type of reinforcement they seek, whether the pursuit of pleasure or the avoidance of pain, relying on self or others for support and nurturing, and behaving in an active and controlling, or more accommodating and reactive, way (Millon, 1996).

There are two features that distinguish a personality disorder: chronic interpersonal difficulties and problems with self and identity. Chronic interpersonal difficulties are "repetitive maladaptive patterns of thoughts, feelings and actions that occur in relationship to others" (Livesley, 2001, p. 10). Problems with self and identity include a failure to develop an integrated sense of identity during adolescence, a poorly integrated sense of self and significant others, and faulty beliefs or thoughts used to process information regarding self and others.

Those people whose personality patterns do not permit consistent mastery of the psychosocial environment can be distinguished from their normal counterparts by:

• Adaptive inflexibility and poor choices of behavior
• A tendency to foster vicious circles
• Tenuous stability under stressful conditions, that is, a tendency to decompensate during times of crisis or stress

See Table 9-2 for a description of maladaptive personality patterns.

Problems of personality thus include stable and consistent traits that are not easily changed, are exhibited inappropriately and in situations in which they are not warranted, and foster vicious cycles of behavior that are difficult to stop and perpetuate and intensify already-present difficulties (Millon, 1981). Daily life activities and interactions cause overwhelming stress. This triggers maladaptive responses, which further heighten the stress and preclude obtaining support or help from others. Thus the vicious circle is put in motion. The individual with a personality disorder lacks the flexibility to choose from a broad range of interper-

Table 9-2.	Maladaptive Personality Patterns
Pattern	*Description*
Adaptive Flexibility	Interpersonal strategies for relating to others, achieving goals, and coping with stress are limited and practiced rigidly. Choices of behavior often do not match the situation in which they are used.
Vicious Circles	Person's choices elicit similar rigid or extreme responses from others. Little understanding of poor choices and how the "wrong" behaviors have "pulled" for other's responses. Consequently, there is little awareness of responsibility for the interactions and inability to change behavior. This sets into motion additional poor choices of behavior and self-defeating sequences with others, which cause already-established difficulties not only to persist but to be aggravated further.
Tenuous Stability	Lack of resilience in conditions perceived as stressful, causing extreme susceptibility to new difficulties and disruptions and reversion to familiar, maladaptive ways of coping. There is lessened control over emotions and a tendency toward developing increasingly distorted perceptions of reality.

Source: Adapted from Millon (1981).

sonal behaviors. He or she may rigidly rely on the same interpersonal behavior or choose an extreme form of behavior that is not warranted in every situation. These poor behavioral choices in turn elicit constricted and extreme responses from others. Finally, the person with a personality disorder is unaware of his or her poor choices and does not understand how the "wrong" behaviors have elicited others' responses. Consequently, there is little awareness of responsibility for the interactions and a resultant inability to change interpersonal behavior (Kiesler, 1986).

An important feature in the disordered personality that complicates understanding and treatment is that what therapists consider abnormal personality traits and patterns generally are perceived as appropriate by the individual. This is often described as an **ego-syntonic** feeling—it "feels right" to the individual. Most people would feel troubled if they were labile, persistently distorted reality, were involved in chaotic and troublesome interactions with others, failed to engage in or were neglected in relationships, and seemed unable to understand or express empathy for others. In these situations, most people would seek help or at least talk to someone they trusted. However, for an individual with a personality disorder, it seems that these traits and patterns are not overly disturbing, troublesome, or strange. Chaos may seem strangely untroubling and part of everyday life. This may be because an individual's strategies and behavior have been determined by haphazard and casual events in the environment to which he or she has been exposed. "The particulars and coloration of many pathological patterns have their beginnings in the offhand behaviors and attitudes to which the child is incidentally exposed" (Millon, 1996, p. 112). Moreover, some behaviors also feel as if they make sense because they are **"hardwired"** into an individual's neurological makeup

(Ratey, 1995). If certain strategies and behaviors have been learned and have neurological substrates, they will tend to "feel right." In fact, some models discuss borderline personality disorder in particular as a disorder of emotional dysregulation (Koerner & Linehan, 2000; Waltz & Linehan, 1999) and the patterns of personality disorders as learned in early relationships with key figures (Benjamin & Pugh, 2001). Therefore, the behaviors not only feel right to persons with the disorder, but their behavior is the only possible choice based on biological makeup and early patterns learned in relation to significant caregivers. See Table 9-1 for other theories that discuss the etiology of personality disorders.

CASE ILLUSTRATION: Robyn—Borderline Personality Disorder with Disabling Problems

Robyn was pleased with her new love of four months, James. It seemed that this relationship was a dream come true. Since the two met they had spent almost every night together, sometimes going out, but often just spending time alone. Robyn said that she finally felt that she could trust someone.

About four months into the relationship, however, Robyn became enraged and hung up on James after he called to cancel a date because he was required to work overtime (environmental event). *She refused to answer his messages or to answer calls from friends. She even started refusing to leave her apartment for a while* (maladaptive coping response) *and began thinking that maybe James was cheating on her* (distorted thinking). *Robyn began to doubt her perception of the previous four months. She experienced familiar feelings that she could only describe as painful. She began to think that cutting herself would be the only way to release the pain* (further aggravation of difficulties).

Discussion

Robyn demonstrated adaptive inflexibility, poor choices of behavior, tenuous stability, and a tendency to foster vicious circles. Her problems did not necessarily feel strange or "weird" to her. In fact, her choices were the only possible ones that she knew based on her biological makeup or sensitivity (emotional dysregulation) *and patterns developed in early relationships with her significant caregivers.*

THE *DSM-IV* PERSONALITY DISORDERS

Personality disorders are characterized by:

- Their early onset
- Their stable and persistent character
- Their influence on several different domains of behavior, such as, work, relationships, free time

- Their primary expression in an interpersonal context
- A significant degree of disturbance of the personality (Derksen & Sloore, 1999)

The *Diagnostic and Statistical Manual of Mental Disorders (DSM-IV-TR)* (APA, 2000) lists general criteria for a personality disorder and recognizes common features in some of the individual disorders (see Figure 9-1). In the *DSM-IV-TR* **traits** are the major unit for distinguishing the personality disorders. This categorization based on traits differs from the symptom approach that emphasizes structural problems for axis I disorders. This difference is important because it establishes (1) the idea of continuity between normal and disordered personalities, (2) that personality disorders are a combination of traits, and (3) that a hierarchy exists of lower-order traits organized into higher-order **dimensions,** such as neuroticism or extraversion. However, a collection of traits or just extreme traits are not sufficient for the disorder. The diagnosis is applied only when traits are inflexible or maladaptive and cause extreme distress or functional impairment (Livesley, 2001).

A. An enduring pattern of inner experience and behavior that deviates markedly from the expectations of the individual's culture. This pattern is manifested in two (or more) of the following areas:
 (1) cognition (i.e., ways of perceiving and interpreting self, other people, and events)
 (2) affectivity (i.e., the range, intensity, lability, and appropriateness of emotional response)
 (3) interpersonal functioning
 (4) impulse control
B. The enduring pattern is inflexible and pervasive across a broad range of personal and social situations.
C. The enduring pattern leads to clinically significant distress or impairment in social, occupational, or other important areas of functioning.
D. The pattern is stable and of long duration and its onset can be traced back at least to adolescence or early adulthood.
E. The enduring pattern is not better accounted for as a manifestation or consequence of another mental disorder.
F. The enduring pattern is not due to the direct physiological effects of a substance (e.g., a drug of abuse, a medication) or a general medical condition (e.g., head trauma).

Figure 9-1. General Diagnostic Criteria for a Personality Disorder

Source: Reprinted with permission from the *Diagnostic and Statistical Manual of Mental Disorders-Text Revision, Fourth Edition.* Copyright 2000 American Psychiatric Association.

Differences between Axis I and Axis II

1. Axis II disorders are chronic conditions whereas axis I disorders are episodic in nature.
2. Personality disorders reflect more basic emotional dysfunctions and are more deeply rooted than axis I disorders.
3. Personality disorders are more complex and difficult to treat than axis I disorders (Derksen & Sloore, 1999). In fact, personality disorders often share symptoms with axis I disorders or with each other. This co-occurrence with other disorders is often called comorbidity (Loranger, 2000; Gelder, Lopez-Ibor, & Andreasen, 2000). Personality disorders are usually associated with other disorders such as substance abuse or addiction, eating disorders, post-traumatic stress syndrome due to childhood abuse and neglect, anxiety disorders, and a tendency for self-abuse and mutilation. Currently, information points to childhood abuse and neglect as occurring in a high percentage (59–70%) of individuals with personality disorders. A large minority of those with eating disorders have a personality disorder, and 40% of those with a personality disorder also have bulimia. Between 36% and 76% of those with anxiety disorders are estimated to also have a personality disorder (mostly avoidant, dependent, obsessive-compulsive, schizotypal, or paranoid). In addition, some studies (listed in Ruegy & Frances, 1995) support a clinical impression that there is a connection of cluster B and chronic pain, conversion (symptoms that affect motor or sensory functioning that cannot be explained by neurological or physical conditions [APA, 2000]), and somatoform symptoms (a variety of physical complaints, such as chronic fatigue, gastrointestinal symptoms or loss of appetite, that cannot be explained by any known physical condition [APA, 2000]).

The individual personality disorders can be grouped or "clustered" according to similar features (see Table 9-3). The three clusters follow a dimensional perspective, that is: They are based on traits or dispositions—a permanent inclination to behave a certain way (Gelder, Lopez-Ibor, & Andreasen, 2000). Currently, popular dimensional models of personality disorders are based on the supposition that we all share the same personality structure but differ in our combination of traits. For example, we all have dimensions of neuroticism, extraversion, openness to experience, agreeableness, and conscientiousness, though we each may fall on different places on a continuum that represents each dimension. How we express each dimension depends on our particular combination of traits. See Table 9-3 for a brief explanation of the various traits and dimensions of these models.

Personality disorder clusters have also been described based on other dimensions (Millon, 1996). These other clusters are also described in Table 9-4. (See Table 9-5 for a more detailed list of essential features, the clinical picture, and general interpersonal approaches for the individual disorders [Sadock & Sadock, 2000] according to their *DSM-IV* clusters.)

Table 9-3. Dimensional Models

Five-Factor Model (Costa & MaCrae)

Neuroticism—chronic level of emotional adjustment, includes traits of anxiety, hostility, depression, self-consciousness, impulsivity, vulnerability.

Extraversion—quantity and intensity of preferred interpersonal interactions, activity level, need for stimulation, capacity for joy, includes traits of warmth, gregariousness, assertiveness, activity, excitement seeking, positive emotions.

Open to experience–active seeking and appreciation of experiences for their own sake; includes the traits of fantasy, aesthetics, feelings, actions, ideas, values.

Agreeableness—kinds of interactions a person prefers along a continuum from compassion to antagonism; includes the traits of trust, straightforwardness, altruism, compliance, modesty, tendermindedness.

Conscientiousness—degree of organization, persistence, control, and motivation in goal-directed behavior; includes the traits of competence, order, dutifulness, achievement striving, self-discipline, deliberation.

Interpersonal (Benjamin)	**Three-Factor Model (Eysenck)**	**Dimensional Assessment of Personality Pathology (Livesley & Walton)**
Dominance-submission	*Extraversion*	*Emotional dysregulation*
Hostility-affection	*Neuroticism*	*Dissocial Behavior*
	Psychoticism	*Inhibitedness*
		Compulsivity

Note: All models cited in Livesley, 2001. The popular five-factor model is described in more detail to aid in understanding the dimensional models (Costa & Widiger, 2002; Livesley, 2001).

Cultural Controversy

Controversies based on gender bias and cultural considerations surround some of the personality disorder diagnoses. For example, at least three times more women than men are diagnosed in inpatient samples. A continuing debate surrounds the issue of gender labeling. Some of the very negative criteria that enable one to make the diagnosis are often considered "normal" female behavior. An example is the following operative definition for inclusion in borderline personality disorder: **affective instability,** marked shifts from baseline mood to depression, irritability, or anxiety. Borderline personality characteristics are accepted as more congruent with male sex roles and therefore more tolerable in men than in women (Gibson, 1990). At the same time, personality characteristics that are more congruent with male sex roles and less so with female sex roles, such as overt aggression, are not included in personality disorders. In other words, we have a diagnosis—borderline personality disorder—that is assigned mostly to women based on impulsive behavior and labile affect, which are traits usually ascribed to females rather than males, but there is no diagnosis (such as "overaggressive personality disorder")

Table 9-4. DSM-IV and Other Personality Disorder Clusters

DSM-IV Classifications

Odd-Eccentric (Cluster A)	Dramatic-Emotional (Cluster B)	Anxious-Fearful (Cluster C)
Paranoid	Antisocial	Avoidant
Schizoid	Borderline	Dependent
Schizotypal	Histrionic	Obsessive-Compulsive
	Narcissistic	

Other Classifications

Pleasure Deficient/Detached	Interpersonally Imbalanced	Structurally Defective	Intrapsychically Conflicted
Schizoid	Dependent	Schizotypal	Obsessive-compulsive
Avoidant	Narcissistic	Borderline	
	Antisocial	Paranoid	
	Histrionic		
Characteristic isolation from external support systems and few interpersonal sources of support; thus disposed to be increasingly isolated, preoccupied, and depressed.	Primarily oriented to others (referred to as dependent) or toward themselves and their own needs (referred to as independent). They either consistently seek out others or are oriented to behave always in their own favor.	Socially incompetent, difficult to relate to, and often isolated, confused, and hostile; thus, they are unlikely to elicit support that can help them be more effective. Personality organization and behavior mitigates against adaptation.	Split between orienting themselves toward others or self and maintaining an independent or dependent stance. Consequently, they often reverse interpersonal behaviors and feel internally divided.

Source: Millon (1996).
Note: Millon (1996) groups the disorders according to dimensions that include both internal and external perspectives; that is, he views the person from what may be happening internally or intrapsychically as well as how he or she interacts with others and believes that both internal personality makeup and external interpersonal behavior combine to manifest the disorder.

assigned mostly to men based on aggressive behavior and angry affect, the traits usually ascribed to males.

In other countries, some of the features of personality disorders may not be considered pathological (Alarcon & Foulks, 1995). Particularly since personality disorders are, by definition, based on interpersonal function, how one is per-

Table 9-5. Essential Features, Clinical Picture, and General Approach for the Various Disorders

	Paranoid	*Schizoid*	*Schizotypal*
Essential Features	Long-standing suspicion and mistrust. Suspect that others are acting to harm or exploit them. Responsibility often refused and assigned to others.	Social withdrawal, discomfort in interactions. Eccentric, constricted emotions. Detached.	Strikingly odd and strange. Difficulty in close relationships. Closest to illusions, like schizophrenia, but not psychotic.
Clinical Picture	Very moralistic, hypersensitive. Can easily spot others' vulnerabilities. Personalize coincidental events. Hypervigilant, tense, humorless. Fear both intimacy and rejection. Emotional detachment, isolated, repeatedly check for evidence of others' malevolent intentions, pathological jealousy.	Aloof, reserved, reclusive in everyday events but may have imagined life of closeness. Solitary hobbies, lack insight and self-identity, difficulty evaluating interpersonal events.	Hypervigilant to others' feelings but not their own. Superstitious, unusual uses and meanings of words. Vague, constricted speech. Concrete thinking, avoid eye contact. Shun relationships. Diminished ability to experience pleasure.
General Approach	Courtesy, honesty, respect, serious, without defensiveness. Gain confidence, avoid early confrontations, make slow, gentle attempts to engage.	Courtesy, honesty, respect. Tolerance of silence and whatever degree of involvement they present. Inititating. Gain therapeutic alliance, sometimes social skills training.	Respect, tolerant attitude. Curiosity but not confrontation or too much fascination with strange beliefs. Careful.

	Borderline	*Narcissistic*	*Histrionic*	*Antisocial*
Essential Features	Pattern of: unstable mood, behavior, relationships, self-image, impulsivity. Affective instability, emotional dysregulation, cognitive perceptual distortions.	Lack of empathy, exaggerated sense of importance or specialness. Indifference to others' feelings. Alternate between idealizing and devaluing. Constant craving for admiration.	Flamboyant, dramatic, excitable, over-emotional. Shallow relationships. Coquettish, aggressively demanding, crave novelty and excitement.	Disregard for or violation of rights of others. Often behavior results in imprisonment or court appearance. Lack of remorse. Irresponsibility. Manipulative.

(continues)

Table 9-5. (continued)

	Borderline	Narcissistic	Histrionic	Antisocial
Clinical Picture	When in crisis may show anger, anxiety, depression and expression of feelings of emptiness. Unpredictable behavior, self-destructive acts, dependent or hostile behavior. May perceive rejection when it isn't warranted. Difficulty being alone and desperate attachments. Easily suggestible, black-and-white thinking, 8–10% will succeed at suicide at the mean age of 37.	Depression not fitting to event. Immature behavior, indifference to others' feelings. Tendency to overreact with rage or shame to perceived criticism. Preoccupation with own feelings of inferiority. Sudden attachment and rejection with others. Chronic envy, anger, and resentment.	Temper tantrums, accusations. Seductive or provocative behavior, though seem unaware of it. Command the center of attention, and will be very disappointed if someone else is more noticeable. Hyperemotional and labile, suggestible, sexualize all relationships.	Seeming lack of anxiety or depression not fitting to the situation. Seem charming to the same sex, manipulative to the opposite sex. Lying, exploitive, apparent easy-going behavior may be interrupted by rage, cruelty, or violence, failure to learn from experience.
General Approach	Focus on the here and now, psychoeducational support, and reality testing in a cognitive-behavioral way. Provide calmness and consistency, without being drawn into rescuing or power struggles.	Setting firm limits, interpreting behavior or understanding and support of idealization. Consistency, matter-of-fact approach.	Identification of one's thoughts and feelings. Do not get caught up in the tendency to embellish emotions. Noncontrolling, consistency, find alternatives to acting out, therapeutic communities, direct confrontation of interpersonal behavior.	Limit setting. Group treatment with peers and self-help groups.

	Avoidant	Dependent	Obsessive-Compulsive
Essential Features	Extreme sensitivity to rejection, extreme shyness. Active isolation from social environment, desire relationships but avoid any chance of disapproval.	Tendency to subordinate one's own needs to those of others. Get others to assume responsibility for major areas of one's life.	Constricted emotions, orderliness, perseverance, stubbornness, indecisiveness and rigidity, difficulty expressing warmth. Attempt to control every uncertainty and one's own thoughts and emotions.

(continues)

Table 9-5. (continued)

	Avoidant	Dependent	Obsessive-Compulsive
Clinical Picture	Intense feelings of inferiority, anxious, insecure, self-critical, distant. Lacks confidence. Uncertain, hypervigilant about rejection. May have an ingratiating, waif-like quality.	Pessimism, self-doubt, fear of expressing feelings, passive. Avoid responsibility. Easier to initiate tasks for someone else than themselves.	Preoccupation with lists, details, procedures, minor problems. Few friends, fear of making mistakes, time spent with rituals. Boring conversation. Unproductive perfectionism, lack spontaneity, controlled affect.
General Approach	Avoidant Respectful, honest, warm, accepting. Reinforce assertiveness and self-esteem, address cognitive distortions.	Dependent Accept initial dependency, but resist assuming responsibility. Gradually expect and require independent problem solving and actions. Use Socratic questioning method. Help to enjoy feeling of independence, social skills training, cognitive restructuring.	Obsessive-Compulsive Accepting of frankly boring conversation. Interrupt when possible. Focus on feelings whenever possible and provide opportunities for spontaneity.

Source: Information adapted from Carrasco & Lecic-Tosevski (2000); Sadock & Sacock (2000).

ceived to behave in the social field brings into play cultural values. For example, in countries outside the United States, the features of schizotypal, avoidant, or dependent personality may have to be much more extreme to be considered deviant. The features are more deviant in the United States, where they are embedded in a more materialistic culture with strong values of individualism. Moreover, some diagnostic criteria, such as paranoia, may be the result of enculturation. For example, members of minority groups, immigrants, and political and economic refugees may act defensively to perceived indifference. Language barriers and general lack of knowledge of the rules of the majority may create guarded behaviors that are misperceived as suspicious. Similarly, a reaction to moving from a small rural area to a large urban one may involve emotional "freezing," which could be misperceived as a schizoid symptom. Alarcon and Foulks call for recognizing cultural contextualization when working with an individual with a personality disorder. This means "to put into a local and cultural perspective each and every behavior presented by a potential patient as well as each and every evaluative technique or clinical approach" (1995, p. 5).

Clinical Picture

Millon (1996) describes personality types according to various other domains (see Table 9-4) that give the clinician a better idea of the features of personality disorders. Table 9-5 also describes essential features and provides clinical descriptions of the disorders.

In a treatment setting the maladaptive patterns and characteristics of people with personality disorders, particularly those diagnoses listed in cluster B (Dramatic-Emotional) can evoke predictable, similar, and troubling responses from the treating therapist or staff. Due to inflexible responses to stress, seemingly minor events may be perceived as very stressful. The individual may respond to a nonexistent problem in what seems to be an immature way. This may happen repeatedly.

Because cluster B disorders may be seen in a clinic setting more often than the others, the following discussion will focus on that cluster.

**CASE ILLUSTRATION: Jean, Lotus, and Casey—
Inflexible Responses to Stress**

When the occupational therapist ended a group 10 minutes early due to an impromptu meeting, Jean (diagnosis: narcissistic personality disorder) became teary and angry, protesting that she was overlooked, no longer felt safe in the group, and could not possibly return. Lotus (diagnosis: schizoid personality disorder) was nonchalant, said nothing, and left unnoticed. Casey (diagnosis: obsessive-compulsive personality disorder) talked about the necessity of cleaning up and ritualistically ordered and reordered the project he had been working on.

Discussion

Jean's, Lotus's, and Casey's responses to stress were each inflexible, however, each person functioned differently in accordance with the symptoms or dimensions of his or her specific disorder.

Individuals may display a capacity to "get under the skin" of others. People may find themselves caught up in the life of the person with a personality disorder. Others may feel "stuck" in thinking too much about the individual. All of which can lead to a sense of failure to help someone. For example, in the case of Jean, Lotus, and Casey, the occupational therapist found himself thinking about them for the rest of the afternoon. He questioned whether he should have ended the group early and if he had adequately explained why he was doing so. He wondered if his treatment was effective. He felt guilty concerning Jean, annoyed concerning Casey, and detached concerning Lotus.

In a treatment setting, the relationships with staff of a person with a personality disorder often become strained or conflictual. A parallel process may happen among the staff. This may be due to an individual's tendency to treat some staff in an idealized way, with intense admiration and complete cooperation, and to treat other staff in a denigrating way, showing disdain and avoidance and acting as if they were almost invisible. This may play into one professional's wishes to be helpful and saving or provoke rejecting behavior and attendant guilt from another for not being helpful enough. Conflict begins when unspoken feelings, such as envy, jealousy, or anger, prompt behavior in which some staff members defend a patient, while others complain about him or her. Working relationships in the staff will be disrupted, and the staff members may turn away from the client. This situation is especially likely to occur with a novice therapist due to lack of experience in understanding the situation, desire to be a "good" therapist and do the right thing, inability to examine his or her own personal motives and needs, or fear of appearing vulnerable when speaking with the other staff members.

When this situation manifests itself with more than one individual or with a staff member, it is called **splitting**. This can be counteracted if the staff members anticipate the splitting process, strive to understand the internal feelings of the client, and recognize that he or she is not acting in this way deliberately. (Think of an approach with the difference between "can't," implying difficulties in biological structure and operations, and "won't," implying deliberate will.) Staff members must also remain aware of their own internal feelings and discuss them openly with each other. They may also model certain responses for the client. Responses should: (1) indicate that no one is all good or bad; rather, each of us has both strengths and limitations; (2) aid the client in becoming aware of the tendency to categorize people in a black-and-white way; and (3) accept the expression of both positive and negative aspects in the client, in oneself, and in other staff members. That is, it is important not to moralize or say that behavior is unacceptable or inappropriate, and rather to provide some understanding of the client's process.

INTERDISCIPLINARY ASSESSMENT AND TREATMENT

Assessment usually consists of self-report inventories, projective techniques, and structured clinical interviews (Clark & Harrison, 2001). Instruments assess both normal and abnormal personalities based on traits or diagnostically based instruments, and based on self-report versus interviews. (All of the following instruments are cited in Clark & Harrison, 2001.) Well-known psychological assessments that are self-report, diagnostically based measures include the Millon Clinical Multiaxial Inventory—III (MCMI–III) and the Minnesota Multiphasic Personality Inventory (MMPI-2). Clinical interviews geared to the *DSM* criteria include the Structured Clinical Interview for DSM-IV Axis II (SCID-II) and the Structured Interview for DSM Personality Disorders-IV (SIDP-IV). Trait-based measures that are self-report include the Inventory of Interpersonal Problems—Personality Disorder Scales (IIP–PD; Pilkonis et al.), NEO-Personality Inventory-Revised (NEO-PI-R; Costa & McCrae), and the Structural Analysis of Social Behavior Intrex Questionnaire (SASB-IQ; Benjamin).

Trait-based measures that are interviews include the Diagnostic Interview for Borderline Patients-Revised (CIB-R; Zanarini et al.). Personality Assessment Schedule (PASl; Tyrer), and the Structured Interview for the Five-Factor Model (SIFFM; Trull & Widiger).

Occupational therapy assessments are not trait- or diagnostically based but are based on occupational functioning in performance areas in contexts. Therefore, occupational therapy assessments add valuable information about individuals that may not be assessed in detail in other measurements. Individuals with personality disorders have difficulty in instrumental activities of daily living, work, leisure pursuits, and social participation, so occupational therapy's emphasis on these areas of occupation in specific environments may provide valuable information to a treatment team. In addition, occupational therapy's emphasis on process, communication and interaction skills, and performance patterns may specify areas of intervention not considered by other disciplines. Finally, the occupational therapy intervention approach of modification or adaptation fits with a major difficulty encountered by people who have personality disorders. (For further information about occupational therapy assessments, see Chapter 17.)

Recent research indicates that manualized therapy programs, particularly those created for borderline personality disorder, are successful (Paris, 2002) as well as intense outpatient psychotherapy, group psychotherapy, and day or therapeutic community treatment. Manualized therapy programs created from cognitive (Koerner & Linehan, 2000) and interpersonal (Benjamin & Pugh, 2001) models of therapy explicitly outline treatment programs of one to two years. These programs have been adopted and found effective in many community mental health settings. Long-term studies of 15 and 27 years (Paris, 2002) find that active psychotherapy improves the natural process of remission sevenfold, but short-term treatment of one year may reduce behaviors such as overdosing, self-harm, and use of hospitalization. Impulsivity is often more likely to change first and emotional dysregulation may take longer to change. Interestingly, these long-term studies showed that borderline symptoms tend to reduce after 15 years, and after 27 years many of the participants did not show borderline symptoms.

Group psychotherapy based on behavioral theories includes social skills training, role playing, and reinforcement used to identify and alter maladaptive behavior. Psychodynamic group therapy clarifies and confronts ego-syntonic traits, and increases capacity to tolerate and integrate emotions, to learn about the impact of one's behavior on others, and to acquire and practice new methods of interacting (Piper & Joyce, 2001).

Day or community treatment or partial hospitalization programs are most effective when they have a high staff to client ratio, a minority of low-functioning clients, clear lines of communication, task-oriented groups, and a routine that everyone is expected to follow.

The aim of treatment is not to modify the personality but to reverse the process by which traits are amplified to disorders. General therapy is teaching clients how to make better use of their personality traits so that traits and

Table 9-6.	General Treatment Suggestions for Personality Disorder Clusters	

Cluster A *Paranoid, Schizoid,* *Schizotypal*	*Cluster B* *Borderline, Narcissistic,* *Histrionic, Antisocial*	*Cluster C* *Avoidant, Dependent,* *Obsessive-Compulsive*
Nondirective cognitive therapy, support to reduce isolation, encourage expressions of emotions, social skills training. Not necessarily capable of sustained intimate relationships so need steady employment in interpersonally undemanding jobs.	Social skills training, cognitive therapy, therapeutic milieu, firm structure, psychoeducation, teach tolerance of interpersonal distress and acting less on impulses, self-management skills, focus on a hierarchy of targeted behaviors. Develop task orientations through employment and less demanding interpersonal contacts through social networks.	Tend to deal with anxiety by avoidance or procrastination so encourage more risks and emotional expressions. Time-limited dynamic therapies are active and confrontational.

Overall Principles: Milieu and group treatments are successful, maladaptive behavior can and should be demonstrated and examined, feedback from peers is very useful, new ways of relating can and should be practiced, individuals can benefit from being helpful to others.

Sources: Paris, 1999; Piper & Joyce, 2001.

therefore individuals become more adaptive. Generally, techniques are designed to modulate emotions to optimal intensities, limit rigid and inappropriate behavior, expand behavior repertoires, develop more satisfying social roles, and establish more stable social networks (Paris, 1999). General suggestions for treatment are listed in Table 9-6. Crisis situations may be precipitated by troubles in relationships and adapting to life changes and also by resultant depression, suicidal thoughts, and impulsive behavior.

Psychopharmacology

Although there have been few studies of pharmacology in those with personality disorders in the last 10 years, research and clinical trials suggest that some personality characteristics are associated with abnormalities in the central nervous system (Markovitz, 2001). About 40% to 50% of personality differences can be explained in terms of heredity (Lopez-Ibor, 2000; Paris, 1999). Furthermore, abnormalities in the central nervous system are associated with behavioral changes, and perhaps some personality traits arise from biological underpinnings. Also, severe psychosocial stress may alter gene expression and life-threatening trauma may set in motion neurobiological changes that continue to affect mood, behavior, memory, and arousal throughout life. In fact, children exposed to both neglect and abuse are presumably prone to both underdevelopment of the hippocampus- and amygdala-mediated memory systems and permanent "branding" of painful memories in the cortex . . . In addition, they are likely to have a "kindled" nervous system, that is, one prone to overreact even to mild stimuli that happen to be reminiscent of the original trauma. (Koenigsberg, Kernberg, Stone, Appelbaum, Yeomans, & Diamond, 2000)

Most studies have been conducted with clients who most frequently present for treatment, for example, those with borderline, antisocial, schizotypal, and avoidant personality disorders. However, the majority of studies concern borderline personality disorder (Markovitz, 2001; Tyrer, 2000). Most medications to treat borderline personality disorder are used to treat the other symptoms of major depression, anxiety, or psychotic episodes. For example, those with avoidant personality disorder may respond to antianxiety medication, with schizotypal to antipsychotics, those with poor impulse control to antidepressives with specific serotonergic action (Lopez-Ibor, 2000). Selective serotonin reuptake inhibitors (SSRIs) seem to be the most promising group of medications to reduce depression, anxiety, impulsivity, and self-injury (Markovitz, 2001). Currently, neurotransmitter studies focus on serotonin, dopamine, and norepinephrine (Ratey, 1995; Ruegy & Frances, 1995). It is believed that serotonin deficits may be implicated in suicide and impulsively violent behavior and may be linked to impulsivity in general.

In fact, drugs are given judiciously due to the potentials for suicide and polydrug abuse. Due to the potential for staff splitting, maintaining a consistent approach and constant, clear communication between and among all treating professionals is a necessity.

Interpersonal Approach

The literature regarding personality disorders indicates that the therapeutic alliance is extremely important to treatment. The elements of a therapeutic alliance are a bond with the therapist, agreement on goals of treatment, and a sense of working together on tasks for addressing important issues. This last element is labeled the *working alliance* and has been identified as the strongest predictor of successful outcome with borderline personality disorder (Clark & Harrison, 2001).

Perhaps the concept of therapeutic alliance comes closest to occupational therapy's intervention of therapeutic use of self defined in the Occupational Therapy Practice Framework (2002). (However, see Chapter 18, which expands the discussion of the therapeutic use of self.)

Table 9-7 lists general interpersonal treatment approaches that are useful guides for all practitioners, including occupational therapists, when interacting with individuals with personality disorders (recognizing however, that each person and performance context is unique). These general interpersonal techniques are culled from supportive, cognitive, psychodynamic, and interpersonal models of

Table 9-7. General Interpersonal Treatment Approaches

Useful Concepts for Interaction

Establish a collaborative stance. Establish agreement on the goals and tasks of therapy and be explicit how the tasks relate to the goals.

Communicate in a conversational style; Provide encouragement that tells the client something about herself, for example, "that took courage." Provide understanding along with advice.

Confront defensive behavior in a supportive atmosphere by focusing on the client's demonstrated behavior instead of your judgment of it.

Provide consistency in the structure of your program and behavior and in limit setting.

Encourage membership in social support groups.

Whenever possible, assist the client to think through the consequences of actions— sometimes called *anticipatory guidance and rehearsal.* That is, together move through situations hypothetically considering possibilities and suggest more appropriate or novel ways to handle the hypothetical situations.

Sincerely express pleasure and enthusiasm in the individual's attempts to change and grow.

---

treatment (Winston, Rosenthal, & Muran, 2001) and grounded in experience. In occupational therapy, activity and daily living groups promote a focus on here-and-now behavior, encourage thinking sequentially and anticipating consequences, and facilitate interpersonal relating, adaptive coping, and realistic thinking. Because problems are manifested in the interpersonal realm, attention to the interpersonal approach is important.

OCCUPATIONAL THERAPY TREATMENT INTERVENTIONS

"More than 50 years ago Allport stated that 'personality is something and personality does something'" (Livesley, 2001, p. 13). Perhaps it can be said that the *DSM-IV-TR* (2000) is concerned with what the personality is, but less attention has been paid to what the personality does, to the functional aspects and adaptations of personality disorders. The adaptations can be described in terms of how people universally solve or negotiate major life tasks or problems. Tasks basic to adaptation are establishing an identity, figuring out where and to whom one belongs, negotiating loss and separation, and establishing where one fits in a hierarchy of family or society. Individuals with personality disorders have difficulty in these life tasks and treatment in general will address these universal life problems.

As was mentioned earlier, there are manualized treatment programs that have been adopted in community mental health. Also, day treatment programs and social skills, psychosocial, and psychoeducational groups have proven successful for personality disorders (Piper & Joyce, 2001; McKenzie, 2001; Ruiz-Sancho, Smith, & Gunderson, 2001).

There are many personality disorders, and each cluster is distinguished by certain features. Discussing expanded treatment for each individual disorder is beyond the scope of this text, however, this section will discuss treatment directed toward the cluster B disorders, which are most often encountered in treatment settings. Generally, in addition to an interpersonal approach, treatment consists of making behavioral, cognitive, and social interventions, such as practicing adaptive coping strategies, learning to think before acting, paying attention to emotional style, learning to develop satisfying relationships, and developing a sense of effectiveness in the world—defined as personal causation (Kielhofner, 2002)—or sense of self-identity. These interventions correspond to the domains described by Millon (1996) and shown in Table 9-3 and to the dimensions listed in Table 9-4.

A common general purpose of an occupational therapy treatment program is to create a safe, interesting, and playful context for treatment (Barris, Kielhofner, & Watts, 1988) through collaboration and establishment of a setting that makes clear, consistent, functional demands within a specific timeframe. The program should allow for spontaneity in work and play and provide a predictable setting in which to practice adult roles, explore adult values and identity, and reflect on one's thoughts, feelings, and behavior. Ultimately, the goal of occupational therapy is to facilitate clients' adaptation in their specific environment (performance context). The program should incorporate treatment that addresses problems in performance skills and patterns stemming from concurrent symptoms (substance abuse, self-mutilation, etc.) and essential features of personality disorders, particularly impulsive and rigid, maladaptive behavior patterns. Occupational therapy can address these issues in the standard occupational performance areas (Instrumental Activities of Daily Living [IADLs], education, work, and social participation).

Leisure

Some individuals with personality disorders lack the ability to gain satisfaction from recreational or leisure pursuits. This may be due to rigid, narrow interests; paranoid or fearful behavior; or fear of closeness. It may be due to a background of growing up where any spontaneous or exploratory behavior was dangerous because it was not approved of by caregivers, or it may be due to an inability to regulate pleasurable feelings or guilt that one is feeling pleasure. It may be due to simply not learning that one can enjoy recreational pursuits because recreation may have involved social activities that clients have shied away from, the pursuits may have been inherently competitive and therefore avoided, or perhaps the clients were so perfectionistic that they held back out of fear they could not meet their own standards.

In other cases, recreational/leisure activities may be one area in which people with personality disorders can feel spontaneous, enjoy some sense of worth for their achievements, and perhaps feel relief from a relentless inner turmoil. For example, Jamal loved words, so he looked forward to playing the game "Dictionary," whereby he realized that he was articulate and had an advanced vocabulary. In this case, leisure activities may demonstrate a strength that can be utilized in treatment. Leisure occupations may also counteract various cognitive beliefs and statements that clients tell themselves, such as, "I enjoy doing things by myself," "I don't deserve to have fun," or "I can't let my guard down." Leisure occupations may provide opportunities to plan sequentially, sustain attention, and anticipate actions.

Psychologically, leisure occupations may provide specific responses to overwhelming feelings and help clients regulate their emotions. Leisure occupations may provide ways in which clients can feel worthwhile and enjoy a sense of accomplishment and competence. In this way they may realize that indeed, some activities can be intrinsically pleasurable and can provide pleasure and meaning even though they are not based on approval. For example, Anais worked out at the gym so that she could gain approval from others. However, in the occupational therapy leisure group, when she carefully monitored her thoughts and feelings while working out, she realized that she also enjoyed the feeling she got after finishing a hard workout.

Socially, leisure occupations can provide avenues in which people can be around others and develop casual relationships in a nonthreatening manner. They can relate to others in a reciprocal fashion, thereby developing a knowledge of empathy, while at the same time enjoying the opportunity to gain attention in an adaptive way.

Work

"There are some data suggesting that occupational difficulties may be associated with personality disorders. In two studies, 23 to 42% of participants with personality disorders were unemployed for 6 months to 4 years" (Mattia & Zimmerman, 2001, p. 110).

Work is often a troublesome area due to a person's shyness and paranoid or fearful behavior on the job. Work may also be troublesome due to a person's difficulties in regulating the expression of emotions while on the job. For example, in a session discussing a return to work, Jill was unable to state why she had been fired from her previous three jobs except that she had had trouble meeting deadlines due to feeling overwhelmed about a new relationship. Trouble with work may be due to difficulties meeting concrete standards of performance or problems in sequencing and anticipating consequences of actions or in utilizing logical thinking. Work situations may seem difficult due to a person's lack of empathy and therefore lack of ability to "read" situations or unwritten rules. People with personality disorders may be underemployed, have jobs for which they are seemingly overqualified, or have an erratic work history. In spite of potential problems, work, like leisure, may be the one area where they may excel and learn to focus solely on objective tasks to the exclusion of other areas of life. For example, cognitively, vocational activities may provide arenas in which participants can learn to anticipate consequences of their actions, problem-solve, develop frustration tolerance, and accept responsibility. Alternately, work may provide opportunities for clients to learn how to regulate emotions, the appropriate times and situations in which to express them, and how to tolerate stress from performance standards.

Work activities could provide arenas in which people can learn social appropriateness and how to get along with others in the workplace.

Social Participation

Current research (Paris, 2002) indicates that over time relationships and social adjustment improve for those with borderline personality disorder. Surprisingly, many participants who improved tended to avoid intimate relationships and concentrate on establishing careers and social networks. In fact, "many who improve find that having less intimate friends, belonging to a social community, or having a pet provides more stability than could have been achieved through intimacy " (p. 319). Due to these findings, occupational therapists should concentrate interventions on community and family interactions and roles.

Self-Care

Usually people with personality disorders are independent in self-care, except perhaps when undergoing acute crises. They possess self-care skills, although at times, due to personality patterns such as impulsivity, they may not use them and they may display poor judgment. For example, even though Jolene had an itemized budget, she felt deprived and so spent half of her one-year student loan on a wardrobe. She rationalized that she needed to have clothes for work when she graduated. Most treatment for self-care, then, would focus on IADLs and how to utilize skills or on motivation and judgment strategies. Often this involves concrete planning and goal setting with built-in rewards or recognizing activities that are valued. It may involve learning how to handle impulsive behavior, such as simply stopping whatever one is doing, breathing deeply, or phoning a friend. It may be learning how to think before acting, such as focusing on self-talk and "changing the tape."

Inner self-care skills—those that concern taking care of the internal self (called the *internal environment* in other chapters of this book) in a psychological/emotional way by utilizing a knowledge of the self and psychological skills in a social environment—may be practiced. Cognitively, an individual focuses on how to think before acting and how to anticipate events in a step-by-step manner. Psychologically, an individual may assume a self-identity, learn values and interests, and practice how to recognize what is pleasurable and interesting for its own sake through exploration and mastery. Socially, being able to work with others helps to develop a capacity for empathy for oneself and others by learning that everyone has strengths and weaknesses. For example, in a group utilizing art media in which the task was to "draw your favorite place" and then tell others about it, Robert was able to wait patiently for his turn. As others discussed their work, he realized that he had similar emotions about his favorite place and that he could understand their statements. He also realized that he valued aspects of nature that brought him tranquillity.

Groups

Groups can be either nonverbal or verbal. Nonverbal groups that provide opportunities to work in the presence of others and relate in a casual way can be nonthreatening and motivating. Working in groups on concrete craft and art projects provides structured ways of utilizing one's strengths, resources, and talents while providing an engaging context in which to explore values and interests. Relaxation and restorative groups provide concrete ways to intervene in impulsive situations or when an individual has the experience of feeling overcome by overwhelming emotions. In addition, clients can explore activities that provide intrinsic pleasure. Verbal groups, particularly those that include action and then reflection on the action, can call on individual problem-solving skills, accessing and delineating of emotions, and recognition of how they interfere maladaptively (such as in work). They can also provide training in social skills and communication and in how to be empathic with others.

CASE ILLUSTRATION: Robyn—Treatment Course for Borderline Personality Disorder

Friends of Robyn who worked with her at a record store became concerned about her when she failed to show up for work for three days. When they went to her apartment, they found that she had not been eating or sleeping and that she had burned herself in two different places on her body. After evaluation in an emergency room, she agreed to psychiatric treatment.

An occupational therapy evaluation with the Allen Diagnostic Module (Allen, Earhart, & Blue, 1993) revealed cognitive functioning of 5.0 (able to cognitively explore the environment, but restricted to overt trial-and-error learning and unable to anticipate consequences). An Occupational Performance History Interview (OPHI) (Kielhofner, 2002; Kielhofner & Henry, 1988; Kielhofner, Henry, Whalens, & Rogers, 1991) revealed that Robyn perceived that she did not have control in any areas of her life, wished for a better job or career, and had a sense that she had troubled relationships. Although recently she had not engaged in hobbies or other forms of recreation, she enjoyed jewelry making and furniture refinishing and had worked out with weights. Based on this information, and in concert with her occupational therapist, Robyn chose to attend the following groups:

1. *The "Coping Skills" group addressed topics such as "stamping out impulsivity," "what to do when you want to hurt yourself," and "bringing tranquillity into your life." The group included education, discussion, paper-and-pencil exercises, and trying out of new behaviors while in the acute setting.*
2. *The "About Work" group included working on small jobs that were time limited and paid, learning about work behaviors and environments, discussing the "unwritten rules" of work, and analyzing and reflecting on each work session.*
3. *The "Becoming Creative with Crafts" group offered a variety of art and craft projects that could be learned and completed in short timeframes.*

Robyn's chosen goals of treatment were to handle her self-mutilating and impulsive behavior, find another job and explore career options, and learn to feel better about herself. She worked individually with an occupational therapist to organize a workout schedule and further explore career options. After one week she had practiced some coping skills. Specifically, when she had the urge to burn herself, she learned that she could stop. At the same time, she began to experiment with making painted picture frames, which became popular on the unit. In the vocational group, she began to realize her problems in following through, and that she created problems in work when she became too attached to co-workers. She began to explore careers that would suit this trait, that is, she explored careers where she could complete short-term tasks instead of long-term projects and where she would not be distracted by too many co-workers.

Prior to discharge, the OTR assisted Robyn in exploring options in the community for continuing her interests and anticipated how she might handle setbacks when she was alone in her own home. In a predischarge review, Robyn stated that she "felt better about herself." She had learned that she could follow through in the art and craft group and, in fact, that she possessed some creativity and originality. She realized that perhaps she could indeed positively affect her environment. In fact, people had asked her to make craft projects for them and she had successfully practiced moderating her impulsive behavior. She decided that she would buy a cat since she could take care of this pet and enjoy loving it but it also could be independent enough to not require too much daily care. She also felt hopeful about finding a new job. Since she had explored her abilities and personality aspects in relation to her career, she realized that she could maintain more control of her own destiny and satisfaction.

Discussion

Robyn's course of treatment demonstrates how occupational therapy, individual and group, in all performance areas is a useful and creative aspect of treatment for a person with a personality disorder.

Summary

Understanding and treating personality disorders is difficult and often daunting to new students and clinicians for various reasons, including an unclear symptomatic picture, different classifications based on personality traits, behavior that alternates between functioning and instability, and problems that involve other people. However, treatment is possible based on an understanding of personality and the therapist's willingness to reflect on his or her own responses. Recent research and detailed treatment programs indicate that those with personality disorders can be successfully treated and live healthy and happy lives.

Disabling personality patterns and traits lead to problems with adapting in most areas of life. Occupational therapy includes an interpersonal approach (for example, a collaborative stance, consistency, and understanding) and interventions in leisure, work, social, and self-care areas. Manualized treatment programs and day treatment, both individual psychotherapy and various supportive group therapies using techniques following various treatment models—behavioral, cognitive, psychodynamic, and interpersonal—provide an optimistic picture for individuals with personality disorders.

Review Questions

1. What are the new developments in research and treatment that lead to successful outcomes?
2. What are dimensional models? How do they explain personality disorders?
3. What universal patterns in living distinguish the behavior of someone with a personality disorder from someone without the disorder?
4. What are useful ways of interacting in a clinical setting with individuals with personality disorders?
5. Why are the work, leisure, and social participation areas of performance particularly important for people with personality disorders?

References

Alarcon, R., & Foulks, E. (1995). Personality disorders and culture. *Cultural Diversity and Mental Health, 1*(1), 3–17.

American Psychiatric Association. (2000). *Diagnostic and statistical manual of mental disorders-Text Revision* (4th ed.). Washington, DC.: Author.

Barris, R., Kielhofner, G., & Watts, J. (1988). *Occupational therapy in psychosocial practice*. Thorofare, NJ: Slack.

Benjamin, L. S., & C. Pugh. (2001). Using interpersonal theory to select effective treatment interventions. In W. J. Livesley (Ed.), *Handbook of personality disorders: Theory, research and treatment* (pp. 414–436). New York: Guilford.

Carrasco, J. L., & Lecic-Tosevski, D. (2000). Specific types of personality disorder. In M. G. Gelder, J. J. Lopez-Ibor, & N. Andreasen (Eds.), *New Oxford textbook of psychiatry* (pp. 927–953). New York: Oxford University Press.

Clark, L. A., & Harrison, J. A. (2001). Assessment instruments. In W. John Livesley (Ed.), *Handbook of personality disorders: Theory, research and treatment* (pp. 277–306). New York: Guilford.

Costa, P. T. J., & Widiger, T. A. (2002). Introduction: Personality disorders and the five-factor model of personality. In J. P. T. Costa & T. H. Widiger (Eds.), *Personality disorders and the five-factor model of personality* (2nd ed., pp. 3–14). Washington, DC: American Psychological Association.

Derksen, J., & Sloore, H. (1999). Psychodiagnostics and indications for treatment in cases of personality disorder: Some pitfalls. In J. Derksen, C. Maffei, & H. Groen (Eds.), *Treatment of personality disorders*. New York: Plenum.

Earhart, C. A., Allen, C. K., & Blue, T. (1993). *Allen Diagnostic Module. The manual*. Colchester, CT: S&S Worldwide.

Gelder, M. G., Lopez-Ibor, J. J., & Andreasen, N. (Eds.). (2000). *New Oxford textbook of psychiatry*. New York: Oxford University Press.

Gibson, D. (1990). Borderline personality disorder: Issues of etiology and gender. *Occupational Therapy in Mental Health, 10*(4), 63–77.

Gunderson, J. G., & Gabbard, G. O. (2001). Personality disorders—Introduction. In G. O. Gabbard (Ed.), *Treatment of psychiatric disorders* (pp. 2223–2225).Washington, DC: American Psychiatric Publishing.

Kernberg, O. (1999). The psychotherapeutic treatment of borderline patients. In J. Dirksen & H. Sloore (Eds.), *Treatment of personality disorders*. New York: Kluwer Academic/Plenum.

Kielhofner, G. (2002). *A model of human occupation: Theory and application* (3rd ed.). Baltimore: Lippincott, Williams & Wilkins.

Kielhofner, G., & Henry, A. D. (1988). Development and investigation of an occupational performance history interview. *American Journal of Occupational Therapy, 42*(8), 489–498.

Kielhofner, G., Henry, A., Whalens, D., & Rogers, E. S. (1991). A generalizability study of the Occupational Performance History Interview. *Occupational Therapy Journal of Research, 11*, 292–306.

Kiesler, D. J. (1986). The 1982 interpersonal circle: An analysis of DSM-III personality disorders. In T. Millon & G. Klerman (Eds.), *Contemporary directions in psychopathology: Towards the DSM-IV.* New York: Guilford.

Koerner, K., & Linehan, M. (2000). Research on dialectical behavior therapy for patients with borderline personality disorder. *The Psychiatric Clinics of North America, 23*(1), 151–167.

Koenigsberg, H. W., Kernberg, O. F., Stone, M. H., Appelbaum, A. H., Yeomans, F. E., & Diamond, D. (2000). *Borderline patients: Extending the limits of treatability.* New York: Basic.

Livesley, W. J. (2001). Conceptual and taxonomic issues. In W. J. Livesley (Ed.), *Handbook of personality disorders: Theory, research and treatment* (pp. 3–38). New York: Guilford.

Lopez-Ibor, J. (2000). Personality disorders. In M. G. Gelder & J. J. Lopez-Ibor (Eds.), *New Oxford textbook of psychiatry* (pp. 919–923). New York: Oxford University Press.

Loranger, A. W. (2000). General clinical description of personality disorders. In M. G. Gelder, J. J. Lopez-Ibor, & N. Andreasen (Eds.), *New Oxford textbook of psychiatry* (pp. 923–926). New York: Oxford University Press.

Markovitz, P. (2001). Pharmacotherapy. In W. J. Livesley (Ed.), *Handbook of personality disorders: Theory, research and treatment* (pp. 475–493). New York: Guilford.

Mattia, J. I., & Zimmerman, M. (2001). Epidemiology. In W. J. Livesley (Ed.), *Handbook of personality disorders: Theory, research and treatment* (pp. 107–123). New York: Guilford.

McKenzie, K. R. (2001). Group psychotherapy. In W. J. Livesley (Ed.), *Handbook of personality disorders: Theory, rersearch and treatment* (pp. 497–526). New York: Guilford.

Millon, T. (1981). *Disorders of personality: DSM-III: Axis II.* New York: Wiley.

Millon, T. (1996). *Disorders of personality: DSM-IV and beyond* (2nd ed.). New York: Wiley.

Millon, T., Meagher, S. E., & Grossman, S. D. (2001). Theoretical perspectives. In W. J. Livesley (Ed.), *Handbook of personality disorders: Theory, research and treatment* (pp. 39–59). New York: Guilford.

Occupational therapy practice framework: Domain and process (2002). *American Journal of Occupational Therapy, 56,* 609–639.

Paris, J. (1994, November). The etiology of borderline personality disorder: A biopsychosocial approach. *Psychiatry, 57,* 316–324.

Paris, J. (1999). A multidimensional approach to personality disorders and their treatment. In J. Derksen, C. Maffei, & H. Groen (Eds.), *Treatment of personality disorders* (pp. 107–117). New York: Plenum.

Paris, J. (2002). Implications of long term outcome research for the management of patients with borderline personality disorder. *Harvard Review of Psychiatry, 10*(6), 315–323.

Piper, W. E., & Joyce, A. S. (2001). Psychosocial treatment outcome. In W. J. Livesley (Ed.), *Handbook of personality disorders: Theory, research and treatment* (pp. 323–343). New York: Guilford.

Ratey, J. J. (Ed.). (1995). *Neuropsychiatry of personality disorders.* Cambridge, MA: Blackwell Science.

Ruegy, R., & Frances, A. (1995). New research in personality disorders. *Journal of Personality Disorders, 9*(1), 1–48.

Ruiz-Sancho, A. M., Smith, G. W., & Gunderson, J. (2001). Psychoeducational approaches. In W. J. Livesley (Ed.), *Handbook of personality disorders: Theory, research and treatment* (pp. 460–474). New York: Guilford.

Sadock, B., & Sadock, H. (2000). *Comprehensive textbook of psychiatry* (7th ed.). Baltimore: Lippincott, Williams & Wilkins.

Tyrer, P. (2000). Drug treatment of personality disorders. In P. Tyrer (Ed.), *Personality disorders: Diagnosis, management and course* (pp. 100–104). Boston: Butterworth-Heinemann.

Waltz, J., & Linehan, M. M. (1999). Functional analysis of borderline personality diosrder behavioral criterion patterns. In J. Derksen, C. Maffei, & H. Groen (Eds.), *Treatment of personality disorders* (pp. 183–205). New York: Kluwer Academic.

Winston, A., Rosenthal, R. N., & Muran, J. C. (2001). Supportive psychotherapy. In W. J. Livesley (Ed.), *Handbook of personality disorders: Theory, research and treatment* (pp. 344–358). New York: Guilford.

Suggested Readings

Effects of Childhood Abuse

Gil, E. (1983). *Outgrowing the pain*. San Francisco: Launch.

Herman, J. (1992). *Trauma and recovery*. New York: HarperCollins.

Miller, A. (1983). *For your own good*. Toronto: McGraw-Hill.

Williams, G., & Money, J. (1980). *Traumatic abuse and neglect of children at home* (abridged). Baltimore: Johns Hopkins University Press.

Borderline and Narcissistic Disorders

Cara, E. (1992). Neutralizing the narcissistic style: Narcissism, self-psychology and occupational therapy, *Occupational Therapy in Health Care*, 8, 2–3.

Gallop, R. (1985). The patient is splitting: Everyone knows and nothing changes. *Journal of Psychosocial Nursing*, 23(4), 6–10.

Hickey, B. (1985). The borderline experience: Subjective impressions. *Journal of Psychosocial Nursing*, 23(4), 24–26.

Kernberg, O. (1975). *Borderline conditions and pathological narcissism*. New York: Aronson.

Kohut, H. (1977). *The restoration of the self*. New York: International Universities Press.

Layton, M. (1995, May–June). Emerging from the shadows: Looking beyond the borderline diagnosis. *Networker*, 35–41.

Miller, A. (1981). *The drama of the gifted child*. New York: Basic.

Miller, S. G. (1994). Borderline personality disorder from the patient's perspective. *Hospital and Community Psychiatry, 45*, 1215–1219.

Shapiro, D. (1965). *Neurotic styles*. New York: Basic.

Obsessive-Compulsive Personality Disorder

Rapoport, J. (1989). *The boy who couldn't stop washing*. New York: Penguin.

Treatment Strategies

Linehan, M. (1993a). *Cognitive behavioral treatment of borderline personality disorder*. New York: Guilford.

Linehan, M. (1993b). *Skills training manual for treating borderline personality disorder*. New York: Guilford.

Simon, S. (1993). *In search of values: 31 strategies for finding out what really matters most to you*. New York: Time Warner.

Tavris, C. (1982). *Anger: The misunderstood emotion*. New York: Simon & Schuster.

Literary Portraits

Allison, D. (1992). *Bastard out of Carolina*. New York: Dutton.

Middlebrook, D. (1991). *Anne Sexton: A biography*. New York: Houghton-Mifflin.

Smiley, J. (1992). *A thousand acres*. New York: Knopf.

Mental Health across the Lifespan

Part IV includes three chapters about the mental health of children, adolescents, and older adults. While the first edition detailed specific psychiatric conditions and discussed general treatment that can be adapted for children and adults, there are also conditions or problems specific to particular age groups. Therefore, these three chapters capture the issues or problems that *can* occur throughout one's life, but are more prevalent at certain times in one's life and require more concentrated occupational therapy interventions.

Much attention is currently being focused on the treatment of children, adolescents, and older adults, and there are many opportunities to develop innovative and dynamic treatment for these groups. Keep in mind while you read that though we may treat certain problems at certain times in one's life, each person is unique and complex, there is growth throughout the lifespan, and individual differences account for variety. The chapters in Part IV provide information that can be used generally for all age groups but is tailored specifically for each unique individual in a certain age range.

Mental Health of Children

William L. Lambert, OTR/L

Key Terms

acting out
consistency
dynamic
latency age
parallel task group

redirection
structure
tic
time-out

Chapter Outline

Implementing Programming for Children
    Evaluation and Assessment
    Intervention
    Examples of Emerging Areas of Practice
Summary and Current Trends

Introduction

Occupational therapy for children with emotional disturbances has been an area of specialization within the profession for many years. Indeed, the practice of occupational therapy with children with mental and behavioral disorders requires specific knowledge of psychiatric disorders and conditions, expertise in normal or typical growth and development, and practice skills unique to this population, its issues, and its concerns.

Those providing care to these children often work in collaboration with other health care professionals such as child psychiatrists, psychologists, social workers, and nurses (Hollander, 2001) or independently as consultants or contract therapists, or through a private practice. The delivery system for providing occupational therapy has changed dramatically in the last two decades. In the past, the primary sites that employed therapists were psychiatric hospitals with children's units or wards, outpatient mental health clinics, partial hospitalization, or day treatment programs (Pratt & Allen, 1989). Currently therapists who treat children with emotional or behavioral problems must think outside the box—or toy box—and move away from medical model/hospital-based treatment to providing therapy in school and community settings not usually thought of as psychiatric, but rather as pediatric (Argabrite Grove, 2002; Burns & Hoagwood, 2002; Hahn, 2000; Lewis, 2002).

This chapter presents an overview of occupational therapy practice with children who are emotionally disturbed. Basic concepts used in providing occupational therapy to children with mental illness are described. Occupational therapy programming is discussed based on experience and on successful interventions used in other settings (Hoffman, 1982; Llorens & Rubin, 1967). Treatment, intervention groups with examples of group protocols, and activities appropriate for this population are presented that may be used in a variety of pediatric settings.

The need to address the psychosocial needs of children in various pediatric settings is becoming more prominently featured in current occupational therapy publications (Florey, 2003; Kaplan & Telford, 1998; Lougher, 2001; Parham & Fazio, 1997). For example, the American Occupational Therapy Association Continuing Education article in the April 2002 issue of *OT Practice* points out that "childhood psychosocial problems that are left untreated often become exacerbated in adolescence and young adulthood" (pp. CE4–CE6) and that children with psychosocial and other disorders must have these needs addressed in occupational therapy in pediatric settings. The article goes on to provide intervention guidelines that have long been treatment objectives in traditional psychosocial settings, such as increasing impulse control; improving frustration tolerance; tolerating transitions; and developing social interaction skills.

DSM-IV Diagnoses

The *Diagnostic and Statistical Manual of Mental Disorders,* Fourth Edition, Text Revision (*DSM-IV-TR*, APA, 2000) lists disorders usually first diagnosed in infancy, childhood, or adolescence. Many of these disorders, such as mental retardation and Tourette's disorder, can continue to cause problems during adulthood. Many disorders that are discussed in other chapters of this volume, such as schizophrenia, major depression, bipolar disorder, and post-traumatic stress disorder may also first be encountered in childhood (Lewis, 2002; Rutter & Taylor, 2002; Sadock & Sadock, 2000). Symptoms of childhood depression include irritability, sadness, social withdrawal, and anhedonia, as well as negative feelings appearing in play (Weingarten-Dubin, 2001). Depression has also been linked to violent behaviors (Bertucco, 2001), and children often exhibit this violent behavior with aggression or **acting out.** Acting out can be defined as the expression of thoughts and feelings through maladaptive behavior instead of recognizing and verbalizing those ideas. Children may express depressive symptoms in other ways, such as anger, as it is cognitively easier for them to be mad than sad.

A difference in the way that children with bipolar disorder present is that their moods may shift many times within the same day or same therapy session. Their presentation is further complicated by frequently also meeting the criteria for attention deficit hyperactivity disorder and oppositional defiant disorder. A family history that includes relatives who have been diagnosed with bipolar disorder greatly assists in making this diagnosis in children. Knowing which medications were beneficial to blood relatives also makes choosing the appropriate medication easier—if Depakote has helped control a parent's bipolar disorder, for instance, it also may be effective with a son or daughter. Figure 10-1 summarizes *DSM-IV* disorders beginning in infancy & childhood.

Common diagnoses of children seen or encountered by occupational therapists in various settings include attention deficit hyperactivity, oppositional defiant, separation anxiety, and conduct disorders. Recently attention has been focused on the occurrence of reactive attachment disorder and pervasive developmental disorder, which include autistic and Asperger's disorders in pediatric areas of practice. Disruptive behavior disorder, which first appeared in *DSM-IV*, provides a helpful provisional diagnosis, as the exact nature of children's mental illness is often hard to pinpoint, especially in its initial presentation.

Two prominent childhood disorders currently receiving attention are attention deficit hyperactivity disorder and reactive attachment disorder. Children with attention deficit hyperactivity disorder often have problematic social interactions with peers, teachers, and authority figures, as well as difficulty in participating appropriately in the classroom and during extracurricular activities ("National Survey Reveals," 2002). Treatment with medications such as Ritalin, Adderall, and Metadate is often at the center of controversy and debate. These

Mental Retardation. This disorder is characterized by significantly subaverage intellectual functioning (an IQ of approximately 70 or below) with onset before age 18 years and concurrent deficits or impairments in adaptive functioning. Separate codes are provided for **Mild, Moderate, Severe,** and **Profound Mental Retardation** and for **Mental Retardation, Severity Unspecified.**

Learning Disorders. These disorders are characterized by academic function that is substantially below that expected given the person's chronological age, measured intelligence, and age-appropriate education. The specific disorders included in this section are **Reading Disorder, Mathematics Disorder, Disorder of Written Expression,** and **Learning Disorder Not Otherwise Specified.**

Motor Skills Disorder. This includes **Developmental Coordination Disorder,** which is characterized by motor coordination that is substantially below that expected given the person's chronological age and measured intelligence.

Communication Disorders. These disorders are characterized by difficulties in speech or language and include **Expressive Language Disorder, Mixed Receptive-Expressive Language Disorder, Phonological Disorder, Stuttering,** and **Communication Disorder Not Otherwise Specified.**

Pervasive Developmental Disorders. These disorders are characterized by severe deficits and pervasive impairment in multiple areas of development. These include impairment in reciprocal social interaction, impairment in communication, and the presence of stereotyped behavior, interests, and activities. The specific disorders included in this section are **Autistic Disorder, Rett's Disorder, Childhood Disintegrative Disorder, Asperger's Disorder,** and **Pervasive Developmental Disorder Not Otherwise Specified.**

Attention-Deficit and Disruptive Behavior Disorders. This section includes **Attention-Deficit/Hyperactivity Disorder,** which is characterized by prominent symptoms of inattention and/or hyperactivity-impulsivity. Subtypes are provided for specifying the predominant symptom presentation: **Predominantly Inattentive Type, Predominantly Hyperactive-Impulsive Type,** and **Combined Type.** Also included in this section are the Disruptive Behavior Disorders: **Conduct Disorder** is characterized by a pattern of behavior that violates the basic rights of others or major age-appropriate societal norms or rules; **Oppositional Defiant Disorder** is characterized by a pattern of negativistic, hostile, and defiant behavior. This section also includes two Not Otherwise Specified categories: **Attention-Deficit/Hyperactivity Disorder Not Otherwise Specified** and **Disruptive Behavior Disorder Not Otherwise Specified.**

Feeding and Eating Disorders of Infancy or Early Childhood. These disorders are characterized by persistent disturbances in feeding and eating. The specific disorders included are **Pica, Rumination Disorder,** and **Feeding Disorder of Infancy or Early Childhood.** Note that Anorexia Nervosa and Bulimia Nervosa are included in the "Eating Disorders" section presented later in the manual (see p. 583).

Tic Disorders. These disorders are characterized by vocal and/or motor tics. The specific disorders included are **Tourette's Disorder, Chronic Motor or Vocal Tic Disorder, Transient Tic Disorder,** and **Tic Disorder Not Otherwise Specified.**

(continues)

Figure 10-1. Disorders Beginning in Infancy, Childhood, or Adolescence

Elimination Disorders. This grouping includes **Encopresis,** the repeated passage of feces into inappropriate places, and **Enuresis,** the repeated voiding of urine into inappropriate places.

Other Disorders of Infancy, Childhood, or Adolescence. This grouping is for disorders that are not covered in the sections listed above. **Separation Anxiety Disorder** is characterized by developmentally inappropriate and excessive anxiety concerning separation from home or from those to whom the child is attached. **Selective Mutism** is characterized by a consistent failure to speak in specific social situations despite speaking in other situations. **Reactive Attachment Disorder of Infancy or Early Childhood** is characterized by markedly disturbed and developmentally inappropriate social relatedness that occurs in most contexts and is associated with grossly pathogenic care. **Stereotypic Movement Disorder** is characterized by repetitive, seemingly driven, and nonfunctional motor behavior that markedly interferes with normal activities and at times may result in bodily injury. **Disorder of Infancy, Childhood, or Adolescence Not Otherwise Specified** is a residual category for coding disorders with onset in infancy, childhood, or adolescence that do not meet criteria for any specific disorder in the Classification.

Figure 10-1. (continued)

and other medications are criticized for being over-prescribed and heavily marketed to parents (Zernike & Peterson, 2001). However, to date there is no evidence of blanket adverse effects, furthermore, stimulants have been shown to be effective for, hyperactivity, impulsivity, and inattention in classrooms (Fonagy, Target, Cottrell, Phillips, & Kurtz, 2002).

Children with attachment disorders can be frustrating to work with and to parent. They present with a high need to be in control, frequently lie without reason, and are described as having poor eye contact except when lying. Interpersonally they may be overly affectionate and inappropriate with others including strangers, or lack interest in others and do not seek attention. They may lack a conscience. Frequently, they hoard or gorge on food in the absence of want. Early experiences with their initial caregivers spur the development of these traits, as well as having a succession of caregivers (Randolph, 1999). Nondirective play therapy and sensory integrative therapy have been identified as efficacious therapeutic interventions (Eshelman, 2002; Florey, 2003; Kaplan & Telford, 1998).

Children may have more than one disorder. For example, children with attention deficit hyperactivity disorder may also have depression, obsessive compulsive disorder, or all three. Children with depression may also have an anxiety disorder, and sensorimotor problems may coexist with many disorders.

The presenting problems encountered by occupational therapists treating children with emotional problems are varied (Florey, 2003; Lewis, 2002; Rutter & Taylor, 2002; Sadock & Sadock, 2000). Some may be specified by the V-codes listed in Figure 10-1. Other "typical" psychosocial stressors may include the parents' divorce; emotional, verbal, physical, and/or sexual abuse; other traumatic events, such as the death of a sibling, parent, or grandparent; and socioeconomic conditions that may be coded according to axis V of the *DSM-IV*. The child may respond to traumatic events by withdrawal, aggressive or atypical behavior, or regression to behavior expected from a younger child. Sometimes the child is confronted by a physical condition such as diabetes, which may limit the child's ability to play and eat what others are eating or require an unusually strict adherence to a medication and blood-monitoring situation (see Chapter 13 for further information regarding psychosocial factors in physical illness). The child may find the illness overwhelming and consequently start acting out at home or become noncompliant with the treatment of the illness in an attempt to exert control.

In other cases a dysfunctional family situation may have led to treatment. Parents sometimes lack the parenting skills required for rearing a normally developing child. In such circumstances, it may be a lack of parental supervision, an inability to set and enforce limits and rules, or the failure to distinguish and differentiate the needs of the parent from the needs of the child. In other situations, parents have placed expectations on children that the latter find overwhelming, such as a parental need to see a child excel in academics or athletics, whether or not the child values these activities. Sociological factors, such as poverty, violence, and crime, may constitute a stressful environment, resulting in depression or anxiety and leading to a need for treatment. Whatever the antecedents that lead to a child receiving professional treatment, the primary reasons are similar to many psychiatric intervention situations. These factors include the following:

- Danger of harming oneself or others
- A breakdown in role functioning, namely, appropriate behavior as a sibling, student, playmate, son, or daughter
- A decrease in obedience to, or compliance with, authority figures
- Social withdrawal
- Increase in aggression or other unacceptable or inappropriate acting-out behaviors, such as fighting, truancy, criminal activities such as theft or vandalism, fire setting, and violence directed toward pets or other animals
- Use of drugs or alcohol
- Stopping medications
- Dropping grades

Other conditions that contribute to emotional problems in children include fetal alcohol syndrome and fetal alcohol effects, which sometimes impair a child's ability to learn from experience or impair the usual responses to medical interventions. The offspring of mothers who used or abused drugs during pregnancy may display a wide range of often unpredictable developmental deficits that complicate treatment and may adversely affect outcomes.

Regardless of the unique circumstances that are part of a child's particular situation, the onset of the illness varies with each child, based on diagnosis, genetic predisposition, level of disability, and equality-of-life factors such as income level, access to health care, and stability of the family situation. Children's emotional problems and the consequences of interpersonal and social impairments become more visible once they reach the age where they can be observed by others at day care, preschool, or the school system setting. At this time difficulties tend to become more evident and families often seek professional, clinical help.

HELPFUL CONCEPTS FOR TREATING CHILDREN

Because children are developing a self-identity and learning how to behave in their social world, concepts such as structure and consistency, interpretation, time-out, limit setting, avoidance of power struggles, modeling, and a consistent team approach are important to keep in mind when working with children. Although some of these concepts are used when working with adults, who presumably have developed some sense of identity and acceptance of social norms, they are particularly important for the developmental period when individuals are learning who they are and how to function successfully in the world.

Structure and Consistency

Two fundamental principles guiding treatment in pediatric psychiatric occupational therapy are **structure** and **consistency**. For individuals with poor impulse control, attention deficits, hyperactivity, or poor response to limits and rules, increasing the amount of structure can improve their response to activity interventions, help them learn how to modulate their own emotions, and assist them in learning appropriate role behavior. The environment itself is used to provide cues to appropriate behavior similar to those used in milieu therapy or therapeutic communities.

Structure can be verbal, such as the tactic of **redirection,** or physical and tangible, depending on the specific activity or equipment used. Activities can begin with the imposition of verbal structure, such as directions and limits or rules regarding the activity. For example, the group leader or therapists may say: "Today in group we are going to share the toys in the playroom. There can be no hitting. If anyone hits someone else, he or she will have to leave the group." This instruction provides an idea or standard that can be referred to throughout the group session to provide structure and consistency. For children, a poster that lists the rules of the group or activity provides an additional reference point that can be used to remind them of the structure (see Figure 10-2).

"Announcements" can be used to start a group. The children can be asked to tell something about themselves or their progress toward therapy goals. They can

Occupational Therapy Group Rules
1. Have Fun
2. Share
3. Listen to Staff
4. Clean Up

Figure 10-2. Rules Poster

be encouraged to share "news" such as upcoming family events, plans for the future (following discharge from therapy), changes in their lives, activities in which they have participated, and the like. Announcements provide the therapist with useful information that may explain the child's response to therapy on that particular day. For example, if a child states, "My mom is taking me to family therapy after OT today," changes in mood or decreases in frustration tolerance might be attributed to anxiety regarding the outcome of the family therapy session later that day. This in turn may enable the therapist to make a successful interpretation that can help the child cope more effectively, learn to express feelings more adaptively, and benefit more from occupational therapy that day.

When conducting groups it is important to ensure that the group begins and ends at the designated times and follows the established routine as much as possible. Naturally, a variety of unpredictable and unavoidable circumstances can interfere with the daily course of programming. For example, a therapist may be sick or on vacation, or special events, such as holiday parties, may take temporary precedence over scheduled programming. In such cases it is important to inform clients of changes in the established consistency. This practice can prevent the eruption of acting-out behavior from a client who may otherwise feel unable to trust the adults and the therapeutic environment responsible for his or her care (see Figure 10-3). A clinical example of acting-out can be seen in the case of a child, Joanie, who was not made aware of the impending absence of the therapist who normally ran her group.

1. To deal with impulsivity, never put anything on the table where you are having a group activity unless you want the children to touch it.

2. Ease transitions, which are frequently difficult for children with mental illness, with a "five-minute warning" before the group ends to prepare them for the change and deal more adaptively with endings.

3. To prevent overstimulation, provide a warm, softly lit environment that is soothing and as free from unwanted noise, disruption, and distractions as possible.

4. Children with emotional disturbances can act out often and produce a considerable amount of maladaptive behavior in therapy. "Catch them being good"— praise positive behavior as often as possible.

5. Maintain an even tone and affect while providing treatment. Your calm demeanor may influence the disruptive child's behavior—at least occasionally!

6. Sometimes groups just fall apart despite the therapist's best efforts and interventions. Don't insist that the activity occur if the children aren't ready to participate. Two effective solutions are to *end group* and *sit quietly and wait for the children to regain control*. Children learn that acting out and disruptive behavior lead to the natural consequence that they lose the opportunity to be involved in the activity. If sitting quietly lasts until the end of group time, they usually realize that their behavior prevented play and say, "Hey, we didn't do anything yet!" Gently remind them that they will need to be in control in the next session if they want the activity to happen.

Figure 10-3.   Six Therapy Tips

CASE ILLUSTRATION: Joanie

When Joanie, 8, arrived in the therapy room, she learned that the group had been changed from an art group to a play group, which caused her to cry, kick, and scream. When an interpretation was made that the child appeared very upset, she blurted out: "I wanted to have art! I have to paint my project so I can give it to my mother!"

Discussion

Had she been informed of the change beforehand, the incident might have been averted and, instead, Joanie might have (1) been able to present her disappointment and concerns calmly, (2) been provided with options for completing her project, and (3) thereby learned how to express her internal feelings and thoughts acceptably.

A point that may be implicitly understood by occupational therapists is that another way to provide structure is through activities themselves. "The child's developmental progression is facilitated by play, games and activities, integral functions of a child's daily life" (Abramson, 1982a, p. 61). An example is making a tile mosaic project in a **parallel task group**. Structure is provided:

- When each client has his or her own project, which encourages work in a specific spot and focuses attention on a personal project
- When an example or sample is provided that may be followed to enhance redirection to task
- When the instructions are clear (e.g., "put tiles in the tray like this"). This encourages following the stated direction
- When steps are graded according to therapy goals (e.g., "pick up each tile and glue it in place")

Children enjoy the structure of individual activities, which can serve as a means of exploring their abilities and skills and possibly learning about their strengths and limitations.

Puppetry, doll play, and drawing provide a technique for dramatizing and externalizing intrapsychic issues. For the older latency-age child, board games may become catalysts for communication and interpersonal relationships . . . At all times, play, games and activities are active experiences, and their focus on productivity and participation offer intrinsic satisfaction for the child: To cultivate those skills necessary to fulfill life roles. (Abramson, 1982a, p. 61)

In general, in planning activities for children or adolescents it should be constantly considered whether:

- The activity chosen is age-appropriate
- The activity is broken down into steps that the child can understand
- The steps are age-appropriate for a child to carry out independently
- The therapist wishes the child to carry out independently or by asking for assistance

For example, if an activity should involve a child sustaining attention to a task, perhaps a tile mosaic project involving the selection of a number of small tiles placed in a trivet is the activity of choice. If improving self-esteem is a consideration, an easy-to-do, foolproof activity such as painting a sun catcher or lacing a small coin purse may do. Where individual play skills are lacking, perhaps the creation and assembly of a toy car that the child can use independently or in conjunction with other children is the activity of choice. In any case, the activity should facilitate developmentally appropriate skills and be fun and intrinsically motivating for the child or adolescent.

Although there are common considerations when choosing an activity for any person, for a child it is particularly important to be mindful of dangerous parts such as sharp edges, toxic chemicals, or toxic paints or parts that can be ingested, such as small wheels found on a toy car for toddlers. Another consideration is whether there are any items that could be used in a suicide attempt or injurious behavior, such as when knives are being used in a cooking group.

Thorough activity analysis, performing sharps counts (number of knives, scissors, etc. used in the group), and limiting the length of string or ribbon provided are ways of ensuring safety both during therapy and afterward when projects are taken home. Depending on the participants presenting problems, copper tooling, for example, may be the wrong activity for a group of aggressive children who may not respond to the structure of the activity or may use the materials inappropriately to harm themselves or others.

Interpretation

Interpretation of, or putting words to, behavior is a therapeutic technique that provides a child with an avenue to express feelings with words, which is more often appropriate than other means such as aggression or acting out. This is often an effective way of de-escalating a child or adolescent who is displaying behavioral problems that result from an inability to use words for self-expression. In the example of Joanie, interpretation involved the therapist identifying to the child in a clear and supportive manner what she observed. Joanie could then better express the behavior's cause (whether the change in routine, a reminder of a **dynamic** within her family, or a feeling she could not identify). The identification of these issues by using interpretation clarifies the situation at hand and teaches a more adaptive coping strategy: the use of words to express feelings and reach acceptable solutions to problems. Activities can be used to provide opportunities to externalize intrapsychic issues or facilitate communication. Once issues have been externalized or communicated, interpretation helps children to understand, learn, cope, and adapt emotionally (Abramson, Hoffman, & Johns, 1979).

Time-Out

Time-out is an intervention technique that results in behavioral changes and increases the child's understanding of her role in a situation. If a child is asked to take time-out for kicking a peer while fighting over a toy, he will learn that aggression leads to the loss of the chance to play. Time-out also provides an opportunity for the adult to teach the child how to share. Thus, the child becomes better able to perceive the situation and learn from it. Similarly, if a child is removed from group for aggression or breaking the rules, she will become better able to think about the situation and learn from it. Time-out is the process of removing a young person from a problematic situation to a specific area away from the group and, at the same time, allowing him or her to think about the behavior that led to removal from the group.

The length of time-out should vary with the individual's age and mental capacities. For example, when a child has provoked a fight with a peer, he will be removed to a time-out chair, a "think about it" area, or another room, where he will be requested to remain for a specified amount of time. Depending on his age, he may be asked to remain in time-out until he can count to 10 or until a minute goes by on a timer. An often-used rule of thumb is one minute per year, that is, a 5-year-old would be placed on a five-minute time-out. However, what may be most effective is for the time-out not to have a specific time in minutes, but last until the child regains control and can effectively process the situation. Using this approach one can avoid situations where the child has regained control, yet had several more minutes of time-out remaining. To be consistent, the adult would have to maintain the time-out until its predetermined parameter, which may allow the child to begin acting out again and not benefit from the experience (Moffit, 1987). Immediately after the time-out the child is most amenable to positive interaction and should be engaged in the activity in a constructive way and then praised for constructive behavior. After the activity, it is important to critically analyze the incident. The child and adult should meet briefly to discuss the behavior that led to the time-out, evaluate whether the intervention was useful for the client, and develop a plan of action that will be utilized in future situations. A plan of action may involve identifying with the client alternative coping strategies (such as a self-assigned time-out) or the use of assertive responses (such as letting a staff person know when he or she is feeling frustrated or agreeing on a "code word" to indicate the need for a behavior change). This process should be kept as brief as possible so that acting-out behavior is not reinforced. When used properly, a time-out can be efficacious in changing maladaptive behavior to that which is more socially appropriate. Time-out should not be conceived of as a punishment, nor should the individual taking a time-out think of it in this way but more as a consequence for problematic behavior or actions. It is important to present the time-out as a way to learn new behavior so that a positive learning experience may occur and negative or maladaptive behaviors may decrease.

Limit Setting

Limit setting involves informing others what is permissible and what is unacceptable; it lets individuals know "how far they can go." Setting limits is especially important for children because they need, and look for, limits, which eventually become internalized as a set of rules that guide socially accepted behavior. The teaching of behavior such as learning to respect the property of others and not taking what doesn't belong to them begins when children are told, in effect, "Thou shalt not steal" (whether this occurs at home, in school, or in a religious setting), and the rule is enforced by the parent. When consistent enforcement of the rule or limit occurs, appropriate behavior will be learned or thus becomes a part of that person's internal code of values, morals, or conscience. Children are protected by rules or limits, such as saying that they may play in the yard but not in the street, or that they must be home before a certain hour. This not only teaches safety and prevents harm, it also shows children that their welfare is the concern of the parent or other adult. Limits that are thus enforced clarify the relationship between the parent (or other adult) and child and teach appropriate role behavior. Limits should be friendly but firm, short, and impersonal. Limits can be put in the context of the group rules, as when the occupational therapist says: "We must share the toys," or, "The house rules say that fighting over what program to watch on TV leads to an early bedtime for everyone." Although setting limits may be interpreted as punishment, if stated in a protective and supportive, friendly, but firm way, it will foster more mature behavior. Naturally, the amount of limit setting depends on the needs of the child and the comfort level of the therapist (Abramson, Hoffman, & Johns, 1979).

An excellent resource for shaping and modifying behavior in children between the ages of 2 and 10 years old is *1-2-3 Magic! Training Your Preschoolers and Preteens to Do What You Want* (1995) by Phelan. *1-2-3-Magic!* develops the child's ability to follow rules and comply with adult authority. Although it is written for parents, any adult working with children who require effective behavior modification could use the concepts.

Therapeutic Use of Relationship

The therapeutic use of relationship entails the development of an individual style that works with clients in a specific way to promote change and growth and help to provide a corrective emotional experience. This is a difficult concept, or "art," to describe. "The art of occupational therapy involves captivating the child through toys, objects, and games or through the therapist's own actions so that the child becomes involved in the therapeutic process. This art is almost intangible" (Kramer & Hinojasa, 1993, p. 443). An occupational therapist responds to a child in a therapeutic manner, conveying appreciation of the child's uniqueness, kindness, love, and understanding; guiding the child through each step of occupational therapy intervention; and encouraging him or her to accomplish the task that has been chosen to meet the treatment goal. Each therapist will develop a unique and personal style or therapeutic personality for working with patients. The therapeutic use of relationship requires providing a new response to an old situation, which enables the client in turn to respond in a new manner that is both adaptive and appropriate. (See Chapter 18 for a further discussion of intersubjectivity and the therapeutic relationship.)

> ### CASE ILLUSTRATION: Kay—The Therapeutic Use of Relationship
>
> *Kay, a client on a children's unit, could not sustain her interest or complete tasks as assigned. During a cooking group, the occupational therapist assigned her the job of chopping vegetables to be put in a salad. However, Kay did not stay with her task, and, moments later, she was in another part of the room engaging in an activity that had been assigned to another child. The young occupational therapist, in a raised voice, told Kay, "You are not where you belong," and asked what was her task. Kay said, "I'm supposed to be chopping vegetables." The therapist said, "You are driving me crazy," to which she responded, "You sound just like my mother: she always says that." At that point, the therapist realized he was not being therapeutic and was indeed responding to Kay in the same manner in which adults had always responded to her. Therefore he acknowledged that fact, apologized for sounding impatient, and redirected Kay to the task at hand (as he should have done previously).*
>
> #### Discussion
>
> *As demonstrated by the therapist in this case, the therapeutic use of relationship involves responding to clients in a way that will guide them onto a new path through developing behaviors that are appropriate and socially acceptable. This involves responding to clients in a different manner than nontherapeutic individuals in past situations.*

Team Approach and Family Involvement

The team concept is particularly essential in providing services and family involvement in treatment is of utmost importance for children because of their roles as family members. Other family members should be consulted and included on the team whenever possible and be a part of treatment goals and decisions. Developmental life roles also are demonstrated to children and adolescents by other professionals such as teachers and education specialists, and other therapists, such as psychologists, speech therapists, psychiatrists or pediatricians, and activity and sports leaders, such as coaches and community activity leaders. Others who participate in a child's life should be regularly consulted. (Naturally, consultation will be with permission of the client or the responsible parent whenever possible.) Contemporary descriptions of the role of occupational therapy show that more than just sensorimotor or neuromuscular skills are being addressed for the child population. Specifically, programs are suggested that include parent-skills training, parent support and education, and facilitation of families' abilities to interact while conducting daily life occupations (Ireys, Dvet, & Sakwa, 2002; Lougher, 2001) as well as assessing play through family narratives (Burke & Schaaf, 1997).

Medications

Even though some medications, such as Ritalin, have received controversial media attention, a variety of other medications are judiciously used in the treatment of children. Medication is often needed to assist the client in gaining control over his or her behavior or stabilizing symptoms so that she or he may more readily participate in therapy. Medication is often selected only after all members of the team including parents and guardians have been consulted or the client has been observed in various settings. The occupational therapist can contribute observations of the client in various life roles or occupational settings.

While medication is often needed to assist the client (and a psychiatrist or family physician is ultimately responsible for prescribing medications), it is important for the occupational therapist and other team members to monitor the medicated client's behaviors and status carefully. The occupational therapist works closely with the individual, and may be the first to observe emerging side effects or changes in behavior. It is particularly important to monitor medications closely in young people because psychoactive medication sometimes interacts with the neurochemistry of the synapses and may interfere with development of new neuron networks and neurologically based competencies (Newton, 1995). Therefore, cognitive and behavioral approaches are usually attempted before a consideration of pharmacology.

CHILD SETTINGS AND PROGRAMS

When considering a program, the need is to always provide the least restrictive environment for the client. The best program will be the most normalized and balanced one, often with the goal of minimizing the need for further intervention. Childrens' programs may be based on a habilitative rather than a rehabilitative approach. Habilitation involves addressing skills and behaviors that were previously unlearned and undeveloped. This is opposed to the rehabilitative approach often used with adults, which focuses on the retrieval of skills clients already have or had prior to their current illness (Lambert, Moffitt, & Rose, 1989).

The role of the registered occupational therapist has been described broadly in the literature. Kent described the OTR working with children with psychosocial dysfunction as a developmental therapist with an assessment role of evaluating functioning level in skills and interests (cited in Sholle-Martin & Alessi, 1990). The OTR's role with children has been described as based on social learning, behavioral, psychoanalytic, systems analysis, and developmental models (Lougher, 2001), as well as the occupational therapy theories of Mary Reilly. Evaluation emphasizes play history, temperament, family dynamics, and patterns of behavior, and treatment modalities include play, behavioral management, sensorimotor integration, values clarification, and activity groups (Reilly, Kielhofner, Ayres, Nelson, Llorens, & Rubin, cited in Sholle-Martin & Alessi, 1990). According to Lambert and Moffitt (1988), OTRs also implement parent-child activity groups to improve parents' ability to interact with their children (cited in Sholle-Martin & Alessi, 1990).

Inpatient hospitalization, long-term residential treatment, outpatient settings, community-based programs, partial hospitalization programs, and school-based settings may all offer opportunities for the therapist. Anywhere there are children there is a possible treatment setting in which their psychosocial needs may be met. Newer developments within the school system and in partial hospitalization programs are discussed here.

School-Based Programs

Following the Columbine High School shootings in April 1999, the mental health needs of children received a great deal of attention from clinicians as well as the mass media. New roles identified for OTs include conducting screenings for "signs and risk factors" among students that "related to conflict and violence" and providing groups to improve appropriate expression of feelings and improving self-esteem (Johansson, 1999).

According to Hill, anger management is a critical focus (cited in Johansson, 1999, p. 9). Being part of a critical incident debriefing team in schools, working with students following a traumatic violent event, has also been identified as a role for therapists working in schools.

School districts are required to meet the special needs of their students in cases where performance in the classroom is affected. Depending on the county and the particular office of education, there may be opportunities for the occupational therapist interested in working to meet the school-aged clients' psychosocial needs. Some counties are meeting the psychosocial needs of severely emotionally disturbed (SED) students through programs offered on public school campuses. Such programs typically provide services through a special education teacher, psychiatrist, and social worker as well as teacher's aides and assistants who work with the clinical staff. Occupational therapists are included in some of these programs and may provide services including assessment, treatment, home programs, school programs, and consultation. In the school-based setting, the goal is to increase the student's function in the special education classroom with the long-term goal of participation in a regular classroom. All treatment goals should indicate progress toward this end. The occupational therapist is able to view students holistically, look at their performance in the classroom, and provide the necessary services for skill development and improved classroom success.

Partial Hospitalization

Partial hospitalization programs are sometimes referred to as day treatment programs. They are another alternative designed to prevent children from entering or staying in an inpatient hospitalization setting. These programs also provide a useful service of transitioning the client from an inpatient to an outpatient setting or to provide an educational experience when the regular school cannot currently meet the needs of the child with a mental illness. Typically, these programs are affiliated with a psychiatric unit or residential program in the community. The clients will attend a program during typical school hours and will receive treatment groups or therapy more intensively than if they were outpatients. The student may attend a program like this to avoid hospitalization or to make necessary adjustments to medication under a supervised setting. As with the school-based program and most treatment programs, the goal is to improve the clients' functioning to the degree to which they can be placed in a less intensive environment.

IMPLEMENTING PROGRAMMING FOR CHILDREN

When developing a program of occupational therapy, it is important to assess the needs of the children, demands of the service delivery system, and structure of the program. For example, if developmental motor lags are an area of concern, sensorimotor groups may be planned. Where play skills are lacking, play groups and opportunities to develop age-appropriate play skills are of prime importance. If children in the treatment setting have difficulty expressing their thoughts and feelings appropriately, programming should address these needs (Lambert, Moffitt, & Rose, 1989; Lambert & Moffitt, 1988).

The second critical step is to look at the service delivery system itself. In acute care settings there is relatively little time to provide treatment before discharge looms. Often it is the role of occupational therapy and the treatment team to begin treatment with the idea that it will be continued outside the hospital setting at school, in a partial hospitalization setting, or in an outpatient office. In a longer-term setting, treatment may be carried out entirely in one place, although because of the frequent changes in health care delivery, there may not be an extended period of time to bring about change. In terms of planning occupational therapy for an existing program, it is important to understand how therapy fits into the current program in terms of philosophy and program needs. This makes an understanding of theory important and flexibility imperative. The therapist must assume a systems approach, involving an awareness of the current program, the service delivery system, and the clients' needs.

In addition to occupational therapy assessments based in specific frames of reference, groups and activities are determined by the developmental needs of individual children. For example, a child may be 12 years old chronologically but function at a three- or four-year-old level, with a limited ability to express feelings in words and impaired cognitive skills secondary to a diagnosis of pervasive developmental disorder or mental retardation. Such a child may be placed in a play group that meets the needs of his or her developmental, age-appropriate level. The child's play and social behavior can be observed at the same time he or she is provided with opportunities for developmentally appropriate play activities. When a child is observed to be playing successfully at a developmentally appropriate level, he or she may then be moved up from a play group to a skills group to learn further personal and social skills (Lambert, Moffitt, & Rose, 1989).

Evaluation and Assessment

General areas of assessment concern the occupational performance areas of self-care and play and also developmental milestone achievement (see Parham & Fazio, 1997 for many assessments of play). Play can be evaluated by observing a child at play and obtaining a play history concerning what toys and games the child chooses. The occupational performance components to be assessed are primarily sensorimotor, cognitive, psychological, and social. Formal evaluations such as the Test of Visual Motor Skills (TVMS), the Good-Enough-Harris Draw-A-Person test, or the Erhhardt Developmental Prehension Assessment (EDPA) may further evaluate adaptive motor skills and coordination as well as a basic assessment of achievement on expected developmental milestones (cited in Asher, 1996). A useful tool for a quick assessment of many components is the Kinetic Self-Image Test (Abramson, 1982b), developed as part of the Initial Play Interview at Mount Sinai Hospital in New York. In this test, the child is asked to draw a picture of himself or herself doing something. Besides data regarding sensorimotor and cognitive components, valuable information such as interests, relationships, and self-concept can be determined.

CASE ILLUSTRATION: Josh—Kinetic Self-Image Assessment

Josh, a newly admitted boy, drew a picture of "me, my mom and Dad going for ice cream." Although the boy was 11 years old, he provided basically stick figures and a poorly drawn house. During the evaluation, Josh kept looking at the clock, and he also asked to go to the bathroom several times. When asked if he had an appointment or was waiting or looking for someone, he said, "I have a family session at 3 o'clock." However, when asked if he was leaving group to see if his parents had arrived, he angrily denied it.

Discussion

This simple assessment can be helpful in determining mental age and motor coordination, what the child is thinking about, and the quality of family or personal functioning and relationships.

CASE ILLUSTRATION: John and Stephen— Kinetic Self-Image Assessment

John, age 10, and Stephen, age 8, were being seen for evaluation during their initial home-based therapy visit. Their parents had recently separated and the boys lived with their mother, who is a nurse. Their father had been described as having bipolar disorder and alcoholism. Divorce is probable and their mother was referred to the therapist by an outpatient child psychiatrist after he evaluated the older child. The mother, concerned with the children's reaction to the separation and pending divorce, wished to provide an outlet for the children's feelings and an arena for them to discuss their concerns. Additionally, she has concerns regarding a strong family history of bipolar disorder and alcoholism on both sides of the family and the possibility of these disorders emerging in the children. In the initial session, the Kinetic Self-Image Assessment was used to assess the boys. Each was asked to draw a picture of himself doing something. John drew a picture of "playing ball with my dad." Of note was a tall tree drawn in the center of the paper separating the boy from the father. Stephen drew a picture of "John and me playing catch." It included birds, trees, and a yellow sun.

Discussion

Clearly, John's relationship with his father and spending time with him are important and his concern about the separation is evident in the picture. For Stephen, the focus of the picture was playing with his brother and with its details and pleasant presentations indicates either a more positive approach to family dynamics or denial of the current situation.

Intervention

Play is often referred to as the work of the child; it is generally defined as the way children learn basic skills and resolve intrapersonal and interpersonal conflicts.

> From a child's play we can gain understanding of how he sees and construes the world[;] . . . play refers to a young child's activities characterized by freedom from all but personally imposed rules, . . . by fantasy involvement and by the absence of any goals outside of the activity itself. (Bettelheim, 1987, p. 15)

It is helpful to distinguish play from games because the latter are a predominant occupation of older children and adolescents. Games are usually competitive, and they have agreed-upon rules that are imposed externally. Games require that the activity be pursued in a prescribed manner, without one's personal fantasy, and there is often a goal, such as winning, outside the activity (Bettelheim, 1987). With the basic acceptance of the importance of play (and later, games) as treatment (Kaplan & Telford, 1998), and also with the recognition of play as the predominant occupation of childhood, it is the primary occupation used in pediatrics and the primary activity used in pediatric groups (Abramson et al., 1979; Hoffman, 1982; Lambert and Moffitt, 1988; Parham & Fazio, 1997; Sholle-Martin & Alessi, 1990). In fact, "play therapy has become the main avenue for helping young children with their emotional difficulties" (Bettelheim, 1987, p. 15).

Play is also the primary mode of evaluating children, which is done through specific assessments and interviews and by ongoing observation. There are various ways to initially evaluate and continue to observe play. Some useful categories to think about while observing play are (C. Grandison, personal communication, January 28, 1997):

- Developmental or stage of play, such as solitary, exploratory, parallel, project, or cooperative (Hoffman, 1982): a 2-year-old can be expected to engage mostly in parallel play, whereas a 10-year-old can be expected to cooperate with other children in play.
- Entrance to play: for example, does a child hesitate to play or quickly bolt toward the toys?
- Initiation toward play: that is, (1) does a child initiate play independently or wait for someone to start with, and (2) is the same pattern consistent throughout play?
- Energy level: what is the level of energy of the child at play and does it change within or over sessions? Is it the same with or without structure? Is it the same with a parent present?
- Body movement and use of space: that is, does the child know where others are? Does he or she define a small area or fill up every space? Does the child use furniture?
- Emotional tone: that is, what is the emotional tenor to the play (e.g., is it angry or sad?) and does it remain the same over time?
- Materials: what materials does the child gravitate toward and how are they used?
- Symbolic nature of play: for example, does the child use objects and play symbolically? What are the themes of play, and are they consistent throughout?

An ongoing, regularly scheduled play group also provides information as to the child's current developmental level of play as reflected in the choice of toys, games, and peers while engaged in play.

There are various play scales (Asher, 1996), play classifications (Florey, 1968), and histories that include other observations and categories. The Knox Play Scale (Reilly, 1974) uses categories of space and material management, imitation, and type of participation. Another play observation looks at toys chosen, time of participation, quality of interaction with the toy, language, and social qualities to play. There is an emphasis on the play's developmental level (e.g., solitary, exploratory, parallel, etc.) and theme (such as aggressive, destructive, nurturing, etc.). A Parent-Teacher Play Questionnaire (Scutta & Schaaf, 1989) elicits information from others concerning a child's favorite toy, choices of toys, playmates, preferred locations for play, and any changes in the past week.

Groups.   Play group is a nondirective group that occurs most easily in the occupational therapy playroom. On an acute inpatient unit such a play group has been particularly efficacious for early **latency age** children. "[It] is a valuable diagnostic tool as well as a developmentally appropriate way for the children to interact with their peers and to deal with potentially stressful situations" (Abramson, Hoffman, & Johns, 1979, p. 391). The group's protocol is illustrated in Figure 10-4.

NAME OF GROUP: Occupational Therapy Play Group

DESCRIPTION: Play is an important part of a child's development. Children learn, express themselves, and develop interpersonal interaction skills through play. Through play, children are able to express inner feelings and conflicts in a non-threatening way. This group's primary goal is to evaluate skills and provide an adequate environment where the children's dynamics, developmental level of play and socialization skills can be observed and practiced.

THERAPIST NAME: William Lambert, OTR/L

TITLE: Occupational Therapist

GOALS:
1.) Provide a stimulating environment where the children will be motivated to play.
2.) Encourage peer interaction through play.
3.) Provide insightful interpretations related to the play when appropriate.
4.) Allow the children to work through dynamic issues through the play.
5.) Encourage the highest developmental level of play and interpersonal interaction possible.

ENTRANCE CRITERIA:
1.) Group members are selected by the OTR according to their developmental levels of play.
2.) Five children is an optimal number of group members.
3.) Patient has appropriate level of privileges.
4.) Patient has been medically cleared by physician.

GROUP RULES:
1.) Have fun
2.) Share
3.) Listen to staff
4.) Clean up

FORMAT:
Group meets two times per week for 45 minutes with two leaders: the OT and a member of the nursing staff.

EXIT CRITERIA:
1.) Change in level of privileges.
2.) Change in developmental status.
3.) Discharge from the hospital.

Figure 10-4. Play Group Protocol

The room includes toys, water and sand play areas, dress-up clothes for fantasy play, and a table and chairs. It serves to encourage the development of play skills, which in turn facilitates the development of social skills. The play group also has the goal of providing an arena whereby children may resolve conflicts and issues that led to their current problems and dysfunction. For example, two children may use dolls to express anger at parents who abused them. They may also recreate arguments or scenes they observed in the home. For example, by using toy sharks, a child may safely and appropriately show anger or jealousy toward a sibling or peer by "eating" him or her during water play or "burying" him or her in the sandbox. A game like Sorry helps increase frustration tolerance, and a game like Twister develops not only laterality but also the ability to be close to others appropriately and respect body space. Beanbag toss games are an appropriate outlet for anger and aggression and also provide the opportunity to engage in turn taking and mild competition. Candyland, Life, and Connect Four are just a few of the many readily available childhood games that can be used or adapted to develop many different skills and prompt conversation and discussion. Inherent in many childhood games such as "Duck, Duck, Goose," "Musical Chairs," and "Dodge Ball" is a focus on developing a variety of basic abilities. "Rolling Dodge Ball" can be played in place of the conventional game. This adaptation involves rolling rather than throwing the ball at peers. This increases safety and prevents the game from becoming overly aggressive.

There are countless ways in which play can help children learn new skills and accomplish treatment goals. For example, it is more efficacious to ask children to try to clean up the entire playroom before you can count to 10 than it is to just command them to clean up the playroom because "it's time to end group." Turning an activity into a game or play, as in this example, is often more effective than other approaches. It is also congruent with the philosophy of occupational therapy and the general approach of using play as a treatment modality. The active experiences of play and the focus on productivity and participation offer intrinsic satisfaction for a child's needs. Aside from conflict resolution, play also offers children the additional ability to work on treatment goals of improving impulse control, developing cognitive skills, mastering the environment, and developing age-appropriate social interactions. Through the mastery of tasks, latency-aged children will be able to benefit from the successful interaction with objects and people in occupational therapy group and gain mastery over themselves in the process.

Creative task groups also serve as highly effective interventions with latency-aged children. The use of tiles to make mosaics, wood projects such as creating a bookshelf or making a toy car, painting sun catchers, or participating in seasonal activities such as carving a pumpkin or baking Christmas cookies offer children rewarding experiences. In addition, the experiences teach appropriate interaction and cognitive skills, such as the ability to follow directions, increase attention span and concentration, complete tasks, and share material. Comments made about the projects often provide a valuable additional perspective on a child's emotions and concerns. Copper tooling is a highly successful creative task project. Children frequently ask, "Can I do more than one?" or after successful completion of the project, they will ask, "Can we do copper tooling projects again?" They may remark, "It's fun to do—it's easy to make." Indeed, the steps of copper tooling are easy to grade according to the therapeutic purposes of the group.

Of course, it is important to take precautions such as removing the solution as soon as all group members have used it and conducting the group in a well-ventilated area.

Most often, creative tasks are provided as part of a parallel task group. This structure provides opportunities to develop appropriate interpersonal interactions on a limited basis, share through the use of supplies that are common to the group activity, and develop impulse control by waiting to follow the steps and to see the project through to completion.

Group goals may include learning how to follow simple, step-by-step verbal directions; sharing materials and space; interacting without being intrusive; sustaining an increasing attention span; and developing impulse control. Other information that can be gained through the use of a simple craft project includes dynamic information such as who the gift or project is to be given to, and, therefore, who is important in the child's life.

Skill development group assists older children who have adequate play and social skills and need to improve problem-solving, coping, and communication skills. See the group's protocol in Figure 10-5. Group topics and discussion focus on common problems and situations that children face as well as the specific problem areas that led to treatment.

NAME OF GROUP: Occupational Therapy Skill Development Group

DESCRIPTION: A developmental task group for children who have developed basic play and social skills and need to acquire skills in cognition, interpersonal interactions and self-expression.

THERAPIST NAME: William Lambert, OTR/L

TITLE: Occupational Therapist

GOALS:
1.) To improve cognitive skills such as:
    a.) problem-solving
    b.) organization of thoughts
    c.) ability to follow directions
2.) To improve interpersonal interaction skills and facilitate sharing cooperation.
3.) To improve ability to express thoughts and feelings appropriately.

ENTRANCE CRITERIA:
1.) Group members are selected by the OTR according to developmental need.
2.) Patient should be on appropriate level of privilege to attend groups.
3.) Patient is medically cleared by physician.
4.) Five to seven children is the optimal number of group members.

GROUP RULES:
1.) Have fun
2.) Share
3.) Listen to staff
4.) Clean up

FORMAT:
Group meets two times per week for 45 minutes with two leaders: the OT and a member of the nursing staff. Activities will be planned to develop specific skills through the use of games and creative tasks.

EXIT CRITERIA:
1.) Change in level of privileges
2.) Discharge from hospital

Figure 10-5. Skills Development Group Protocol

- Soft lighting to provide a calming atmosphere.
- Area rugs or carpet to play on.
- Colorful but not overstimulating room.
- Adequate tables and chairs. These do not need to be child-sized except for younger preschool-age children. Most latchkey-age children can use a conventional-sized table and chairs.
- Materials should be easy to clean.
- An area for water play and larger gross motor groups is ideal, but be adaptive! A bathtub or utility sink can do as needed or on a regular basis, depending on funding, facility, and frequency of use.
- Craft paper in large rolls can be used for many purposes—to cover the table for a craft activity, to do body tracings, to make murals and drawings, and so on. This inexpensive investment goes a long way and lasts a long time!

Figure 10-6. Tips for Creating an Effective Playroom or Therapy Area

While a variety of activities can be used in the skills development group, including crafts, therapeutic board games are frequently used. "Stress Strategies" is a game used to develop coping skills, and "The Talking, Feeling and Doing Game" (Lambert, Moffitt, & Rose, 1989) facilitates the expression of thoughts and feelings. Both are examples of games that are effective in meeting treatment goals. Because they use a board game format, children are usually willing to participate and an appropriate amount of structure is provided. Children are often happy to have an outlet for their unexpressed feelings and thoughts and view the game as a safe and nonthreatening means of personal expression. See Figure 10-6 for ways to assure that the environment supports effective group and individual interventions.

CASE ILLUSTRATION: The Talking, Feeling, and Doing Game

Seven children ages 8 to 12 years old are playing the game with the occupational therapist, a member of the nursing staff, and an OT student. Sam rolls the dice, lands on a yellow space, and selects a "feeling" card, which reads: "Name three things that could cause a person to be angry." He pauses and then says, "Being told to shut up, being hit, and being lied to." Dave lands on a white space and selects a "talking" card, which reads, "What kind of work does your father do? What do you think about that kind of job?" Dave answers, "He fixes trucks," although he does not mention that his father is in prison. "I'm going to race motorcycles when I grow up," he says when asked what he thinks of his father's job. Christine rolls the dice and also lands on a white space. Her card asks, "What is the best thing you can say about your family?" She replies, "They bring me candy and lots of things." John lands on a red space and picks a "doing" card, which reads, "Skip across the room and then return to your seat." He says, "I'm not doing that," but he agrees to take another card. This one asks him to pretend that he is having an argument with someone and to tell the group what it is about. "I'm arguing with Melissa. She won't share," John replies. The therapist then rolls and lands on a "feeling" space. His card reads, "When was the last time you cried?" He says, "I cried when my dad died." Then he talks about how crying is helpful in expressing feelings of sadness. Linda and Rhonda, the other adults in group, reinforce what the therapist has said. This helps the children talk about their feelings and express them appropriately.

Discussion

This game promotes, through talking, the expression of what is on children's minds. The game facilitates the expression of feelings, promotes the discussion of personal problems, and can explore family dynamics without threat and in a manner that matches the children's emotional age. It is important to have a good working knowledge of the children to lead a game such as this effectively.

There are ever-increasing numbers of blended and nontraditional families in the United States (Waterman, 2001). The traditional family may no longer be constituted of a biological mother and father with biological siblings. Children and adolescents may be adopted and raised by extended families, grandparents, relatives, stepparents, or family friends. Whoever the child or adolescent considers to be "family" may be permitted to join in treatment, as is often the case in the parent-child activity group (Lambert, 1990).

The parent-child activity group (Lambert, 1990) involves engaging the parents of the emotionally disturbed child in an activity with the child. It is held weekly in the occupational therapy room, where families usually work on a project together with the goal of completing it in one session. This group improves the parent-child interaction by engaging them together in a pleasurable, successful activity, something that may not otherwise be possible due to the child's illness. The therapist provides encouragement and support and models appropriate caregiver behavior such as setting limits on inappropriate actions and giving praise for desirable ones. The OTR assists parents in differentiating between behavior that is maladaptive and behavior that is typical for the child's developmental level. Beyond providing occupational therapy for families and their disturbed children, the OTR is able to provide those involved in the child's treatment with information about family interactive patterns, the child's response to therapy with the parents, and how well the parents are implementing what they are being taught about how to interact with their child. The parent-child activity has expanded the scope of occupational therapy in the hospital setting to areas traditionally reserved for individual and family therapists. By providing information on how the child behaves and the outcomes of the session, occupational therapy has enhanced the team's ability to see the child and family more globally and respond with more integrated treatment for both.

Examples of Emerging Areas of Practice

Therapists have been challenged to follow clients into the community, to consider consulting as an alternative to direct service, and to find new sources of funding, including cash (Kautzmann, 1998; Kornblau, 1999; Learnard, 1998; Richert, 1998). Clinicians need to present occupational therapy outcomes (Richert, 1998) and market to the needs of clients and community agencies. As the location of care moves out of the hospital and lengths of stay become increasingly shorter, one arena for therapists is to go into private practice and consider private pay for reimbursement of services through community-based practice (Dorman and Helfrich, 2001; Ramsey, Best, Merryman, Learnard, & Scheinholtz, 1998).

Following are examples of emerging areas of practice that can be implemented by using the inpatient interventions described earlier in this chapter in the community through private practice. These interventions include consultation and direct service for a foster care agency and home-based therapy and are reimbursed through the therapist's private practice. Both involve a family-centered approach and a fee-for-service format for payment (cash or check). Traditional forms of reimbursement such as private insurance or managed care companies are *not* utilized or accepted. This arrangement also adds an increased measure of confidentiality and the therapist, family, or agency can determine the number of sessions. Private clients can be seen for cash for what may not be much more than some insurance providers require as a co-payment.

Occupational Therapy Services for a Foster Care Agency.   Providing occupational therapy services for a foster care agency brings unique and rewarding challenges and illustrates a new role for occupational therapy in the community in a nontraditional practice setting. The child in foster care can be assisted in adapting to various situations through occupational therapy intervention that increases the child's ability to function in an age-appropriate manner at his or her current level of development. Intervention is aimed at reducing the number of times that a child's life is interrupted so that agency goals of successful pre- and postadoptive placements can be achieved, as well as smoothing a child's transition from a foster care placement to reunification with the biological parent(s) and birth family (Barney, personal communication, March 10, 2003; Derdeyn & Lamps, 2002; Nickman, 2000).

Frequently the long-term goal of foster care is to have the children reunified with their family of origin. Some states, such as California, may also pursue adoption at the same time that family reunification is attempted. Therefore, having consistent therapy that focuses on children's functioning may help them negotiate this difficult adoption or reunification situation.

CASE ILLUSTRATION: Reunification—The Rinaldo Family

Jose, age 5, lives with his mother, Rosalita, age 27, in a large city. They have just successfully completed family-based therapy sessions with the occupational therapist, which was an essential piece of their reunification plan. Now Rosalita and Jose will again have Juan, Sophia, Carlos, and Jesus back in the home. Currently Juan, age 10, lives in a foster care home. Sophia, age 8, Carlos, age 6, and Jesus, age 3 1/2, live in another foster care home. Reunification will be facilitated through two separate intervention strategies. First, parent-child activity sessions with the entire family will be conducted by the occupational therapist once a month. Second, the OT will schedule sibling groups between the family sessions to reacquaint the brothers and sisters with each other. Rosalita and Jose arrive for their scheduled parent-child activity on Saturday morning, and join the other siblings and the OT at the OT office. The initial intervention is for the children and mother to play together using the toys in the room, and later to make pudding to have for dessert, which will follow a lunch provided by the foster care agency. The OT begins the activity by asking, "Juan, why don't you be a big brother and help your little sister and brothers by being in charge of pouring the milk?" This intervention occurs once the therapist notices that Rosalita appears overwhelmed and makes no attempt to organize the task. The OT then notices Jesus crawling for the door and retrieves him. "Sophia, will you keep an eye on Jesus so he doesn't get into trouble?" suggests the OT. Eventually Rosalita opens the pudding package after reading the directions to the children, several of whom are not paying attention, and begins giving her children various tasks to complete. The OT moves to the periphery of the room to facilitate the mother taking charge of the situation and to assess the parent-child interaction. Once the pudding has been spooned into cups and put in the refrigerator, the OT cues the family to clean up the dishes. The family is given time to socialize as they wait for pizza to be delivered. The younger children fight over a toy but the mother redirects them to share. Juan, as usual, is quiet and isolative. Rosalita picks up the toddler and attempts to engage Jesus in play with nearby toys. Jose engages in spontaneous play with his younger brothers and wrestles with them. Sophia, who had been drawing, starts to cry, as she feels left out. The OT suggests ways for her to ask her siblings to play with her, such as asking them to come draw with her or to play a game.

Discussion

Occupational therapy groups were used to facilitate reunification of several siblings living in different foster care homes with their biological mother and an additional sibling residing with her. Sibling groups based on the play-group format refamiliarize the siblings with each other during sessions employing play, games, and arts and crafts in addition to developing and building relationships and interactions among the children and provide opportunities for professional observation and assessment. The sibling groups were used in conjunction with a parent-child activity that occurred during the biological mother's scheduled monthly visit with all of her children, a vital part of the reunification process. This group used activities such as making pudding and simple meals, arts and crafts, structured play, and games designed to reinforce roles of mother, older brother, sister, younger brothers, and toddler with the therapist serving as facilitator. These groups were used to promote appropriate parent-child interactions and establish filial roles. The groups also provided a therapeutic milieu for the mother and children to meet each other in a safe setting for not only interaction but also expression of feelings regarding present and future visitation (Barney, personal communication, March 10, 2003).

The therapist provided role modeling and suggestions for improving parenting skills. He also solicited the mother's feedback as to how she perceived the reunification process to be progressing. The therapist also provided the foster care agency with ongoing reports and his assessment of family functioning and helped determine when reunification would occur. Following 21 months of occupational therapy intervention, the family was reunited and continues to live together. While therapy progressed well across time, other factors, such as the mother finding an appropriately sized home, having the home approved, and various bureaucratic requirements lengthened the reunification process. This case illustrates how the luxury of time and many ongoing sessions can exist when traditional reimbursement sources are not used (Lambert, 2003).

Foster Care Agency—Expert Witness. In another case of family reunification, the mother failed to attend any of the scheduled parent-child activity sessions. During groups with the occupational therapist, the siblings consistently expressed their desire to remain in the preadoptive foster home and to be adopted by their foster parents. At the custody hearing, the report of the children's desire to be adopted and to have the biological mother's rights terminated to facilitate their adoption was presented to the judge and served as an objective outside opinion as well as an expert witness. In chambers, the children corroborated the therapist's testimony and the judge ruled for termination based on the children's statements, the occupational therapist's evidence, and that of others involved in the case. This evidence from various sources paved the way for adoption in an appropriate home for these children (Lambert, 2003).

Testifying in court is a unique experience (Rosen, 2002). Some suggestions when testifying are to remember to always address the judge as "your honor" and answer only the questions you are asked succinctly and specifically. The more information volunteered, the more opportunities the opposing side's attorney has to discredit your testimony.

In court hearings to involuntarily terminate parental rights of children in foster care who want to be adopted by their foster parents the responsibilities of the therapist are specific. They are to assess the children through information from interviews and therapy sessions. Then in court the therapist presents, her or his clinical opinion regarding what outcome the children want, their feelings regarding the termination, and what outcome she or he recommends based on her or his area of expertise and clinical experience.

Being a witness in court includes being a developmental specialist, child advocate, and clinical expert regarding children's behavioral and emotional health through the eye and lens of occupational therapy.

Foster Care Agency—Direct Service. The occupational therapist provides other services for the foster care agency including family intervention and troubleshooting regarding developmentally appropriate rules and activities for children in foster care. This is especially important in instances where the foster parents require direction and instruction to smooth family difficulties and deal adaptively and appropriately with the children and their diverse issues, presenting problems, and diagnoses.

With the aid of occupational therapy intervention, a foster care or preadoptive home placement can remain consistent and reduce the number of times that a child's life is interrupted (Barney, personal communication, March 10, 2003). Minimizing interruptions is imperative to the mental health of children in the foster care system (Waterman, 2001).

Home-Based Occupational Therapy. Occupational therapists have been encouraged to develop new strategies for serving the mental health needs of children and their families (Mental Health Needs of Children and Youth, Dorman & Helfrich, 2001). Therefore, home-based intervention has been cited as a growing area of practice and uses the natural setting of the home to assess and treat areas of behavior, family dynamics, and parent-child interactions (Case-Smith, 2001; Pratt & Allen, 1996). Interventions can include anger management, social skills training, and parent-child activities. The parent-child activity discussed previously in this chapter and in foster care case interventions above is also part of a home-based approach with the added dimension of using the family home as a treatment setting. This provides an "in vivo" environment (Shultz et al., 2001) to observe situations and interactions that affect therapy outcomes but are not able to be observed in other settings. For example, the 24-hour television, the dog running through the house barking because of a thunderstorm, a younger sibling who intrudes on the session with his brother and steals game board pieces, dinner late or burning provide real-life situations and stressors that can be observed and used as intervention points in therapy.

Upon referral from a child psychiatrist, occupational therapists may see children and their families in their own homes to address the variety of psychosocial deficits and problems that led the children and their families to seek professional help. Again, the duration and length of therapy is determined largely by the family and the therapist, with direction provided by the referring psychiatrist. The occupational therapist must possess an extensive background in providing psychosocial interventions to children with emotional disturbances and their families and be able to practice autonomously. An additional benefit to this practice setting is that there is rarely a missed appointment, although a family may forget about the scheduled visit. Receiving payment upon conclusion of the session eliminates the need for billing, and seeing children and their families in their homes eliminates the need for renting office space. However, it does include other expenses that should be taken into account when billing, such as mileage and increased wear and tear on one's car. Also, like many other home health therapists, one's car becomes a clinic where supplies are kept, and for a pediatric therapist the car becomes a traveling collection of toys, games, and other therapy supplies.

SUMMARY AND CURRENT TRENDS

The various conditions of children with mental illnesses include *DSM IV-TR* (APA, 2000) axis I diagnoses such as depression, bipolar, and post-traumatic stress disorders, in addition to disorders first diagnosed in infancy and childhood, such as attention deficit hyperactivity, oppositional defiant, and disruptive behavior disorders. When connecting behavior and diagnosis, genetic predispositions to mental illness and the symptoms and presenting problems of the disorders should be considered as well as environmental psychosocial stressors such as family dysfunction, abuse, trauma, neglect, violence, and poverty. Developmental-level and age-appropriate tasks should also be considered when working with children with emotional disturbances.

Useful concepts to consider when working with this population are structure and consistency, redirection, interpretation of behavior, time-out, a personal therapeutic style, a team approach, and the use of psychotropic medications.

When implementing a program it is important to consider the needs of the consumers, the demands of the service delivery system, and the structure of the current or planned program. Various assessments, including observation, are useful tools for occupational therapists planning therapeutic interventions. Intervention for children can be based primarily on play and include nondirective play, skill development, creative tasks, and parent-child activity groups.

"Sicker and quicker" has become an often-used phrase when describing the trend toward offering less time for therapy for children who may have very severe emotional problems. As managed care often replaces traditional insurance and reimbursement programs, timeframes for therapy are becoming shorter and inpatient hospitalizations are being curtailed in favor of community-based care. Unfortunately, cost containment may also limit access to occupational therapy unless therapists make the transition from traditional hospital and medical model practice settings to emerging areas of practice and community-based care. In an attempt to bring their expertise to these other arenas of the continuum of care, therapists need to "think outside the box," or perhaps "outside of the toy box in the clinic," and explore new ways of providing therapy to this population. These new ways include, but are not limited to, foster care, home, public, and private school settings, and in unfamiliar territory in any of the variety of agencies and programs already in place that provide services to children with and without identified disorders.

Children in need of services to remediate mental and behavioral pathology and develop and integrate new skills can be found everywhere—in the hospital, the school, at daycare, at home, and in your neighborhood (Forness, Florey & Greene, 1993). As children and often their parents are not always effective self-advocates, it is incumbent upon therapists to advocate appropriate services, including occupational therapy for underserved populations.

Review Questions

1. Name three symptoms of ADHD and one commonly prescribed medication used to treat this disorder.
2. Identify four intervention strategies that can be used to reduce acting-out or behavior problems.

3. What are two creative tasks that are effective in providing structure?
4. Identify three common games that can be used therapeutically with children with mental illness.
5. Identify two play activities that provide age-appropriate outlets for feelings and thoughts in children.

References

Abramson, R. M. (1982a). Therapeutic activities for the hospitalized child. In L. Hoffman (Ed.), *The evaluation and care of severely disturbed children* (pp. 61–69). New York: SP Medical & Scientific Books.

Abramson, R. M. (1982b). Developmental and diagnostic assessment. In L. Hoffmann (Ed.), *The evaluation and care of severely disturbed children* (pp. 37–44). New York: SP Medical & Scientific Books.

Abramson, R. M., Hoffman, L., & Johns, C. A. (1979). Play group psychotherapy for early latency-age children on an in-patient psychiatric unit. *International Journal of Group Psychotherapy, 29,* 383–392.

American Occupational Therapy Association. (2002, April 18). The psychosocial deficits of children with regulatory disorders. *OT Practice*, CE4–CE6.

American Psychiatric Association (APA). (2000). *Diagnostic and statistical manual of mental disorders*. Text Revision (4th ed.). Washington, DC: APA.

Argabrite Grove, R. E. (2002, March 25). Embracing our psychosocial roots. *OT Practice*, 21–25.

Asher, I. E. (1996). *Occupational therapy evaluation tools: An annotated index* (2nd ed.). Bethesda, MD: American Occupational Therapy Association.

Benoit, W. (2000). Foster care. In B. J. Sadock & V. A. Sadock. (Eds.), *Kaplan and Sadock's comprehensive textbook of psychiatry* (7th Ed., pp. 2873–2877). Philadelphia: Lippincott Williams & Wilkins.

Bertucco, M. (2001, May/June). Bad behavior. *Psychology Today, 28.*

Bettelheim, B. (1987, March). The importance of play. *Atlantic Monthly,* 35–46.

Block, B. M., Arney, K., Campbell, D. J., Kiser, L. T., Lefkovitz, D. M., & Speer, S. K. (1991). American Association for Partial Hospitalization, Child and Adolescent Special Interest Group: Standards for child and adolescent partial hospitalization programs. *International Journal of Partial Hospitalization, 7*(1), 13–21.

Bruce, M., & Borg, B. (1993). *Psychosocial occupational therapy: Frames of reference for intervention* (2nd ed.). Thorofare, NJ: Slack.

Burke, J. P., & Schaaf, R. C. (1997). Family narratives and play assessment. In L. D. Parham & L. S. Fazio (Eds.), *Play in occupational therapy for children* (pp. 67–85). St. Louis, MO: Mosby.

Burns, B. J., & Hoagwood, K. (2002). *Community treatment for youth: Evidence-based interventions for severe emotional and behavioral disorders*. New York: Oxford University Press.

Chess, S., & Thomas, A. (1984). *Origins and evolution of behavior disorders: From infancy to early adult life*. New York: Brunner/Mazel.

Derdeyn, A. P., & Lamps, C. A. (2002). Adoption. In M. L. Lewis (Ed.), *Child and adolescent psychiatry: A comprehensive textbook* (pp. 1266–1274). Philadelphia: Lippincott Williams & Wilkins.

Dorman, W., & Helfrich, C. (2001). *Psychosocial competence and its impact on function in children and youth*. Paper presented at the meeting of the American Occupational Therapy Association, Philadelphia.

Dryfoos, J. G. (1992). Adolescents at risk. A summary of work in the field: Programs and policies. In D. Rogers & E. Ginzberg (Eds.), *Cornell University Medical College Seventh Conference on Health Policy* (pp. 128–141). Boulder: Westview.

Eshleman, L. (2002, June). *Treatment approaches*. Paper presented at the Reactive Attachment Disorder conference sponsored by the Milton S. Hershey Medical Center College of Medicine, Scranton, PA.

295

Florey, L. L. (1968). *A developmental classification of play*. Unpublished master's thesis, University of Southern California, Los Angeles.

Florey, L. (2003). Psychosocial dysfunction in childhood and adolescence. In E. B. Crepeau, E. S. Cohn, & B. A. B. Schell (Eds.), *Willard and Spackman's occupational therapy* (10th ed., pp. 731–744). Philadelphia: Lippincott Williams & Wilkins.

Fonagy, P., Target, M., Cottrell, D., Phillips, J., & Kurtz, Z. (2002). *What works for whom?: A critical review of treatments for children and adolescents*. New York: Guilford.

Forness, S., Florey, L., & Green, S. (1993). *Hidden in plain sight: Children with behavior disorder in school systems*. Paper presented at the 73rd annual conference of the American Occupational Therapy Association, Seattle, WA.

Hahn, C. (2000, October 23). Building mental health roles into a school system practice. *OT Practice*, 14–16.

Hoffman, L. (1982). *The evaluation and care of severely disturbed children*. New York: SP Medical & Scientific Books.

Hollander, E. (2001). *Professional handbook of psychotropic drugs*. Springhouse, PA: Springhouse.

Ireys, H. T., Devet, K. A., & Sakwa, D. (2002). Family support and education. In B. J. Burns & K. Hoagwood (Eds.), *Community treatment for youth: Evidence-based interventions for severe emotional and behavioral disorders* (pp. 154–175). New York: Oxford University Press.

Johansson, C. (1999, August 5). O. T. prescription for school violence. *OT Week*.

Kaplan, C., & Telford, R. (1998). *The butterfly children: An account of non-directive play therapy*. New York: Churchill Livingstone.

Kautzmann, L. (1998). *Managed behavioral healthcare: Opportunities and challenges for practice*. Paper presented at the meeting of the American Occupational Therapy Association, Baltimore.

Kornblau, B. (1999). *Expanding your practice in an era of health care reform*. Paper presented at the meeting of the American Occupational Therapy Association, Indianapolis, IN.

Kramer, P., & Hinojosa, J. (1993). *Frames of reference for pediatric occupational therapy*. Baltimore: Williams & Wilkins.

Lambert, W. (2003). *Family-centered mental health OT with foster care children*. Paper presented at the meeting of the Pennsylvania Occupational Therapy Association, Pittsburgh, PA.

Lambert, W. (1990). *Parent-child activity: Assessment and treatment of families*. Paper presented at the Pennsylvania Occupational Therapy Association Annual Conference, Philadelphia.

Lambert, W., & Moffitt, R. (1988). *A collaborative approach to developmental group in child psychiatry*. Paper presented at the Pennsylvania Occupational Therapy Association Annual Conference, State College, PA.

Lambert, W., Moffitt, R., & Rose, J. (1989). *Therapeutic use of toys and games in child psychiatry*. Paper presented at the Pennsylvania Occupational Therapy Association Annual Conference, Hershey, PA.

Learnard, L. T. (1998). *Occupational therapy consultation and rehabilitative services*. Paper presented at the meeting of the American Occupational Therapy Association, Baltimore.

Lewis, M. L. (Ed.). (2002). *Child and adolescent psychiatry: A comprehensive textbook*. Philadelphia: Lippincott Williams & Wilkins.

Llorens, L., & Rubin, E. (1967). *Developing ego functions in disturbed children: Occupational therapy in milieu*. Detroit: Wayne State University Press.

Lougher, L. (Ed.). (2001). *Occupational therapy for child and adolescent mental health*. New York: Churchill Livingstone.

Moffit, R. (1987). *Guidelines for reinforcing socially acceptable behaviors and extinguishing inappropriate, maladaptive behaviors*. Unpublished manuscript.

Morrison, J. (1995). *DSM-IV made easy: The clinician's guide to diagnosis*. New York: Guilford.

National Survey Reveals Impact of ADHD. (2002, January 28). *Advance for Occupational Therapy Practitioners*, 42.

Nickman, S. L. (2000). Adoption. In B. J. Sadock & V. A. Sadock (Eds.), *Kaplan and Sadock's comprehensive textbook of psychiatry* (7th ed., pp. 2868–2872). Philadelphia: Lippincott Williams & Wilkins.

Offer, D., & Schonert-Reichl, K. (1992). Debunking the myths of adolescence: Findings from recent research. *Journal of the American Academy of Child and Adolescent Psychiatry, 31*, 1003–1013.

Papalia, D. E., & Olds, S. W. (1992). *Human development*. New York: McGraw-Hill.

Parham, L. D., & Fazio, L. S. (Eds.). (1997). *Play in occupational therapy for children*. St. Louis, MO: Mosby.

Phelan, T. W. (1995). *1-2-3 Magic! Getting your preschoolers and preteens to do what you want*. Glen Ellyn, IL: Child Management.

Pratt, P., & Allen, A. (1989). *Occupational therapy for children* (2nd ed.). Baltimore: Mosby.

Ramsey, R., Best, L., Merryman, B., Learnard, L., & Schienholtz, M. (1998). *Payment and programming for occupational therapy in behavioral health care*. Short course presented at the meeting of the American Occupational Therapy Association, Baltimore.

Randolph, E. (1999). *Children who shock and surprise: A guide to attachment disorders* (3rd ed.). Salt Lake City, UT: RFR.

Reilly, M. (Ed.). (1974). *Play as exploratory learning*. Beverly Hills, CA: Sage.

Richert, G. (1998). *Cutting edge response to systems change; Community-based consultation: Expanding mental health services*. Paper presented at the meeting of the American Occupational Therapy Association, Baltimore.

Rosen, D. N. (2002). Testifying in court: A trial lawyer's perspective. In M. L. Lewis (Ed.), *Child and adolescent psychiatry: A comprehensive textbook* (pp. 1309–1314). Philadelphia: Lippincott Williams & Wilkins.

Rutter, M., & Taylor, E. (Eds.). (2002). *Child and adolescent psychiatry* (4th ed.). Oxford: Blackwell Science.

Sadock, B. J., & Sadock, V. A. (Eds.). (2000). *Kaplan and Sadock's comprehensive textbook of psychiatry* (7th. ed.). Philadelphia: Lippincott Williams & Wilkins.

Scutta, C., & Schaaf, R. C. (1989, October). *A time for play?* Paper presented at the Pennsylvania Occupational Therapy Association Annual Conference, Hershey, PA.

Sholle-Martin, S., & Alessi, N. E. (1990). Formulating a role for occupational therapy in child psychiatry: A clinical application. *American Journal of Occupational Therapy, 44*(10), 871–882.

Shultz, S., et al. (2001). *Issues in specific populations and intervention strategies: Behavioral disorder practice model*. Paper presented at the meeting of the American Occupational Therapy Association, Philadelphia.

Thomas, A., & Chess, S. (1986). The New York longitudinal study: From infancy to early adult life. In R. Plomin & J. Dunn (Eds.), *The study of temperament: Changes, continuities, and challenges*. Hillsdale, NJ: Erlbaum.

Waterman, B. (2001). Mourning the loss builds the bond: Primal communication between foster, adoptive, or stepmother and child. *Journal of Loss and Trauma, 6*, 277–300.

Weingarten-Dubin, J. (2001, May/June). More than a mood. *Psychology Today*, 26.

Zernicke, K., & Peterson, M. (2001, August 19). School's backing of behavior drugs comes under fire. *New York Times National Edition*, 1, 30.

Suggested Reading

Banus, B. S., Kent, C. A., Norton, Y., Sukiennicki, D. R., & Becker, M. L. (1982). *The developmental therapist* (2nd ed.). Thorofare, NJ: Slack.

Berger, K. S. (1994). *The developing person through the lifespan* (3rd ed.). New York: Worth.

Bingham, M., Edmondson, J., & Stryker, S. (1983). *Choices: A teen women's journal for self-awareness and personal planning*. Santa Barbara, CA: Advocacy.

Blake, J. (1990). *Risky times: How to be AIDS-smart and stay healthy: A guide for teenagers*. New York: Workman. (Spanish version published in 1993)

Byrne, K. (1987). *A parents' guide to anorexia and bulimia*. New York: Henry Holt.

Case-Smith, J. (2001). *Occupational therapy for children* (4th ed.). Baltimore: Mosby.

Freud, A. (1967). *The ego and the mechanisms of defense*. New York: International Universities Press.

Gil, E. (1983). *Outgrowing the pain: A book for and about adults abused as children*. New York: Dell.

Hall, C. S. (1982). *A primer of Freudian psychology*. New York: Harper & Row.

Heron, A. (Ed.). (1994). *Twenty writings by gay and lesbian youth*. Boston: Alyson.

Hunter, M. (1990). *Abused boys: The neglected victims of sexual abuse*. New York: Ballantine.

Levy, B. (1993). *In love and in danger: A teen's guide to breaking free of abusive relationships*. Seattle: Seal.

McCoy, K., & Wibbelsman, C. (1992). *The new teenage body book*. New York: Body/Perigee.

New Games Foundation. (1976). *The new games book*. Garden City, NY: Doubleday.

Outward Bound, USA. (1981). *Learning through experience in adventure based education*. New York: Morrow.

Stein, M. B., Hyde, K. L., & Monopolis, S. J. (1991). Child and family outreach services as an adjunct to child and adolescent mental health treatment. *International Journal of Partial Hospitalization*, 7(1) 69–75.

Steiner, H. (1995). *Treating adolescents*. San Francisco: Jossey-Bass.

Vogler, R., & Bartz, W. (1992). *Teenagers and alcohol*. Philadelphia: Charles.

Mental Health of Adolescents

Susan Haiman, MPS, OTR/L, FAOTA

William L. Lambert, OTR/L

Barbara Jo Rodrigues, MS, OTR/L

Key Terms

adolescent

mentor

redirection

temperament

transitional services

Chapter Outline

Introduction

It is often difficult to believe that normal **adolescent** development is not necessarily a period punctuated with turmoil and anguish. But the majority of adolescents actually negotiate the transition to adulthood with little difficulty. It is those adolescents whose difficult behaviors or symptoms bring them to the attention of school counselors, mental health professionals, or the legal system that have gained the most notoriety (Lewis, 2002; Rutter & Taylor, 2002).

Mental health is a major public health challenge in the world (Manikam, 2002). One study revealed that mental health problems are responsible for as much as 11% of the burden of disease worldwide. Children and adolescents were reported to be at special risk, particularly those who have poor nurturing or live in poverty. Fifteen to 20% of children and adolescents have mental health problems worldwide.

Adolescents in the United States are not immune to pressures on their mental health (Cohen & Caffo, 1998; Schwab-Stone & Briggs-Gowan, 1998). They are exposed to violence, either real or on television, video games, and the Internet, drugs, and the loss of family and community milieus that guided traditional methods of initiation into adulthood. At the same time mental health needs of children and adolescents are not a priority in most countries. Psychopathology in adolescents arises from a complex interaction of the characteristics of the teen, such as psychological, genetic, and biological factors and of the environment, such as parent, sibling, family, and peer relations, peer and neighborhood, and school and community factors in a larger social cultural context. "Manifestations of psychological dysfunction are indications of problems in living, not symptoms of disease process" (Manikam, 2002, p. 5).

Until the early 1990s, the hospital was the primary site for treatment of mental illnesses in general, whether it be on a small inpatient unit or in a large state hospital. Today radical changes in the health care system have resulted in much of the hospital intervention occurring in short-term settings, whenever possible. Residential treatment facilities for adolescents traditionally have provided long-term treatment, but there has also been an increase in the need for day treatment, special education settings, and group homes as well as intervention in the juvenile penal and detention system. This chapter presents an overview of occupational therapy practice with adolescents with a focus on settings where occupational therapy is or could be delivered as a critical service.

ADOLESCENT DEVELOPMENT

The period of adolescence is a time in which there is a great deal of transition, learning, and growth (Austrian, 2002; Bukatko & Daehler, 2001; King, 2002; Lefrancois, 2001; Pearce, 2003; Rice & Dolgin, 2002; Rutter & Taylor, 2002). Changes are occurring physically, emotionally, and socially as an adolescent moves from childhood to adulthood. As teenagers move through this period they begin to assume new roles with increasing independence from the adults in their lives. This transition to adulthood requires increasing cognitive, intellectual, social, language, and motor skills that are essential for adult living. This is typically a process in which the adolescent moves in and out of new and old roles rapidly. These changing roles sometimes make it difficult for parents and clinicians to know how to treat individuals, as either children, adolescents, or adults. On the one hand, adolescents need to be provided with opportunities to learn how to assume independence in a responsible way. On the other hand, they must learn to comply with expectations that are not too demanding, restrictive, or permissive. Work and life roles must be experienced so that behavior can be developed for self-identification and emotional independence. These tasks become more complex in an industrialized Western society in which there are few rituals or religious ceremonies that indicate the rite of passage from childhood to adulthood. (There are some exceptions such as the Bar/Bah Mitzvah for Jewish teens, and on a lesser scale, Confirmation for Catholic teens.) Unlike the ritual ordeals of more traditional societies, which presented youths with challenges that enabled them to prove themselves as adults and join their society, modern times have seen the increase in unhealthy behaviors that could be considered as substitutes for rituals. The experimentation with substance use or sexual behavior at an earlier age with more than one partner are maladaptive and threatening to physical and mental health. Yet these behaviors are more and more common among early adolescents at all socioeconomic levels. Also, adolescence has been lengthened, lowering the age of entrance to the period as well as raising the exit age. For example, 10- and 11-year-old girls are often beginning puberty, are encouraged to wear makeup, adolescent clothes, and teenage jewelry, and to present themselves as "sexy," yet 22- to 24-year-olds may still be living at home and have trouble participating in the economy as self-supporting, independent adults (Newton, 1995).

There may also be role performance confusion, for example, in the United States, a person 18 or older is able to vote, own property, and participate in military wars, but cannot legally drink alcohol or obtain a loan from a bank for financing his or her own car or housing. Therefore, this time period can be filled with uncertainty, fear, anxiety, or ambivalence, and change can be extremely difficult for the emerging adolescent. The teenager may sometimes want to be both a responsible adult who makes autonomous decisions and a child who is not expected to be as responsible as an adult. Though an adolescent may mistakenly believe he or she has acquired the maturation and skills necessary for adult responsibility, at the same time he or she may feel out of control of changes taking place in his or her own body (King, 2002).

Although typically this period is described as a tumultuous period for all teens, some (Arnett, 1999; Block, 1991; King, 2002; Offer & Schonert-Reichl, 1992) suggest that tumult is not necessarily the norm. The idea that normal adolescence consists of rebellion, stress, conflict, and trouble is particularly noted in biological and psychodynamic theories (Papalia & Olds, 1992; Sigelman & Shaffer, 1995). While this is a popular framework for clinicians working with adolescents, there are researchers who have identified adolescent personalities, which do not show the pathological or disturbed behavior that is considered normal in adolescence. In fact, three paths of development from adolescence to adulthood have been described (Offer & Schonert-Reichl, 1992). The first identifies a smooth, consistent transition with little conflict. The second identifies a "surgent growth" including spurt periods with minor conflicts and difficulty. A third path discusses "tumultuous growth" involving behaviors and problems considered "normal" by many developmental theorists. Adolescents from this third path of growth often come from crisis-oriented families with some evidence of pathology. Yet, it is adolescents with this third path of growth, who have been mistaken for the norm. Additionally, those who study **temperament** (Chess & Thomas, 1984; 1996; 2002) find that if adolescents' temperaments "fits" within their developmental trajectory, they could go through adolescence in a relatively nontroubled mode. These findings suggest that disturbance and conflict are indeed pathological rather than normal for this life period.

There are many normal developmental tasks for the healthy, growing adolescent:

- Accept physical changes in the body, such as changing voice and size, hair growth, maturing body parts and genitals, menstruation, acne, perspiration
- Establish more adult relationships with others
- Develop sexual orientation
- Develop social roles
- Develop executive functions such as the cognitive functions of judgment, abstract reasoning, coping and problem-solving skills
- Establish a personal philosophy and unique values and attitudes

These developments will influence life in all areas of occupational performance in family, school, work, church, and peer group activities. The adolescent is anxious to try out "adult" roles. He or she often requires consistent direction, guidance, structure, and limits provided by others (parents, teachers, treatment staff) to take on roles that are congruent with developing maturity.

DIAGNOSES AND PRESENTING PROBLEMS

The *Diagnostic and Statistical Manual IV*—Text Revision (*DSM-IV-TR*) lists disorders usually first diagnosed in infancy, childhood, or adolescence (APA, 2000). Many of these disorders, such as mental retardation or Tourette's disorder, can influence development of adaptive occupational performance throughout the person's lifetime (Mash & Wolfe, 2003). Alternatively, there is no clear distinction between childhood and adult disorders. Disorders such as schizophrenia or mood disorders can also first be encountered in adolescence or may develop early but not be formally diagnosed until adulthood (APA, 2000; Lewis, 2002; Morrison, 1995; Rutter & Taylor, 2002; Sadock & Sadock, 2000). Figure 11-1 summarizes *DSM-IV-TR* disorders that may begin in adolescence.

Adolescents seen by occupational therapists in American mental health settings commonly have the diagnoses of mood, anxiety, substance-related, eating, conduct, oppositional defiant, and separation anxiety disorders. Also, adolescents living in violent environments who have witnessed acts of terror or persistent abuse may also have post-traumatic stress disorder.

Other disorders described in the *DSM-IV-TR*, such as mental retardation and pervasive developmental disorders or attention deficit/hyperactivity disorders, may commonly be seen by occupational therapists in school, after school, and in private clinics or general hospitals that are not specifically designated as mental health settings. Today, occupational therapists in school-based practice are just as likely to encounter adolescents with "hidden disabilities" for which limited mental health resources are available. Alternatively, the occupational therapist may be able to engage in early identification of adolescents who are at risk for mood disorders and/or suicide.

Presenting problems encountered by occupational therapists treating adolescents with emotional problems are varied. Axis IV of the multiaxial diagnostic system is of particular interest to occupational therapists because it focuses on psychosocial functioning in context. Accurate assessment of axis IV information can aid in the development of thorough intervention plans based on history and current levels of function. (See Chapter 5 for further discussion of diagnosis.) The previous chapter addressing the mental health of children discussed a myriad of stressors linked to presenting problems. All of these still apply to adolescents but in addition, there is an increased incidence of presenting problems regarding gender identity, violence, and substance abuse (Lewis, 2002; Whyte, 2000; Rutter & Taylor, 2002).

HELPFUL CONCEPTS FOR TREATING ADOLESCENTS

The helpful concepts of structure and consistency, limit setting, therapeutic relationship, and a team approach that were discussed in the previous chapter for work with children also have relevance to the adolescent population. Rather than repeat the descriptions of each concept, the reader is encouraged to review

Disorders Diagnosed in Childhood or Adolescence

Conduct Disorder. The individual violates rules, age-appropriate norms, or the rights of others, evidenced by aggression against people or animals, property destruction, lying or theft, or seriously violating rules. The symptoms cause impairment in job, school, or social life. Adolescent onset is included if there are not problems before age 10. Severity, such as mild, moderate, or severe, is also coded. This is a common precursor to antisocial personality disorder.

Parent-Adolescent Relational Problems. A V-code (meaning there is no disorder or condition on axis I or II—not a mental disorder, but a presenting problem) used when a parent and adolescent have problems getting along.

Sibling Relational Problems. A V-code used for difficulties between siblings.

Problems Related to Abuse or Neglect. A V-code used to cover difficulties that arise from neglect or from physical or sexual abuse.

Adult Psychiatric Disorders That Can Be Diagnosed in Adolescence

Substance-related disorders include disorders related to abusing chemicals, including alcohol, side effects of medication, or a toxin. In adolescents these disorders are most often divided into *Substance Use Disorder* (substance dependence and substance abuse) or *Substance-Induced Disorders* (such as substance intoxication).

Mood Disorders. Major depressive episode is a period of at least two seeks during which there is depressed mood or loss of pleasure or interest in almost all activities. Sadness is present and in adolescents there may be irritability. Also present may be hypersomnia, psychomotor retardation, and delusions.

Bipolar Disorder I is characterized by both manic and mixed manic and depressive episodes. Approximately 10% to 15% of adolescents with recurrent major depressive episodes go on to develop bipolar I disorder.

Cyclothymic Disorder is characterized by numerous periods of hypomanic and depressive symptoms that do not last long enough to meet criteria for either major depressive episode or bipolar disorder. This disorder often begins in early life and is thought to reflect a temperamental disposition to other mood disorders.

Anxiety Disorders are found in children and adolescents and include such diagnoses as *Specific Phobia, Social Phobia, Obsessive Compulsive Disorder,* and *Generalized Anxiety Disorder.* In children and adolescents, generalized anxiety disorder is often expressed as excessive worries over the quality of performance even when it is not being judged.

Eating Disorders are severe disturbances in eating behavior. The most common disorders are *Anorexia Nervosa* and *Bulimia.* Popular culture has drawn attention to these disorders as they affect young women in their pursuit of idealized images of thinness and as they affect young men in their pursuit of athletic goals.

Multiaxial diagnoses require occupational therapists to attend to all five axes, but for adolescents they should attend especially to axis IV, which lists psychosocial and environmental problems.

Figure 11-1. Disorders Diagnosed in Adolescents (Adapted from American Psychiatric Association (2000). *Diagnostic and Statistical Manual of Mental Disorders,* Fourth Edition, Text Revision. Washington, DC, American Psychiatric Association)

Chapter 10 and to apply the concepts to the adolescent examples and case illustrations provided here.

Structure and Consistency

Structure and consistency can help adolescents who have difficulty following rules and who have poor impulse control and difficulty modulating their emotions. The therapist can provide structure by simply stating the rules of an activity or group. This introduction provides an idea or standard that can be referred to throughout the group. For adolescents, a brief discussion of what the rules mean for each participant or periodic reminders will serve to reinforce the structure; a graphic reinforcement that is age-appropriate is also handy. Depending on the group, the teenagers might elect their own "rule keeper" for each session or time period, although setting oneself up in this group role may in fact create distance between the client and his or her peers.

CASE ILLUSTRATION: Providing Structure for Felicita

Lang, an occupational therapist, worked for a religious organization that sponsored a youth group for teens at risk of dropping out of school due to their impoverished situations and family pressure to help out. For Mexican Independence Day, the adolescents were going to make a piñata that could be used by the younger children at their celebration party. At the start of the group he stated, "Today in group we are going to share the supplies to begin building a piñata for the Mexican celebration. There can be no name-calling, foul language, or threatening behavior. If anyone engages in such behavior toward anyone else, he will have to leave the group." As the teens began planning who would assume which roles, Felicita became angry and started to "diss" another member. Three or four of the other youth intervened and reminded her of the group rules.

Discussion

Providing structure by stating the rules explicitly at the beginning of the group enabled the group members to manage other members who were acting out.

In another clinical example, choosing someone to be the time-keeper demonstrates both the capacity for adolescents to act out creatively and to challenge the practitioner's authority and the need to reinforce structure and limits by encouraging the clients to reflect on their actions.

CASE ILLUSTRATION: Alya—The Watch-Changer

During this same group session concerning planning for and making the piñata for the celebration, Alya, a 15-year-old girl, asked Lang, "What time is it?" The leader, wanting to encourage a group member to take responsibility for monitoring the time, said, "How about my lending you my watch, and you can be the time-keeper today?" Happily she accepted the watch, dutifully announced when it was time for group to end, and returned the watch to the practitioner. Upon returning with the group to the central lounge area, Lang noticed a 20-minute discrepancy between his own watch and the wall clock. It seemed his watch was now 20 minutes fast. Checking the time with other staff, he realized the client had surreptitiously changed the watch to speed up the end time of the group! Lang sought out Alya later in the day and said that although he thought that she really did a pretty good job of fooling him, he now wondered whether he could trust Alya in the future. He also wondered if it was fair that the group ended early for all of her friends who were having fun making the piñata.

Discussion

Lang dealt with Alya's behavior by a direct approach, some degree of "respect" for her ability to fool the practitioner, and feedback about the impact of the behavior and the attribute of trustworthiness—both issues of concern to this client, who trusted few in her world.

As described in Chapter 10, another way to provide structure is through activities themselves. For example, jewelry making or burning CDs can be structured activities that are age-appropriate and offer a sense of accomplishment and satisfaction. While many adolescents are impulsive in their approach to tasks, some amazing results occur when there is just the right fit between the task and the interest or motivation of the person. Such a fit was demonstrated when in another group Lang offered small premolded plaster Christmas ornaments for painting with acrylic paints. Some of the most inattentive adolescents, who often flitted from one activity to the next, with constant **redirection,** could be found carefully painting elves and Santas, for themselves and their family, during the period between Thanksgiving and Christmas. Capturing the "child" in each adolescent with the wonder of the holiday season, and offering an object with meaning yet a great deal of structure seemed like just the magic that is often occupational therapy. It makes the best use of environmental demands, meaning, and participation.

Limit Setting

For adolescents who are more cognitively advanced and bigger than children, setting limits can be more complex and a therapist may need to be flexible in her or his response. When setting limits during an intervention session, it is particularly important to consider "Why am I asking for this limit to be maintained?" Is this a safety consideration, a limit necessary for maintaining a therapeutic environment, or a response to disruptive and irritating behavior? If the behavior is compromising safety in an emergency way, then limits must be placed immediately and follow-through must occur prior to any further incident. Interventions and policies set forth by the facility must be initiated to eliminate any further compromise of safety or risk to the client or others. Such was the case when an adolescent with a history of fire setting intentionally pulled the fire alarm while he was an inpatient. The staff was faced with the unusual paradox of addressing the offense of signaling a false alarm, and the "progress" the young man had made in *not* setting a fire!

If the behavior is one that destroys the therapeutic environment, such as name calling or sexual comments, the clinician may make some choices regarding his or her intervention and consequences for the behavior. The therapist will base the intervention on the program rules or policy, which may include a time-out or missing the next group or activity, or the therapist may have the opportunity to choose a response to this behavior based on his or her rapport with the adolescent, interventions that have worked in the past, and the developmental level of the group. The therapist may choose to not comment on the behavior but at the same time utilize the opportunity by asking participants in the group to comment on their peer's behavior, thereby encouraging assertive responses to this intrusive behavior.

CASE ILLUSTRATION: Jonnie—Peer Limit Setting

A group for teens who attended an alternative high school focused on behaviors that were necessary to get and to maintain a job. Vy, the occupational therapist, had conducted the group for about four weeks and it had run smoothly, with participants staying on task. However, during this group that dealt with appropriate dress, one of the teens, Jonnie, started making comments about the girls in the group after one of them suggested that pants that hung well below a boy's waist, such as the ones that Jonnie wore, would be barriers to getting a job. Jonnie's comments were sexual in nature, suggesting that the girls were probably really interested in his "booty." Vy asked the other group members how they felt about Jonnie's comments. Other boys in the group thought that Jonnie was "being stupid." Jonnie ceased his comments and was able to contribute to the small problem-solving group that he was part of.

Discussion
Vy utilized a strategy in the group of asking other members to comment on one participant's behavior as a way of setting limits.

Some useful methods in setting limits that have stood the test of time can be taken from the popular assertiveness movement of the 1970s. They include the "broken record" technique and the "rule of five" (Alberti & Emmons, 1995; Jakubowski & Lange, 1978; Smith, 1975). The broken record method is when a limit and a direction are repeated until the desired response results. Slight variations can be allowed in this method to address adolescents and to reassure them that you are listening. However, you are also repeating the main directive that needs to be followed.

The rule of five is particularly useful when the adolescent is not able to reason due to developmental age or escalating behavior and loss of impulse control with the potential for continued escalation. The directive statement to the client should have no more than five words in it with no more than five letters in each word. The goal at this point is to "keep it simple." It is more directive in an effort to establish control immediately and is often utilized in escalating situations. Consistent limits and consequences help adolescents to know that they will not be "harmed" by each other's behavior, will be guided in maintaining self-control, and will learn to modulate feelings and emotions appropriate to various situations and contexts. They also rely on limits to reassure them that the environment is consistent and has set expectations of occupational performance.

Avoiding Power Struggles

Because of the developmental tasks of adolescents, which include identification with peer groups, increasing autonomy, and ambivalence about autonomy versus independence (Erikson, 1968; Greenberg, Haiman, & Esman, 1987; King, 2002; Whyte, 2003), power struggles are more likely to occur with teens. The following is an example of a potential situation in which there could be a standoff between therapist and client. However, the therapist's nondefensive behavior avoids a power struggle.

CASE ILLUSTRATION: Avoiding a Power Struggle with Roberto

Initially, the occupational therapist, Mariko, presented the "group project" in a way that promoted a power struggle, by stating, "Since July 4th is coming, today we will make a huge American flag to hang at our picnic! Each of you will select an area to work on and we can have a team effort to celebrate the day." When group members began to "moan" about the assignment, Mariko realized she had not been very client-centered in her approach. This could have led to a big power struggle when, Roberto, a 15-year-old male said, "I don't want to do something so lame!" Mariko answered, "Well, the one 'given' for this hour is that we all work on projects together. It would be great if everyone could participate in some way. Do you have any suggestions?" Roberto said "Yep! What about if each of us designs his own flag to fly on Independence Day?" Mariko, after thinking about it, stated, "Interesting idea. What do the rest of you think?" The group members all enthusiastically agreed with Roberto's idea. So, the group embarked on designing and presenting their own flags, a true demonstration of "Declarations of Independence" accomplished in the most age- and role-consonant fashion. The most ironic outcome: the young man who raised the initial objection to work in the group designed and completed his personal American flag!

Discussion

The therapist defused a potential power struggle by: (1) recognizing her mistake, (2) acknowledging it to the group, and (3) asking the teens for their input.

Providing adolescents with a choice within a group setting is beneficial for many reasons. In many settings much power and control has been stripped away when individuals are no longer in their own environment or are in a restrictive environment. A person may be in the setting because of an action in which he or she was not able to maintain control and may feel a great deal of remorse and guilt, though not express it openly. The therapist's task is to help the individual regain self-confidence and the ability to modulate emotions and regulate behavior.

Therapeutic Use of Relationship

It is important to provide ample opportunity for exploration of adult roles, opportunity to identify with "healthy" role models, and the chance to experience much of what peers outside the mental health system are experiencing. Thus, any practitioner must be "tuned in" to what is normative in an adolescent's world, regardless of the "adult" perspective or judgment. The following cases illustrate how therapists can use the therapeutic relationship to role-model genuine behavior and also to understand teens' behaviors from their perspective.

CASE ILLUSTRATION: Jumbe—Name Calling

In one session the OTR, Moses, inquired about the extent of name calling, believing it to be a precursor to potentially more aggressive acting out.

Moses: I guess I don't understand the names you guys call each other. Can you explain it to me?
Jumbe: We don't expect you to understand.
Moses: I was a kid once, and I don't remember that being part of how friends treated each other.
Jumbe: You didn't grow up in a neighborhood like ours.
Moses: What kind of neighborhood do you think I came from?
Jumbe: A quiet one.
Moses: Oh, I think maybe I misinterpreted your interactions as being hurtful to each other, when clearly they are not.
Jumbe: This means we like each other, man!

Discussion

In this instance, rather than setting a clear limit, the OT got a window into the lives and culture of the group and of the ideas the group harbored about him and his different background. True or not, the perceived differences can be utilized if openly acknowledged as ways in which culture impacts behavior.

CASE ILLUSTRATION: John—Therapeutic Use of Relationship

John, a client in an adolescent after-school program, was a young man with impulsive behavior who could not sustain interest or complete a task as assigned. He also was hearing impaired and often sought tactile contact with adults by coming too close, touching them, and otherwise challenging personal boundaries. While not dangerous, this behavior, particularly when occurring during group activities, was especially annoying to the therapist. On one occasion, during the transition from OT to school, the young man came up behind Jennifer, the occupational therapist, and was so close he was literally "breathing down her neck." When Jennifer was surprised by this, she raised her voice and told the client, "Stop it! I don't like people touching me!" It took only one second to realize she was not being therapeutic and was indeed responding in anger, rather than being able to define the "problem behavior" in a helpful way or set a reasonable limit. The therapist acknowledged this and apologized to John while saying she would think of some way that he could get his tactile needs satisfied in a way that did not adversely affect people.

Discussion

In this case being therapeutic in the relationship involved understanding the client and his needs, being genuine, and role-modeling how to correct words spoken out in anger.

Therapeutic use of relationship involves responding to clients in a way that will guide them in new paths to develop behaviors that are desired and socially acceptable. This is different than responding to the clients in the same manner as nontherapeutic individuals in past situations. Often adolescents behave in ways that will provoke familiar responses, getting others to treat them in a way that reflects how they feel about themselves (Greenberg, Haiman, & Esman, 1987). The imperative for the occupational therapist is to be able to reflect on his or her own experiences and not to replicate those of the adolescent. (See Chapter 18 for further discussion of the therapeutic use of relationship.)

Adolescents in psychosocial settings may have experienced emotional, physical, and sexual abuse or neglect. An adolescent may experience many emotions surrounding abuse and neglect, yet be unaware of them or unable to express them directly. Sometimes, emotions may be displaced toward a therapist, particularly if the therapist can be trusted not to retaliate or withdraw (Glaser, 2002; Greenberg, Haiman, & Esman, 1987). For teens this behavior may be more apparent because a major task of the adolescent is to establish one's own identity apart from adults and authority figures. It is important to maintain the therapeutic role, understand the young person, and respond in ways that indicate your wish to understand him or her. You may help the individual to find other ways of coping by providing alternative responses than those of previous hurtful adults, by providing opportunities to express emotions that assist in modulating them, by putting words to feelings, and by providing age-appropriate opportunities to explore and master self and environment.

More often than with other age groups, and particularly in a period when young people experience many more threats in their environment, such as drugs, violence, abuse, terrorism, and rape (Hoffman, 2001; LaGreca, Silverman, Vernberg,

& Roberts, 2002), working with teens necessitates that beliefs be set aside and an understanding, empathic attitude be adopted (Department of Occupational Science and Occupational Therapy, USC 2003). For example, young teens may be sexually active, become pregnant, or develop sexually transmitted diseases. A young woman may be alone in deciding whether to terminate a pregnancy, give a baby up for adoption, or raise the child. Even though your beliefs and values may dictate the decision that you would make for yourself, you are ethically obligated to assume a neutral attitude and assist the individual to come to her own conclusion. Adolescents may be addicted to drugs or alcohol, or may be responsible for violence or self-mutilation. Moral judgments have to be suspended so that teenagers can reflect and think about their lives in a context of support (Greenspan, 2002), and so that therapists can provide the best possible intervention emanating from the needs of the client. One way of suspending judgment and providing treatment that is driven by an understanding of the clients needs is to know your own thoughts, feelings, values, and biases, and by acknowledging and accepting emotions and thoughts evoked in yourself when working with teenagers. As a therapist you will then be able to provide respect, empathy, genuineness, sensitivity, and warmth to adolescents who perhaps have not received enough of these responses. A single factor that has been described as accounting for the difference between an adolescent from a troubled environment with stressed socioeconomic levels becoming a "troubled" or "healthy" adult in terms of mental health, substance use, and criminal behavior is the presence of "a caring adult" to provide support, responsibility, and advocacy for the young person (Michaelson & Nakamura, 2001; Rhodes, 2002). Support and advocacy can be natural roles for an occupational therapist or certified occupational therapy assistant working with adolescents.

Team Approach

Just as with children, the team approach is essential in providing services for the adolescent because his or her life role is as a family member. Therefore, family members should be consulted and included whenever possible. Just as with children, as adolescents move through the life cycle, there are many adults with whom they have extensive contact. Some of these are found as they traverse normative developmental pathways, while others come into their lives when they enter the mental health service arenas. These adults are mentioned in Chapter 10, and include professional educators, therapists, and sports leaders (Call & Mortimer, 2001; Fritz et al., 1993). Any of those who engage regularly with a troubled adolescent can provide a wealth of information about occupational performance and be a wonderful resource for planning and community support (Kirshner, O'Donoghue, & McLauglin, 2002). Naturally, consultation will be with permission of the client, or the responsible parent, whenever possible. As with children, more than just sensorimotor or neuromuscular skills are being addressed for this population, even within the school setting. Thus, the OT is also a resource to the school based-team.

Medications

The use of some medications with children has received much attention in the media (Fonagy et al., 2002); medications are also helpful in the treatment of adolescents with specific psychiatric illnesses. These medications are only effective if a complete diagnostic work-up has been done and all medical records examined to determine if symptoms might be caused by a medical condition. Medication is often needed to assist clients in gaining control over their mood, thinking, or behavior, or in stabilizing symptoms such as impulsivity, so that clients are more resilient and able to participate in their own recovery. Medication is not offered freely but is often selected with input from all team members or after much observation of the client in various contexts. The occupational therapist can contribute her or his observations of clients in various life roles or performance contexts.

CASE ILLUSTRATION: Mark—Use of Medications

Mark, an usually high-achieving 16-year-old, began to complain of having no friends, inability to concentrate, low energy, and loss of interest in track, a previously loved sport, as well as other after-school activities. As his irritability increased, huge family fights erupted in the home. After going out one night, getting drunk, and crashing the family car into a tree, Mark was admitted to the hospital for treatment of his broken leg and other injuries. The occupational therapist on the acute medical unit evaluated his rehabilitation needs. The Occupational Profile indicated a young man who was disappointed in all areas of his own role engagement and felt unable to fully participate in his own life, even before the accident. Moreover, he was reluctant to envision participation in OT or physical therapy in order to prepare for a return home. Suspecting that such disengagement in occupational performance was the result of depression and that the "accident" may have in fact been a suicide attempt, a psychiatric evaluation was suggested. After two weeks on a standard antidepressant and short-term psychotherapy, Mark returned for outpatient rehabilitation of his badly broken leg. The OT, meeting him in the hallway saw a vivacious, engaged, and motivated young man anxious to get on with therapy to return to track practice.

Discussion

Judicious consultation with the treatment team and the use of one medication, in conjunction with psychotherapy brought about the desired change in a client's behavior and facilitated more adaptive functioning. A variety of medications can be used, depending upon the clinical needs of the individual adolescent. They may vary from setting to setting and even from doctor to doctor.

While medication is often needed to assist clients, and the psychiatrist is ultimately responsible for prescribing medications, it is important for the occupational therapist and other team members to be knowledgeable about medications and their side effects and to monitor behaviors and status of the client carefully. The occupational therapist, working closely with the individual on medications, may be the first to observe emerging side effects or changes in behavior. It is particularly important to monitor medications closely because sometimes when psychotropic medication is used with a young person, it interacts with the neuro-chemistry of the synapses and may interfere with development of new neuron networks and neurologically based competencies (Newton, 1995). Therefore, cognitive and behavioral approaches are usually considered very carefully and attempted before pharmacology. If pharmacology is utilized, close monitoring is highly recommended (Fonagy et al., 2002).

ADOLESCENT SETTINGS AND PROGRAMS

When considering a program, the need is to always provide the least restrictive environment for the client. The best program will provide the client with the most normalized and balanced program, always with the goal of the client no longer requiring intervention. Adolescent programs may be based on a facilitative rather than a rehabilitative approach (Delgado, 2002; Kirshner et al., 2002; Michaelson & Nakamura, 2001; Sadock & Sadock, 2000). Habilitation means addressing skills and behaviors that are yet to be learned or are undeveloped as opposed to a reha-bilitation that may be used with adults that would focus on the retrieval of skills that the clients already have or have had in the past (Lambert, Moffitt, & Rose, 1989). The challenge is to intervene while addressing the ongoing developmental issues of adolescence, so normative adaptation is facilitated as much as possible (Burns & Hoagwood, 2002).

The role of the occupational therapist or occupational therapy assistant has been described broadly in the literature. In working with adolescents with psy-chosocial dysfunction, the occupational therapist has been described as a devel-opmental therapist, with an assessment role of evaluating functioning level in skills and interests (Sholle-Martin & Alessi, 1990). The OTR's role with adoles-cents has been described as based on nonoccupational therapy theories, such as social learning, cognitive-behavioral, psychoanalytic, and developmental mod-els. Occupational therapy offers many theoretical approaches that incorporate these principles but adds the critical focus on the meaning and use of occupation. Those models that focus on occupation include, but are not limited to the Human Occupation (Kielhofner, 2002), the Ecology of Human Performance (Dunn, Brown, & McGuigan, 1994), Occupational Adaptation (Schkade & Schultz, 1992; Schultz & Schkade, 1992), Canadian Model of Occupational Performance (Townsend, 1997), and the Person-Environment-Occupation (Law et al., 1996) models. In addition, the occupational behavior theories of Mary Reilly (1974) are still pertinent, with evaluation emphasizing play history, temperament, family relationships, and patterns of behavior. Occupational therapy goals may include interventions focusing on occupational and vocational exploration, social skills development, humor and creative expression, play, behavioral management, sensorimotor processing, values clarification and occupational role identification and enhancement (Reilly, Kielhofner, Ayres, Nelson, Llorens, & Rubin, cited in Sholle-Martin & Alessi, 1990). In occupational therapy the range of interventions might include but not be limited to those listed in Table 11-1.

Inpatient hospitalization, long-term residential treatment, outpatient settings, community-based programs, partial hospitalization programs, and school-based settings may all offer opportunity for the therapist (Lewis, 2002; Rutter & Taylor, 2002; Sadock & Sadock, 2000). Anywhere there are adolescents there is a possible treatment setting in which their psychosocial needs may be met.

At the dawn of the twenty-first century, traditional medical model settings in which occupational therapy practitioners work with adolescents have diminished. In many of the hospital and residential settings, OTs have been replaced by recreation and creative arts therapists. Yet there are new horizons in which occupational therapists with vision may be able to create roles where none previously existed. The evidence of need in these areas can be found in the newspapers, in accounts of adolescent substance abuse, suicide, violent acting out, and the issue of youth in the criminal justice system. As recently as 2001, a residential treatment center for male adolescent sex offenders hired its second occupational therapist, the first having been promoted to program manager! The Surgeon General's report (2001) offers a comprehensive overview of the state of the art of interventions for adolescents and is a virtual directory of arenas where occupational therapy may be able to offer valuable services.

Treatment of adolescents has been affected by changes in mental health care delivery just as that of the adult population. In recent years acute hospital admissions have shortened and even long-term residential settings have much shorter lengths of stay. This is as much due to a decrease in resources as trends toward efforts to keep the teen integrated into the family and community, rather than removal from the home and separation from family by "parent-ectomy," unless for reasons of abuse. This is a result of new views developed in the 1990s that parents do not cause mental illness and in fact are an important resource for the ongoing care and management of the adolescent's care, progress, and medications.

Table 11-1. Interventions for Adolescents

Activity	Function
Sports	Encourage cooperation, modulate competition, learn the value of rule following, and focus appropriate release of physical energy
Fitness/Exercise	Address issues of body image and wellness, and engage in relevant social and cultural normative activity
Vocational exploration	Identify and pursue transitional goals and interests
Life skills	Fulfill adult role performance currently or in the near future
Social skills	For those adolescents who have mild developmental disorders of early childhood or simply do not "fit" with peers

Case Management

The move toward a more "ecological" orientation offers opportunities for occupational therapy as case managers capable of facilitating the empowerment of both adolescent and family (Evans & Armstrong, 2002; Lehman et al., 2002). Some of the skills the occupational therapist can both assess and intervene to help adolescents acquire are "choice making; problem solving; goal setting and goal attainment; self-observation, self-evaluation and self reinforcement; internal locus of control" (Lehman et al., 2002, p. 135). Simultaneously, there is a need for a service coordinator who can help adolescents and their families make choices based on the best fit between the person, the resources and opportunities in the environment, and roles and occupations. Thus the occupational therapist is well positioned to assure that the services fit the client, not that the client fits into a single template of services.

School-Based Programs

School districts are required to meet special needs of their students when the students' performance in the classroom is affected. Depending on the county and the office of education, there may be opportunities for the occupational therapist interested in working to meet the school-aged clients' psychosocial needs. Some counties are meeting the psychosocial needs of their severely emotionally disturbed (SED) students through programs offered on public school campuses. They typically have a special education teacher, psychiatrist, and social worker providing services as well as teacher aides and assistants that work with the clinical staff. Occupational therapists are included in some of these programs and could provide services including assessment, treatment, home programs, school programs, or consultation services. In the school-based setting the goal is to increase the student's function in the special education classroom with the long-term goal of the student participating in a regular classroom. All treatment goals should indicate progress toward this end. The occupational therapist is able to view the student holistically, look at her or his performance in the classroom, and provide the necessary services for skill development and improved classroom success. A review of effective outcomes (Roth & Fonagy, 1996) revealed that "any therapy, including consultation to . . . teachers, was more helpful than none" (p. 317).

An especially vital role for occupational therapy may be in the provision and formulation of **transitional services** and facilitation of meeting students' goals as they move from school to work or from adolescence to young adulthood. Lehman et al. (2002) write about the need for transitional services to be client-centered, empowering, and assuring support as vulnerable youth seek appropriate resources and relationships to move on the next developmental challenge. An occupational therapist could easily fill the role of resource coordinator in a transitional services model that matches client and family with resource and unearths resources where no obvious ones exist.

If not as a resource coordinator, the OTR can provide valuable prevocational exploration experiences, as adolescents enter the work (or volunteer force), seeking jobs to add to their support, structure their time, pay for luxuries, or explore options before further training and education. Helping to determine the best person-environment-occupation fit is a unique occupational therapy skill, as demonstrated by the following case.

CASE ILLUSTRATION: Vicki—Role Transition

Vicki was a 17-year-old girl who attended a private high school for adolescents with psychiatric illness. As in many such settings, her local district paid for her special education. The teachers, psychiatrist, and social workers on the team were anxious for her to find "meaningful work," but all reports were that Vicki failed most vocational tasks at school and had identified no real "interest." An occupational therapist in a work adjustment program was consulted. A thorough review of neuropsychological testing revealed that Vicki had problems with motor planning, bilateral integration, and crossing the midline. No one ever had designed vocational experiences that either addressed these deficits or enabled her to develop adaptive strategies to compensate for them. Thus, during the evaluation interview, the OT determined that Vicki loved flowers, especially arranging them. The OT invited Vicki to join the flower shop program, where she experienced success at a loved occupation for the first time. Suddenly, Vicki had a new view of herself, working in a flower shop!

Discussion

Occupational therapy services are vital for assisting adolescents to transition from a student to a worker role.

Partial Hospitalization Programs

As with children, partial hospitalization programs are another way to prevent adolescents from entering or staying in an inpatient hospitalization setting (see Kiser, Heston, & Pruitt, 2002 for more information on partial hospitalization programs). They also facilitate transitions from an inpatient to an outpatient setting. As with children, the clients attend a program during typical school hours and receive treatment groups or therapy more intensively than if they were outpatients. A partial hospitalization program may avoid hospitalization or enable adjustments to medication in a supervised setting. One of the goals of partial hospitalization is to improve adolescents' functioning to the degree to which they can be placed in a less intensive environment. The adolescent in this program, however, may not be attending school, may be in need of transitioning back into the school system, or may require assistance in becoming emancipated or will need life skills training.

IMPLEMENTING PROGRAMS

When developing a program of occupational therapy, it is important to assess the needs of the clients and the service delivery system. Using the Occupational

Therapy Practice Framework (2002) will help the practitioner formulate sound clinical reasoning to assure programmatic goals fit with the goals, philosophy, and context of the service delivery setting.

Evaluation

In order to facilitate each adolescent's "engagement in occupation to support participation in contexts," the evaluation process must be concerned with the following considerations based on the Occupational Therapy Practice Framework (2002):

- Performance areas of occupation
- Performance skills
- Performance patterns
- Context
- Activity demands
- Client factors, such as body structure and functions

These can be observed/evaluated though standardized testing or observation, by obtaining a thorough performance history, and from identifying the goals, values, hopes, and satisfaction with occupational performance of the adolescent and his or her family. (See Chapter 17 for further information regarding assessments.) Formal evaluations that are discussed in Asher (1996) and Hemphill-Pearson (1999) offer a wide range of opportunities to assess not only the person, or client factors, but the environment as well. A useful tool for a quick assessment of the body functions is the Kinetic-Self Image Test (mentioned in the previous chapter) which was developed as part of the Initial Play Interview at The Mount Sinai Hospital in New York. The adolescent is asked to draw a picture of himself or herself doing something. Besides information regarding sensorimotor and cognitive components, valuable information such as interests, relationships, and self-concept can be determined.

Occupational Therapy Intervention

Play is often referred to as the work of the children, but playfulness is an inherently useful quality when struggling with the vicissitudes of adolescence because just as with children, playfulness and creativity may offer ways in which adolescents learn basic skills and resolve intra- and interpersonal conflicts. It is helpful to distinguish play from games (see Chapter 18 for further information about games), because games are a predominant occupation of preadolescents and adolescents. Games are usually competitive, and there are agreed upon rules that are imposed externally. Games require that the activity be pursued in a proscribed manner, without one's personal fantasy and often there is a goal, such as winning, outside of the activity. With the basic acceptance of the importance of play (Morrison & Metzger, 2001; Parham & Fazio, 1997) (and later, games) as an intervention strategy, and the recognition of playfulness as an adaptive strategy, the world of potential occupational contexts in which adolescents can be engaged opens wide. In fact, creativity and emotional expression may serve as one avenue through which adolescents can explore their emotional difficulties (Lougher, 2001).

While some adolescents may be quite articulate in defining their occupational role performance, others may be best evaluated through specific assessments and interviews and by ongoing observation. There are various ways to initially evaluate and continue to observe engagement in occupations. Some useful categories to think about (Lougher, 2001) while observing are:

- Personal presentation
- Activity accomplishment
- Group skills, such as tolerance of others, acceptance of rules, level of participation
- Relationship with adults
- Relationship with peers
- Symbolic nature of creative expressions in art or other projective activities. What are the expressed themes in writing, drawing, collage making, and the like? Are they consistent throughout?

Groups

A creative arts group is a nondirective group that occurs in the occupational therapy space. Therapy in a group "(playing or talking about emotional issues) is very effective and also economical" (Roth & Fonagy, 1996, p. 317). The room includes art supplies, craft kits, a CD player, a computer workstation loaded with games, a sink, water, and a table and chairs. It serves to encourage the development of cognitive, sensorimotor, and social skills. The group also has the goal of providing an arena whereby adolescents may seek to resolve interaction problems and confront issues that led to current problems and dysfunction. Adolescents may use journal writing, painting, and other expressive media to express feelings. They may re-create arguments or scenes they observed in the home. A game like Sorry helps increase frustration tolerance while Twister develops not only laterality but also the ability to be close to others appropriately and respect body space. The choice to use this game depends greatly on the impulsivity of the group, as it challenges boundaries and requires intimate body contact. Other board games are an appropriate outlet for anger and aggression, and also provide the opportunity to engage in turn taking and mild competition.

Participating in seasonal activities, such as carving a pumpkin or making pies for Thanksgiving and cookies for Christmas or decorations for women's or African American history month, offer rewarding experiences. These seasonal activities facilitate development of an internal locus of control as adolescents learn they can have an impact on making a holiday season positive through their own efforts and resources. Comments made about projects often provide valuable, additional perspective on an adolescent's emotions and concerns. Tie-dyeing is a highly successful creative task project. Adolescents frequently want to do more and indeed the steps of the activity are easy to grade according to the therapeutic purposes of the group. Some of the reasons this project appeals to adolescents are:

- The adolescent has the necessary fine motor skills required
- The adolescent enjoys the repetitive nature of motor task activities
- It is completed in one session
- Regardless of artistic talent, an adolescent can turn out a reasonable fac-simile of the sample project, a fact that bolsters self-esteem
- The adolescent creates a "cool" item that can be worn to school or the mall

Two aspects of tie-dyeing that often concern others outside of occupational therapy are the mess and the space to safely dry t-shirts or sheets without risk of theft. It is important to keep these personal effects in a safe area that is not accessible to others. The adolescents are informed of the concerns about spillage and security at the onset of the group and generally they accept the firm limits. Many want to send their project home to their family members, particularly if the family has been involved in the group. Additionally, the smell given off from the chemical, liver of sulfur, presents brief periods of laughter and off-color remarks by the adolescent, depending on the maturity of the group members. A way to deal with this situation is simply to acknowledge the smell.

Most often creative tasks are provided as part of a parallel task group. This structure provides opportunities to develop appropriate interpersonal interactions on a limited basis, share through the use of supplies that are common to the group activity, and develop impulse control by waiting to follow the steps and to see the project through to completion.

Group goals may include learning how to follow simple step-by-step verbal directions, sharing materials and space, interacting without being intrusive, sustaining and increasing attention span, and developing impulse control. Other information that can be gained even through the use of a project includes who the gift or project is to be given to, whether that be a mother, an aunt, or someone that the adolescent has just met, and, therefore, who is important in the adolescent's life.

A skills development group is provided for older adolescents who have social skills and need to improve problem-solving, coping, and communication skills. (See the group's protocol in Figure 11-2.) Group topics and discussion focus on common problems and situations that adolescents face as well as the client's specific problem areas that led to treatment.

A variety of activities can be used in this group, including crafts, therapeutic board games, and a wide range of art materials. "Stress Strategies" (Lambert, Moffitt, & Rose, 1989) is a game to develop coping skills, and "Creative Arts through the Ages" (Haiman & Green, 1998) which facilitates expression of thoughts and feelings, are two examples of interventions that are effective in meeting goals. Because they use a format that does not directly ask for emotional expression, ado-

NAME OF GROUP: Occupational Therapy Creative Arts Group

DESCRIPTION: Expression is an important part of an adolescent's development. Adolescents learn, express themselves, and develop interpersonal skills through a wide range of media. Through crafts, computers, games, and the like, adolescents are able to express inner feelings and conflicts in a nonthreatening way. This group's primary goal is to evaluate skills and provide an environment where the adolescents' occupational performance can be observed and practiced.

THERAPIST NAME: Susan Haiman, MPS, OTR/L, FAOTA

TITLE: Occupational Therapist

GOALS:

1. Provide a stimulating environment where the adolescents will be motivated to explore options for engagement.
2. Encourage peer interaction through shared projects, games, and the like.
3. Provide feedback related to behavior.
4. Encourage use of existing cognitive and social skills and development of new ones.

ENTRANCE CRITERIA:

1. Group members are selected by the OT according to ability to tolerate working in a setting with peers and with some degree of noise and distraction.
2. Ten is an optimal number of group members.
3. Client has been medically cleared by physician.
4. Client is able to define one reason for attending the group.

GROUP RULES:

1. Have fun.
2. Share.
3. Listen to staff.
4. Clean up.

FORMAT: Group meets two times per week for 45 minutes with two leaders —the OT and a member of the nursing staff.

EXIT CRITERIA: Goals are met as reported by adolescent, family, or team members.

Figure 11-2.   Occupational Therapy Department Group Protocol

lescents are usually willing to participate, and an appropriate amount of structure is provided. Adolescents are often happy to have an outlet for their unexpressed feelings and thoughts and view the group as a safe and nonthreatening means of personal expression. The following case study illustrates additional creative arts groups in which teens can have fun expressing themselves.

CASE ILLUSTRATION: Creative Arts through the Ages

Seven adolescents, ages 12 to 16 years old, view the film Romeo and Juliet with Cynthia, the occupational therapist. There is much giggling about the complex, unfamiliar language. The selected scene deals with Romeo's suicide upon finding Juliet "dead." After the initial discomfort with the language, Cynthia facilitates a discussion of several critical adolescent themes: gangs, parental approval of mates, suicide, striving for autonomy. Recognizing many of the themes and normal struggles with varied solutions, the clients can talk about their feelings and explore potential solutions they might have available for appropriate expression of feelings, other than acting out.

Discussion

Adolescents are willing to discuss contemporary, personal themes when they can view them through another creative medium.

Family Involvement

The Weekend Planning Activity group (Haiman, 1989) involves engaging the parents of the emotionally disturbed adolescent in an activity with their adolescent. It is held weekly in a partial hospital program and it is a chance to work with parents to facilitate age-appropriate normal socialization during the hours when the program is not in session. Since many adolescents do not have transportation and/or are in need of supervision, together they can plan for an afternoon activity that parents are willing to help organize, supervise, and, at times, subsidize. The optimal balance sought by the therapist is to allow adolescents to plan without too much control from adults. This group improves the parent-adolescent interaction by engaging in a pleasurable, successful activity together, something that may not have been possible due to the adolescent's illness. The therapist provides encouragement and support, and models appropriate caregiver behavior such as setting limits on inappropriate actions and giving praise for desirable behavior. He or she assists parents in differentiating between what is maladaptive behavior and what are typical behaviors for the adolescent's developmental level. Beyond providing occupational therapy for families and their disturbed adolescents, the OT is able to provide the treatment team with information about family interactive patterns, and about the ease with which community reintegration with parental support will be maximized. By providing information on how and what the adolescent is doing during this group, occupational therapy enhances the team's ability to see the adolescent and his or her family within a broadened context and respond with more integrated treatment for the families and clients involved.

Just as with any client, the family is important to the adolescent (Ireys, Devet, & Sakwa, 2002; Roth & Fonagy, 1996). Although the teenager may be establishing a self-identity that is autonomous from the family, the family is still the pertinent shaper of values and interests and represents the primary foundation from which the adolescent can establish an individual identity (Brinthaupt & Lipka, 2002). Just as play is the overall occupation of childhood and individual play activities are formative, the overall occupation of adolescence is to form an identity that includes school and work as well as play or leisure. Educational, vocational, and leisure activities are all extremely formative. Along with the family, the peer group assumes a role as a pertinent shaper of values and interests. Therefore, when working with adolescent clients, the intervention process must include their peers. Since the essential developmental process occurring for this age group is establishing independence and an autonomous identity, sometimes interpreted as different from the family, the adolescent often relies heavily on peers.

In any setting, the "milieu" is a powerful tool because it allows the group to assume responsibility and empowers individuals in the group to make decisions for the good of the whole. An example of utilizing the milieu as an intervention tool is to have the adolescent group define the rules for their program, with staff guidance that is nondidactic but asks the group members to reflect on the process and think for themselves. The OT is included as a member of the milieu and also can duplicate the process in occupational therapy. For example, the group can make decisions, such as what modalities will be used for the week, where the group will go on the weekly outing, what will be made in cooking group, and so on.

Because the family is the primary foundation from which the individual is able to build self-identity, parental and family factors are essential to consider (Slee, 2002). There may be demands by parents for the adolescent to take on a role of independence before he or she is developmentally able, or to become a caretaker of siblings, a task disproportionately interfering with developmental tasks of the period. Conversely, a parent may inadvertently keep the adolescent in a dependent role and may reinforce childish behaviors. Either of these situations may result in a disruption of the normal developmental tasks for the adolescent, leading to frustration at the least or acting out in negative ways at the most. The adolescent may sever communication and set out to prove he or she is independent. Parents and teens may conflict, though, in fact, what the adolescent needs are differing degrees of security, limits, and responsibilities appropriate to various situations. Conflicts with parents may often occur around social life, such as customs or family traditions, home responsibilities, school and grades, social values and morals, use of the telephone or family car, and family rules. To help teens learn social values and appropriate behavior in society, parents must maintain consistent behavior while at the same time providing a flexible caring, communicative environment with the expression of love, trust, and the respect for privacy. The task of parenting an adolescent is not easy!

When an adolescent enters the mental health system as "the client," the family and the individual should be helped to realize the **family is a system** in itself, that is, each family member affects and is affected by each other. The adolescent may become the identified client, but the family may have to acknowledge how the family as a whole, or system, may fit into the creation and also the solution of the problems that may be expressed in the identified client. Therefore, the family should be informed about, included, and involved as much as possible in treatment. Occupational therapy can involve the family, particularly when focusing on activities that may be shared by a family.

As stated in Chapter 10, numbers of blended and nontraditional families in the United States are increasing (Waterman, 2001). The traditional family may no longer be a biological mom and dad with biological siblings. Adolescents may be adopted and raised by extended families, grandparents, relatives, stepparents, or family friends (see Nickman, 2000, and Benoit, 2000 for more information on adoption and foster care). Whoever the adolescent considers to be his or her "family" may be considered to join in treatment, as is often the case in the parent-adolescent activity group (Lambert, 1990) previously described.

Because of the adolescent task of establishing independent self-identity, and learning about vocational and leisure interests and values, **mentors** may become important during this developmental time. Therefore, it is particularly important that staff in any setting be aware of the symbolic nature that their relationship and interactions may have for guiding adolescents in their quest for establishing independent values and interests in occupational areas and components.

Occupation-Based Interventions

For adolescents, care must be taken to choose modalities suited to their developmental age. As mentioned previously, games are often appropriate, due to their externally imposed parameters and rules, opportunity for competition, and achieving a goal other than the game itself. Those modalities and games that offer ease of adaptation and creativity are useful due to the varied developmental age ranges possible in a group of teenagers. Because the peer group is so important, success-oriented activities that provide a sense of mastery and self-confidence are key to increasing the adolescent's willingness to participate.

As was stated earlier, generally the more opportunity for the group participants to be a part of the decision making, the more sense of cooperation will be developed and the smoother the group sessions will go. In fact, an ongoing theme in working with adolescents is helping the adolescent move cognitively and behaviorally from a style of decision making and coping that is guided only by outside pressure to a style that becomes internally self-initiated based on integrated and flexible thinking and social norms and mores (Newton, 1995). Therefore, OT intervention should encourage the adolescent to move from an emotion-focused problem-solving style, which can be more impulsive and rigid, to a more mature, flexible, thoughtful, and reflective style.

Some theorists (Kohlberg, cited in Cole, 1998 and Sigelman & Shaffer, 1995) suggest three levels and six stages of moral development, any of which may be found to operate in adolescents. They note that motivation to move to the next level is created by experiences that contradict former beliefs and bring into question one's own reasoning. Occupational therapists can encourage growth in moral reasoning by exposing group members to reasoning at a higher level by encouraging role taking and role reversal (Bruce & Borg, 2002). Developmental learning can be accomplished through introducing moral dilemmas for discussion and problem solving (Cole, 1998) or, in other words, utilizing concepts of values clarification (Simon, Howe, & Kirschenbaum, 1995). By using an occupational therapy knowledge base of activity analysis occupational therapists can assist teenagers in developing this cognitive learning process. Table 11–2 lists some developmental goals, modalities, and specific activities that are grounded in these ideas when treating adolescents.

Table 11-2. Interventions for Adolescents

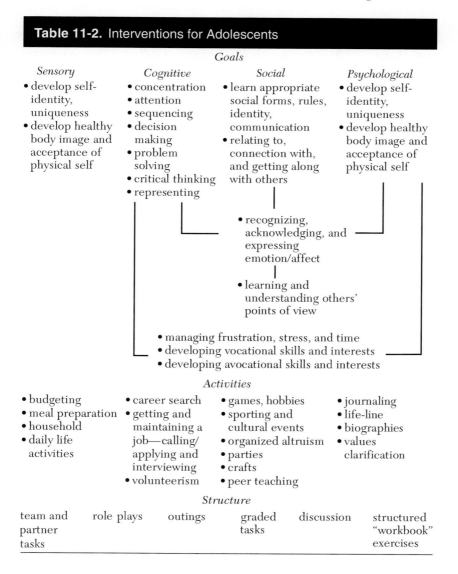

Goals

Sensory	Cognitive	Social	Psychological
• develop self-identity, uniqueness • develop healthy body image and acceptance of physical self	• concentration • attention • sequencing • decision making • problem solving • critical thinking • representing	• learn appropriate social forms, rules, identity, communication • relating to, connection with, and getting along with others	• develop self-identity, uniqueness • develop healthy body image and acceptance of physical self

• recognizing, acknowledging, and expressing emotion/affect

• learning and understanding others' points of view

• managing frustration, stress, and time
• developing vocational skills and interests
• developing avocational skills and interests

Activities

• budgeting • meal preparation • household • daily life activities	• career search • getting and maintaining a job—calling/ applying and interviewing • volunteerism	• games, hobbies • sporting and cultural events • organized altruism • parties • crafts • peer teaching	• journaling • life-line • biographies • values clarification

Structure

team and partner tasks	role plays	outings	graded tasks	discussion	structured "workbook" exercises

Specific activities meet more than one developmental goal and utilize more than one occupational performance skill or habit pattern (Fleming, 1994). For example, it is impossible to work on social skills without considering cognitive abilities, self-esteem, and communication skills. Activities improve skills in more than one area. For example, meal preparation may be utilized for training and assessment in areas of cognition (following a recipe), socialization (with a group format), and independent living (safety in the kitchen).

Team Building

One specific form that is extremely useful in working with adolescents, particularly for developing social and relational skills, cognitive reasoning, and self-awareness, is team building. It includes experiential activities, such as a ROPES course (Voight, 1988) or Outward Bound program (Godfrey, 1980). While these programs vary, the basic premise is to have the group, faced with what seems to be an impossible task initially, successfully mobilize a team to accomplish the tasks presented. The tasks are conquered throughout a day or several days while the participants face increasing fears that demand increasingly complex problem solving and teamwork. This modality is excellent in developing a young group of peers into a team that supports and cares for each other and recognizes the value of cooperation, enhances individual strengths, develops leadership roles, and encourages creative group problem solving. The key to utilization of team building is activity analysis and facilitator training. The therapist must have the training required for this specific program working with this specific age and population. Many elements of the challenging tasks may need to be adapted to meet the needs of the group, so activity analysis is essential.

CASE ILLUSTRATION: Team-Building Group

"There is a huge spider that lives underground. She has built this web in front of you and your group must get to the other side of it." The group is standing in front of a six-foot-square spider web made from ropes and elastic cords with holes of various sizes and shapes; the number of holes must equal or exceed the number in the group. "There is no way to go under or around this web and once someone goes through a hole in the web another person may not; if the web is touched, the spider will come out of the ground and eat the group." Obviously, this is not a true situation and, therefore, humor and fun can be brought into the task. As the group works to solve this situation the facilitator listens and allows the group to process and progress together. A key element of the facilitator of these groups is that the facilitator knows how to let the group work and at what point to intervene before the group becomes totally frustrated.

Discussion

With training in facilitation, occupational therapists can use their knowledge of activity analysis and grading activities to utilize team building to provide a rich and developmentally corrective experience for adolescents.

Creative Expression

These modalities are useful for the adolescent who is attempting to establish an understanding of changing emotions and thoughts that are often happening in his or her life at this stage. Creative expressive activities may be verbal or nonverbal and may include art, crafts, movement, dance, music, song writing, singing, poetry, writing, or using a journal or diary. Due to the expressive nature of these modalities an adolescent may initially be uncomfortable or shy in sharing with the group. One useful method of encouraging sharing is to begin with dyadic interaction. Ask the adolescent to choose at least one person in the group with whom to share his or her work. This method also shows respect for the individual's desire for privacy. Consider establishing the trust, safety, and security of the group by including discussions about confidentiality and reassurance that "what is shared with the group stays within the group." This is a time to facilitate the process of individuals in a group establishing their own rules and standards for their group. Teaching and role-modeling mutual respect as well as giving assurance that work will not be "analyzed" for hidden meaning and that creative talent will not be judged are useful in establishing an environment of creative sharing.

An example of a creative expression activity with a focus is a "Life Line." One variation of this activity is to ask the group to "indicate your life on this piece of paper. You can use symbols, words, or drawings. Include events that are important to you, or things that you remember as you were growing up and things that you would like to happen or may occur in your future." Have supplies available and offer encouragement that "there is no right or wrong way to complete this task." Figure 11-3 is an example of a life line created by an adolescent female diagnosed with a severe eating disorder.

Summary and Current Trends

There are various diagnoses and presenting problems of adolescents that include *DSM-IV-TR* (APA, 2000) disorders such as depression and eating disorders, in addition to disorders first diagnosed in infancy, childhood, or adolescence. Environmental psychosocial stresses, such as family dysfunction, abuse, neglect, violence, and poverty, as well as developmental stages and tasks should be considered when treating adolescents.

Useful concepts to consider when working with adolescents are structure and consistency, feedback on the impact of behavior, time-out, limit setting, use of the therapeutic relationship, and team approach. When implementing a program consider the needs of the clients, the demands of the service delivery system, and the structure of the current or planned program. Various assessments are useful for occupational therapists (Asher, 1996; Hemphill-Pearson, 1999).

Intervention for adolescents is based primarily on the occupational contexts of school, family, and leisure (play), and can include creative tasks, communication skill development, and problem-solving strategies. Intervention for adolescents is based on the developmental task of establishing self-identity and involves

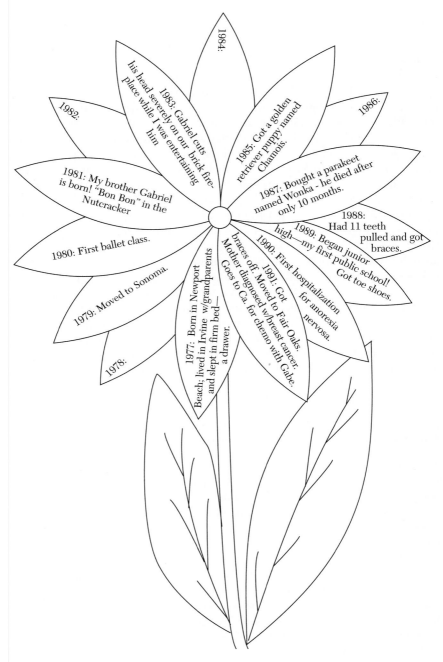

Figure 11-3. Life Line

issues of the peer group and the family. Intervention may include team building and self-expression, based on areas of occupation and performance skills and patterns, particularly those focusing on cognitive, psychological, and social skills.

Unfortunately, cost containment limits access to occupational therapy, if therapists do not make the transition from hospital to community-based practice. Since adolescents cannot usually be effective self-advocates due to their age and status, especially in a "bottom-line" driven economic climate, it is important for therapists to advocate appropriate services for adolescents, including occupational therapy. Unfortunately, not all hospitals and localities currently offer occupational therapy and other mental health services to adolescents who require them. Addressing the needs of this population may include an increased focus on the public school setting, where OT continues to be a strong presence. Adolescents in need of occupational therapy for emotional disturbances can be found everywhere, in the hospital, in the school, and in your neighborhood (Forness, Florey, & Greene, 1993). Therapists will, most likely, need to become stronger advocates for their clients, as well as their profession, to meet the need for community mental health treatment for adolescents.

Review Questions

1. What do the terms *acting out* and *setting limits* mean? Why are they important in working with adolescents?
2. What are the most likely diagnoses of adolescents that you may encounter in a mental health setting?
3. What or who constitutes the system or environment of an adolescent that must be considered in treatment? In what community settings are you most likely to treat adolescents?
4. Why are expressive and team-building groups important for adolescents?
5. What is the underlying base of intervention for adolescents and why is it so important?

References

Abramson, R. M. (1982a). Therapeutic activities for the hospitalized adolescent. In L. Hoffman (Ed.), *The evaluation and care of severely disturbed children*. New York: SP Medical & Scientific Books.

Abramson, R. M. (1982b). Developmental and diagnostic assessment. In L. Hoffman (Ed.), *The evaluation and care of severely disturbed children* (pp. 37–44). New York: SP Medical & Scientific Books.

Alberti, R., & Emmons, M. (1995). *Your perfect right* (7th ed.). San Luis Obispo, CA: Impact.

American Psychiatric Association. (2000). *Diagnostic and statistical manual of mental disorders*-text revision (4th ed.). Washington, DC: American Psychiatric Association.

Arnett, J. (1999). Adolescent storm and stress, reconsidered. *American Psychologist, 54*, 317–326.

Asher, I. E. (1996). *Occupational therapy evaluation tools: An annotated index* (2nd ed.). Bethesda, MD: American Occupational Therapy Association.

Austrian, S. G. (Ed.). (2002). *Developmental theories through the life cycle*. New York: Columbia University Press.

Barrows, C. (1996). Clinical interpretation of "Predictors of Functional Outcome Among Adolescents and Young Adults With Psychotic Disorders." *American Journal of Occupational Therapy, 50*(3), 180–183.

Benoit, M. B. (2000). Foster care. In B. J. Sadock & V. A. Sadock (Eds.), *Kaplan and Sadock's comprehensive textbook of psychiatry* (7th ed., pp. 2873–2877). Philadelphia: Lippincott Williams & Wilkins.

Bettelheim, B. (1987, March). The importance of play. *Atlantic Monthly,* 35–46.

Block, B. M., Arney, K., Campbell, D. J., Kiser, L. T., Lefkovitz, D. M., & Speer, S. K. (1991). American Association for Partial Hospitalization, Child and Adolescent Special Interest Group: Standards for child and adolescent partial hospitalization programs. *International Journal of Partial Hospitalization, 7*(1), 13–21.

Brinthaupt, T. M., & Lipka, R. P. (Eds.). (2002). *Understanding early adolescent self and identity: Applications and interventions.* Albany: State University of New York Press.

Bronfenbrenner, U. (1979). *The ecology of human development.* Cambridge, MA: Harvard University Press.

Brown, C., & Harwood, K. J. (1992). Neuropathology in schizophrenia: Implications for occupational therapy. *Occupational Therapy in Health Care, 8*(2/3), 117–133.

Bruce, M., & Borg, B. (2002). *Psychosocial occupational therapy: Frames of reference for intervention* (3rd ed.). Thorofare, NJ: Slack.

Bukatko, D., & Daehler, M. W. (2001). *Child development: A thematic approach* (4th ed.). Boston: Houghton Mifflin.

Burns, B. J., & Hoagwood, K. (2002). *Community treatment for youth: Evidence-based interventions for severe emotional and behavioral disorders.* New York: Oxford University Press.

Call, K. C., & Mortimer, J. T. (2001). *Arenas of comfort in adolescence: A study of adjustment in context.* Mahwah, NJ: Erlbaum.

Chess, S., & Thomas, A. (1984). *Origins and evolution of behavior disorders: From infancy to early adult life.* New York: Brunner/Mazel.

Chess, S., & Thomas, A. (1996). *Temperament: Theory and practice.* New York: Brunner/Mazel.

Chess, S. & Thomas, A. (2002). Temperament and its clinical implications. In M. Lewis (Ed.). *Child and adolescent psychiatry: A comprehensive textbook* (pp. 220–227). Philadelphia: Lippincott Williams & Wilkins.

Cohen, D. J., & Caffo, E. (1998). Developmental psychopathology and child mental health services: Risk and protective factors in children, families, and society. In J. G. Young & P. Ferrari (Eds.), *Designing mental health services and systems for children and adolescents: A shrewd investment* (pp. 3–13). Philadelphia: Brunner/Mazel.

Cole, M. B. (1990). Group dynamics in occupational therapy (2nd ed.). Thorofare, NJ: Slack.

Delgado, M. (2002). *New frontiers for youth development in the twenty-first century: Revitalizing and broadening youth development.* New York: Columbia University Press.

Delman, J., & Jones, A. (2002). *Voices of youth in transition: The experience of aging out of the adolescent public mental health service system in Massachusetts: Policy implications and recommendations.* Dorchester, MA: Consumer Quality Initiatives.

Department of Occupational Science and Occupational Therapy. (2003). *OT for young adults and youth at-risk. University of Southern California.* Retrieved Marcyh 10, 2003, from http://www.usc.edu/hsc/ihp/ot/facultypractice.htm.

Dryfoos, J. G. (1992). Adolescents at risk. A summary of work in the field: Programs and policies. In D. Rogers & E. Ginzberg (Eds.), *Cornell University Medical College Seventh Conference on Health Policy* (pp. 128–141). Boulder: Westview.

Dunn, W., Brown, C., & McGuigan, A. (1994). The ecology of human performance: A framework for considering the effect of context. *American Journal of Occupational Therapy 48*(7), 595–607.

Erikson, E. H., (1968). *Identity: Youth and crisis.* New York: Norton.

Evans, M. E., & Armstrong, M. I. (2002). What is case management? In B. J. Burns & K. Hoagwood, *Community treatment for youth: Evidence-based interventions for severe emotional and behavioral disorders* (pp. 39–68). New York: Oxford University Press.

Fleming, M. H. (1994). Conditional reasoning: Creating meaningful experiences. In C. Mattingly & M. H. Fleming, *Clinical reasoning: Forms of inquiry in a therapeutic practice* (pp. 197–235). Philadelphia: F. A. Davis.

Florey, L. L. (1968). *A developmental classification of play.* Unpublished master's thesis, University of Southern California, Los Angeles.

Fonagy, P., Target, M., Cottrell, D., Phillips, J., & Kurtz, Z. (2002). What works for whom? A critical review of treatments for children and adolescents. New York: Guilford.

Forness, S., Florey, L., & Green, S. (1993). *Hidden in plain sight: Children with behavior disorder in school systems.* Paper presented at the 73rd annual conference of the American Occupational Therapy Association, Seattle, WA.

Fritz, G. K., Mattison, R. E., Nurcombe, B., & Spirito, A. (1993). *Child and adolescent mental health consultation in hospitals, schools, and courts.* Washington, DC: American Psychiatric Association.

Glaser, D. (2002). Child sexual abuse. In M. Rutter & E. Taylor (Eds.), *Child and adolescent psychiatry: A comprehensive textbook* (pp. 340–358). Oxford: Blackwell Science.

Godfrey, B. (1980). *Outward bound: Schools of the possible.* New York: Doubleday.

Greenberg, L., Haiman, S., & Esman, A. (1987). Countertransference—its impact on the hospital treatment of adolescents. In Sherman Feinstein (Ed.), *Adolescent psychiatry,* (Vol. 15, pp. 316–331). Chicago: University of Chicago Press.

Greenspan, S. I. (2002). *The secure child: Helping children feel safe and confident in a changing world.* Cambridge, MA: Perseus.

Haiman, S. (1990). Selecting group protocols: Recipe or reasoning? *Group protocols: A psychosocial compendium.* Binghamton, NY: Haworth.

Haiman, S., & Greene, S. (1998). Occupational therapy. In J. D. Noshpitz, N. E. Alessi, J. T. Coyle, S. I. Harrison, & S. Eth (Eds.), *Handbook of child and adolescent psychiatry* (Vol. 6). New York: Wiley.

Heaven, P. L. (2001). *The social psychology of adolescence.* Basingstoke: Palgrave.

Hemphill-Pearson, B. (1999). *Assessments in occupational therapy in mental health.* Thorofare, NJ: Slack.

Hoffman, A. M. (Ed.). (2001). *Teen violence: A global view.* Westport, CT: Greenwood.

Hoffman, L. (1982). *The evaluation and care of severely disturbed children.* New York: SP Medical & Scientific Books.

Ireys, H. T., Devet, K. A., & Sakwa, D. (2002). Family support and education. In K. J. Burns & K. Hoagwood (Eds.), *Community treatment for youth: Evidence-based interventions for severe emotional and behavioral disorders* (pp. 154–175). New York: Oxford University Press.

Jakubowski, P., & Lange, A. (1978). *The assertive option: Your rights and responsibilities.* Champaign, IL: Research Press.

Kaplan, H., & Sadock, B. (1995). *Comprehensive textbook of psychiatry* (6th ed.). Baltimore: Williams & Wilkins.

Kielhofner, G. (2002). A model of human occupation: Theory and application (3rd ed.). Philadelphia: Lippincott Williams & Wilkins.

King, R. A. (2002). Adolescence. In M. L. Lewis (Ed.), *Child and adolescent psychiatry: A comprehensive textbook* (pp. 332–342). Philadelphia: Lippincott Williams & Wilkins.

Kirshner, B., O'Donoghue, J. L., & McLaughlin, M. (Eds.). (2002). *Youth participation: Improving institutions and communities.* San Francisco: Jossey-Bass.

Kiser, L. J., Heston, J. D., & Pruitt, D. B. (2002). Child and adolescent partial hospitalization and ambulatory behavioral health services. In M. L. Lewis (Ed.), *Child and adolescent psychiatry: A comprehensive textbook* (pp. 1083–1090). Philadelphia: Lippincott Williams & Wilkins.

LaGreca, A., Silverman, W. K., Vernberg, E. M., & Roberts, E. M. (Eds.). (2002). *Helping children cope with disasters and terrorism.* Washington, DC: American Psychological Association.

Lambert, W. (1990). *Parent-child activity: Assessment and treatment of families.* Paper presented at the Pennsylvania Occupational Therapy Association Annual Conference, Philadelphia.

Lambert, W., & Moffitt, R. (1988). *A collaborative approach to developmental group in child psychiatry.* Paper presented at the Pennsylvania Occupational Therapy Association Annual Conference, State College, PA.

Lambert, W., Moffitt, R., & Rose, J. (1989). *Therapeutic use of toys and games in child psychiatry.* Paper presented at the Pennsylvania Occupational Therapy Association Annual Conference, Hershey, PA.

Law, M., Cooper, B., Strong, Stewart, D., Rigby, P., & Letts, L. (1996). Person-environment-occupation model: a transactive approach to occupational performance. *Canadian Journal of Occupational Therapy, 63*, 9–23.

Lefrancois, G. (2001). *Of children: An introduction to child and adolescent development* (9th ed.). Belmont, CA.: Wadsworth/Thomson Learning.

Lehman, C. M., Clark, H. B., Bullis, M., Rinkin J., & Castellanos, L. A. (2002). Transition from school to adult life: Empowering youth through community ownership and accountability. *Journal of Child and Family Studies, 11*(1), 127–141.

Lewis, M. L. (Ed.). (2002). *Child and adolescent psychiatry: A comprehensive textbook*. Philadelphia: Lippincott Williams & Wilkins.

Llorens, L., & Rubin, E. (1967). *Developing ego functions in disturbed children: Occupational therapy in milieu*. Detroit: Wayne State University Press.

Lougher, L. (Ed.) (2001). *Occupational therapy for child and adolescent mental health*. New York: Churchill Livingstone.

Manikam, R. (2002). Mental health of children and adolescents. In N. Singh, T. H. Ollendick, & A. N. Singh, *International perspectives on child and adolescent mental health (Vol. 2): Selected proceedings of the Second International Conference on Child and Adolescent Mental Health, Kuala Lumpur, Malaysia* (pp. 1–36). Amsterdam, NY: Elsevier.

Mash, E. J., & Wolfe, D. A. (2003). Disorders of childhood and adolescence. In G. Stricker & T. Wideger (Eds.), *Handbook of psychology: Clinical psychology* (Vol. 8, pp. 27–63). New York: Wiley.

Mental Health: A Report of the Surgeon General. (1999). http://www.surgeongeneral.gov/library/mentalhealth/home.html.

Michaelson, M., & Nakamura, J. (Eds.). (2001). *Supportive frameworks for youth engagement*. San Francisco: Jossey-Bass.

Morrison, C. D., & Metzger, P. (2001). Play. In Jane Case-Smith (Ed.), *Occupational therapy for children* (4th ed., pp. 528–545). St. Louis, MO: Mosby.

Morrison, J. (1995). *DSM-IV made easy: The clinician's guide to diagnosis*. New York: Guilford.

Newtown, M. (1995). *Adolescence: Guiding youth through the perilous ordeal*. New York: Norton.

Nickman, S. L. (2000). Adoption. In B. J. Sadock & V. A. Sadock (Eds.), *Kaplan and Sadock's comprehensive textbook of psychiatry* (7th ed., pp. 2868–2872). Philadelphia: Lippincott Williams & Wilkins.

Occupational Therapy Practice Framework: Domain and Process. (2002). *American Journal of Occupational Therapy, 56*, 609–639.

Offer, D., & Schonert-Reichl, K. A. (1992). Debunking the myths of adolescence: Findings from recent research. *Journal of the American Academy of Child and Adolescent Psychiatry, 31*, 1003–1013.

Office of Juvenile Justice and Delinquency Prevention. (1995). *Guide for implementing the comprehensive strategy for serious, violent and chronic juvenile offenders*. Washington, DC: U.S. Department of Justice.

Papalia, D. E., & Olds, S. W. (1992). *Human development*. New York: McGraw-Hill.

Parham, L. D., & Fazio, L. S. (Eds.). (1997). *Play in occupational therapy for children*. St. Louis, MO: Mosby.

Pearce, J. C. (2003). *From magical child to magical teen: A guide to adolescent development*. Rochester, VT: Park Street.

Reilly, M. (Ed.). (1974). *Play as exploratory learning*. Beverly Hills, CA: Sage.

Rhodes, J. E. (2002). *Stand by me: The risks and rewards of mentoring today's youth*. Cambridge, MA: Harvard University Press.

Rice, P. F., & Dolgin, K. G. (2002). *The adolescent: Development, relationships, and culture* (10th ed.). Needham Heights, MA: Allyn & Bacon.

Roth, A., & Fonagy, P. (1996). *What works for whom: A critical review of psychotherapy research*. New York: Guilford.

Rutter, M., & Taylor, E. (Eds.). (2002). *Child and adolescent psychiatry* (4th ed.). Oxford: Blackwell Science.

Sadock, B. J., and Sadock, V. A. (Eds.). (2000). *Kaplan and Sadock's comprehensive textbook of psychiatry* (7th ed.). Vols. 1–2. Philadelphia:O Lippincott Williams & Wilkins.

Scalletti, R. (1999). A community development role for occupational therapists working with children, adolescents and their familes: A mental health perspective. *Australian Occupational Therapy Journal, 46*(2), 43–51.

Schkade, J. K., & Schultz, S. (1992). Occupational adaptation: Toward a holistic approach for contemporary practice, Part 1. *American Journal of Occupational Therapy, 10*(46), 829–837.

Schultz, S., & Schkade, J. K. (1992). Occupational adaptation: Toward a holistic approach for contemporary practice, Part 2. *American Journal of Occupational Therapy, 10*(46), 917–925.

Schwab-Stone, M. E., & Briggs-Gowan, M. J. (1998). The scope and prevalence of psychiatric disorders in childhood and adolescence. In J. G. Young & P. Ferrari (Eds.), *Designing mental health services and systems for children and adolescents: A shrewd investment* (pp. 15–25). Philadelphia: Brunner/Mazel.

Schwab-Stone, M. E., Henrich, C., & Armbruster, P. (2002). School consultation. In M. L. Lewis (Ed.), *Child and adolescent psychiatry: A comprehensive textbook* (pp. 1361–1369). Philadelphia: Lippincott Williams & Wilkins.

Scott, M. A., Snowden L., & Libby, A. M. (2002). From mental health to juvenile justice: What factors predict this transition? *Journal of Child and Family Studies, 11*(3), 299–311.

Scutta, C., & Schaaf, R. C. (1989, October). *A time for play?* Paper presented at the Pennsylvania Occupational Therapy Association Annual Conference, Hershey, PA.

Sholle-Martin, S., & Alessi, N. E. (1990). Formulating a role for occupational therapy in child psychiatry: A clinical application. *American Journal of Occupational Therapy, 44*(10), 871–882.

Sigelman, C. K., & Shaffer, D. R. (1995). *Life-span human development* (2nd ed.). Pacific Grove, CA: Brooks/Cole.

Simon, S. B., Howe, L. W., & Kirschenbaum, H. (1995). *Values clarification: A handbook of practical strategies for teachers and students* (Rev. ed.). New York: Warner.

Slee, P. T. (2002). *Child, adolescent and family development* (2nd ed.). New York: Cambridge University Press.

Smith, M. J. (1975). *When I say no I feel guilty.* New York: Dial.

Strong, S., Rigby, P., Stewart, D., Law, M., Etts, L., & Cooper, B. (1999). Application of the person environment–occupation model: A practical tool. *Canadian Journal of Occupational Therapy, 66*(3), 122–133.

Surgeon General. (2001). *Youth violence: A report of the Surgeon General.* Retrieved August 25, 2003 from, http://www.surgeongeneral.gov/library/youthviolence/chapter3/sec1.html#development.

Thomas, A., & Chess, S. (1977). *Temperament and development.* New York: Brunner/Mazel.

Thomas, A., & Chess, S. (1986). The New York longitudinal study: From infancy to early adult life. In R. Plomin & J. Dunn (Eds.), *The study of temperament: Changes, continuities, and challenges.* Hillsdale, NJ: Erlbaum.

Townsend, E. (Ed.). (1997). *Enabling occupation: An occupational therapy perspective.* Ottawa: Canadian Association of Occupational Therapists.

Voight, A. (1988). The use of ropes courses as a treatment for emotionally disturbed adolescents in hospitals. *Therapeutic Recreation Journal, 12*(2), 57–64.

Waterman, B. (2001). Mourning the loss builds the bond: Primal communications between foster, adoptive, or stepmother and child. *Journal of Loss and Trauma, 6,* 277–300.

Whyte, J. (2000). Adolescent development. In A. M. Hosin (Ed.), *Essays on issues in applied developmental psychology and child psychiatry* (pp. 335–379). Lewiston, NY: Edwin Mellen.

Suggested Reading

Banus, B. S., Kent, C. A., Norton, Y., Sukiennicki, D. R., & Becker, M. L. (1982). *The developmental therapist* (2nd ed.). Thorofare, NJ: Slack.

Berger, K. S. (1994). *The developing person through the lifespan* (3rd ed.). New York: Worth.

Bingham, M., Edmondson, J., & Stryker, S. (1983). *Choices: A teen women's journal for self-awareness and personal planning.* Santa Barbara, CA.: Advocacy.

Blake, J. (1990). *Risky Times: How to be AIDS-smart and stay healthy: A guide for teenagers*. New York: Workman.

Barber, B. K. (2002). *Intrusive parenting: How psychological control affects children and adolescents*. Washington, DC: American Psychological Association.

Block, B. M., Arney, K., Campbell, D. J., Kiser, L. J., Lefkovitz, P. M. & Speer, S. K. (1991). American Association for Partial Hospitalization, Adolescent and Adolescent Special Interest Group: Standards for adolescent and adolescent partial hospitalization programs, *International Journal of Partial Hospitalization, 7*(1).

Booth, A., & Crouter, A. C. (Eds.) (2001). *Does it take a village? Community effects on children, adolescents, and families*. Mahwah, NJ: Erlbaum.

Byrne, K. (1987). *A parents guide to anorexia and bulimia*. New York: Henry Holt.

Calvert, S. L., Jordan, A. B., & Cocking, R. R. (Eds.). (2000). *Children in the digital age: Influences of electronic media on development*. Westport, CT: Praeger.

Capacchione, L. (2001). *The creative journal for teens: Making friends with yourself* (2nd ed.). Franklin Lakes, NJ: Career Press.

Cunningham, A. (2002). Social skills intervention for teens with ADHD. *OT Practice, 7*(20), 10–14.

Freud, A. (1967). *The ego and the mechanisms of defense*. New York: International Universities Press.

Gil, E. (1983). *Outgrowing the pain: A book for and about adults abused as children*. New York: Dell.

Gilligan, C. (1979). Woman's place in man's life cycle. *Harvard Educational Review, 49*, 431–446.

Gilligan, C. (Ed.). (1991). *Women, girls and psychotherapy: Reframing resistance*. New York: Haworth.

Gilligan, C., Lyons, N. P., & Hammer, T. J. (Eds.). (1990). *Making connections: The relational worlds of adolescent girls at Emma Willard School*. Cambridge, MA: Harvard University Press.

Hall, Calvin S. (1982). *A primer of Freudian psychology*. New York: Harper & Row.

Heron, A. (Ed.). (1994). *Twenty writings by gay and lesbian youth*. Boston: Alyson.

Hunter, M. (1990). *Abused boys: The neglected victims of sexual abuse*. New York: Ballantine.

Korb-Khalsa, K. L., Azok, S. D., & Leutenberg, E. A. (1990). *Life management skills I*. Beachwood, OH: Wellness Reproductions.

Korb-Khalsa, K. L., Azok, S. D., & Leutenberg, E. A. (1991). *Life management skills II*. Beachwood, OH: Wellness Reproductions.

Korb-Khalsa, K. L., Azok, S. D., & Leutenberg, E. A. (1994). *Life management skills III*. Beachwood, OH: Wellness Reproductions.

Korb-Khalsa, K. L., Azok, S. D., & Leutenberg, E. A. (1995). *S E A L S + plus/self-esteem and life skills*. Beachwood, OH: Wellness Reproductions.

Kundanis, R. M. (2003). *Children, teens, and mass media: The millennial generation*. Mahwah, NJ.: Erlbaum.

LeCroy, C. W., & Daley, J. (2001). *Empowering adolescent girls: Examining the present and building skills for the future with the Go Grrrls Program*. New York: Norton.

Lerner, R. M. (2002). *Adolescence: Development, diversity, context, and application*. Upper Saddle River, NJ: Prentice-Hall.

Levy, B. (1993). *In love and in danger: A teen's guide to breaking free of abusive relationships*. Seattle: Seal.

McCoy, K., & Wibbelsman, C. (1992). *The new teenage body book*. New York: BodyPress/Perigee.

Melia, M. A., & Weikert, K. (1987). Evaluation and treatment of adolescents on a short-term unit. *Occupational Therapy in Mental Health, 7*(2), 51–66.

Michael, R. T. (Ed.). (2001). *Social awakening: Adolescent behavior as adulthood approaches*. New York: Russell Sage Foundation.

Mortimer, J. T., & Larson, R. W. (2002). *The changing adolescent experience: Societal trends and the transition to adulthood*. New York: Cambridge University Press.

Nelson, R. R., & Condrin, J. L. (1987). A vocational readiness and independent skills program for psychiatrically impaired adolescents. *Occupational Therapy in Mental Health, 7*(2), 22–38.

Newton, N. A., & Sprengle, K. (Eds.) (2000). *Psychosocial interventions in the home: Housecalls*. New York: Springer.

New Games Foundation. (1976). *The new games book*. Garden City, NY: Doubleday.

O'Reilly, P., Penn, E. M., & deMarrais, K. (Eds.) (2001). *Educating young adolescent girls*. Mahwah, NJ: Erlbaum.

Outward Bound, USA: Learning through experience in adventure based education. (1981). New York: Morrow.

Poikolainen, K. (2002). Antecedents of substance abuse in adolescence. *Current Opinion in Psychiatry, 15*(3), 242–245.

Remocker, A. J., & Storch, E. T. (1979). *Action speaks louder: A handbook of nonverbal group techniques*. New York: Churchill-Livingstone.

Stein, M. B., Hyde, K. L., Monopolis, S. J. (1991). Adolescent and family outreach services as an adjunct to child and adolescent mental health treatment. *International Journal of Partial Hospitalization, 7*(1).

Steiner, H. (1995). *Treating adolescents*. San Francisco: Jossey-Bass.

Vogler, R., & Bartz, W. (1992). *Teenagers and alcohol*. Philadelphia: Charles Press.

CHAPTER 12

Mental Health of the Older Adult

Anne MacRae, PhD, OTR/L

Key Terms

aging in place
dementia
elder abuse
geriatric
in vivo

lifestyle redesign
Medicare
quality of life
somatic
well elderly

Chapter Outline

Introduction

This chapter, while focusing on the mental health issues of aging, by necessity addresses the health of the older adult from a broad perspective. The interdependence of context with physical and mental health is even more pronounced in the elderly than in the general population. Furthermore, as discussed throughout this chapter, there are several external factors that confound the ability to address psychiatric or psychological problems of this age group.

Many occupational therapists have long held the belief that the medical model is insufficient to meet all of the health-related needs of the world's population. Nowhere is that more evident than in meeting the needs of the older adult. The health conditions of this population are more likely to be of a chronic nature and, as Yerxa states, "the medical approach of fix and cure is inadequate for those who must live out their lives with the triple challenge of handicap, social stigma and environmental unfriendliness" (2000, p. 198). As will be shown in this chapter, the mental as well as physical health of the older population is explicitly contingent on physical, social, and personal contexts. The medical profession has attempted to address the specific issues of aging with the development of specialties in **geriatric** medicine and psychiatry. However, the complexity of health maintenance and treatment in the older population is best met through a coordinated interdisciplinary approach that also addresses multiple contexts (APA Working Group on the Older Adult, 1998).

THE DEMOGRAPHICS OF AGING

According to the Administration on Aging (AoA), the population of older adults (age 65+) in the United States in the year 2000 totaled 35 million people. By the year 2030, this population is expected to more than double to about 70 million (2002). The worldwide demographic changes are even more dramatic.

> The number of persons aged 60 years or older is estimated to be 629 million in 2002 and is projected to grow to almost 2 billion by 2050, at which time, the population of older persons will be larger than the population of children (0–4 years) for the first time in human history. (United Nations Secretariat, 2003, p. 1)

This rise in numbers of older adults will have significant effects on all areas of human and societal function, including economics and family life (Ineichen, 1998). To provide effective care for this population, all health professionals will need to expand their focus beyond a medical model and become advocates for change in social, economic, and health care policies and systems.

In 2000, 27% of older persons in the United States assessed their heath as fair or poor, compared to 9% for all persons (AoA, 2002). Self-report of health has repeatedly been shown in the literature to have a high correlation to disability and function (AoA, 2002; Han, 2002). Clearly, the health care needs of this population are significant. However, this data also shows that the majority of older people are healthy and probably active and productive members of their communities. This group is commonly referred to as the **well elderly.** Some of the factors that help the older adult stay healthy are obvious and are tied to known morbidity factors of the general population (smoking, diet, management of preexisting health conditions, etc.). Interestingly, however, many of the factors identified in the promotion of elder health are related to the psychological and social well-being of the individual, which is discussed throughout this chapter.

PSYCHIATRIC DIAGNOSIS

It is widely reported in the literature that older adults have a much lower incidence of all psychiatric diagnosis, excluding cognitive disorders, than any other age group (APA Working Group on the Older Adult, 1998; APA, 2000; AGS, 1993). However, such statistics must be viewed with caution for several reasons.

1. Most older adults receive their health care through a primary physician or a general medicine clinic or institution. There is a serious lack of training and administrative support in these settings for identifying symptoms of mental illness and making appropriate referrals (AGS, 1993; Jervis, 2002; Reynolds, 1995; Smith, 2001).
2. There is generally a greater concern in the older population than in the general population about the stigma of mental illness and therefore treatment specified as "psychiatric" or "psychological" is often avoided (APA Working Group, 1998; Davis, Moye, & Karel, 2002; Reynolds, 1995).
3. The majority of older adults in the United States are at least partially dependent on **Medicare** (a government-sponsored health care payment program, primarily for those over age 65), which is woefully inadequate in reimbursement for mental health. The consequence of this is twofold: the individual avoids such treatment and the health care providers are often unwilling to diagnose and treat conditions that may not be reimbursable (AGS, 1993).
4. Presentation of psychiatric illness in the elderly is often different than in younger people and is therefore difficult to diagnose. Most notably is the tendency of the elderly to emphasize and describe **somatic** (physical) concerns rather than emotional concerns (APA Working Group, 1998; Sadock & Sadock, 2003; Tune, 2001). This often leads to both under-recognized psychiatric illness and unnecessary medical treatment.

Even in cases where the individual may not meet the full criteria for a psychiatric disorder, many psychiatric symptoms may be found in the elderly population due to general medical conditions or life stressors (Tune, 2001). Many of these symptoms (described in Table 12-1) are treatable if recognized. These psychiatric symptoms are sometimes seen in **dementia**, but may also be indicative

Table 12-1. Presentation of Psychiatric Symptoms in Older Adults

Psychiatric Condition	*Diagnostic Issues*
Anxiety	Anxiety disorder is less common in older adults than in younger adults (Schaub & Linden, 2000). However, anxiety is a common symptom associated with other medical and psychiatric conditions (Smith, Sherrill, & Colenda, 1995), as well as changes in environment and other life stressors. New onset of anxiety in older adults may also be associated with medication side effects and drug withdrawal (Flint, 2001). Clients living alone may be more prone to a "phobic type" anxiety (Schaub & Linden, 2000).
Depression	The presentation of depression in the elderly is generally markedly different than in a younger population and is therefore under-diagnosed (Brodaty, Luscombe, Parker, Hickie, & Mitchell, 1997; Peach, Koob, & Kraus, 2001). Lack of energy, anhedonia, poor concentration, and psychomotor disturbance are commonly shared symptoms in depression, dementia, and many general medical conditions (Forsell & Winblad, 1998). People with vascular dementia are more likely to have depressive symptoms than people with Alzheimer's dementia (Ballard, Neill, O'Brian, McKeith, Ince, & Perry, 2000).
Mania	Diagnosis of bipolar disorder in the older adult is not common but may be diagnosed if an earlier incidence of a depressive episode was present. It is hypothesized that the incidence of changed polarity of depressive illness increases with age (Young, 1997). Mania may also be a symptom of cognitive disorders or confused with the irritability and lability found in dementia and delirium (APA, 2000).
Psychosis	Psychotic symptoms are associated with a myriad of different psychiatric and medical disorders. However, it is also found in both vascular dementia and dementia of the Alzheimer's type. The presentation of psychosis in people with dementia is sufficiently different from psychotic disorders such as schizophrenia that it is theorized to be a distinct syndrome (Leroi, Voulgari, Breitner, & Lyketsos, 2003).
Substance Abuse	The prevalence of alcohol abuse in older adults appears to be lower than in the general population. However, due to physiologic changes in the aged, use of alcohol may be more detrimental to overall health (APA Working Group, 1998). Alcohol or other substance abuse is also commonly found in depression and/or as a maladaptive coping strategy. Alcohol abuse impairs memory and information processing and so may go unrecognized in the early stages of dementia and yet cause significant functional deterioration. Toxicity from over-the-counter and combinations of prescribed medication also can cause both serious medical consequences as well as cognitive impairments that may erroneously lead to a diagnosis of early dementia (Hall, 2002).

of a separate and distinct disorder that too often goes undiagnosed and therefore untreated. "About 10 to 15 percent of all patients who exhibit symptoms of dementia have potentially treatable conditions. The treatable conditions include systemic disorders. . .; vitamin deficiency; medications; and primary mental disorders, most notably, depression" (Sadock & Sadock, 2003, p. 1322).

CASE ILLUSTRATION: Mr. Sorensen—Differential Diagnosis— Depression and Dementia

Mr. Sorensen is a widower who lives in an elder assisted living facility. His wife of 42 years who visited him every day suddenly passed away and the family had to put their aging dog to sleep because no one was able to care for him. The staff noted that Mr. Sorensen was not eating well and was spending more time alone. He was generally noncommunicative and often appeared confused. He needed prompting to get out of bed in the morning and supervision to complete personal care.

Discussion

Grief and multiple losses are common in the elderly and can lead to depression if not addressed. The staff at the facility may not realize the magnitude of Mr. Sorensen's personal losses and dismiss his current behavior as to be expected. Mr. Sorensen may indeed have a progressive dementia but the life stressors he is enduring certainly warrant intervention, including counseling and/or medication, for what may be a treatable depression.

CASE ILLUSTRATION: Mrs. DeVaughn—Differential Diagnosis—Toxicity and Dementia

Mrs. DeVaughn has been displaying increased confusion, memory loss, and irritability. Her daughter, Edna, arranged for a home health care team to evaluate her safety in the home. She fully expected that a recommendation will be made for Mrs. DeVaughn to move to a supervised living situation because of what her daughter sees as deteriorating dementia. Mrs. DeVaughn refused to let the visiting nurse go over her medications with her, but agreed to let the occupational therapist help her organize her bathroom and kitchen cabinets "just to make things easier." The OT found 14 prescription medications prescribed by five different medical specialists as well as her primary care physician. She also found a plethora of over-the-counter medications as well as herbal supplements. The OT contacted the case managing nurse, who arranged with the MD to have Mrs. DeVaughn hospitalized so her medicines could either be discontinued, reduced, or changed. Within three days, Mrs. De Vaughn's mental status markedly improved and, much to her daughter's surprise, she was able to return to independent living.

Discussion

While physicians and pharmacists have increased their awareness of drug interactions and symptoms and methods for tracking medical prescriptions are much improved, the problems associated with using multiple health care providers still exists. The older adult tends to trust health care providers and is unlikely to question a prescription or offer information about other medications unless specifically asked. The occupational therapist is in an ideal role to evaluate actual medication regimes in the home by addressing daily living habits and routines and can then coordinate with the team for treatment recommendations. In any case of suspected dementia, it is vital that all other, often treatable, causes are ruled out. In the case of Mrs. DeVaughn, there may have also been a metabolic or general medical condition, such as decreased kidney function, that would increase the likelihood of toxicity (increased concentration of substances because of decreased elimination).

All of the symptoms and disorders listed in Table 12-1 are described in depth in various chapters of this book. However, unique to the elderly population (at least in terms of high incidence) is dementia, an emotionally, socially, and physically devastating condition, which therefore warrants further discussion.

Dementia

Dementia is a syndrome identified by the presence of multiple cognitive deficits. (For further information and definitions of cognitive deficits, see Chapter 14.) The *Diagnostic and Statistical Manual* (APA, 2000) lists three criteria for diagnosis:

1. Memory impairment
2. At least one other cognitive impairment including aphasia, apraxia, agnosia, or disturbance in executive functioning
3. Significant impairment in social or occupational functioning and a significant decline from a previous level of functioning

As previously discussed, there are many other symptoms associated with the presence of dementia, but they are not diagnostic criteria and the presentation of dementia varies significantly with the individual and the stage of the condition.

Dementia may be caused by a wide variety of conditions, including degenerative disorders of the central nervous system such as Parkinson's disease or Huntington's disease; cardiac disorders, which may result in vascular dementia; metabolic disorders such as diabetes that may result in vascular dementia or uncontrolled thyroid conditions; nutritional, especially vitamin, deficiencies; toxicity or drug-related, such as substance-induced dementia; brain tumors, trauma, and infections, most notably Creutzfeldt-Jacob Disease (CJD) and human immunodeficiency virus (HIV). From a medical viewpoint, it is critical to determine the underlying reason for the dementia, as many of the aforementioned conditions can be medically treated or at least controlled. However, more than half of all diagnosed dementia is caused by Alzheimer's disease, a progressive condition for which there is no known cure.

Vascular dementia and Alzheimer's are both strongly age-related, with the prevalence approximately doubling every five years from age 60 through 90 (Jorm, 1990). With the worldwide demographic changes previously discussed, the incidence of these dementias is sure to rise, perhaps dramatically. Alzheimer's Disease International (2000) projects that the number of people with dementia will rise to 34 million by 2025, almost doubling the estimated 18 million people with dementia in 2000.

Alzheimer's disease is progressive and often very difficult to diagnose in its early stages; therefore, the diagnosis may be made retrospectively. The relatively minor memory problems consistent with early stages of Alzheimer's disease may be found in any older adult and is not necessarily indicative of pending decline.

Table 12-2 outlines the stages of the disease as described by Reisberg, Ferris, and Crook (1983) in the Global Deterioration Scale. The staging is helpful in anticipating common reactions and behaviors and adjusting intervention to address them.

MENTAL HEALTH ASSESSMENT

All health care providers should be cognizant of the presence of psychiatric disorders, particularly ones that are too often overlooked, such as depression and substance abuse. Simple screening tools may identify treatable conditions. The most commonly used depression screen for older adults is the Geriatric Depression Scale (GDS), originally designed by Yesavage and now in the public domain; it is often updated and is currently translated into over 20 languages. The short version (Shiekh & Yesavage, 1986) probably has the most widespread usage. The GDS has shown to be a reliable and cost-effective screening tool, especially when used in conjunction with other tests (Peach, Koob, & Kraus, 2001). There are several screening tools used to identify geriatric alcohol abuse. One of the most popular is the Short Michigan Alcoholism Screening Test-Geriatric Version (MAST-G) (University of Michigan Alcohol Research Center, 1991).

Given the global effects of dementia on the individual and her or his family, it is important to arrive at a working diagnosis as early as possible. There are several specific assessments to screen, diagnose, and classify the stages of Alzheimer's disease as well as other dementias. Commonly used ones are the Alzheimer's Disease Assessment Scale (ADAS) (Rosen, Mohs, & Davis, 1984); the Alzheimer's Disease Functional Assessment and Change Scale (ADFACS) (Galasko et al., 1997); and the Disability Assessment for Dementia (DAD) Scale (Gelinas, Gauthier, & McIntyre, 1999).

Occupational Therapy Assessment

Assessment of the overall mental health of older adults is often appropriately conducted as an interdisciplinary effort. The focus of the interdisciplinary assessment

Table 12-2. Clinical Course of Alzheimer's Disease

Stage	Description	Examples of Performance and Behaviors
Stage 1	No Cognitive Decline	Normal functioning—occasional lapses of memory.
Stage 2	Very Mild Cognitive Decline	No deficits noted in occupational or social roles. However, the individual may express concern over "forgetfulness." Often forgets names or misplaces objects.
Stage 3	Mild Cognitive Decline	Immediate recall is impaired and agnosia may be present. Because of decreased performance in demanding employment and social situations, it is in this stage that family, friends, and co-workers may recognize a problem. Anxiety over performance is common at this stage, but there is usually significant denial as well.
Stage 4	Moderate Cognitive Decline	Deficits are now obvious, including poor concentration, decreased knowledge of recent and current events, and difficulties traveling alone (especially to unfamiliar places) and in handling personal finances. The individual usually remains orientated to time and familiar places and persons. There is often a withdrawal from new or challenging situations and the person generally will still be in denial of the seriousness of her or his condition.
Stage 5	Moderately Severe Cognitive Decline	Individuals at stage 5 generally need assistance to live safely. They are likely to forget important phone numbers or emergency procedures and are frequently disoriented to time or place, but usually will remember own name and names of close friends and family. The person begins to have problems with multistep daily living activities, such as dressing, but does not need assistance with many personal care tasks such as eating or toileting.
Stage 6	Severe Cognitive Decline	The individual occasionally forgets spouse's name or the names of other significant people in his or her life. Retains some sketchy knowledge of past life, but is largely unaware of recent events and experiences. Disoriented to time and place. Sleep patterns are frequently disturbed. There is often marked personality/emotional changes in this stage that may include delusions, obsessiveness, anxiety, agitation, apathy, and, occasionally, violent behavior.
Stage 7	Very Severe Cognitive Decline	Profound physical symptoms such as incontinence and limited mobility (may be unable to walk). Communication is severely impaired and may be limited to grunting. Needs assistance with all personal care.

Source: Adapted from the *Global Deterioration Scale* by Reisberg, Ferris, & Crook, 1983.

corresponds with many of the traditional domains of occupational therapy (OT), therefore, OT assessments, especially those that focus on cognition, occupation, environment, and social relations, are valuable for this population. Figure 12-1 is a select list of assessments that focus on these areas; most but not all, were designed by occupational therapists.

Many other assessments that are described throughout this book can also be used with the older adult population, and readers are encouraged to explore a wide variety of assessments to fit the individual needs of particular clients. A key element of OT assessment is the skill to perform functional evaluations, either through formal assessment or task analysis, **in vivo,** or in the client's natural environment. A study by Hoppes, Davis, and Thompson (2003) on the environmental effects on the assessment of people with dementia concluded that "while it may be time consuming to assess clients in specific settings of interest, this may be the only

---

Title of Assessment and Author(s)/Source

Activity Index & Meaningfulness of Activity Scale (Gregory, 1983; Nystrom, 1974)

Assessment of Communication and Interaction Skills (ACIS) (Forsyth, Salamy, Simon, & Kielhofner, available through MOHO Clearinghouse)

Assessment of Living Skills and Resources (ALSAR) (Williams et al., 1991)

Assessment of Motor and Process Skills (AMPS) (Fisher, 2002; available only to therapists who have received training)

Cognitive Performance Test (CPT) (Burns, Mortimer, & Merchek, 1994)

Community Integration Measure (McColl, Davies, Carlson, Johnston, & Milnnes, 2001)

Contextual Memory Test (Toglia, available through Therapy Skill Builders)

Kitchen Task Assessment (Baum & Edwards, 1993)

Leisure Interest Profile for Seniors (Henry, research version available from the University of Massachusetts Medical Center, Boston)

Lowenstein Occupational Therapy Cognitive Assessment-Geriatric (LOTCA-G) (Elazar, Itzkovich, & Katz, available through Maddack, Inc.)

Mini Mental State Exam (MMSE) (Folstein, Folstein, & McHugh, 1975)

Multidimensional Functional Assessment Questionnaire (Duke University Center for the Study of Aging and Human Development, 1978)

Rivermead Behavioral Memory Test (Wilson, Cockburn, & Baddeley, 1985)

Routine Task Inventory (Heimann, Allen, & Yerxa, 1989)

Test of Orientation for Rehabilitation Patients (TORP) (Deitz, Tovar, Beeman, Thorn, & Trevisan, 1992)

Figure 12-1. Assessments for Use with Older Adults: A Selective List with a Focus on Cognition, Occupation, Environment, and Social Relations

valid way to determine abilities to function in those settings" (p. 401). In Chapter 2, a case illustration was given (Uyen) where the in-clinic assessment overestimated the client's functional capabilities. The next case illustration demonstrates the opposite situation.

CASE ILLUSTRATION: Mrs. Ayala—In Vivo Assessment

Mrs. Ayala is a 76-year-old woman with a history of vascular disease who was recently hospitalized for a transient ischemic attack (TIA). The hospital interdisciplinary team determined that she had a moderate level of dementia, most likely of the vascular type. The hospital-based occupational therapist performed a kitchen assessment in the OT clinic to determine Mrs. Ayala's safety and functional abilities in activities of daily living. During the assessment it was noted that Mrs. Ayala became quite agitated and confused. She did remember to turn off the electric range top, but then placed a plastic bowl on the burner. The OT needed to intervene to prevent the bowl from melting and then provided moderate assistance to complete the task safely.

The hospital-based team recommended that after discharge Mrs. Ayala not be allowed to stay at home alone. She lives with her daughter's family, but all family members are either at work or school during the day. The family refused to consider placement for her outside the home but did agree to home health care services.

The home health occupational therapist received the discharge notes from the hospital-based therapist. Therefore, she was quite surprised when arriving at Mrs. Ayala's home to find her in the kitchen alone successfully making Pancit (a traditional Filipino meal made of rice stick noodles, vegetables, and shrimp or meat) as well as homemade lumpia (egg rolls) for her family's dinner. When the OT expressed her concern, Mrs. Ayala laughingly replied, "I've been doing this all of my life!"

Discussion

In her own home, Mrs. Ayala demonstrated a much higher functional ability than previously seen in the hospital. She was able to perform cooking tasks that were actually much more complicated than what was asked of her during the hospital evaluation. The familiarity of the tools (such as a gas range instead of an electric one) and the layout of the kitchen often help people with memory or other cognitive deficits perform tasks automatically. The cultural familiarity with the items being prepared is also an important factor. A third, critical factor is being able to preserve an important and meaningful role as a contributing member of the family.

Quality of Life Assessment

Life satisfaction or **quality of life** assessment is now very much a part of interdisciplinary evaluation and is recognized as a significant outcome of treatment by both the World Health Organization (WHO, 2001) and the Occupational Therapy Practice Framework (2002), as well as many other OT and health care organizations around the world. Despite this recent focus, there is little agreement in the literature on a definition of quality of life. According to Alzheimer's Disease International (ADI, 2000), "quality of life is a much broader concept than either health or disease. It is rather difficult to define as everyone has their own ideas" (p. 1). Some key elements identified by ADI as common elements and areas needing assessment are:

- Mobility
- Social relations
- Affording and obtaining necessities
- Living independently
- Occupations (occupying one's time)
- Comfort
- Self-esteem
- Satisfaction with daily activities
- Sources of pleasure

The important point in a quality of life assessment is to recognize the individual and subjective nature of the responses. Clients will have interests and priorities in life that may be quite different than what the therapist thinks is important. A truly client-centered approach with active listening is essential for a meaningful quality of life assessment.

CASE ILLUSTRATION: Professor Fujiyama's Quality of Life

Dr. Fujiyama is an emeritus professor of neurobiology at a prestigious university. He is in the early to moderate stage of Alzheimer's disease. All of his adult life he took immense pride in his intellectual ability and is having great difficulty in adjusting to his memory lapses and generally decreased function. He became withdrawn and is often irritable. The home health occupational therapist wanted to engage him in self-care activities but met with great resistance. The OT decided to change her approach and offered to work with him on "cognitive" activities. She showed the doctor some interactive computer programs on biology and engaged him in several pencil and paper tasks using memory strategies. Eventually he started asking questions about cognitive rehabilitation and the theories behind her choice of activities for him. He developed an interest in using the computer and researching web sites about Alzheimer's disease.

The OT would leave worksheets and suggested activities for the professor after every visit and upon her return he would confidently show the OT his completed "homework." Although Dr. Fujiyama continued to avoid most activities of daily living (ADLs) and depended on his wife or an aide to perform such tasks, his affect was brighter, he had less angry outbursts, and he appeared more engaged and interested in life.

Discussion

Although the OT was unable to engage Dr. Fujiyama in many of the traditional activities used by home health therapists, she was able to adjust her intervention to include tasks that were personally meaningful and appropriately challenging to the professor. This provided a quality of life to this client that could not be found in more "conventional" therapy.

Quality of life should be a focus in all occupational therapy assessment but it has particular significance for the older adult, as the more conventional outcomes of restoration, rehabilitation, or improvement of function may not be realistic goals. This presents one of the many challenges for occupational therapists working with the older adult, as functional "progress" is often the basis for reimbursement and conventional rehabilitation may be viewed by employers as the only OT services that should be offered. Occupational therapists need to advocate for a broadening of their role in many settings and engage in research that demonstrates the long-term cost-effectiveness of quality of life intervention.

OCCUPATIONAL THERAPY INTERVENTION

Intervention for the older adult, as with assessment, is best provided with a holistic and coordinated approach that includes professionals as well as family, caregivers, and other significant individuals. However, for the purposes of this chapter, the discussion is limited to the interventions most frequently used by occupational therapists. Depending on the condition being addressed, the expected outcomes may include restoration of function and rehabilitation, but goals addressing quality of life, prevention, and adaptation are also crucial for the older adult population.

Occupation

The overarching purpose of occupational therapy is to promote the "engagement in occupation to support participation" (Occupational Therapy Practice Framework, 2002). A study conducted by Aubin, Hachey, and Mercier (1999) suggests that "perceived competence in daily tasks and rest, and pleasure in work and rest activities are positively correlated with subjective quality of life. The influence of occupation and its meaning on quality of life, an occupational therapy assumption, is supported by these results" (p. 53). A critical review of 23 other studies concurred:

> Occupation has an important influence on health and well-being. Ranging from physiological to functional outcomes, it is clear that the performance of everyday occupations is an important part of everyday life. Withdrawal or changes in occupation for a person have a significant

impact on a person's self-perceived health and well-being. (Law, Stein-wender, & Leclair, 1998, pp. 89–90)

In another critical review that specifically addressed activity programs for people with dementia, Law et al. (1999) reported that four well-designed studies using rigorous methods "support the use of activity groups for older persons with dementia for improving their well being, communication, mental status and emotional state" (p. 4). However, it was also noted that limited data was available and further research is indicated.

The positive effects of occupation are not only seen in clients but in their caregivers as well. In a study conducted by Baum (1995), it was found that "individuals who remained active in occupation demonstrated fewer disturbing behaviors, required less help with basic self care, and their carers experienced less stress" (p. 59).

Although considerable research is now being conducted on the effects of occupation, it is difficult to draw generalizations. In order for occupation to be effective as an intervention, it must be personally meaningful and present an appropriate level of challenge. A task that is overly simple may be seen as demeaning yet an overly complex task may promote feelings of failure. In order for occupation to be used as a therapeutic modality (rather than a simple diversion), an occupational therapist chooses the activity or occupation with the client but may also need to adapt it to meet specific goals and provide "just the right" challenge for the client. Occupations or activities used by occupational therapists are often commonplace in daily life, therefore, an erroneous conclusion may be drawn by administrators that occupation-based groups may be competently and less expensively conducted by para- or nonprofessionals. While some diversional activities groups are helpful and welcomed by the older adult, a groundbreaking three-year well elderly study conducted by Clark et al. (1997) concluded that "superior outcomes can be expected when an activity-centered intervention is administered by professional therapists as opposed to being conducted by nonprofessionals" (p. 1325).

CASE ILLUSTRATION: The Occupations of Mr. Hatfield

Mr. Hatfield is a retired factory worker who is currently being evaluated for depression and dementia. He reports to the occupational therapist that the only thing that he ever liked doing was fishing but he can't drive his truck to the pier anymore. Through further conversation, the OT learns that Mr. Hatfield always tied his own flies for fly fishing and she asks him to teach her the craft. He wrote a shopping list of all the supplies that he needed and together they shopped for supplies and continued to tie fancy fishing flies for several sessions. Mr. Hatfield seemed to enjoy the sessions and reminisced about past great fishing trips. However, he clearly still missed his prime occupation of actually going fishing. The occupational therapist helped Mr. Hatfield contact a local volunteer organization to find a fishing companion willing and able to accompany and transport Mr. Hatfield to local fishing spots. A successful match was made and a trip was planned for the following week. His volunteer companion also told Mr. Hatfield that there was a fly tying club over in the next town and he would be glad to take him to a meeting. Although Mr. Hatfield remained somewhat forgetful and he needed guidance to perform many tasks, his affect greatly improved.

Discussion

Although Mr. Hatfield's interests seem limited, his passion for fishing opened up possibilities for new leisure and social pursuits and provided the motivation to engage in cognitively challenging activities such as constructing a craft and shopping for supplies. The need to teach an activity (to the occupational therapist) also provided a sense of purpose and an opportunity to demonstrate mastery and competence.

Environmental Support and Adaptation

Understanding the context of treatment is critical to the occupational therapy process. (See Chapter 2 for further discussion.) Environment plays a vital role in both the overall functioning and the quality of life of the older adult. In the United States and in other parts of the world, the preference of older adults is to remain in their homes or communities for as long as possible. A phenomenological study conducted in Scandinavia "showed that moving to sheltered housing meant for a majority of participants that their self image changed from being self reliant and independent to becoming dependent and perceiving themselves and their care to be a burden" (Sviden, Wikstrom, & Hjortsjo-Norberg, 2002, p. 10). To meet the needs of the older population and honor their choices, facilitating **aging in place** has become a focal point of treatment both for "humanistic reasons and to minimize health care costs" (Horowitz, 2002, p. 1). As discussed in Chapter 2, occupational therapists are specifically trained in environmental adaptation that addresses the physical, social, emotional, spiritual, and cognitive contexts. Given the often complex needs of the older adult, this holistic view of the environment is essential for successful intervention.

CASE ILLUSTRATION: Mrs. Christie—The Meaning of Home

Mrs. Christie lives in a large Victorian home in the city where she raised her four children. After her husband passed away, her grown children, all with families of their own, wanted her to move to a smaller home or apartment, out in the suburbs, closer to them. Two of the four children also offered to have her move in with them. Although Mrs. Christie freely admits that she has slowed down "quite a bit," she still feels quite able to care for herself. Her biggest functional change has been to give up driving. She has groceries delivered or walks to the corner store and either takes a taxi or has a friend drive her to appointments. Mrs. Christie's children all exclaim that the house is too much work for her and they think she would be safer out of the city. Also, if she was in the suburbs they could check up on her more frequently. She steadfastly resists, stating that she would miss her friends and her garden.

Discussion

Many older adults freely choose to move to a low maintenance residence or move in with family; however, many others wish to stay in a familiar place. While the concerns expressed by Mrs. Christie's children could be realistic, they fail to take into account the personal meaning of home. In some cultures, such as the Anglo-American culture of Mrs. Christie, independence is highly prized and moving in with one's children may be seen as an imposition or failure (even if invited).

A familiar home often provides a sense of community. It is likely that Mrs. Christie knows her neighbors, grocer, church minister, and pharmacist. She has also shown the ability to be adaptive, maintaining her mobility in the community without driving. Her home is a place full of memories and favorite occupations such as gardening. Intervention geared toward helping Mrs. Christie stay as independent as possible in her own home and doing the things she likes to do, rather than encouraging her to abandon her home, would be preferable.

The social context of the environment includes the roles of caregivers and family as well as the individual client and it is often appropriate for the OT to include them in direct treatment as well as provide education, training, and support. Research also indicated that friends of both the older adult and the caregivers provide valuable emotional and social support (Lilly, Richards, & Buckwalter, 2003) and should be included in assessment and treatment as needed. Evaluating the needs of the caregiver and facilitating coping and caregiving strategies as well as empowering caregivers are vital roles of the occupational therapist (Baum, 1991; Gitlin, Corcorcan, & Leinmiller-Echhardt, 1995; Wallens & Rockwell-Dylla, 1996). As an older adult declines in function the role of the caregiver increases, thereby increasing her or his stress. If supported by outside services, the caregiver may be more effective and be provided necessary education. The cost-effectiveness of a family approach to treatment is due to the ability of the older adult to remain in the home rather than being moved to an institutional placement.

The occupational therapist, along with the social worker, plays a critical role in reconnecting an isolated individual with her or his community by making appropriate referrals to community and social groups and by facilitating the ability to access social support systems. These community referrals may also benefit the caregiver by providing support and respite. (See Appendix B for resources.)

Although aging in place is preferred by many older adults and has many advantages, care must be taken not to assume that one's home is always the ideal living situation. For many people the responsibility of home management is not possible or is overly stressful. According to the AoA (2002), 30% of older adults (primarily women) live alone. In the case of Mrs. Christie that was clearly her choice and she was still actively involved in her community and had a social support network. However, for many older adults, living alone can be a frightening and lonely experience. A move to a socially active senior residence or with family may ease the loneliness as well as provide necessary support.

Another aspect of the environmental conditions that must be evaluated is the potential for **elder abuse.** Although there have been scandals involving abuse and neglect in nursing facilities, the sad truth is that most elder abuse occurs in the home, usually inflicted by a family member. It is estimated that 10% of people over the age of 65 have been abused (Sadock & Sadock, 2003). This may be an underestimation, as victims of elder abuse rarely report such incidences and they are not likely to be seen in public where others may report their concerns.

CASE ILLUSTRATION: The Abuse of Mr. Dempsey

Mr. Dempsey is an 82-year-old former prizefighter with Parkinson's disease and dementia. His once strong physique is now quite frail. Mr. Dempsey is unable to walk, eat, or use the toilet without assistance, and he is sometimes incontinent. Mr. Dempsey lives with his son, Charlie, in a small, run-down flat. Charlie greatly resents having to "clean up Dad's messes and put up with his babbling." However, Charlie is out of work and depends on his father's social security check for income. Charlie's resentment often turns to rage, especially when he has been drinking. On several occasions, he has punched his father, but more often, Charlie ignores his father's physical needs, sometimes forgetting to feed him or change his clothes and bedsheets.

Discussion

Elder abuse can take many forms and it is not uncommon for the abuser to financially benefit from the relationship. Victims are usually either incapable of reporting the crime or are too frightened to do so. There is also a high incidence of denial from both the abuser and victim. Assessment of potential elder abuse requires strong observation skills and an understanding of the physiology of age-related diseases. The level of force needed to injure a frail person is minimal and the consequences of improper care can lead to a myriad of serious health consequences. In the United States, it is required that all health professionals report suspected abuse to Adult Protective Services.

Behavioral Techniques and Humanistic Philosophy

Behavioral techniques used by both professionals and caregivers can greatly increase the comfort and safety of not only the older adult but also those around her or him as well. Figure 12-2 outlines helpful behavioral strategies for dealing with people with dementia. However, conflict can occur between a behavioral approach, which emphasizes safety of the older adult, and a humanistic philosophy, which emphasizes choice and respect for the older adult. "Older people may be so protected by their carers that they are prevented from achieving fulfillment in their lives. There can be a temptation to stop someone attempting anything

Aggression & Anger
- Assure individuals who behave aggressively that they are okay—that you understand that they cannot help themselves.
- Speak in a well-modulated voice.
- Offer food or drink (it is difficult to eat and be angry at the same time).
- Position yourself about four or five feet away.
- Sit or stand a little to the side rather than face them directly. You're less intimidating to them this way.
- Be prepared to accept some insults and verbal abuse.
- Ask yourself if too much is being expected of them.

Catastrophic reactions
- Reduce confusion with memory aids and highly structured routines.
- Simplify everything, e.g., decision-making, leisure activities.
- Assist them one step at a time. Reinforce each successful step.
- Stop and give those that are confused a chance to calm down.
- Reassure.
- Gently holding a person's hands, patting on the arm or gently rocking can be soothing, along with quiet music.
- Accept the behavior as a response to dementing illness, beyond the control of the impaired person.
- Distract, if possible.

Confusion
- Provide a nightlight to help the person see and locate familiar things and prevent falls in the dark; protect against wandering
- Consider the side effects of some sedatives and cold remedies as well as prescribed drugs.
- Encourage reminiscence. Gently assist with keeping facts reasonably accurate and related to the past.
- Use communication rich in reminders, cues, gestures and physical guiding (if appropriate) to increase personal awareness. Keep explanations simple.
- Avoid unrealistic promises.
- Keep your mood and responses consistent.
- Provide special personal space filled with familiar things where the confused person can go, rest and feel safe and secure.
- Ask permission if something must be moved or changed: This helps to establish feelings of trust and control.
- Overprotection leads to feelings of helplessness and boredom. Provide reminders, directions, adequate time and praise for self-care efforts on an adult level.

(continues)

Figure 12-2.   Approaches to Problem Behaviors

Source: [Author unknown], [Handout on managing problem behaviors in people with dementia] (Presented at a workshop on dementia, Palo Alto Veterans' Administration Medical Center, Palo Alto, CA).

- Schedule respite care regularly in the caregiving routine so it becomes accepted and predictable.

Depression
- Respond to the impaired person with kind firmness.
- Try to rebuild self-esteem through reminiscence, participation in activities and decisions. Notice pictures and momentos. Ask about them and listen.
- Alert the person's doctor, medications may help.
- Spend time with them. Do not ignore quiet, uncomplaining people.
- Encourage them to talk freely.
- Be familiar with the factors that predispose people to depression. They include problems with: health, living situation, losses, and a family history of depressive illness.
- A gentle touch with a reassuring smile projects a caring attitude.

Hoarding, rummaging behavior — Because of memory loss, demented people frequently look for something that is "missing": rooms, clothes, personal items. These things may not look familiar so they are constantly looking for familiar things.
- Don't scold or try to rationalize with the person.
- Distract the impaired person when he/she is somewhere he/she is not supposed to be.
- Learn the impaired person's hiding places.

Sundowner's syndrome — This occurs when impaired people become confused, restless and insecure late in the afternoon and after dark.
- Set up a rigid daily routine. It will reduce anxiety about decision making and what happens next.
- Alternate activity with programmed rest.
- Reduce all stimuli during rest periods.
- Strive to keep daily activities within the person's coping ability.
- Prepare the impaired person for special events so it doesn't come as a shock.
- Take an inventory of the person's daily experience. Consider bright lights, noise from TVs, radios, and conversations, visitors and special events, odors from miscellaneous sources, and the stimulation of personal contact with the caregiver.

Suspiciousness, distrust — Occurs most often with people with dementia when they cannot make sense of what is happening.
- Be honest.
- Avoid grand gestures and promises that cannot be carried out.
- Go to the person when you have forgotten something and apologize.
- Do not argue about or rationally explain disappearances of the person's possessions.
- Offer to look for an item if the person says that it is missing.
- Learn the person's favorite hiding places.

Figure 12-2. (continued)

which may result in harm" (Poole, 1997, p. 371). Care must be taken to prevent over-management of the client's life, as "appropriate risk taking is a normal part of everyday life and adds quality to the subjective experience" (Poole, 1997, p. 371). The charter of principles of Alzheimer's Disease International (2000) emphasizes the importance of a humanistic, client-centered approach with the following statements: "A person with dementia continues to be a person of worth and dignity, and deserving of the same respect as any other human being" and "people with dementia should as far as possible participate in decisions affecting their daily lives and future care" (p. 1).

CASE ILLUSTRATION: Mrs. Christie—One Year Later

The family arguments about Mrs. Christie living alone have escalated. In the past year she has fallen off a step stool while reaching for something in a high cabinet; gotten lost while shopping, although she was able to call a neighbor for help; and was hospitalized once for dehydration. She said the doctors told her to stop drinking so much tea and start drinking more water, which she says she now does.

Mrs. Christie's oldest daughter is especially upset by what she sees as her mother's "stubbornness" and takes the drastic move to apply to the courts to be named her conservator. After a comprehensive psychiatric and physical evaluation, the courts turn down the daughter's request, stating that Mrs. Christie is aware of the consequences of her actions and is competent to make her own decisions. The psychiatric team recommends family counseling for the mother and daughter to be able to make compromises regarding Mrs. Christie's activities and minimize the family stress.

Discussion

Mrs. Christie is asserting her right of free choice and her daughter's well-meaning but misguided attempts to control her mother's actions have created considerable distress. Family intervention, including psychological counseling and occupational therapy, can help this family understand the mother's needs and yet develop adaptive strategies in daily activities to ease the worry of the daughter and increase Mrs. Christie's safety in the home and community.

Prevention and Health Maintenance

A phenomenological study with elderly Swedish women (Hedelin & Strandmark, 2001) found that "the essence of mental health is the experience of confirmation, trust and confidence in the future, as well as a zest for life, development, and involvement in one's relationship to oneself and to others" (p. 9). This finding concurs with the criteria for quality of life and eloquently gives us important guidelines for prevention and health maintenance interventions for the older adult.

Although occupation is the cornerstone of occupational therapy intervention, the well elderly study by Clark et al. (1997) suggests that activity or "keeping busy" alone is insufficient for health maintenance or promotion. Rather, a systematic application of OT principles is needed, which includes highly individualized programs (even when conducted in a group setting); instruction in life management skills; and choice of occupations that are viewed as meaningful and health promoting. This study showed significant results of preventative occupational therapy in many areas, including improvement in general mental health and physical functioning as well as increased social functioning and activity, vitality, and life satisfaction. Based on this study a plethora of programs are now being developed in **lifestyle redesign**, "an intervention model that promotes quality of life in well elders" (Jackson, Mandel, Zemke, & Clark, 2001, p. 5).

Although substantial evidence that shows the effectiveness of OT in prevention and health maintenance now exists, the traditional medically oriented model often does not allow occupational therapists to utilize their full repertoire of skills. OTs must be proactive in advocating for change in health care systems and in increasing professional recognition in order to provide necessary and meaningful intervention for the large older adult population.

Summary

In 2000, the American Occupational Therapy Association (AOTA) estimated that 37% of all occupational therapists in the United States worked with older adults. However, given the demographic data provided in this chapter, that number is certainly rising. Although the majority of older adults are well elderly, the devastating and global effects of chronic and mental illness in the older population have significant consequences for the individual, family, and society as a whole.

Occupational therapists have a unique role in preserving and fostering mental as well as physical health of the older adult. The emphasis on meaningful occupation in context that is focused on quality of life issues and prevention as well as restoration of function is a critical component of health care for the older adult.

Review Questions

1. How will the expected increase in the number of older adults affect occupational therapy as a profession?
2. What difficulties are there in determining accurate psychiatric diagnosis in the older adult population?
3. Which psychiatric disorders may be mistaken for dementia?
4. How does engagement in occupation benefit the older adult?
5. What are the benefits and limitations of aging in place?

References

Administration on Aging (AoA). (2002). *A profile of older Americans: 2002*. U.S. Department of Health and Human Services.

Alzheimer's Disease International (ADA). (2000, September). *World Alzheimer's Day Bulletin*. Author.

American Geriatric Society (AGS). (1993). *Mental health and the elderly position statement.*

American Occupational Therapy Association (AOTA). (2000). *"2000' membership invoice questionnaire.* Bethesda, MD: Author.

American Psychiatric Association (APA). (2000). *Diagnostic and statistical manual* (4th ed.-text revised). Washington, DC: Author.

APA Working Group on the Older Adult. (1998). What practitioners should know about working with older adults. *Professional Psychology: Research and Practice, 29*(5), 413–417.

Aubin, G., Hachey, R., & Mercier, C. (1999). Meaning of daily activities and subjective quality of life in people with severe mental illness. *Scandinavian Journal of Occupational Therapy, 6,* 53–62.

Ballard, C., Neill, D., O'Brian, J., McKeith, I. G., Ince, P., & Perry, R. (2000). Anxiety, depression and psychosis in vascular dementia: Prevalence and associations. *Journal of Affective Disorders, 59,* 97–106.

Baum, C. M. (1991). Addressing the needs of the cognitively impaired elderly from a family policy perspective. *American Journal of Occupational Therapy, 45*(7), 594–606.

Baum, C. M. (1995). The contribution of occupation to function in persons with Alzheimer's disease. *Journal of Occupational Science, 2,* 59–67.

Baum, C., & Edwards, D. (1993). Cognitive performance in senile dementia of the Alzheimer's type. *American Journal of Occupational Therapy, 47,* 431–436.

Burns, T., Mortimer, J. A., & Merchak, P. (1994). Cognitive performance test: A new approach to functional assessment in Alzheimer's disease. *Journal of Geriatric Psychiatry and Neurology, 7*(1), 46–54.

Brodaty, H., Luscombe, G., Parker, G., Wilhelm, K., Hickie, I., Austin, M. P., & Mitchell, P. (1997). Increased rate of psychosis and psychomotor change in depression with age. *Psychological Medicine, 27,* 1205–1213.

Clark, F., Azen, S., Zemke, R., Jackson, J., Carlson, M., & Mandell, D., et al. (1997). Occupational therapy for independent-living older adults: A randomized controlled study. *Journal of the American Medical Association, 278,* 1321–1326.

Davis, M. J., Moye J., & Karel, M. J. (2002). Mental health screening of older adults in primary care. *Journal of Mental Health & Aging, 8*(2), 139–149.

Deitz, J. C., Tovar, V. S., Beeman, C., Thorn, D. W., & Trevisan, M. S. (1992). The test of orientation for rehabilitation patients: Test-retest reliability. *Occupational Therapy Journal of Research, 12*(3), 172–185.

Duke University Center for the Study of Aging and Human Development. (1978). *Multidimensional functional assessment: The OARS methodology.* Durham, NC: Author.

Flint, A. J. (2001). Core concepts in geriatrics: Anxiety disorders. *Clinical Geriatrics, 9*(11), 21, 24–5, 28–30.

Folstein, M., Folstein, S., & McHugh, P. (1975). Mini mental state: A practical method for grading the cognitive state of patients for the clinician. *Journal of Psychiatric Research, 12,* 189–198.

Forsell, Y., & Winblad, B. (1998). Major depression in a population of demented and non-demented older people: Prevalence and correlates. *Journal of the American Geriatrics Society, 46*(1), 27–30.

Galasko, D., Bennett, D., Sano, M., et al. (1997). An inventory to assess activities of daily living for clinical trials in Alzheimer's disease: The Alzheimer's disease co-operative study. *Alzheimer's Disease and Associated Disorders, 11* (suppl. 2), S33–39.

Gelinas, I., Gauthier, L., & McIntyre, M. (1999). Development of a functional measure for persons with Alzheimer's disease: The Disability Assessment for Dementia. *American Journal of Occupational Therapy, 53,* 471–481.

Gitlin, L., Corcorcan, M., & Leinmiller-Echhardt, S. (1995). Understanding the family perspective: An ethnographic framework for providing occupational therapy in the home. *American Journal of Occupational Therapy, 49,* 802–809.

Gregory, M. D. (1983). Occupational behavior and life satisfaction among retirees. *American Journal of Occupational Therapy, 37,* 548–553.

Hall, C. (2002). Special considerations for the geriatric population. *Critical Care Nursing Clinics of North America, 14*(4), 427–434.

Han, B. (2002). Depressive symptoms and self-rated health in community-dwelling older adults: A longitudinal study. *Journal of the American Geriatrics Society, 50*(9), 1549–1556.

Hedelin, B., & Strandmark, M. (2001). The meaning of mental health from elderly women's perspectives: A basis for health promotion. *Perspectives in Psychiatric Care, 37*(1), 7–14.

Heimann, N. E., & Allen, C. K. (1989). The routine task inventory: A tool for describing the functional behavior of the cognitively disabled. *Occupational Therapy Practice, 1*(1), 67–74.

Hoppes, S., Davis, L. A., & Thompson, D. (2003). Environmental effects on the assessment of people with dementia: A pilot study. *American Journal of Occupational Therapy, 57*(4), 396–402.

Horowitz, B. P. (2002). Occupational therapy home assessments: Supporting community living through client-centered practice. *Occupational Therapy in Mental Health, 18*(1), 1–17.

Ineichen, B. (1998). The geography of dementia: An approach through epidemiology. *Health and Place, 4*(4), 383–394.

Jackson, J., Mandel, D., Zemke, R., & Clark, F. (2001). Promoting quality of life in elders: An occupation-based occupational therapy program. *World Federation of Occupational Therapists (WFOT) Bulletin, 43*, 5–12.

Jervis, L. (2002). Contending with "problem behaviors" in the nursing home. *Archives of Psychiatric Nursing, 16*(1), 32–38.

Jorm, A. F. (1990). *The epidemiology of Alzheimer's disease and related disorders*. London: Chapman & Hall.

Law, M., Steinwender, S., & Leclair, L. (1998). Occupation, health and well-being. *Canadian Journal of Occupational Therapy, 65*, 81–91.

Law, M., Stewart, D., Letts, L., Pollock, N., Bosch, J., Philpot, A., & Westmorland, M. (1999). *Effectiveness of activity programmes for older persons with dementia*. Hamilton, ONT: Occupational Therapy Evidence Based Practice Research Group.

Leroi, I., Voulgari, A., Breitner, J., & Lyketsos, C. (2003). Epidemiology of psychosis in dementia. *American Journal of Geriatric Psychiatry, 11*(1), 83–91.

Lilly, M. L., Richards, B. S., & Buckwalter, K. C. (2003). Friends and social support in dementia caregiving: Assessment and intervention. *Journal of Gerontological Nursing, 29*(1), 29–36.

McColl, M. A., Davies, D., Carlson, P., Johnston, J., & Milnnes, P. (2001). The community integration measure: Development and preliminary validation. *Archives of Physical Medicine and Rehabilitation, 82*, 429–434.

Nystrom, E. P. (1974). Activity patterns and leisure concepts among the elderly. *American Journal of Occupational Therapy, 28*, 337–345.

Occupational Therapy Practice Framework: Domain and Process. (2002). *American Journal of Occupational Therapy, 56*(6), 614–639.

Peach J., Koob, J. J., & Kraus, M. J. (2001). Psychometric evaluation of the Geriatric Depression Scale (GDS): Supporting its use in health care settings. *Clinical Gerontologist, 23*(3/4), 57–68.

Poole, J. (1997). Older people. In J. Creek (Ed.), *Occupational therapy and mental health* (pp. 357–375). London: Churchhill Livingstone.

Reisberg, B., Ferris, S. H., & Crook, T. (1983). Global Deterioration Scale. In B. Reisberg (Ed.), *A guide to Alzheimer's disease*. New York: Free Press.

Reynolds, C. (1995). Recognition and differentiation of elderly depression in the clinical setting. *Geriatrics, 50* (suppl. 1), S6–S11.

Rosen, W. G., Mohs, R. C., & Davis, K. L. (1984). A new rating scale for Alzheimer's disease. *American Journal of Psychiatry, 141*, 1356–1364.

Sadock, B. J. & Sadock, V. A. (2003). *Kaplan and Sadock's synopsis of psychiatry: Behavioral sciences, clinical psychiatry*. Lippincott Williams & Wilkins.

Schaub, R. T., & Linden, M. (2000). Anxiety and anxiety disorders in the old and very old—Results from the Berlin Aging Study (BASE). *Comprehensive Psychiatry, 41*(2), suppl. 1, 48–54.

Shiekh, J., & Yesavage, J. (1986). Geriatric Depression Scale: Recent findings in development of a shorter version. In J. Brink (Ed.), *Clinical gerontology: A guide to assessment and intervention*. New York: Howarth.

Smith, J. (2001). *Do occupational therapists address psychosocial issues with geriatric patients?* Unpublished master's thesis. San Jose State University.

Smith, S. L., Sherrill, K. A., & Colenda, C. C. (1995). Assessing and treating anxiety in elderly persons. *Psychiatric Services, 46*(1), 36–42.

Sviden, G., Wikstrom, B. M., & Hjortsjo-Norberg, M. (2002). Elderly person's reflections on relocating to living at sheltered housing. *Scandinavian Journal of Occupational Therapy, 9*, 10–16.

Tune, L. (2001). Assessing psychiatric illness in geriatric patients. *Clinical Cornerstone. 3*(3), 23–36, 62–6.

United Nations Secretariat. (2003). *Population ageing 2002.* United Nations, Population Division, Department of Economic and Social Affairs. (Wall Chart).

University of Michigan Alcohol Research Center. (1991). Short Michigan Alcohol Screening Test—Geriatric Version (Short MAST-G). Ann Arbor: University of Michigan.

Wallens, D., & Rockwell-Dylla, L.(1996). Client and family—practitioner relationships. In O. Larson, R. Stevens-Ratchford, L. Pedretti, & J. Crabtree (Eds.), *Role of occupational therapy with the elderly* (pp. 826–855). Bethesda, MD: AOTA.

Williams, J. H., Drinka, T. J. K., Greenberg, J. R., Farrell-Holtan, J., Euhardy, R., & Schram, M. (1991). Development and testing of the assessment of living skills and resources (ALSAR) in elderly community-dwelling veterans. *Gerontologist, 31*(1), 84–91.

Wilson, B., Cockburn, J., & Baddeley, A. (1985). *The Rivermead Behavioral Memory Test.* Suffolk: Thanes Valley Test.

World Health Organization (WHO). (2001). *International classification of functioning, disability and health* (ICF). WHO.

Yerxa, E. (2000). Confessions of an occupational therapist who became a detective. *British Journal of Occupational Therapy, 63*(5), 192–199.

Young, R. C. (1997). Bipolar mood disorders in the elderly. *Geriatric Psychiatry, 20*(1), 121–136.

Suggested Readings

Abram, S. W., Beers, M., & Berkow, R. (2000). *Merck manual of geriatrics* (3rd ed.). Whitehouse Station, NJ: Merck.

Bartels, S. J., Dums, A. R., Oxman, T. E., Schneider, L. S., Arean, P. A., Alexopoulos, G. S., & Jeste, D. V. (2002). Evidence-based practices in geriatric mental health care. *Psychiatric Services, 53*(11), 1419–1431.

Bonder, B., & Wagner, M. (2001). *Functional performance in older adults* (2nd ed.). Phiadelphia: F. A. Davis.

Butler, R., Lewis, M., & Sunderland, T. (1998). *Aging and mental health.* Essex: Pearson, Allyn & Bacon.

Corcoran, M. (2004). *Geriatric issues in occupational therapy: A compendium of leading research.* Bethesda, MD: American Occupational Therapy Association.

Kane, R., Ouslander, J., & Abrass, I. (1999). *Essentials of clinical geriatrics* (4th ed.). Columbus, OH: McGraw-Hill Professional.

Larson, K. O., Stevens-Ratchford, R., Pedretti, L., & Crabtree, J. (Eds). (1996). *The role of occupational therapy with the elderly* (2nd ed.). Bethesda, MD: American Occupational Therapy Association.

Lewis, S. C. (2003). *Elder care in occupational therapy* (2nd ed.). Thorofare, NJ: Slack.

Mandel, D., Jackson, J., Zemke, R., Nelson, L., & Clark, F. (Eds.). (1999). *Lifestyle redesign: Implementing the well elderly program.* Bethesda, MD: American Occupational Therapy Association.

Sadavoy, J. (2004). *Comprehensive textbook of geriatric psychiatry* (3rd ed.). New York: Norton.

Mental Health with Physical Disorders

Part V includes four chapters that address psychosocial concerns across a spectrum of conditions, including a broad look at physical disability of various etiologies, brain injury, chronic pain, and substance abuse. Clients with dysfunction related to these conditions may or may not be seen in traditional "mental health" settings. Unfortunately, the psychosocial, cognitive, and behavioral issues discussed in these chapters are too often under-recognized or inadequately treated, yet they have been repeatedly reported to have significant impact on an individual's functional outcome with intervention.

The authors of these chapters advocate for an occupation-based approach that addresses the various psychosocial issues through assessment and intervention regardless of treatment setting. Occupational therapists are in the ideal role to both advocate for these services and educate team members and families, as our generalist background provides the holistic and comprehensive perspective to look beyond the treatment setting boundaries.

CHAPTER 13

Psychosocial Issues in Physical Disability

Heidi McHugh Pendleton PhD, OTR/L, FAOTA

Winifred Schultz-Krohn PhD, OTR/L, BCP, FAOTA

Key Terms

adaptation

adjustment

coping strategies

International Classification
  of Function, Disability,
  and Health (ICF)

life satisfaction

quality of life

self-concept

Chapter Outline

Introduction

You wake up in the morning, get out of bed, stretch, search for your glasses, and begin the process of getting ready for your day. The act of translating intention, such as getting ready for the day, into action, requires physical abilities. These physical abilities are considered a critical component of human occupation. Fisher and Kielhofner (1995) note "that merely having the desire to perform a task is not sufficient; the individual must also have the underlying capacity needed to perform" (p. 83). Understanding the importance of physical ability in the engagement in occupation and its impact on psychosocial functioning and well-being forms the foundation for this chapter. Individuals who have a physical disability may have significant problems engaging in, or resuming engagement in, personally desirable and cherished occupations. The results of this inability or decrease in ability to participate in occupation can lead to significant psychosocial problems, including depression, anxiety, poor coping ability, altered body image, decreased or altered sense of self, decreased self-esteem, and withdrawal from social interaction, to name just a few typical responses (Hughes, Swedlund, Petersen, & Nosek, 2001; Kemp & Kraus, 1999; Novotny, 1991; Tate & Forchheimer, 2001; Tzonichaki & Kleftaras, 2002).

It has been charged by many occupational therapists (OTs) that those therapists who are working with persons with physical disabilities seldom address these psychosocial issues directly or adequately. It seems that intervention priority is given to the amelioration of the client's physical and occupational performance problems (Gutman, 2001a; Smith, 2001). It may be that the OTs regard any intervention that is aimed at restoring the person's physical or functional ability to participate in occupation as simultaneously addressing her or his psychosocial problems, thus speculating that the psychosocial problems will be remediated if the individual is successful in resuming his or her occupational performance. The problem is not that simple—the psychosocial issues confronting people with physical disabilities are complex, need to be explicitly recognized by the individual as well as those working with him or her, and must be addressed directly with appropriate occupational therapy psychosocial intervention. This chapter addresses the psychosocial issues frequently encountered by a person who has a physical disability.

The **International Classification of Functioning, Disability, and Health (ICF)** is used as a framework to understand the relationship of the psychosocial issues to physical disability in this chapter. The cultural and societal factors that influence the experience of physical disability are presented, followed by a discussion of the concept of self and how it is affected in the presence of physical disability. Several models useful for understanding **adjustment** to life with physical disability are explicated and then the concept of **quality of life** with physical disability is explored.

OCCUPATIONAL THERAPY AND THE INTERNATIONAL CLASSIFICATION OF FUNCTIONING

The World Health Organization's (WHO) ICF helps the occupational therapist understand the complexity of having a disability (WHO, 2001). The ICF has "moved away from being a 'consequences of disease' classification to become a 'components of health' classification"—progressing from impairment, disability, and handicap to body functions and structures, activities, and participation (WHO, 2001, p. 4). The term *body structures* refers to the anatomical parts of the body while *body functions* refers to a person's physiological and psychological functions. Also considered in this new model is the impact of environmental and personal factors as they relate to functioning. The ICF has adopted a universal model that considers health along a continuum where there is a potential for everyone to have a disability.

The ICF also provides support for OTs to address specifically activity and activity limitations encountered by persons with disabilities (WHO, 2001). This document also describes the importance of participation in life situations, or "domains," including learning and applying knowledge; general tasks and task demands; communication; movement; self-care; domestic life areas; interpersonal interactions; major life areas associated with work, school, and family life; and community, social, and civic life—all historically familiar areas of concern and intervention to OT. Although a physical disability may compromise a person's ability to climb stairs or dress, the ICF redirects the service provider to also consider activity limitations that may result in restricted participation in desired life situations. A problem with a person's bodily structure, such as an absent or severely contracted limb, is recognized as a potentially limiting factor but that is not the focus of intervention.

Occupational therapy intervention provided for people with physical disabilities should extend beyond a focus on recovery of physical skills to address the person's engagement, or active participation, in occupations. This viewpoint is the cornerstone of the Occupational Therapy Practice Framework (2002). Such active participation in occupation is dependent upon the client's psychosocial well-being, which must be simultaneously addressed through the occupational therapy intervention. This orientation is congruent with the emphasis of the ICF.

Figure 13-1 depicts the relationships and interrelationships among cultural and societal expectations with activities, participation, and prioritized occupations as viewed through the lens of the ICF. This figure represents a synthesis of the Occupational Therapy Practice Framework and the ICF where prioritized occupations are influenced by cultural and societal expectations and occur as a

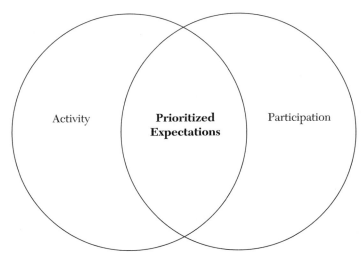

Figure 13-1.   Cultural and Societal Expectations

product of the individual's ability to engage in an activity that promotes participation in a desired life situation.

CULTURAL AND SOCIETAL FACTORS

The process of adjusting to a physically disabling condition occurs over time and is influenced by cultural and societal expectations (Charmaz, 1995). A person who has sustained a stroke may be willing to expend energy to propel a wheelchair but relies on others to help with meal preparation. In this situation, the person prioritizes independent mobility over independent meal preparation. The importance of independence in daily activities is heavily biased by Western cultural norms and is not a universally accepted priority (Williams & Ispa, 1999). Many cultures accommodate a person's disability by expecting family members to assume the primary caregiving role. The individual with a disabling condition is not expected to become independent because family members are responsible for the care of the person. In this cultural orientation an acceptable societal role is being dependent upon others. Not only may the dependence on others be acceptable to the society but additionally be regarded as preferable, a measure of the esteem with which the family honors the individual.

Culture influences a person's ability to cope or adjust to a disabling condition (Hampton & Marshall, 2000). One culture may place great importance on independence whereas another culture is focused on group cohesiveness. For example, the cultural orientation of the United States is considered individualistic in nature whereas China has a collectivistic orientation. The terms *individualistic* and *collectivistic* are often used when differentiating cultural perspectives (Brice & Campbell, 1999; Ohbuchi, Fukushima, & Tedeschi, 1999). An individualistic orientation places personal pursuits and individual achievement above group gains. A collectivistic culture emphasizes the benefit of action for the group and individual achievements are minimized.

These differing cultural orientations can contribute to the coping methods used when an individual is faced with a disabling condition (Hampton & Marshall, 2000). Even the concept of a disability has been described as "an artifact of culture and an identity responsive to material conditions" (Frank, 2000, p. 168). Often routines and habits must be substantially revised in the face of a disabling condition. The degree to which a person is able to modify his or her routines to meet the challenge of a disability is also influenced by culture (Gallimore & Lopez, 2002).

Bonder (2001) describes a comparison of weavers from the United States and Guatemala. In Guatemala, particularly in the Mayan culture, the occupation of weaving carries a rich history and traditionally specified methods are used to engage in this activity. A Mayan woman was no longer able to sit on the floor to weave using the traditional method in this village. A suggestion was made to sit on a stool as a modification to the activity. This altered method of performing the weaving activity was rejected because it would compromise the meaning of weaving. In the United States, weaving has a personal meaning but does not carry the comparable cultural significance as in the Mayan culture in Guatemala. A woman in the United States, unable to use her left arm after a stroke, modified the activity of weaving to continue with this personally meaningful occupation.

Culture defines what is an ideal routine (Gallimore & Lopez, 2002). The acceptability of a routine is not solely related to the end product but is also strongly rooted in cultural norms. For example, a young mother, who is physically limited by multiple sclerosis, may be very willing for her 3-year-old daughter to spend time with her mother or mother-in-law during the day but wants her daughter to be home in the evening. Although the effort of getting her daughter ready for bed may be exhausting, this is a culturally endorsed routine that defines part of this woman's role as a mother.

Confounding and contributing to a person's psychosocial response to disability—depression, anxiety, decreased **self-concept**/self-worth—are the societal attitudes of those around him or her. These were undoubtedly the same views he or she once held toward those who have disability but now must be faced as referring to oneself. Noted among these views, reactions, or beliefs that society attributes to those with disabilities are that life must now be a tragedy because of having a disability, that one is now the object of pity, and even that it would be understandable if the person were to consider suicide (Wright, 1983; Yerxa, 2001; & Hockenberry, 1995). The person with a disability may alternately experience being the recipient of society's stares or being invisible (Murphy, 2001). For those who have a physical disability, there is almost a universal experience of being stigmatized by society (Goffman, 1963). Many also endure the beliefs of others that some personal action or attribute of the individual caused the disability. The effects of these cultural and societal responses on individuals with disabilities significantly influence self-concept, as will be explored in the following section.

CONCEPT OF SELF

A discussion of the construction of self is helpful for understanding the potential psychosocial impact of a physically disabling condition. Charmaz (2002) describes the concept of self as constructed from habits that often occur with minimal or no reflection or intention by the person. These habits are referred to as the "taken-for-granted ways" a person manages her or his daily life and how that person interacts with others in a variety of settings (p. S32). A person may engage in a habitual pattern of interacting with loved ones and this pattern may become firmly established over the years.

The pattern or habit does not necessarily serve a clear function but instead is a unique feature of that person's behavioral repertoire. The daughter who begins every conversation with her mother by saying "But Mom . . ." The son who always drops his school bag by the front door instead of taking it all the way to his room only to retrieve it later when he needs to begin his homework. The mother who can't fathom brushing her hair before she has had her first cup of coffee. The father who must read the comic pages of the newspaper before reading any other portion of the paper. These habits form the self and may be considered as a "signature of self." When this signature of self, these habitual actions or behaviors, are disrupted by illness or disease, the person may feel a disruption in the integrity of self (Charmaz, 1995). The concept of self may be very strongly formed and resistant to change, even when a physically disabling condition prohibits engaging in specific behaviors or habits.

Clients with chronic disabling conditions, particularly those with a progressive course, present a significant challenge to the occupational therapy practitioner (OT). Although the OT may be able to devise clever and creative strategies to accomplish daily activities, these modifications may be viewed by a client as confirmation that the previous self is disintegrating (Charmaz, 1995).

CASE ILLUSTRATION: Ms. Kaminsky—Preserving the Concept of Self

Ms. Kaminsky is a 58-year-old woman with chronic obstructive pulmonary disorder (COPD) and severe shortness of breath. As the OT, you have made several suggestions regarding energy conservation techniques and methods to manage her daily activities. This woman would habitually blow on her tea three times before taking a sip. You suggest that after she brews the tea she allows the tea to cool slightly before drinking it or that she add a small ice cube or ice chips to cool the tea instead of blowing on it. She becomes distressed at these suggestions and refuses to drink tea.

Discussion

The habit of blowing on her tea was part of her signature of self and now that habit is no longer available to her. Although her dyspnea makes it virtually impossible for her to effectively blow on her tea to cool it, she refuses alternate methods. She actively tries to maintain previous habits to avoid reconfiguring her sense of self as a disabled person, a person with limited respiratory capacity.

For some people, at the onset of chronic physical disability it becomes clear that they will experience disruption of their daily lives and be forced to alter and redefine their sense of self. These individuals are likely to approach rehabilitation, including OT intervention, with motivation and resolve to maximize their remaining capabilities, learn to compensate for their disabilities, and in many instances, craft a compromise or novel concept of self. However, for many other people at the onset of physical disability, this clarity regarding changed abilities comes over a period of extended time coupled with the experience of actually "doing" or "trying" those occupations and activities that customarily contribute to their sense of self. Charmaz (2002) suggests that "until people view their daily habits as undermined and experience themselves as changed, they will maintain the concept of self established earlier" (p. S31). Many individuals with acute onset (or even progressive onset) chronic disability may not have had sufficient time to experience themselves as changed and may therefore initially view occupational therapy as irrelevant and unnecessary. In fact, as was observed by Charmaz, the very activities, which commonly comprise the OT intervention confront the individual's habitualized self-concept and are experienced as negative. Shortened rehabilitation stays, lack of third-party payment for ongoing or outpatient therapy, as well as a society with limited social and temporal support contexts for people with disability may further compromise the individual's establishment of satisfactory performance of everyday occupations and resulting satisfactory self-concept.

Penny, the participant described in Clark's (1993) Slagle lecture, aptly exemplifies the aforementioned experience and, as Clark so eloquently writes, demonstrates " that rehabilitation can be experienced by the survivor as a rite of passage in which the person is moved to disability status by experts and therapists and then abandoned" (p. 1068). Following the sudden onset of a brain aneurysm, Penny, a 47-year-old professor and department chair in the school of education at a large university, experienced occupational therapy negatively. Penny described sitting in her wheelchair waiting in line for her turn for therapy, dutifully performing the routines they showed her and then being returned to the line to wait to go back to her room. She seemed to regard the occupational therapy interventions aimed at relearning self-care and other activities as comprising her customary routines as "little stuff," unchallenging, purposeless, and a waste of time. She felt "angry and resentful," wishing that "she would be able to set goals for herself so she could have a sense of progress toward something and the therapists, like personal coaches, would work with her to achieve them" (p. 1071).

Within the course of Penny's narrative Clark observes that the rehabilitation program seems to serve as a "rite of passage" to the survivor of a disabling condition, "carrying the person from one stage of life to the next" (1993, p. 1072). During this rite of passage the person is stripped of her old status (old self) and then transitions to the status of the disabled. In this transitional, or "liminal" state "one is betwixt and between, neither what one was nor what one shall become" (Moore, 1992, p. 133). When this phase is completed, the participant begins the task of reentering the world from which she has been separated (Clark, 1993, p. 1072). Penny indeed experienced this status of liminality as evidenced by her feeling disconnected from her former self—a self who was a revered academician, an accomplished skier, world traveler, gourmet cook, and treasured friend. Her experience in rehabilitation suggested that those providing treatment, regardless of their "kind and caring demeanor" supported this liminal status by seemingly stripping Penny of her prior status and relegating her to the status of the next client waiting in the line for treatment.

Once discharged, Penny felt ill-equipped with the tools to adapt to her changed self within her old familiar environment. She observed that occupations were important because they marked the new you versus the old you. During their collaboration, Clark encouraged Penny to recount her occupational history, identifying the childhood and later life occupations that had previously contributed to her success in life, that is, composing her life to that point, and then, "coached" Penny in recycling these occupations to recompose her life (Clark, 1993). Penny reached back to her past, retrieving those familiar friendship strategies that were previously so adaptive for her and reestablished cherished rituals. Old friends and new friends, including Clark, facilitated Penny's concoction of a new persona, that of a proper eccentric professor, by joining her as she collected her accoutrements (including a British walking stick) and in celebrating her victories. Penny served as the primary change agent in determining her quality of life and her story of reconfiguring her self-concept using occupation is also consistent with and illustrative of other models of **adaptation** to disability, as will be evident in the following discussions.

MODELS OF ADAPTING TO PHYSICAL DISABILITY

A physically disabling condition may be chronic and relatively stable in nature, such as a congenital disorder, or, over time, the individual may be faced with a progressive loss of function. Physically disabling conditions may also occur rapidly, as is seen with a traumatic injury or accident, but then result in a chronic, and sometimes progressive, loss of function. Literature differentiates the **coping strategies** employed by persons faced with either a traumatic injury or acute illness and those faced with a chronic physically disabling condition (Charmaz, 1983; 2002; Davidhizar, 1997; Morse & O'Brien, 1995). Whether clients experience a chronic or traumatic onset of a physically disabling condition, they will require the expertise of an occupational therapy practitioner in helping them create a new sense of self regardless of the physical limitations they face.

Chronic Disabling Conditions

When a person is faced with a chronic disabling condition, particularly one associated with progressive deterioration in physical abilities, coping or adapting to the changes is an ongoing process (Charmaz, 1995). Adults and children faced with chronic physically disabling conditions must construct a sense of self with a body that does not consistently and accurately respond to their demands. This lack of reliable control over one's body is further compromised by the cultural and societal expectations that one should have control over the body. The lack of bowel and bladder control after the age of 2 or 3 years is considered unacceptable and yet many individuals with spina bifida, multiple sclerosis, and Parkinson's disease have incontinence (Cate, Kennedy, & Stevenson, 2002; Roe, 2000; Schultz-Krohn, Foti, & Glogoski, 2001).

Three stages have been identified in the process of adapting to a chronic physically disabling condition, but the OT should not assume that a client smoothly progresses through these stages in a linear manner. Charmaz (1995, p. 657) has described these three stages as represented in Table 13-1.

The first stage of coping is marked by the person's appreciation of his or her altered physical condition (Charmaz, 1995). Some clients fight against the experience of this new relationship between their body and their concept of self. They may reject any form of adaptive equipment because it is a symbol of an altered body. Clients may deny that previous physical abilities are no longer available to them (Katz, Fleming, Keren, Lightbody, & Hartman-Maeir, 2002). A client with severe rheumatoid arthritis may persist in attempting to wash windows in her home even though lifting her arms above her head produces severe fatigue and pain.

A chronic and progressively disabling condition requires frequent reappraisals of physical abilities. Each time a person experiences a new loss of motor control or function, such as the deterioration of fine motor skills due to the progression of multiple sclerosis or Parkinson's disease, he or she must adjust to an altered sense of bodily control. Control over the body was previously a "taken-for-granted" experience that now, with deterioration of function, requires reappraisal and revisions

Table 13-1. Adapting to a Chronic Disabling Condition	
Stage and Label	*Description*
Stage 1: Experience and Definition of Impairment	Ongoing appraisal and acknowledgment of his or her altered physical condition.
Stage 2: Bodily Adjustment and Identity Trade-Offs	Identifies commitments and responsibilities associated with previous roles. Commitments and responsibilities are meshed with the changed physical abilities and require the person to make an identity trade-off. Creates a new identity through negotiating his or her personal needs, the expectations and needs of significant others, and the demands of the environment.
Stage 3: Surrendering to the Changed Body (Embracing the Changed Body)	Accepts the physical changes and incorporates these changes into a new concept of self. Develops respect for the limitations of the body instead of constantly trying to change the body functions.

Source: Adapted from Charmaz, 1995.

(Charmaz, 1995, p. 662). Initially, "people with chronic illnesses may make firm separations between their impaired bodies and their self-concepts" (p. 663). The illness or disabling condition may be viewed as an enemy that must be battled (Huttlinger et al., 1992). This stance underlies a hope for clients "to regain their past identities" and abilities, such as complete control over their bodies to perform according to past experiences (Charmaz, 1995, p. 663). This position may be held for an extended period of time and compromises the client's ability to accept modifications and adaptations that would allow successful completion of everyday tasks.

The concept of self and the use of body should not be viewed as separate entities but as intimately connected, influencing each other to produce an integrated person (Charmaz, 2002). That does not mean a person with a disabling condition cannot achieve an integrated self, but instead, that a progressive physically disabling condition requires frequent adjustments to the relationship between the body and self. When a person experiences a progressive deterioration of physical abilities, the reliance on the use of the body is severely compromised. Each new episode or loss of function requires adjustment and often includes adjusting to a change in physical appearance. The previous model of the physical body disintegrates and a new model must be developed (Charmaz, 1995). This new body structure may be unacceptable by societal standards. Absent or severely contracted limbs as well as extraneous and involuntary movements are barely tolerated by society (Frank, 2000; Novotny, 1991; Varni & Setoguchi, 1991). The person with a physical disability is expected to adjust to an undependable body, the structure and/or function of which is usually not endorsed by society.

Charmaz (1995) differentiates between struggling *against* a disorder or illness and struggling *with* a disorder or illness. A struggle against the disorder is seen as a lack of acceptance of the changed body. A struggle with the disorder reflects a degree of acceptance and an attempt to reconfigure a concept of self with an altered physical ability as was seen in Penny's successful struggle to resume her academic role with a new persona of an eccentric professor with a proper British cane. The acceptance of a changed body and efforts to mesh this body with self require energy. Occupational therapists need to be aware of the efforts expended by people with physical disabilities as they work on integrating the changed body with the concept of self. As a person reconfigures his or her concept of self integrated with a self-appraisal of the changed body, the person moves to the next stage of coping.

The second stage of coping with a physical disability requires revising identity goals due to the change in physical ability (Charmaz, 1995). This stage requires careful consideration of the social context for the person. Returning to driving after a person sustains a cerebrovascular accident (CVA) may be an important identity goal as a symbol of independence but may require substantial trade-offs to achieve this goal.

For example, a young man sustained a CVA due to a ruptured aneurysm, resulting in severe loss of function on his right arm and leg. During OT he expressed a primary goal of being able to drive. He had previously driven a motorcycle and a sports car with a manual transmission. He described himself as a "biker with a hotrod" but now resigned himself to learning to drive an "old man's car" (a car with an automatic transmission) with modifications to the controls to allow him to drive using only his left hand and leg. This change in identity goals was significant for this young man. Although for his OT it was rewarding to see him regain his ability to drive, it was also important to note and address his frequent comments about his feelings of loss that he had to sell his motorcycle. He viewed himself as damaged and experienced a loss of social standing within his social network. The following example illustrates the key elements of this stage of adapting to a chronic disabling condition.

> ### CASE ILLUSTRATION: Ms. Shapiro—Adapting to a Chronic Disabling Condition

Ms. Shapiro, a 30-year-old woman, had a clear identity of herself as a full-time professional, wife, and mother of two young children but after being diagnosed with multiple sclerosis was required to make modifications to this identity. Multiple sclerosis is chronic and progressive, marked by exacerbations and remissions of symptoms where the progression of the disease is unpredictable (Dyck, 2002). Her symptoms included weakness, visual problems, and tremors. The unpredictable nature of multiple sclerosis placed Ms. Shapiro in a position where she needed to make identity trade-offs (Charmaz, 1995; Murphy, 1987). She was no longer able to work a demanding, but rewarding, full-time professional job and fulfill the expectations of caring for her children. She was faced with reducing her work hours and enlisting the help of her husband in the care of their children and with the household chores.

Mr. Choi, her husband, also a working professional, did not feel ready to accept the full responsibilities for household upkeep but did take on the responsibility of grocery shopping. He did rearrange his busy work schedule to help with the children every morning. This couple worked on a budget and they were able to hire a person to help clean the house. The interactions between this husband and wife resulted in the wife further reducing her work hours to continue as the primary caregiver for their children.

Discussion

Ms. Shapiro traded her role as a professional to continue in her role as a mother. The result of being diagnosed with multiple sclerosis and understanding the impact of the disease not only affected her identity roles but role expectations of her husband and children, necessitating trade-offs in roles and identities. These trade-offs were not made unilaterally but the decisions of which roles to relinquish and how to reconfigure identity roles was the product of interaction between this woman's priorities and the expectations of her husband and children.

The final stage of adapting to impairment requires the person to accept the physical changes brought about by the illness or disorder and to incorporate these changes into the concept of self (Charmaz, 1995; 2002; Davidhizar, 1997). This stage is not to be confused with people who become resigned to physical changes and give up hope for any positive outcomes. The hallmark of this stage is acceptance of the physical changes and a willingness to work within the confines of the changed body. Davidhizar (1997) cites several works where **life satisfaction** is not directly correlated with severity of physical disability. A person with greater physical limitations has fewer options available to engage in life situations, however, primarily due to environmental barriers.

Those with physical disabilities who stop pushing their physical body to improve find they can still exercise choice (Charmaz, 1995). The choice may be directed to different occupations that can be accomplished within the confines of the changed body. The struggle often faced by individuals during this stage is not the denial of symptoms or the false hopes of recovery, but instead, individuals are now confronted with social labels and interactions that stigmatize and restrict their choices (Dyck, 2002).

Surrendering to the changed body allows a new construction of self with routines and habits that support the new self (Charmaz, 2002). Accepting the changed body and prioritizing routines and habits appears to be expressed somewhat differently between men and women. Women tend to respond by decreasing their responsibilities to those around them and "relinquishing the super-mom image on which their self-concepts had been predicated" (p. S38). Men tend to prioritize personal relationships in routines and habits during this final stage of adapting to a changed body.

Adapting to a physical disability should not be construed as a step-by-step process whereby a client passes through one stage to another (Charmaz, 1995; 2002; Davidhizar, 1997; Dyck, 2002). Those faced with a chronic disabling condition, particularly one that is progressive in nature, may revisit any of the above stages during the course of their lifetime. The OT must be sensitive to the psychosocial support each client requires; understanding the adaptation process aids in providing meaningful occupational therapy intervention to those who have a chronic physical disability. When a person is faced with an acute onset of a physical disability, such as a spinal cord injury, traumatic brain injury, CVA, or amputation, the adaptation process is initially different from the above description due to the acute nature (Morse & O'Brien, 1995). Refer to Table 13-2 for specific details of the process of adapting to the acute onset of a physically disabling condition.

Acute Onset of Disabling Conditions

Adapting to lasting bodily changes resulting from an acute trauma has been described as a four-stage process by Morse and O'Brien (1995). The first stage was labeled as "vigilance: becoming engulfed" (p. 887). This stage occurred at the initial point of injury or acute illness and continued until the individual "relinquished self to caregivers . . . or when they lost consciousness" (p. 887). Many of the individuals reported a separation of the subjective body and the objective body. They experienced an internal sense of calmness contrasted with their outward behavior of screaming and distress. This was often reported when severe pain was present. The stage of vigilance ended when the person surrendered care to another, often in an emergency room.

Table 13-2.	Adapting to Acute Onset Disabling Conditions	
Stage and Label	*Environmental Circumstance*	*Description*
Stage 1: Vigilance: Becoming Engulfed	Site of onset of the acute condition, such as CVA or trauma, such as a spinal cord injury.	Encounters a separation between the experience of the body and emotions. This stage ends as the person relinquishes control to others or loses consciousness.
Stage 2: Disruption: Taking Time Out	Hospital/acute care	Experiences a disruption in reality orientation. Significant others are critical to provide an anchor to reality regarding self in the midst of the unfamiliar and disorganizing environment.
Stage 3: Enduring the Self: Confronting and Regrouping	Acute care/acute rehabilitation services	Reality orientation improves and the person becomes aware of an abrupt change in physical ability.
Stage 4: Striving to Regain Self: Merging the Old and New Reality	Rehabilitation	Tests the limits of the changed bodily functions. Revises and reformulates life goals with respect to the changed body. Creates a new sense of self.

Source: Adapted from Morse & O'Brien, 1995.

The second stage was identified as "disruption: taking time out" (Morse & O'Brien, 1995, p. 890). During this stage, individuals experienced a disruption in reality, often describing feeling as if they were in a fog. There was a great need for significant others to be present and to provide a "safe haven in a confusing nightmare" (p. 890). The role of significant others was not merely for support but served as an orienting force in a chaotic environment. Significant others were seen as the anchor for individuals who sustained an acute injury to "remind them who they were and gave them a sense of self" in the disordered world of an acute care hospital setting (p. 891).

The third stage, "enduring the self: confronting and regrouping," was marked by an improvement in reality orientation (Morse & O'Brien, 1995, p. 891). As reality orientation improved, the implications of the acute injury or illness began to be recognized. Many participants in this study experienced severe physical pain, but reported that the realization of the severity of the changed body was more difficult than the pain endured. The abrupt change signified a loss of physical control of their bodies and the environment and a dependence on others for even mundane routines. This stage was seen as the time when individuals were first faced with learning the severity of their physical limitations. One individual described how being alone produced feelings of panic and fear due to the lack of physical ability.

Those who sustained an acute injury resulting in a chronic physically disabling condition described the need for others as a support during this stage. Here the support provided was not merely as an assist to control the environment but also for encouragement. Many discussed how the encouragement from therapists and significant others helped them endure the arduous process of healing from injuries and acute illness. Several individuals described how even small gains achieved during the therapy sessions were interpreted as evidence that they could recover previous physical abilities. This also reflects the lack of acceptance of changed physical abilities (Katz et al., 2002). Although Morse and O'Brien (1995) discuss that this preserved sense of hope to reclaim previous abilities may have helped individuals with the initial healing process from burns, amputations, and spinal cord injuries, they also acknowledge that individuals "refused to accept the permanence of the damage" by holding on to the faith the medical miracles would return them to their previous selves (p. 893).

The final stage was called "striving to regain self: Merging the old and the new reality" (Morse & O'Brien, 1995, p. 893). During this stage, the rehabilitation services provided helped individuals test the limits of their newly altered bodies. Through the course of rehabilitation "the more an individual tried to do, the more he or she realized what he or she could not" do (p. 894). This stage was marked by frustration in attempting to regain previously taken-for-granted tasks such as walking and feeding oneself by using new strategies that confirm an altered body. Life goals had to be revised and reformulated due to this changed body. Many individuals reported feelings of exhaustion as they developed new routines and determined the physical limits of their newly altered bodies. Individuals who had sustained a spinal cord injury reported the amount of energy and effort they expended to complete even simple self-care tasks (Manns & Chad, 2001). The energy expenditure then limited their participation in other activities.

Individuals who sustain a traumatic injury or illness resulting in persistent physical disabilities adapt to their changed bodies and create a new sense of self. This occurs through an appraisal of their current physical capabilities. The need to decide what activities to pursue and what activities to discontinue is similar to the stage identified by Charmaz (1995) as identity trade-offs. The stages of adapting to a physically changed body, whether from an acute injury or illness or due to a chronic and often progressive condition, are provided here to help the OT understand the process of adaptation. This process should be incorporated into the intervention plan and addressed as part of the occupational therapy services provided.

LIFE SATISFACTION AND QUALITY OF LIFE

The concepts of life satisfaction and quality of life are very important when discussing the psychosocial issues of physical disabilities and adapting to limitations in body functions and structures. Life satisfaction is considered to be the subjective component of an individual's overall quality of life (Tzonichaki & Kleftaras, 2002). How satisfied an individual is with his or her life may include such factors as satisfaction with family life, engagement in leisure activities, vocational pursuits, self-care, and sexual expression. Satisfaction does not require the same level of participation from each individual but instead reflects the person's value regarding his or her level of participation in various life situations.

> ### CASE ILLUSTRATION: Sam's Satisfaction in Life
>
> *Sam, a 9-year-old boy with spina bifida, used a wheelchair for mobility. He participated on a wheelchair soccer team using a large ball, had his own collection of video games, talked to other boys about how "gross" girls are, and reported being very satisfied with his life with the exception of school. Sam hated school. He had visual perceptual deficits necessitating modifications and accommodations to his educational program. Although he was unable to walk, did not have bowel and bladder control, and had visual perceptual deficits, Sam reported feeling satisfied with his overall life, particularly during summer vacation. He was quick to add that more video games would make his life better.*
>
> #### Discussion
>
> *Sam was able to participate in the activities he deemed important. Success in school was not a priority in Sam's life even though his parents were concerned with his performance in his educational program. Life satisfaction, from Sam's perspective, meant being able to get together with friends to play video games or wheelchair soccer. His ability to engage in these life situations was unencumbered by his diagnosis and he viewed his life as quite satisfying.*

Quality of life includes life satisfaction along with overall physical and emotional health and functional status (Manns & Chad, 2001). The appraisal of quality of life is not generated solely from the individual's perspective but includes participation in activities. For example, a teenager with spastic cerebral palsy may be unable to control his arms or legs to participate in everyday activities and family members may report the need to provide assistance for dressing and bathing him (McCarthy et al., 2002). The need for others to complete basic self-care tasks for a teenager reflects the lack of physical control he experiences, thereby compromising his overall quality of life. Activity limitations and problems in participation in life situations are included when discussing the quality of life for the individual. On the other hand, Derek, a 25-year-old college senior and student body president, who has high-level quadriplegia, is unable to physically perform any ADL. However, Derek is so adept at conveying his needs and preferences to his personal care attendant that a dinner partner quickly becomes unaware of the attendant's presence during the meal. In fact, Derek is in control and a very active participant in his self-care and social activity. In this instance the concept of participation is reconfigured and likely contributes positively to Derek's quality of life.

Of particular relevance to occupational therapy is what clients report as contributing to their quality of life and life satisfaction. Over 20 years ago Burnett and Yerxa (1980) found that individuals with disability, while satisfied with their performance of personal activities of daily living, after discharge from rehabilitation felt ill prepared for functioning in the home and community. In response, Pendleton (1990) investigated OTs' use of independent accident living skills training (ILST) and found that OTs working in rehabilitation centers with clients with physical disabilities frequently placed more emphasis on therapeutic exercise and self-care training than on the skills needed for independent living and those associated with life satisfaction. These skills are often identified as the instrumental activities of daily living but embrace more than meal preparation and time concepts. Independent living skills require the OT to include a client's participation in preferred occupations, which involves not only the environment in which these occupations take place but the socialization that supports engagement in these occupations. More recent studies indicate that those individuals with disability who report high quality of life and life satisfaction regarded socialization (friendship), leisure, and productive occupations as most responsible for their reported high quality of life and life satisfaction (Hammel, 1995; Pendleton, 1998). In fact, for the four participants in Pendleton's qualitative study of the friendships of successful women with physical disability, friendship supported participation in occupation and participation in occupation in turn facilitated their friendship.

A preponderance of the literature regarding psychosocial issues of physical disability for those with a variety of chronic disabling conditions (whether acute, progressive, or congenital onset) describes using an individual's perceived quality of life or life satisfaction as a measure of the person's success in adapting to or overcoming the emotional consequences of these diagnoses. Self-reported absence of depression, anxiety, and suicidal ideation is deemed evidence of mental health, which is frequently equated with high quality of life and life satisfaction (Kemp & Krause, 1999; Tate & Forchheimer, 2001). Adaptation to disability, and consequently satisfaction with life, is found to be related to many factors, including the individual's age, gender, cause of onset, developmental stage at onset, culture, ethnicity, religious and familial beliefs, meaning and value of the abilities lost, previous life experiences and coping styles, life stressors, and support and response of family and friends (Novotny, 1991; Antonak, Livneh, & Antonak, 1993). Also of significance is the therapeutic competence and attitudes toward disability of the health care professionals involved in their care (Novotny, 1991). One can see the importance and interrelatedness of these factors affecting psychosocial adjustment and well-being when examining the life stories of any client with a disability.

CASE ILLUSTRATION: Jenny—Age 16

Jenny has paraplegia as a result of an automobile accident she experienced at the age of 16. She was driving at the time of the accident without her parents' permission and without a driver's license. These circumstances caused Jenny guilt and anxiety and the perceived notion that the disability was a punishment for her disobedience. Furthermore, as a sophomore attending a small town high school, at an age when body image and self-concept are fragile without the chal-

lenge of disability, she did not want to return to classes, where she believed she would now be regarded negatively. Friends seemed to reinforce her beliefs when they phoned her for rides to the mall (soon after she obtained a car with hand controls) but never asked her to join them once they arrived.

Discussion

All of these factors contributed to Jenny's feelings of low self-esteem, stigma, depression, and a resulting perceived low quality of life. Factors affecting her more favorably were her loving and supportive family, her previous academic and social successes, adequate financial resources, and a comprehensive rehabilitation program at a major SCI treatment center. Regardless of the diagnosis these factors are crucial to anticipating and understanding the psychosocial ramifications of disability for a particular client like Jenny and ultimately providing the appropriate OT intervention.

SPECIFIC PSYCHOSOCIAL ISSUES WITH SELECT DISABILITIES

In the following sections the psychosocial issues common to three major categories of physical disability will be briefly discussed. Discussion will focus upon selected diagnoses from each of the categories and be illustrated by vignettes or client stories that depict real-life examples of characteristic psychosocial responses to the particular disability. An accompanying table (Table 13-3), showing expected psychosocial issues associated with specific diagnoses, commonly used assessments, and suggested OT interventions, is provided. However, this table is not intended to be an exhaustive listing of all the possible psychosocial problems for each disability, assessments, or intervention, but rather, a simple tool to be used by the OT to inspire or jog one's thinking when confronted with the psychosocial issues experienced by clients with various diagnoses. With few exceptions, the psychosocial issue described for one diagnosis could be included with each diagnosis listed. However, for the purpose of this table, only the main problems represented repeatedly in the relevant literature are included. If, for example, when working with a client with a spinal cord injury it is hoped that the viewer of this table would peruse the categories listed for other diagnoses and consider whether any of these have implications, or applications, for her or his current client.

Chronic Disorders with an Acute Onset

By its very definition—sudden onset—psychosocial coping with this type of physical disability is experientially different than coping with progressive or congenital chronic disability. Individuals with such disability initially experience shock accompanied by high anxiety and fear for their very survival. Once survival becomes more certain their shock segues into denial of the ramifications of or the very existence of the disability (Antonak, Livneh, & Antonak, 1993; Gutman,

Table 13-3. Psychosocial Issues, Assessments, and Interventions

Diagnosis	Frequently Expected Psychosocial issues	Commonly Used Assessments	Suggested Interventions
Spinal cord injury	Depression Anxiety Decreased coping Decreased self-concept Loneliness Vulnerability to abuse—especially in women	Occupational Performance History Interview (OPHI) (Kielhofner et al., 1998) Canadian Occupational Performance Measure (COPM) (Law et al., 1994) Activity Configuration (Cynkin & Robinson, 1990) Beck Depression Inventory (BDI) (Beck et al., 1961) Beck Anxiety Inventory (BAI) (Beck, Epstein, Brown, & Steer, 1988) Occupational Self-Assessment (OSA) (Baron, Kielhofner, Goldhammer, & Wolenski, 1999) Ways of Coping Questionnaire (Folkman & Lazarus, 1987)	Stress management Coping skills training Education on social connectedness Education on depression awareness Education addressing sexuality Education on the connection between occupation and emotional health
Acquired amputation	Altered body image Loss of identity/sexuality Anxiety/fear of the unknown or rejection Low self-worth Self-repulsion Phantom pain Grief Loss of sense of wholeness/decreased self-concept Depression Anger	COPE Inventory (Carver, Scheier, & Weintraub, 1989) Acceptance of Disability Scale Reactions to Impairment and Disability Inventory (RIDI) (Livneh & Antonak, 1990) Prosthesis Evaluation Questionnaire (PEQ) (Legro, Smith, del Aguila, Larson, & Boone, 1998) Trinity Amputation Prosthetic Experience Scales (TAPES) (Gallagher & MacLachlan, 2000) COPM	Coping skills training Active decision making/active problem solving Education re: disability in a timely and factual manner Adequate preparation Pre-op peer discussion Peer support groups Opportunities for social involvement
Traumatic brain injury (Also see Chapter 14)	Depression Reduced insight Denial Personality changes	Assessment of Communication and Interaction Skills (Salamy, et al., 1993) Occupational Role History (Florey & Michelman, 1982) Role Checklist (Oakley, 1986)	Education in coping strategies for both client and family Collaborative goal setting with client

(continues)

Table 13-3. (continued)			
Diagnosis	*Frequently Expected Psychosocial issues*	*Commonly Used Assessments*	*Suggested Interventions*
	Decreased social competence	Life History Interview (Moorhead, 1969)	Intrapersonal skills groups—activity based with peer support
	Anger, hostility, aggressiveness, behavioral disinhibition, sex offending, impulsivity, risk taking	OPHI OSA Sickness Impact Profile (SIP) (Gibson et al., 1975)	Life skills group classes
	Confusion	Glasgow Assessment Scale (GAS) (Livingston & Livingston, 1985)	Interpersonal skills group—personal boundaries and limit setting
	Decreased self-awareness	Portland Adaptability Inventory (PAI) (Lezak, 1987)	
	Decreased insight		Long-term Psychosocial Rehabilitation Groups (PSR)—club like group activities aimed at skills needed for psychosocial rehab
	Anxiety, agitation		
	Women—high incidence of being sexually abused pre-injury and highly vulnerable to victimization post-injury		
Cerebral vascular accident	Depression	Geriatric Depression Scale (Sheikh & Yesavage, 1986)	Involve client in goal setting and selecting interventions
	Anxiety	Older Adult Health and Mood Questionnaire (Kemp & Adams, 1995)	Realistic approach, particularly in setting goals
	Decreased motivation to initiate activity	Mini Mental Status (Folstein et al., 1975)	Relaxation training
	Isolation, loneliness	Interest Checklist (Rogers, 1988)	Exploration and education in coping skills
	Emotional lability	COPM	Socialization and support groups
	Fear of falling		One on one discussion re: depression, anxiety or any other observed psychosocial issue
Multiple Sclerosis (MS)	Depression	BDI	Social support groups
	Cognitive changes	COPM OSA Expanded Disability Status Scale (EDSS) (Paty, Willoughby, & Whitaker, 1992) Fatigue Impact Scale (FIS) (Fisk, Pontefract, Ritvo, Archibald, & Murray, 1994)	Diagnostic support groups Energy conservation

(continues)

Table 13-3.   (continued)

Diagnosis	Frequently Expected Psychosocial issues	Commonly Used Assessments	Suggested Interventions
		Multiple Sclerosis Quality of Life Inventory (MSQLI) (Ritvo, Fischer, Miller, Andrews, Paty, & LaRocca, 1997)	
Parkinson's Disease (PD)	Depression Social isolation Decreased facial expressiveness	BDI COPM OSA Unified Parkinson's Disease Rating Scale (UPDRS) (Hoehn & Yahr, 1967) Parkinson's Disease Questionnaire (PDQ-39) (Peto, Jenkinson, Fitzpatrick, & Greenhall, 1995)	Social support groups Environmental supports to facilitate control Activity/exercise groups for psychosocial support
Huntington's Disease	Depression Suicide	BDI COPM OSA Unified Huntington's Disease Rating Scale (UHDRS) (Huntington Study Group, 1996)	Environmental modifications to support control Social support groups
Cerebral palsy	Dependency Behavioral problems Risk for social isolation	Disability Inventory (PEDI) (Haley, Coster, Ludlow, Haltiwanger, & Andrellos, 1992) School Function Assessment (SFA) (Coster, Deeney, Haltiwanger, & Haley, 1998)	
Spina bifida	Dependency Risk for social isolation	PEDI SFA	

2001a). Researchers and individuals who have written about their experience of disability point out that often it isn't until a year or more after the onset of their disability that the psychosocial issues become paramount and the search for the physical or miraculous cure recedes into a less prominent position (Gutman, 2001a; Hockenberry, 1995, Price-Lackey & Cashman, 1996). It therefore becomes a challenge to the OT to address the psychosocial issues while meeting the client's emotional readiness to contemplate such issues.

In the following sections the psychosocial issues of several diagnoses associated with acute onset will be discussed. The reader will undoubtedly note the commonalities and the differences inherent in how each psychosocial issue is experienced among the diagnoses. It is also important to keep in mind the personal, cultural, and social demographics of each client and the import of that perspective on how each psychosocial issue might be uniquely experienced.

Spinal Cord Injury. At the onset of spinal cord injury (SCI) many individuals experience situational depression, anxiety, decreased coping skills, and altered self-concept (Galvin & Godfrey, 2001; Hughes, Swedlund, Petersen, & Nosek, 2001; Kemp & Kraus, 1999). Incidence of depression is increased and various studies suggest that 30% to 40% develop a depressive disorder while 20% to 25% experience anxiety. Suicide rates are two to six times higher than in the community population and substance abuse is almost twice as high for individuals with SCI (46%) than in the community population (25%), though those with SCI demonstrated a higher incidence of substance abuse prior to injury (Galvin & Godfrey, 2001). Divorce rates are significantly higher (four out of five marriages dissolve within the first two years) and there is generally a decrease in financial and employment opportunities. The incidence of depression, anxiety, and suicidal ideation four to six years after onset of injury appears to be no greater for those with SCI than for the community population. Quality of life and life satisfaction among persons with SCI were found to also mirror that of the general population with the exception of satisfaction with sexuality, physical condition, and leisure activities (Benony, Daloz, Bungener, Chahraoui, Frenay, & Auvin, 2002). In another study, mobility and perceived health were found to be predictors of quality of life and life satisfaction for participants with SCI (Putzke, Richards, Hicken, & De Vivo, 2002).

CASE ILLUSTRATION: Jim—Confronting Abrupt Change

Jim, a 30-year-old race car champion, sustained an SCI at the C6 level during a competition. Jim's concept of self is that of an athlete skilled and accomplished in a sport known for its daredevil aspects. He is also accustomed to the adulation of his fans, especially the women, who are attracted to his good looks and success. Much of his body image, self-concept, and self-esteem are dependent upon his view of himself as a physically capable race car professional. His sexuality is also highly defined by this self-concept. It is anticipated that after rehab he will use a wheelchair for mobility, be able to drive an adapted van, and accomplish most of his self-care activities using a tenodesis hand splint. Plans are for him to move back to his home where he will require part-time assistance for his bowel and bladder care, bathing, and home maintenance. He is very depressed and expresses anxiety about his social life. Next to his hospital bed he has a photo of his crashed race car and talks about his accident with visitors and rehab staff.

Discussion

Jim's concept of self is clearly being challenged, particularly with regards to his sexuality. His behavior seems consistent with that expected at the stage of adaptation previously described as "enduring the self: confronting and regrouping."

While he is grappling with the abrupt changes in his physical abilities, the occupational therapist working with Jim will be challenged to help him explore his previously successful occupational strategies and reconfigure them in crafting a new self to meet his new reality.

It has been found that the longer one lives with a SCI positively correlates with an increasing feeling of life satisfaction (Kemp & Krause, 1999). However, those who are aging with an SCI are likely to experience onset of new physical problems, including osteoporotic changes, fatigue, pain, weakness, low endurance, significantly increased incidence of heart disease (and at a significantly earlier age than their peers), and a decreased level of independence in activities of daily living (ADLs) and instrumental activities of daily living (IADLs), also known as home and community skills. There is a concomitant increase in depression as individuals contemplate what these extensions of their disabilities mean for their futures. Kemp and Krause (1999) found that these individuals reported significantly lower life satisfaction than that of their nondisabled peers or counterparts. Interestingly, the problem areas that were most responsible for their dissatisfaction with life were not primarily at the level of their body structures or routine activity performance (ADLs and IADLs) but rather at no longer being able to participate in valued work, social, and favored leisure occupations.

Women with SCI experience the psychosocial sequelae of disability somewhat differently than men with SCI. Tate and Forsheimer (2001) found that while women with SCI reported higher life satisfaction than men with SCI, they had lower mental health related quality of life and were likely to experience qualitatively more severe problems of poor body image, lower self-concept, and feelings of increased vulnerability, especially those women who required personal assistance. They explained that women with SCI were at higher risk for abuse, both physical (neglect) and emotional, as well as at risk for financial exploitation. They also found that the participants who had a longer time since the onset of injury reported better quality of life outcomes.

CASE ILLUSTRATION: Jenny—Age 52

Jenny, the 16-year-old girl with paraplegia described in an earlier example, is now a 52-year-old successful college professor who is happily married and typifies the problems associated with aging with an SCI. She has bilateral carpal tunnel syndrome and her shoulders are very painful after years of pushing her wheelchair and transferring to and from the bottom of a tub (which she was taught to do in OT). Her image of herself as the attractive, active, and competent woman in the sporty wheelchair is constantly being challenged as she now times her departure from the campus to coincide with that of other colleagues so that she can get a push to her car. She spent their vacation money to remodel the bathroom with a roll-in shower and purchased a van with a lift (not in her self-image either), eschewing her custom of always driving something sporty. Of most concern to Jenny is the fatigue she experiences, necessitating that she go to bed early every night and spend the weekend catching up on her rest. In order to preserve her much loved employment she is increasingly forgoing many of her favorite leisure and social occupations and only engaging in those ADLs and IADLs that are essential. She is very anxious about what the future holds considering she is this limited at only 52. With uncharacteristic sadness she expresses that she thought she had already made the difficult adjustment when she was 16.

Discussion

Jenny's new situation is reminiscent of that described earlier in Charmaz' three-stage model of adaptation to a progressive chronic disability. Review that model with Jenny's experience in mind. Note also that Jenny's 36-year experience of SCI suggests few of the aforementioned problems of particular concern to women with SCI. However, she worries about what will happen to her should her physical and functional capabilities continue to decline or if she outlives her spouse or he becomes ill and they both require the help of a personal care attendant. If her fears are realized an older and widowed Jenny may be seeking OT intervention for help with her challenged concept of self as well as her declining physical and functional capabilities.

Acquired Amputation. Depression is a major psychosocial sequelae of acquired amputation (whether lower or upper extremity) and experienced by approximately 28% to 35% of the population (Desmond & MacLachlan, 2002; Fitzpatrick, 1999; Livneh, Antonak, & Gerhardt, 1999; Novotny, 1991; Rybarczyk, Nyenhuis, Nicholas, Cash, & Kaiser, 1995; Varni & Setoguchi, 1991; Walters & Williamson, 1998). For some individuals the failure to resume a self-perceived satisfactory life was found to have more to do with both the individual's and societal attitudes toward amputation than to the loss of the limb itself (Fitzpatrick, 1999; Walters & Williamson, 1998). In a study of people with lower extremity amputations, Rybarczyk, Nyenhuis, Nicholas, Cash, and Kaiser (1995) found that poor body image and perceived social stigma resulting in social discomfort accounted for approximately 40% of the clinical depression experienced. The average length of time since amputation for their participants was 17 years, which suggested to the researchers that depression was both a short-term and a long-term adjustment problem following lower limb amputation.

Fitzpatrick (1999) observed that those individuals whose amputations are the result of a traumatic event (such as war, horrific accidents, or cancer), in which threat of death or actual death of others occurs, may be subject to post-traumatic stress disorder (PTSD). This is an anxiety disorder where the traumatic event is repeatedly relived and the emotional impact reexperienced and should be addressed before a chronic emotional disorder develops. Given the nature of the cause of many of the acute onset diagnoses it may behoove the occupational therapist to be alert to the possibility of PTSD when working with any of these clients.

Approximately 80% of persons with amputations experience the phenomenon of phantom limb (sensory perception of the amputated limb) that seldom interferes long-term with psychosocial adjustment to the changed body and eventually becomes incorporated into the individual's body image. Phantom pain, on the other hand, while experienced by fewer of this population, is a more serious problem with little or no remedy (Desmond & MacLachlan, 2002). Management of this pain is important for the person to be able to participate in important life activities and occupations such as sexual expression and was found to be associated with resuming sexual activity (Walters & Williamson, 1998). Furthermore, sexual satisfaction was found to be a predictor of quality of life and thus contributed to psychosocial adjustment for persons with amputations. Achieving social and sexual satisfaction after amputation may further imply that the individual has been able to satisfactorily incorporate his or her new body image with residual limb(s) and developed coping strategies for handling stigma (Desmond & MacLachlan, 2002).

Consider the example of a young woman who is a part-time model, athlete, and participant runner and jumper in the Para Olympics. This articulate and physically attractive woman, who has bilateral lower extremity amputations, expresses to a television audience that she regards her various prosthetic legs (running legs, modeling legs, and legs for every day) as "art," "engineering marvels," and "really beautiful." Images of her running with her black S-shaped metal legs ("shaped like the hind leg of a cheetah") with shoes attached, footage of her as she struts the fashion show runway in Paris, and home movies of her and her boyfriend resting after a race—her with her prostheses off and her residual limbs exposed—seem to be indicators that she has reframed her body image and society's standards of beauty into a new and satisfactory self-concept.

Traumatic Brain Injury.   The psychosocial problems associated with traumatic brain injury (TBI) are not dissimilar to those of the previously discussed acute onset diagnoses but the clients' response to them is further complicated by their concomitant problems with cognition and perception (Gutman, 2001b). The average age at onset is 15 to 30 years old, with the incidence in males three times higher than in females (Bell & Pepping, 2001). There is a high incidence of depression, which may not be solely a reaction to the loss of body structures and functions or activity limitations but may also be a response to biological changes in the neuroreceptors of the temporal and frontal lobes of the brain (Antonak, Livneh, & Antonak, 1993). Antonak, Livneh, and Antonak (1993) note that there is frequently a preexisting history of substance abuse and risk-taking behaviors characteristic of the males who sustain TBI. Females who sustain TBI were found to have frequently had a preinjury history of childhood sexual abuse and adult alcoholism and the resulting social and behavioral problems associated with each which need to be taken into account when coupled with the new problems (Gutman & Swarbrick, 1998). For both genders after injury there is often internalized anger caused by guilt and blaming oneself for the injury whereas externalized hostility is observed in those who blame others for their injury although there is debate over whether the hostile behavior is organically based or an attempt at coping (Antonak, Livneh, & Antonak, 1993).

An overwhelming issue is the client's decreased or unsatisfactorily altered concept of self, which is a long-term consequence of decreased social roles and social isolation. Many experience the loss of roles of dating, marriage, intimacy, and even the perceived adult role of living independently (Gutman, 2001a, b). Behavioral problems frequently limit job opportunities and the resulting circumstances and environment for social interaction and friendship (Vandiver & Christofero-Snider, 2000).

Antonak, Livneh, and Antonak (1993) note that there needs to be an intellectual acceptance or acknowledgment of one's impairment and a gradual reintegration of the new body image and functioning into one's self-concept. Eventually, for most people with physical disability, there is an emotional acceptance of the disability with "integration of one's impairment into one's self concept coupled with behavioral adaptation and social reintegration into the new life situation" (p. 89). However, emotional problems are frequently not perceived by individuals with TBI, who characterize their problems as physical and cognitive whereas family members are more likely to report the psychosocial problems as more prevalent (Antonak, Livneh, & Antonak, 1993). Follow-up studies and personal accounts conducted two to seven years after onset suggest that the majority of individuals with TBI continue to have problems with psychosocial issues (Price-Lackey & Cashman, 1996; Vandiver & Christofero-Snider, 2000).

Price-Lackey and Cashman (1996) tell the compelling story of Cashman's more than five-year struggle reconfiguring her self-concept through graded participation in a previously valued occupation after a traumatic brain injury. Cashman, a 30-year-old freelance journalist with an impressive eclectic academic and employment career, was driving on a mountain road when her car was backed into by a large truck. She never lost consciousness and even signed a waiver at the crash site saying that she had suffered no repercussions from the impact. Her brain injury symptoms developed later that day as she attempted to pay for her groceries at the checkout counter and had no idea what to do with the checkbook. The psychosocial issues she confronts echo those described above and one can see the significant repercussions as one by one she is unable to maintain her job, loses her house, is forced to move in with relatives, and focuses her efforts in trying to recoup some of her former skills. Though her writing never reaches its preinjury caliber, she is able to develop cognitive and coping strategies to attend graduate school in a new career trajectory that capitalizes on her current skills. (See Chapter 14 for further discussion of TBI.)

Cerebrovascular Accident.　Cerebrovascular accident (CVA) is the most common physical disability diagnosis addressed by occupational therapy. There are a myriad of body structures and functions that can be affected by CVA, and each individual client may experience some or many of them to varying degrees of severity or impact on satisfactory participation in an occupation. Typical psychosocial issues may include depression, which is thought to be highly underreported, and anxiety, which is frequently associated with a fear of falling and not being able to get up—reminiscent of the onset of CVA (Smith, 2001). Other psychosocial issues include a decreased motivation to initiate activity, social isolation and loneliness, and emotional lability. Mr. Kelley's story exemplifies how the various psychosocial effects of stroke might be experienced and addressed by occupational therapy.

CASE ILLUSTRATION: Mr. Kelley—The Psychosocial Effects of Stroke

Mr. Kelley is an 82-year-old retired accountant who lives with his wife of 50 years in their own home close to the homes of his three grown children. Since age 62 he has "made a career out of retirement," enjoying daily golf, bowling, watching sports on television, and attending lectures and meetings of his college alumni group and a senior men's social organization. He is a master bridge player and plays couples bridge with his wife at weekly dinner/bridge games and keeps current with the tax laws so that he can volunteer to assist seniors at the local senior center in preparing their tax returns. He attends church on Sundays and drives his wife (who does not drive) to her various appointments and errands. They travel frequently and are very involved with their children and grandchildren.

While on one of their trips Mr. Kelley sustained a CVA and initially had weakness in his left side and some neglect which rather quickly resolved. After a one-week nursing home stay, where he relearned his ADLs, he returned home and sat in front of TV with his exercise equipment. He confided that he felt "a little blue." His wife felt trapped in the house ("he never leaves") and fondly reminisced about the days when he left early in the morning and came home later in the afternoon ready to take her out to dinner. Fortunately the home health OT sized up the situation and together with Mr. Kelley set goals for resuming his participation in his occupational life. Mr. Kelley's depression was discussed and strategies for handling it were developed.

Additional OT intervention was aimed first at relearning the chores he customarily performed around the house. Next the OT explored his bridge and tax skills and he discovered, to his relief, that he still had those capabilities. She then referred him to a community college based post-stroke program, where that OT worked with him on resuming his golfing and social dancing skills in time for his 50th anniversary celebration. A referral to another OT confirmed his ability to drive safely and two years after his stroke he was able to volunteer at the post-stroke program and reengage in many of his pre-stroke activities though his golfing was not at the level of proficiency he previously enjoyed— though his game was now more in concert with those of his daughters and new golfing partners.

Discussion

Mr. Kelley's story exemplifies the gamut of psychosocial issues typically associated with the experience of having a CVA, including depression, decreased concept of self, and seemingly decreased motivation to initiate activity. The strategies his OT taught him to cope with his depression enabled him to practice and participate in previously loved occupations, which in turn helped to quell his anxiety and fear of falling. Repeated success in performance of his preferred occupations helped him to craft an acceptable, though changed, self-concept.

Progressive Physical Disorders

Individuals who experience a progressive loss of reliable body function through a degenerative disease process require the OT to consider how this deterioration can compromise sense of self (Charmaz, 2002). Previously established habits are no longer effective and a person is faced making continuous trade-offs as function is lost. Within the general category of progressive chronic physical disorders two specific diagnoses will be described to illustrate the impact of this deterioration of function. Additionally, specific psychosocial issues are addressed.

Parkinson's Disease.   Individuals with Parkinson's disease (PD) present with a progressive loss of motor control. Eventually, the person is dependent upon others for all personal care (Gaudet, 2002; Schultz-Krohn, Foti, & Glo-goski, 2001). The loss of physical function is associated with a degeneration of portions of the basal ganglia, resulting in a substantial reduction in neurotrans-mitters within the brain (Olanow, Jenner, Tatton, & Tatton, 1998).

Approximately 50% of individuals diagnosed with PD are also diagnosed with depression (Pollak, 1998). This depression is not merely reactive to the severity of symptoms or the chronic and progressive nature of the disease but appears to be related to a serotonergic deficit (Duvoisin & Sage, 1990). The depression seen in individuals with PD is similar to that in individuals without PD who have depression. An additional characteristic problem seen with individuals who have PD is decreased facial expressiveness, known as the "masked face" (Pollak, 1998). This "masked face" begins unilaterally but, as the disease progresses, there is a loss of facial expressions on both sides of the face (Duvoisin & Sage, 1990).

CASE ILLUSTRATION: The Masked Face of Mr. Sanchez

Mr. Sanchez is a 61-year-old man diagnosed with PD. He owned a small construction company but needed to retire last year due to the progression of PD. His eldest son assumed the responsibility of running the company. Mr. Sanchez has a very good relationship with all his children and they all live in the area. His children are married and he takes great pleasure in spending time with his grandchildren now that he has retired. The progression of PD, particularly the masked face, has made it very difficult for Mr. Sanchez to smile when his young grandchildren come to see him. The grandchildren interpret this lack of facial responsiveness as indifference to their presence and often ask their mother, "Why doesn't Grandpa like us?" The grandfather overheard this question and began to limit the amount of time he spent with his grandchildren to coincide with when his medications are working.

Discussion

Mr. Sanchez had experienced the loss of a worker role when he had to retire from his position as the boss of his own company. He reconfigured his sense of self to be the loving grandfather, always available to visit his grandchildren. Now that role was being revised since Mr. Sanchez's grandchildren were misinterpreting

his masked face as indifference. He self-limited that role to coincide to his med-
ication schedule, confirming how the disease process of PD was dominating his
occupational configuration.

Individuals with PD often limit social participation because they are embarrassed about decreased facial expressions and movement disorders (Gaudet,
2002). The decrease in activity and participation is not just a product of the loss of
motor control but the ability to adapt to the progressing loss of function and the
interpretation of the loss of function by others.

Huntington's Disease.   Huntington's disease (HD) is a fatal degenerative
neurological disease that is characterized by progressive disorders of both voluntary and involuntary movement in addition to significant deterioration of cognitive
and behavioral abilities (Phillips & Stelmach, 1996). The initial symptoms vary but
are most often reported as changes in behavior, cognitive function, and unusual
movements of the hands (Wiederholt, 1995). Emotional and behavioral changes
are often the earliest symptoms of HD (Folstein, 1989). The movement disorder,
known as chorea, is sometimes mistaken for intoxication, particularly because of
the gait disturbances associated with HD. The initial cognitive changes may be
seen as forgetfulness or difficulties concentrating on tasks. During the initial
stages of HD, a client may experience difficulties maintaining adequate work performance. Family members often identify the initial behavioral changes seen in
the person with HD as increased irritability or depression. Irritability and depression may be inappropriately attributed to the decline in work performance rather
than the disease process. As HD progresses, depression often worsens and suicide
is not uncommon (Wiederholt, 1995). Clients with HD are frequently hospitalized due to various psychiatric problems, including depression, emotional lability,
and behavioral outbursts. Although the loss of function may contribute to the
client's level of depression, depression is clearly identified as a specific characteristic of HD (Folstein, 1989).

Chronic Congenital Nonprogressive Disorders

Individuals with congenital physically disabling conditions must adapt to a body
that is unable to meet cultural and societal expectations. Developmental motor
skills are not attained within the expected timeframes, and for some are never
attained. Congenital physically disabling conditions may be nonprogressive in
nature, such as cerebral palsy and spina bifida, or progressive, such as Rett's syndrome (Rogers, Gordon, Schanzenbacher, & Case-Smith, 2001). The following
will address two common congenital disorders that are considered nonprogressive. Even though cerebral palsy and spina bifida are considered nonprogressive
in nature, as environmental demands increase in complexity, the child with either
of these disorders may fall farther behind peers in performance. Of further significance is the understanding that the child with a congenital disorder is positioned within a family with expectations, hopes, and dreams. As the child grows
and additional developmental milestones are unmet, families, and particularly

parents, may feel socially isolated and overwhelmed by the care of the child and express loss of identity (Helitzer, Cunningham-Sabo, VanLeit, & Crowe, 2002).

Cerebral Palsy. Children with cerebral palsy (CP) present with limited motor control that can compromise mobility, self-care, and social participation (Beckung & Hagberg, 2002). These activity limitations obviously impact the child's occupational pursuits, but families are also influenced by these limitations (Helitzer et al., 2002). Children with CP were found to have a much higher frequency of behavioral problems such as disruptive behaviors and hyperactivity (McDermott et al., 1996). There was also a higher frequency of self-care dependency, surpassing what would be expected from their activity limitations due to problems with body function. The dependency frequently seen with children with CP is not solely related to problems in controlling movements. Children who have motor problems expend significant energy attempting even simple tasks such as feeding or dressing themselves.

Karen is a 12-year-old girl who has CP. The family system finds it easier to provide consistent support to help Karen dress instead of having her develop the habits to be able to dress independently. Karen has been able to complete some dressing tasks during OT intervention sessions but complains that it takes too much time. As a result of this family pattern of interacting with Karen, she has continued to be dependent on others to complete dressing tasks, past the expected age where it is culturally and socially endorsed to require assistance. This compromised her ability to attend "sleep-overs" at her friend Susie's house because of the imposition it would place on Susie's parents to dress Karen for bed and then in the morning.

Understanding the impact of limited motor control on social participation and making informed decisions regarding energy expenditures should be included in OT intervention for individuals with CP. OT services should also address the child's developmental trajectory and prepare the child for adolescent and adult roles (King, Cathers, Polgar, MacKinnon, & Havens, 2000). King et al. interviewed 10 older adolescents with CP regarding their perceptions of success in life. These teenagers described three key features related to being successful "in life: being believed in, believing in yourself, and being accepted by others" (p. 734). The concepts of independence in self-care and control of movements were not included in the themes. These teenagers placed a much higher value on interdependence and interactions with others than on independence in personal care. OT services provided to children and adolescents who have CP typically focus on developing independent functional skills. Unfortunately, this emphasis does not help adolescents with CP meet their goal of a successful life. King and associates argues that adolescents with CP "need opportunities to participate that will provide supportive relationships, belief in themselves, and a sense of community belonging" (p. 746).

Spina Bifida. Children with spina bifida, or myelomeningocele, have associated psychosocial issues that require careful consideration when developing an OT intervention plan. The high incidence of hydrocephalus, incontinence, sensory loss, and orthopedic surgeries is stressful for both the individual with spina bifida and the family (Cate, Kennedy, & Stevenson, 2002). Mothers of children with spina bifida reported a compromised sense of competence as a parent and less satisfaction in their role (Hombeck et al., 1997). Appleton et al. (1997) reported that individuals with spina bifida were at a greater risk for experiencing depression, social isolation, and low self-worth.

CASE ILLUSTRATION: Sandy—Social and Psychological Support

Sandy is a 15-year-old and attends a public high school. Sandy has myelomeningocele and has had over 10 surgeries, including revisions to her ventriculoperitoneal shunt placed to reduce the risk of hydrocephalus. She uses a manual wheelchair for mobility and manages her own bowel and bladder program. Sandy uses an intermittent self-catherization program and has been allowed to use the nurse's office at the school for privacy on a daily basis. She lives with both parents and her 17-year-old sister who attends the same high school. Her sister plays on the varsity soccer team and is in the marching band. Sandy is also in the marching band but to play her instrument, the flute, she requires assistance from her friend to push her wheelchair. Through the use of environmental accommodations within the school Sandy is included in many activities and is allowed to participate according to her interest level. Her one comment is that it would be nice to date but doesn't see that happening soon. She laughs and says her father is over-protective but then adds that no boys are interested in dating a girl in a wheelchair.

Discussion

The psychosocial issues faced by Sandy are common to children and adolescents with spina bifida. Borjeson and Lagergren (1990) asked teenagers with myelomeningocele to identify their concerns and half listed social and psychological issues as a greater concern than physical issues. Unfortunately, the majority of services provided these adolescents focused on the physical aspects of myelomeningocele and failed to provide the psychosocial support these teenagers needed.

Summary

The experiences of the OT clients described throughout this chapter should represent a resounding call to occupational therapists to redouble their efforts to thoroughly consider and effectively address the psychosocial challenges of their clients with physical disabilities. Due to time and space limitations many diagnoses commonly treated by occupational therapists working with clients with physical disabilities were not directly addressed. Those diagnoses that were discussed exemplify a model of how psychosocial issues associated with any physical disability diagnosis can be recognized, researched, assessed, and addressed by occupational therapy in its commitment to empower the whole person to engage in occupation to support satisfactory participation in life (Occupational Therapy Practice Framework, 2002).

Review Questions

1. What are the differences between adapting to physical limitations that occur from a chronic illness or condition and adapting to physical limitations resulting from an acute injury or illness?
2. What is the difference between the terms *life satisfaction* and quality of life as is used in the literature addressing physical disabilities?
3. How do cultural and societal factors influence adaptation to a physical disability?
4. Identify three reasons for an OT to assess and provide intervention to directly address psychosocial issues for clients with physical disabilities.
5. Name three psychosocial issues of concern to those with physical disabilities and describe appropriate OT interventions to address those issues.

References

Adams, D. L. (1969). Analysis of a life satisfaction index. *Journal of Gerontology, 24*, 470–474.

Antonak, R. F., Livneh, H., & Antonak, C. (1993). A review of research on psychosocial adjustment to impairment in persons with traumatic brain injury. *Journal of Head Trauma Rehabilitation, 8*(4), 87–100.

Appleton, P. L., Ellis, N. C., Minchom, P. E., Lawson, V., Boll, V., & Jones, P. (1997). Depressive symptoms and self-concept in young people with spina bifida. *Journal of Pediatric Psychology, 22*, 707–722.

Baron, K., Kielhofner, G., Goldhammer, V., & Wolenski, J. (1999). *The Occupational Self Assessment (OSA)(Version 1.0)*. Model of Human Occupational Clearinghouse. Chicago: University of Illinois at Chicago.

Beck, A. T., Epstein, N., Brown, G., & Steer, R. A. (1988). An inventory for measuring clinical anxiety: Psychometric properties. *Journal of Consulting and Clinical Psychology, 56*, 893–897.

Beck, A. T., Ward, C. M., Mendelson, M., Mock, J., & Erbaugh, J. (1961). An inventory for measuring depression. *Archives of General Psychiatry, 4*, 561–571.

Beckung, E., & Hagberg, G. (2002). Neuroimpairments, activity limitations, and participation restrictions in children with cerebral palsy. *Developmental Medicine and Child Neurology, 44*, 309–316.

Bell, K. R., & Pepping, M. (2001). Women and traumatic brain injury. *Physical Medicine and Rehabilitation Clinics of North America, 12*(1), 169–182.

Benony, H., Daloz, L., Bungener, C., Chahraoui, K., Frenay, C., & Auvin, J. (2002). Emotional factors and subjective quality of life in subjects with spinal cord injuries. *American Journal of Physical Medicine and Rehabilitation, 81*, 437–445.

Bonder, B. (2001). Culture and occupation: A comparison of weaving in two traditions. *Canadian Journal of Occupational Therapy, 68*, 310–319.

Borjeson, M. C., & Lagergren, J. (1990). Life conditions of adolescents with myelomeningocele. *Developmental Medicine and Child Neurology, 32*, 698–706.

Brice, A., & Campbell, L. (1999). Cross-cultural communication. In R. L. Leavitt (Ed.), *Cross-cultural rehabilitation* (pp. 83–94). London: W. B. Saunders.

Burnett, S. E., & Yerxa, E. J. (1980). Community based and college based needs assessment of physically disabled persons. *American Journal of Occupational Therapy, 34*, 201–207.

Carver, C. S., Scheier, M. F., & Weintraub, J. K. (1989). Assessing coping strategies: A theoretically based approach. *Journal of Personality and Social Psychology, 56*, 267–283.

Cate, I. M. P., Kennedy, C., & Stevenson, J. (2002). Disability and quality of life in spina bifida and hydrocephalus. *Developmental Medicine and Child Neurology, 44,* 317–322.

Charmaz, K. (1983). Loss of self: A fundamental form of suffering in the chronically ill. *Sociology of Health and Illness, 5,* 168–195.

Charmaz, K. (1995). The body, identity, and self: Adapting to impairment. *Sociological Quarterly, 36,* 657–680.

Charmaz, K. (2002). The self as habit: The reconstruction of self in chronic illness. *Occupational Therapy Journal of Research, S22,* S31–S41.

Clark, F. (1993). Occupation embedded in a real life: Interweaving occupational science and occupational therapy. *American Journal of Occupational Therapy, 47*(12), 1067–1078.

Coster, W., Deeney, T. Haltiwanger, J., & Haley, S. (1998). *School Function Assessment (SFA): User's manual.* San Antonio, TX: Psychological Corporation.

Cynkin, S., & Robinson, A. M. (1990). *Occupational therapy and activities health: Toward health through activities.* Boston: Little, Brown.

Davidhizar, R. (1997). Disability does not have to be the grief that never ends: Helping patients adjust. *Rehabilitation Nursing, 22,* 32–35.

Desmond, D., & MacLachlan, M. (2002). Psychosocial issues in the field of prosthetics and orthotics. *Journal of Prosthetics and Orthotics, 14*(1), 19–22.

Duvoisin, R. C., and Sage, J. I. (1990). The spectrum of Parkinsonism. In S. Chokroverty (Ed.). *Movement disorders.* New Brunswick, NJ: PMA.

Dyck, I. (2002). Beyond the clinic: Restructuring the environment in chronic illness experience. *Occupational Therapy Journal of Research, S22,* S52–S60.

Fisher, A., & Kielhofner, G. (1995). Mind-brain-body performance subsystem. In G. Kielhofner (Ed.), *A model of human occupation theory and application* (2nd ed., pp. 83–90). Baltimore: Williams & Wilkins.

Fisk, J. D., Pontefract, A., Ritvo, P. G., Archibald, C. J., & Murray, T. J. (1994). The impact of fatigue on patients with multiple sclerosis. *Canadian Journal of Neurological Sciences, 21,* 9–14.

Fitzpatrick, M. C. (1999). The psychologic assessment and psychosocial recovery of the patient with an amputation. *Clinical Orthopaedics and Related Research, 361,* 98–107.

Florey, L., & Michelman, S. M. (1982). The occupational role history. *American Journal of Occupational Therapy, 36*(5), 301–308.

Folkman, S., & Lazarus, R. S. (1987). *The Ways of Coping Questionnaire.* Palo Alto, CA: Consulting Psychologists Press

Folstein, M. F., et al. (1975). Mini-mental state: A practical method for grading the cognitive state of patients for the clinician. *Journal of Psychiatric Research, 12*(3), 189–198.

Folstein, S. E. (1989). *Huntington's disease: A disorder of families.* Baltimore: Johns Hopkins University Press.

Frank, G. (2000). *Venus on wheels.* Los Angeles: University of California Press.

Gallagher, P., & MacLachlan, M. (2000). Development and psychometric evaluation of the Trinity Amputation and Prosthesis Experience Scales (TAPES). *Rehabilitation Psychology, 45,* 130–154.

Gallimore, R., & Lopez, E. M. (2002). Everyday routines, human agency, and ecocultural context: Construction and maintenance of individual habits. *Occupational Therapy Journal of Research, S22,* S70–S79.

Galvin, L. R., & Godfrey, H. P. D. (2001). The impact of coping on emotional adjustment to spinal cord injury (SCI): Review of the literature and application of a stress appraisal and coping formulation. *Spinal Cord, 39,* 615–627.

Gaudet, P. (2002). Measuring the impact of Parkinson's disease: An occupational therapy perspective. *Canadian Journal of Occupational Therapy, 69,* 104–113.

Gibson, B. S., et al. (1975). The Sickness Impact Profile: Development of an outcome measure of healthcare. *American Journal of Public Health, 65,* 1304–1310.

Goffman, E. (1963). *Stigma: Notes on the management of spoiled identity.* Upper Saddle River, NJ: Prentice-Hall.

Gutman, S. A. (2001a). The psychosocial sequelae of traumatic brain injury, part I: Identification. *OT Practice, 6*(3), 1–8.

Gutman, S. A., (2001b). Traumatic brain injury. In L. W. Pedretti & M. B. Early (Eds.), *Occupational therapy: Practice skills for physical dysfunction* (pp. 671–701). St. Louis, MO: Mosby.

Gutman, S. A., & Swarbrick, P. (1998). The multiple linkages between childhood sexual abuse, adult alcoholism, and traumatic brain injury in women: A set of guidelines for occupational therapy practice. *Occupational Therapy in Mental Health, 14*(3), 33–65.

Haley, S. M., Coster, W. J., Ludlow, L. H., Haltiwanger, J. T., & Andrellos, P. J. (1992). *Pediatric Evaluation of Disability Inventory (PEDI): Development, standardization and administration manual.* Boston: New England Medical Center Hospitals.

Hammel, K. W. (1995). Spinal cord injury; quality of life; occupational therapy: Is there a connection? *British Journal of Occupational Therapy, 58*(4), 151–157.

Hampton, N. Z., & Marshall, A. (2000). Culture, gender, self-efficacy, and life satisfaction: A comparison between Americans and Chinese people with spinal cord injuries. *Journal of Rehabilitation, 66*, 3–25.

Helitzer, D., L., Cunningham-Sabo, L., D., VanLeit, B., & Crowe, T. K. (2002). Perceived changes in self-image and coping strategies of mothers of children with disabilities. *Occupational Therapy Journal of Research, 22*, 25–33.

Hockenberry, J. (1995). *Moving violations: War zones, wheelchairs, and declarations of independence.* New York: Hyperion.

Hoehn, M. M., & Yahr, M. D. (1967). Parkinsonism: Onset, progression and mortality. *Neurology, 17*, 422–427.

Hombeck, G. N., Gorey-Ferguson, L., Hudson, T., Seefeldt, T., Shapera, W., Turner, J., & Uhler, J. (1997). Maternal, paternal, and marital functioning in families of preadolescents with spina bifida. *Journal of Pediatric Psychology, 22*, 167–181.

Hughes, R. B., Swedlund, N., Petersen, N., & Nosek, M. A. (2001). Depression and women with spinal cord injury. *Topics in Spinal Cord Injury Rehabilitation, 7*(1), 16–24.

Huntington Study Group. (1996). Unified Huntington's Disease Rating Scale: Reliability and consistency. *Movement Disorders, 11*, 136–142.

Huttlinger, K., Krefting, L., Drevdahl, D., Tree, P., Baca, E., & Benally, A. (1992). "Doing battle": A metaphorical analysis of diabetes mellitus among Navajo people. *American Journal of Occupational Therapy, 46,* 706–711.

Katz, N., Fleming, J., Keren, N., Lightbody, S., & Hartman-Maeir, A. (2002). Unawareness and/or denial of disability: Implications for occupational therapy intervention. *Canadian Journal of Occupational Therapy, 69*, 281–292.

Kemp, B. J., & Adams, B. (1995). The older adult health and mood index: A new measure of depression for older persons. *Journal of Geriatric Neurology and Psychiatry, 8*, 162–167.

Kemp, B. J., & Kraus, J. S. (1999). Depression and life-satisfaction among people ageing with post-polio and spinal cord injury. *Disability and Rehabilitation, 21*(5/6), 241–249.

Kielhofner, G., Malinson, T., Crawford, C., Nowak, M., Rigby, M., Henry, A., & Walens, D. (1998). *The Occupational Performance History Interview (Version 2.0)(OPHI II).* Model of Human Occupational Clearinghouse. Chicago: University of Illinois at Chicago.

King, G. A., Cathers, T., Polgar, J. M., MacKinnon, E., & Havens, L. (2000). Success in life for older adolescents with cerebral palsy. *Qualitative Health Research, 10*, 734–749.

Law, M., et al. (1994). *The Canadian Occupational Performance Measure* (2nd ed.). Ottawa: CAOT Publications Ace.

Legro, M. W., Smith, D. G., del Aguila, M., Larson, J., & Boone, D. (1998). Prosthesis evaluation questionnaire for persons with lower limb amputations: Assessing prosthesis-related quality of life. *Archives of Physical Medicine and Rehabilitation, 79*, 931–938.

Lezak, M. D. (1987). Relationship between personality disorders, social disturbance, and physical disability following traumatic brain injury. *Journal of Head Trauma Rehabilitation, 2*(1), 57–59.

Linkowski, D. (1987). *The Acceptance of Disability Scale.* Washington, DC: George Washington University.

Livingston, M. G., & Livingston, H. M. (1985). The Glasgow Assessment Schedule (GAS): Clinical and research assessment of head injury outcome. *International Rehabilitation Medicine, 7,* 145–149.

Livneh, H., & Antonak, R. F. (1990). Reactions to disability: An empirical investigation of their nature and structure. *Journal of Applied Rehabilitation Counseling, 21*(4), 13–21.

Livneh, H., Antonak, R. F., & Gerhardt, J. (1999). Psychosocial adaptation to amputation: The role of sociodemographic variables, disability-related factors and coping strategies. *International Journal of Rehabilitation Research, 22*, 21–31.

Manns, P. J., & Chad, K. E. (2001). Components of quality of life for persons with a quadriplegic and paraplegic spinal cord injury. *Qualitative Health Research, 11*, 795–811.

McCarthy, M. L., Silberstein, C. E., Atkins, E. A., Harryman, S. E., Sponseller, P. D., & Hadley-Miller, N. A. (2002). Comparing reliability and validity of pediatric instruments for measuring health and well-being of children with spastic cerebral palsy. *Developmental Medicine and Child Neurology, 44*, 468–476.

McDermott, S., Coker, A. L., Mani, S., Krishnaaswami, S., Nagle, R. J., Barnett-Queen, L. L., & Wuori, D. F. (1996). A population-based analysis of behavior problems in children with cerebral palsy. *Journal of Pediatric Psychology, 21*, 447–463.

Moore, A. (1992). *Cultural anthropology: The field study of human beings.* San Diego, CA: Collegiate.

Moorhead, L. (1969). The occupational history. *American Journal of Occupational Therapy, 23*, 329–334.

Morse, J. M., & O'Brien, B. (1995). Preserving self: From victim, to patient, to disabled person. *Journal of Advanced Nursing, 21*, 886–896.

Murphy, R. F. (2001). *The body silent.* New York: W. W. Norton.

Novotny, M. P. (1991). Psychosocial issues affecting rehabilitation. *Physical Medicine and Rehabilitation, Clinics of North America, 2*(2), 373–393.

Oakley, F. M. (1986). The role checklist. *Occupational Therapy Journal of Research, 6*(3), 157–169.

Occupational Therapy Practice Framework: Domain and Process. (2002). *American Journal of Occupational Therapy, 56*, 609–639.

Ohbuchi, K., Fukushima, O., & Tedeschi, J. T. (1999). Cultural values in conflict management. *Journal of Cross-Cultural Psychology, 30*, 51–71.

Olanow, C. W., Jenner, P., Tatton, N. A., & Tatton, W. G. (1998). Neurodegeneration and Parkinson's disease. In J. Jankovic & E. Tolosa (Eds.), *Parkinson's disease and movement disorders* (3rd ed.). Baltimore: Williams & Wilkins.

Paty, D., Willoughby, E., & Whitaker, J. (1992). Assessing the outcome of experimental therapies in multiple sclerosis. In R. A. Rudick & D. E. Goodkin (Eds.), *Treatment of multiple sclerosis trial design, results, and future perspectives.* London: Springer-Verlag.

Pendleton, H. McH. (1990). Occupational therapists' current use of independent living skills training for adult inpatients who are physically disabled. In J. Johnson & E. Yerxa (Eds.), *Occupational science: The foundations for new models of practice* (pp. 93–108). Binghampton, NY: Haworth.

Pendleton, H. McH. (1998). *Establishment and sustainment of friendship of women with physical disability: The role of participation in occupation.* Doctoral dissertation, University of Southern California, Los Angeles. Available through UMI.

Peto, V., Jenkinson, C., Fitzpatrick, R., & Greenhall, R. (1995). The development and validation of a short measure of functioning and well-being for individuals with Parkinson's disease. *Quality of Life Research, 4*, 241–248.

Phillips, J. G., and Stelmach, G. E. (1996). Parkinson's disease and other involuntary movement disorders of the basal ganglia. In C. M. Fredericks & L. K. Saladin (Eds.), *Pathophysiology of the motor systems.* Philadelphia: F. A. Davis.

Pollak, P. (1998). Parkinson's disease and related movement disorders. In J. Bogousslasky & M. Fisher (Eds.), *Textbook of neurology.* Boston: Butterworth Heinemann.

Price-Lackey, P., & Cashman, J. (1996). Jenny's story: Reinventing oneself through occupation and narrative configuration. *American Journal of Occupational Therapy, 50*(4), 306–314.

Putzke, J. D., Richards, J. S., Hicken, B. L., & De Vivo, M. J. (2002). Predictors of life satisfaction: A spinal cord injury cohort study. *Archives of Physical Medicine and Rehabilitation, 83*, 555–561.

Ritvo, P. G., Fischer, J. S., Miller, D. M., Andrews, H., Paty, D., & LaRocca, N. G. (1997). *Multiple Sclerosis Quality of Life Inventory (MSQLI): A user's manual.* New York: National Multiple Sclerosis Society.

Roe, B. (2000). Effective and ineffective management of incontinence: Issues around illness trajectory and health care. *Qualitative Health Research, 10*, 677–690.

Rogers, J. (1988). The NPI interest checklist. In B. Hemphill (Ed.), *Mental health assessment in occupational therapy.* Thorofare, NJ: Slack.

Rogers, S. L., Gordon, C. Y., Schanzenbacher, K. E., & Case-Smith, J. (2001). Common diagnosis in pediatric occupational therapy practice. In J. Case-Smith (Ed.), *Occupational therapy for children* (4th ed., pp. 136–187). St. Louis, MO: Mosby.

Rybarczyk, B., Nyenhuis, D. L., Nicholas, J. J., Cash, S. M., & Kaiser, J. (1995). Body image, perceived social stigma, and the predictions of psychosocial adjustment to leg amputation. *Rehabilitation Psychology, 40*(2), 95–110.

Salamy, M., et al. (1993). *Assessment of communication and interaction skills.* Model of Human Occupational Clearinghouse. Chicago: University of Illinois at Chicago.

Schultz-Krohn, W., Foti, D., & Glogoski, C. (2001). Degenerative diseases of the central nervous system. In L. W. Pedretti & M. B. Early (Eds.), *Occupational therapy: Practice skills for physical dysfunction* (pp. 702–729). St. Louis, MO: Mosby.

Sheikh, J. I., & Yesavage, J. A. (1986). Geriatric Depression Scale (GDS): Recent evidence and development of a shorter version. *Clinical Gerontologist, 5*, 165–173.

Sherer, M., Maddux, J. E., Mercandante, B., Pentice-Dunn, S., Jacobs, B., & Rogers, R. W. (1982). The Self-Efficacy Scale: Construction and validation. *Psychological Reports, 51*, 663–671.

Simpson, G., Blaszczynski, A., & Hodgkinson, A. (1999). Sex offending as a psychosocial sequela of traumatic brain injury. *Journal of Head Trauma Rehabilitation, 14*(6), 567–580.

Smith, J. A. (2001). *How do occupational therapists address psychosocial issues with geriatric patients?* Unpublished master's thesis, San Jose State University, San Jose, CA.

Tate, D. G., & Forchheimer, M. (2001). Health-related quality of life and life satisfaction for women with spinal cord injury. *Topics in Spinal Cord Injury Rehabilitation, 7*(1), 1–15.

Tyerman, A., & Humphrey, M. (1984). Changes in self-concept following severe head injury. *International Journal of Rehabilitation, 7*, 11–23.

Tzonichaki, I., & Kleftaras, G. (2002). Paraplegia from spinal cord injury: Self-esteem, loneliness, and life satisfaction. *Occupational Therapy Journal of Research, 22*, 96–103.

Vandiver, V. L., & Christofero-Snider, C. (2000). TBI club: A psychosocial support group for adults with traumatic brain injury. *Journal of Cognitive Rehabilitation, 18*(4), 22–27.

Varni, J. W., & Setoguchi, Y. (1991). Psychosocial factors in the management of children with limb deficiencies. *Physical Medicine and Rehabilitation Clinics of North America, 2*(2), 395–404.

Walters, A. S., & Williamson, G. M. (1998). Sexual satisfaction predicts quality of life: A study of adult amputees. *Sexuality and Disability, 16*(2), 103–115.

Wiederholt, W. (1995). Parkinson's disease and other movement disorders. In *Neurology for non-neurologists* (3rd ed.). Philadephia: Saunders.

Williams, D., & Ispa, J. M. (1999). A comparison of the child-rearing goals of Russian and U.S. university students. *Journal of Cross-Cultural Psychology, 30*, 540–546.

World Health Organization. (2001). *International classification of functioning, disability and health (ICF).* Geneva: Author.

Wright, B. (1983). *Physical disability: A psychosocial approach* (2nd ed.). New York: Harper & Row.

Yerxa, E. J. (2001). The social and psychological experience of having a disability: Implications for occupational therapy. In L. W. Pedretti & M. B. Early (Eds.), *Occupational therapy: Practice skills for physical dysfunction* (pp. 470–492). St. Louis, MO: Mosby.

CHAPTER 14

The Cognitive, Behavioral, and Psychosocial Sequelae of Brain Injury

Shawn C. Phipps, MS, OTR/L

Key Terms

abstract thinking
anosognosia
confabulation
demotivational syndrome
diffuse axonal injury
disinhibition
executive functions

generalization
Glasgow Coma Scale
initiation
neuroplasticity
perseveration
post-traumatic amnesia
Rancho Los Amigos Levels
    of Cognitive Functioning

Chapter Outline

Introduction
Diagnosis and Etiology

Introduction

Each year, an estimated 2 million Americans sustain a traumatic brain injury (TBI) (Sadock & Sadock, 2003) and the incidence is probably higher in Europe and Africa (Bruns & Hauser, 2003). More than 50,000 people die as a result of TBI and of those who survive, 80,000 annually experience the onset of long-term disability (Thurman et al., 1999). It has also been suggested that there is significant risk for a second or third head injury after an initial TBI, but the reports are inconsistent and the prevalence needs to be further researched. However, the literature is in agreement that a person with a TBI has at least a 15% to 20% chance of sustaining another head injury (Gutman, 2001). Currently, there are an estimated 5.3 million Americans (more than 2% of the U.S. population) who are living with long-term disabilities resulting from a TBI (CDC, 2001).

The cost of TBI is estimated to be $48.3 billion annually in the United States (CDC, 2001), and the emotional, behavioral, social, perceptual, and physical sequelae following brain injury are even more costly to the individuals, their families, and the society at large. In traditional rehabilitation settings, there has been a historical overemphasis on the physical impairments impacting occupational performance following brain injury, which can include hemiplegia, visual-perceptual dysfunction, and sensory disturbances. Remediative and compensatory occupational therapy approaches have traditionally focused on improving motor control, visual/perceptual skills, sensory awareness, basic and instrumental activities of daily living, community reentry, prevocational skills, and driving skills. However, this chapter addresses the cognitive, behavioral, and psychosocial sequelae of brain injury as these are often the most disabling, stressful, and costly aspects of TBI. A client with brain injury presents with a complex clinical picture that often affects every area of occupation, including basic and instrumental activities of daily living, education, work, play, leisure, and social participation. In order to effectively assist the person with brain injury to reengage in daily occupations and to reintegrate into home, community, and work environments, the occupational therapist is challenged to provide holistic, client-centered care that integrates assessment and treatment of both the physical and psychosocial dimensions of the person to support participation in the context of his or her environment (Occupational Therapy Practice Framework, 2002). It is also important to consider the performance skills (e.g., motor skills, process skills, and communication/interaction skills), performance patterns (e.g., habits, routines, and roles), activity demands, and client factors (e.g., affective, cognitive, and perceptual mental functions) that impact the person's ability to participate in her or his cultural, physical, social, personal, spiritual, temporal, and/or virtual context.

DIAGNOSIS AND ETIOLOGY

"Head trauma most commonly occurs in people 15 to 25 years of age and has a male-to-female predominance of approximately 3 to 1" (Sadock & Sadock, 2003, p. 361). Among young people, motor vehicle as well as sports and recreation accidents are among the leading causes of TBI. Although exact figures are difficult to determine, some of these accidents are a result of engaging in high-risk behaviors or due to drug or alcohol abuse. Violence, including self-inflicted gunshot wounds, accounts for at least 10% of all TBI (Winkler, 2001). Low income has also been associated with a higher incidence of TBI (Bruns & Hauser, 2003) although the relationship between injury and socioeconomic status is not clear. Although adolescents and young adults have the highest incidence of TBI, the second largest representative group is the elderly, primarily due to falls (Bruns & Hauser, 2003; Pulaski, 2003; Radomski, 2002). Older adults typically show less complete recovery from brain injury than their younger counterparts (Rothweiler, Temkin, & Dikmen 1998).

According to the World Health Organization (2001), diagnostic information should be elicited with regard to the functioning and disability of the individual. The model of functioning and disability describes a dynamic process of evaluating impairments with body functions and structures, activity limitations, and participation restrictions, as well as personal and environmental factors that affect functioning and social participation in the fabric of daily life. For the occupational therapist evaluating a person with a brain injury, a thorough understanding of these components will strengthen the quality of the intervention plan designed to rehabilitate a person to the highest level of functioning.

A medical diagnosis of brain injury is confirmed by specialized imaging studies using magnetic resonance imaging (MRI) and computed tomography (CT) scans, once the bruising or lesion has formed on the brain. The physician is often able to predict possible cognitive, behavioral, visual-perceptual, language, and physical impairments based on the location of the lesion in the brain. However, **diffuse axonal injury,** which results from the tearing and shearing of the axons of the nerve fibers throughout the brain due to the bouncing of the brain inside the skull, is not visible on imaging studies. Therefore, the physician is required to diagnose the brain injury based on observable signs and symptoms, such as the level of consciousness, cortical posturing, cognition, and behavior.

Figure 14-1 shows the six main lobes of the brain and their functional responsibilities. This can also assist the occupational therapist in predicting the functional and clinical problems that may present with the client based on information on the area of the brain that is damaged. Depending on the type and amount of external force impacting the brain, one functional area, various areas, or all areas of the brain can be affected. Because each brain injury is unique, the clinical picture can vary greatly from person to person.

The *Diagnostic and Statistical Manual of Mental Disorders,* fourth edition, text-revised (*DSM-IV-TR*) (American Psychiatric Association, 2000) categorizes brain injury under the axis I clinical disorders as "Dementia Due to Head Trauma" (p. 164). The most prominent impairment noted following brain injury is **post-traumatic amnesia,** or short- or long-term memory deficits resulting from concussion or head trauma. Other impairments include "aphasia, attentional problems, irritability, anxiety, depression or affective lability, apathy, increased aggression, or other changes in personality" (p. 164). The clinician should also be aware of substance abuse, chemical dependency, or the effects of intoxication at the time of the brain injury.

There are many types of brain injury with different etiologies and clinical presentations (see Table 14-1). Brain injury is typically categorized by whether the injury is acquired or the direct result of a traumatic event.

PROGNOSIS FOR RECOVERY

Prognosis for recovery following brain injury is dependent on a number of factors, such as age, the size and location of injury to the brain, substance use at the time of injury, the type of injury, the level of consciousness at the time of injury, and the length of coma if loss of consciousness has occurred (Sadock & Sadock, 2003; Leahy & Lam, 1998). The brain is able to recover following TBI due to its **neuroplasticity**, which enables it to reorganize alternate neuronal pathways to compensate for damaged areas. Younger age, more focal points of injury, and short episodes of loss of consciousness have been associated with a more rapid recovery.

The **Glasgow Coma Scale (GCS)** has been traditionally used to evaluate the client's level of consciousness at the scene of the accident and frequently

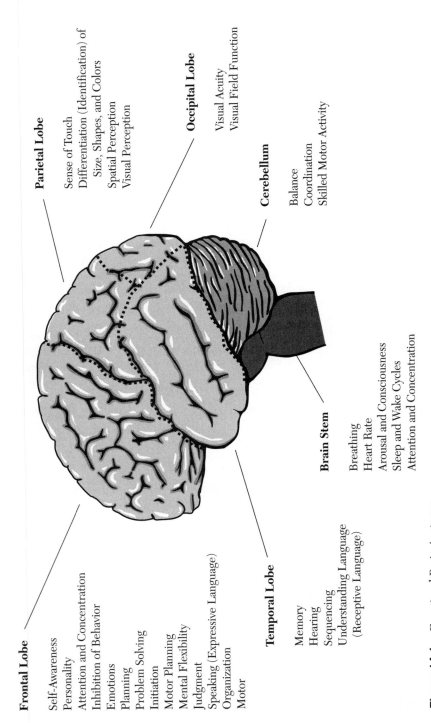

Frontal Lobe

Self-Awareness
Personality
Attention and Concentration
Inhibition of Behavior
Emotions
Planning
Problem Solving
Initiation
Motor Planning
Mental Flexibility
Judgment
Speaking (Expressive Language)
Organization
Motor

Parietal Lobe

Sense of Touch
Differentiation (Identification) of
   Size, Shapes, and Colors
Spatial Perception
Visual Perception

Occipital Lobe

Visual Acuity
Visual Field Function

Cerebellum

Balance
Coordination
Skilled Motor Activity

Brain Stem

Breathing
Heart Rate
Arousal and Consciousness
Sleep and Wake Cycles
Attention and Concentration

Temporal Lobe

Memory
Hearing
Sequencing
Understanding Language
   (Receptive Language)

Figure 14-1. Functional Brain Anatomy

Reprinted with permission of Mary Groves, OTR/L. Copyright 2003.

Table 14-1. Types of Brain Injury

Type of Brain Injury	Definition	Etiology
Traumatic Brain Injury	Insult to the brain that may produce a diminished or altered state of consciousness, which results in an impairment of cognitive abilities or physical functioning. It can also result in the disturbance of behavioral or emotional functioning. These impairments may be either temporary or permanent and cause partial or total functional disability or psychosocial maladjustment.	Caused by an external force; not of a degenerative or congenital nature
Open Head Injury	Injury to the head that results in a skull fracture	Caused by an external force that fractures the skull such as a penetrating gunshot wound
Closed Head Injury	Impact to the head from an outside force, but the skull does not fracture or displace	Caused by an external force that does not fracture the skull
Diffuse Axonal Injury	Injury that occurs because the unmoving brain lags behind the movement of the skull, causing brain structures to tear. There is extensive tearing of nerve tissue throughout the brain. This can cause brain chemicals to be released, causing additional injury.	Caused by shaking or strong rotation of the head or by rotational forces
Concussion	The most common type of brain injury, produced by either closed or open head injuries. The brain receives trauma from an impact or a sudden momentum or movement change. The blood vessels in the brain may stretch and cranial nerves may be damaged. A person may or may not experience a brief loss of consciousness. A concussion may or may not show up on a diagnostic imaging test.	Caused by direct blows to the head, gunshot wounds, violent shaking of the head, or force from a whiplash-type injury
Contusion	Bruise or bleeding on the brain	Direct impact to the head

(continues)

Table 14-1.   (continued)

Type of Brain Injury	Definition	Etiology
Coup-Contrecoup Injury	Contusions that are both at the site of the impact and on the complete opposite side of the brain	Occurs when the force impacting the head is not only great enough to cause a contusion at the site of impact, but also is able to move the brain and cause it to slam into the opposite side of the skull, which causes the additional contusion
Penetration Injury	Sharp object forces hair, skin, bone, and fragments from the object into the brain. A "through-and-through" injury occurs if an object enters the skull, goes through the brain, and exits the skull.	Impact of a bullet, knife, or other sharp object; mostly caused by firearms
Shaken Baby Syndrome	Violent criminal act that causes traumatic brain injury through the whiplash-like motion	Perpetrator aggressively shakes a baby or young child
Acquired Brain Injury	Injury to the brain, which is not hereditary, congenital, degenerative, or induced by birth trauma, which commonly results in a change in neuronal activity, which affects the physical integrity, metabolic activity, or functional ability of the neural cell.	Anoxia, hypoxia, tumors, stroke, and/or neurotoxins, airway obstruction, near-drowning, throat swelling, choking, strangulation, crush injuries to the chest, electrical shock, vascular disruption, heart attack, stroke, arteriovenous malformation (AVM), aneurysm, intracranial surgery, infectious disease, intracranial tumors, metabolic disorders, meningitis, venereal disease, AIDS, insect-carried diseases, brain tumors, hypo/hyperglycemia, hepatic encephalopathy, uremic encephalopathy, seizure disorders, toxic exposure, illegal drug use, alcohol abuse, lead, carbon monoxide poisoning, toxic chemicals, and chemotherapy

Source: Adapted from the Brain Injury Association of America, 2001.

thereafter. Table 14-2 shows the criteria for scoring the client's level of consciousness. A total score of 13 to 15 indicates a mild brain injury; a score of 9 to 12 indicates a moderate brain injury; and a total score of 8 or below indicates a severe brain injury (Gelb, 2000).

The GCS has been used to quantify the severity of the brain injury and to predict long-term outcomes, although more recent studies have shown that the GCS

Table 14-2. Glasgow Coma Scale

Examiner's Test	Patient Response	Score
Eye Opening		
Spontaneous	Opens eyes on own	4
To Speech	Opens eyes when asked to in a loud voice	3
To Pain	Opens eyes when pinched	2
	Does not open eyes when pinched	3
Best Motor Response		
To commands	Follows simple commands	6
To pain	Pulls examiner's hand away when pinched	5
	Pulls a part of body away when pinched	4
	Flexes body part inappropriately to pain	3
	Body becomes rigid in an extended position when examiner pinches patient (decerebrate posturing)	2
	No motor response to pinch	1
Verbal Response		
To speech	Converses appropriately with examiner; oriented to person, place, or time	5
	Appears confused or disoriented	4
	Speaks clearly but makes no sense	3
	Makes incomprehensible sounds	2
	Makes no sound	1

Source: Reprinted from *Introduction to Clinical Neurology, 2nd Edition* (p. 273), by D. J. Gelb, 2000, with permission from Elsevier.

is more effectively used to describe the severity of the brain injury (Bushnik, Hanks, Kreutzer, & Rosenthal, 2003; Zafonte et al., 1996). Therefore, severity of brain injury is not always an indicator of the long-term functional outcomes. For example, a person with a severe brain injury may make a significant recovery and eventually return to work. Conversely, a person with a mild brain injury may have cognitive and psychosocial impairments that prevent him or her from resuming previous roles.

PREMORBID PSYCHOSOCIAL FACTORS

Beyond sex, age, and socioeconomic factors, premorbid psychiatric disturbances (e.g., psychotic disorders, anxiety, depression, and personality disorders) and a history of alcohol and drug abuse have all been associated with increased risk of brain injury as well as increased levels of neurobehavioral disturbances post-TBI (Fann et al., 2002; Hibbard et al., 1998; McGuire et al., 1998; Mooney & Speed, 2001; Ruff, Camenzuli, & Mueller, 1996; Tate et al., 1999). An understanding of premorbid personality features, coping mechanisms, and injury-related psychosocial stressors can assist the occupational therapist in developing an effective treatment plan.

Substance use and abuse is also a contributing factor to the occurrence and reoccurrence of TBI. Alcohol and drugs are estimated to be the primary cause of at least 50% to 75% of all TBIs in the United States. Alcohol- and drug-related TBIs are also associated with more complicated recoveries, longer hospitalizations, longer periods of agitation, and more impaired cognitive function at discharge from rehabilitation. Because so many persons with TBIs have premorbid substance dependency issues and are not effectively treated for these problems during rehabilitation, approximately one-third of those with substance abuse problems will return home to use substances again, which further compromises their cognitive and functional capacities (Gutman, 2001). This places them at a much higher risk of seizures and subsequent head traumas. It is important to educate clients with a TBI and their families on the importance of treatment for substance abuse disorders following acute rehabilitation to prevent future injuries from occurring and to promote recovery.

CASE ILLUSTRATION: David—Premorbid Psychosocial Contributions to TBI

David is a 26-year-old male who sustained a second traumatic brain injury from a motor vehicle accident. Three years ago, he had a brain injury from an assault. He has had a long history of drug and alcohol abuse. David's drugs of choice are amphetamines and alcohol. Over the past 10 years, he has been through three drug and alcohol recovery programs, but has been unable to remain sober.

Discussion

David's long history of substance abuse has placed him at high risk for traumatic brain injury. He is likely to present with more severe cognitive deficits, increased agitation levels, and a poorer functional outcome. He is also at risk for abusing substances following discharge from inpatient acute rehabilitation. In addition to treating David for his brain injury, the treatment team must place a high priority on treating the underlying substance abuse disorder and preventing a third injury. The occupational therapist plays a unique role in helping David reorganize his use of time to participate in healthy, meaningful, and purposeful activity that incorporates his unique interests, values, and roles.

COGNITIVE SEQUELAE FOLLOWING BRAIN INJURY

Due to the fact that cognitive functions are integrated throughout all of the brain centers, all clients with brain injury will have cognitive impairment to varying degrees. The main cognitive impairments are lack of orientation, attention deficits, impaired memory, impaired initiation and termination of activities, impaired insight, impaired judgment, impaired safety awareness, decreased information-processing abilities, and impaired executive functioning and abstract thinking ability. Cognitive skills are hierarchical and successively build from lower order to higher order cognitive functions. Each area of cognition affected by brain injury is presented from lower order to higher order.

Impaired Orientation

Persons with brain injury are often in a state of confusion following their acute injuries. Affected individuals often lose a sense of the passage of time, their external environment, their situation, and even who their family and friends are. As their confusion clears and the recovery process unveils, their orientation improves.

Persons without brain injury are often oriented to who they are (person), where they are (place), what year, month, day, or time of day it is (time), and why they are in the environment they are in (reason). However, a person with brain injury can lose orientation to person, place, time, or reason. Impaired memory and topographical orientation to the environment contributes to this confusion. Individuals with brain injury can have difficulty remembering their identity and the identity of those around them, lose a sense of the passage of time, and have a decreased awareness of themselves in relation to the environment.

Attention Deficits

Attention is a complex, dynamic ability that is regulated by the arousal systems of the brain and the more complex cerebral functions. Attention is important for maintaining concentration and focus on a task in the environment that is relevant at a particular time. It requires alertness, mental flexibility, sustained effort, and the selective ability to screen necessary and unnecessary stimulation from the environment (Katz, 1998). Attention is also imperative for higher-order information processing, such as memory and problem solving. Without attention, information cannot be coded into memory so that the individual can use this information for problem solving in future tasks. Individuals with brain injury may have minimal deficits with attention or severe attention deficits that prevent them from adapting to their environment.

There are four main types of attention that are impacted following brain injury. The simplest form of attention is focused attention, which requires the ability to focus concentration on a task for a sustained period of time without external distractions. Selective attention requires the ability to sustain focus on a task while screening out distractions from the environment, such as noise and conversation. Alternating attention requires a sustained focus on a task while also attending to relevant stimulation from the environment, such as talking on the phone while boiling pasta on the stove. Divided attention is the most unconscious form of concentration that allows an individual to alternate attention between many different tasks (multitasking). Individuals with brain injury may be able to perform tasks using some or all types of attention, but may be impaired with their ability to sustain this attention for the required amount of time for task completion.

Impaired Memory

Impaired short-term memory is the most frequent complaint from individuals with brain injury and can often be the source of long-term disability throughout the lifespan. Memory requires the dynamic ability to code, store, and retrieve relevant past or present information. Memory requires sustained attention to information for temporary storage into short-term memory and encoding into long-term memory. Most clients with brain injury recover long-term memory, but have enduring deficits with short-term memory, which affects their ability to learn and problem-solve through new tasks and occupations.

There are many types of memory that affect an individual's ability to engage in occupation. Declarative memory is required to recall or recite information, such as personal history and experiences, people, language, and rules of social behavior (Katz, 1998). Prospective memory requires the ability to remember future events, such as important deadlines and appointments. Because individuals with brain injury may have significant gaps in memory and are confused about the details pertaining to time, people, and places, they may use **confabulation** to fill in the missing gaps with erroneous information. Confabulation is not an intentional process and is the result of confusion that leads the person with brain injury to unconsciously make sense out of the broken pieces of information and control his or her thought processes.

Because individuals with brain injury tend to have significant short-term memory deficits related to declarative and prospective information, it is important for the occupational therapist to assist the client in engaging in familiar occupations that tap into procedural memory, which is the subcortical memory of skill and task performance. Procedural memory is responsible for assisting clients with significant memory deficits to engage in familiar tasks without recalling the steps involved. Most occupations that are performed prior to the brain injury can be accessed using procedural memory, particularly those tasks performed since early childhood.

Impaired Initiation and Termination of Activities

Survivors of brain injury tend to have difficulty starting and ending activities throughout their day. **Initiation** refers to the ability to begin an activity at an appropriate time in the day to accomplish a goal. This ability is impaired primarily by damage to the frontal lobe of the brain. The client may require verbal cues from caregivers to begin the activity. Conversely, the client may have difficulty terminating an activity after starting by perseverating on a task that is no longer productive. **Perseveration** refers to the inability to disengage from an activity and reengage in a more appropriate activity. Perseveration may also be a constant thought pattern that permeates the individual's mind and keeps the person from engaging in more appropriate activity.

Impaired Insight, Judgment, and Safety Awareness

Individuals with frontal lobe damage from brain injury often present with impaired insight into their limitations and disabilities. Impaired insight does not result from denial as a coping mechanism. Individuals with frontal lobe damage have a cognitive impairment, also referred to as **anosognosia,** which inhibits them from recognizing or acknowledging deficits in cognition, perception, or mobility (Unsworth, 1999). Without appropriate levels of insight, the person with brain injury tends to exhibit poor judgment in decision making, which can lead to poor safety awareness. For example, an individual with poor mobility, visual neglect, and poor insight may underestimate the time required to cross a busy street and will cross without using the crosswalk.

Impaired Information Processing

Following brain injury, individuals tend to require an increased amount of time to process information during social conversations, activities of daily living, and information from the external environment. The delayed speed in processing information is the result of a variety of factors, including decreased alertness, impaired perceptual skills, decreased attention, decreased memory, and an increased time for the brain to encode information before processing. It may appear as if the client is not responding or processing information at all, but with increased time, the client will often be able to answer the question or complete a task.

Impaired Executive Functions

Executive functions are higher-order cognitive processes that are controlled primarily by the frontal lobe. Executive functions enable a person to identify a problem, plan a strategy for problem solving, develop goals for the future, and modify a plan of action based on information from the environment (Burgess et al., 1998). Individuals with brain injury tend to have difficulty, particularly in the early stages of learning, in identifying problems, planning, goal-setting, and using mental flexibility to modify a plan of action based on information received from the external environment. Impaired executive functions can often be the most disabling part of brain injury, since executive functions are essential for problem solving, planning for the future, being effective in a work environment, and managing oneself safely in the home and community.

Impaired Abstract Thinking and Integration of New Learning

Clients with brain injury tend to also have difficulty using **abstract thinking** to critically reason and use analytical methods to infer relationships between ideas and filter irrelevant details from relevant information (Burgess et al., 1998). Clients with brain injury may not be able to understand analogies, jokes, or inferences.

Because individuals with brain injury tend to think on the most concrete level, this prevents **generalization** of cognitive and functional skills to a variety of different environments, thus limiting the amount of new learning that can occur. This is why it is often difficult for a client with brain injury to carry a skill learned in the acute hospital environment to the home environment. It is critical for occupational therapists working with clients with brain injury to assess the environment that the client is returning to and to treat in this environment as much as possible.

CASE ILLUSTRATION: Tony—Cognitive Sequelae Following TBI

Tony is a 33-year-old male who sustained a traumatic brain injury from a penetrating gunshot wound to the right frontal lobe. Tony is only oriented to person. He is only oriented to his own name. He is unable to recall the date, place of hospitalization, or the reason he is in the hospital. Tony also presents with a short attention span, and is only able to engage in a simple activity for 30 seconds before losing attention to the task. Tony has good recall of his life before the brain injury, but is unable to recall new information after a five-minute delay. Tony has difficulty initiating activity and after beginning an activity, he has difficulty transitioning to a new activity. Tony demonstrates poor safety awareness, and states that he is ready to leave the hospital. The occupational therapist has provided Tony with a memory log to help him remember important dates, people, and appointments. The occupational therapist has also structured the environment to reduce noise and distractions to assist Tony in processing information effectively and engaging in activities with a longer period of sustained attention.

Discussion

Tony demonstrates classic cognitive impairments with orientation, attention, short-term memory, initiation and termination of activity, judgment, safety awareness, and information processing. Tony will also have deficits with higher-order executive functions and abstract reasoning due to the fact that he is unable to attend to tasks for long periods of time and store information into long-term memory. His organization, time management, and planning ability will most likely be compromised due to the lower-order cognitive impairments. In addition to providing a memory log and restructuring the treatment environment, the occupational therapist can begin treatment by focusing on concrete, one-step tasks that tap into procedural memory, which is responsible for assisting clients with significant memory deficits to engage in familiar tasks without recalling the steps involved. Most occupations that are performed prior to the brain injury can be accessed using procedural memory, particularly those tasks performed since early childhood. Basic activities of daily living, simple leisure tasks, and basic home management are examples of activities that can be used to tap into procedural memory. Each task can be upgraded or downgraded to the individual's cognitive level.

BEHAVIORAL SEQUELAE FOLLOWING BRAIN INJURY

The behavioral sequelae following brain injury are sometimes the most challenging aspects of client management. Many of the behavioral syndromes are temporary and part of the recovery process, while others can persist in some degree throughout the lifespan. The main behavioral sequelae following brain injury are agitation, aggression, disinhibition, hypersexual behaviors, demotivational syndrome, and inappropriate emotional responses.

Agitation and Aggression

Agitation and aggression are the most common behavioral sequelae following brain injury. Agitation is typical of those clients in the Rancho Los Amigos Cognitive Level IV stage of recovery—Confused and Agitated (Hagen, Malkmus, & Stenderup-Bowman, 1973). Because of their level of confusion and inability to process sensory information from the environment correctly, clients in this stage may display decreased frustration tolerance, and be socially inappropriate, restless, impulsive, verbally combative, and physically assaultive. Clients in this stage can also escalate very quickly into an aggressive and combative state, and it is important to work with a team of other professionals to manage these behaviors early in the recovery process. This stage of recovery is also the most frightening for families, who often have never seen their loved one verbally or physically assault another human being. It is important to educate family members and staff that this is a normal part of the recovery process and is rarely permanent.

Disinhibition

Clients with frontal lobe damage tend to also exhibit impulsive, perseveratory behavior that often disinhibits them from making inappropriate verbal remarks and causes them to participate in unsafe activities. For example, **disinhibition** is observed with a client who states that a therapist is "fat" or "ugly." The normal filters that we use to screen our behaviors in response to social norms become void. In addition, the client with brain injury may also perseverate on tasks that are nonpurposeful, inappropriate, or unsafe. It is as if the client has no control over participation in these activities. It is often difficult to confront the individual, which can sometimes provoke agitation or inappropriate verbal remarks.

Hypersexual Behaviors

Individuals with brain injury can also have difficulty controlling sexual urges that can lead to inappropriate sexual advances with treatment staff, friends, and even family members. Because the therapeutic relationship between an occupational therapist and his or her client is one of respect, tolerance, and trust, some clients will misinterpret this relationship as a sexual advance on behalf of the staff member. Other times, the client purely has a sexual urge and is not able to inhibit his or her desires. Negative behaviors, such as masturbation in a public area, touching, fondling, sexual remarks, and sometimes intercourse with other clients, take place in treatment settings where there is little structure and supervision.

Demotivational Syndrome

Apathy and disinterest in previous occupations can sometimes result from frontal lobe damage following head trauma. For some clients, the **demotivational syndrome** is the result of a lack of initiation and sustained participation in activity, and for others it can be an outright refusal to participate in previously enjoyed activities. Depression can also be a contributing factor to the lack of motivation to participate in everyday activities. It is important to consult with the treatment team to differentiate between major depression and demotivational syndrome from brain injury.

Inappropriate Emotional Responses

Emotional lability, decreased affect (flat), or increased affect (euphoria) can result following brain injury. A client may laugh, cry, or scream out of proportion to the environmental stimulus. Those clients with left hemisphere damage tend to have increased levels of depression and emotional lability, from euphoric to flat (Ownsworth, 1998). It is important to note that a person may appear to be depressed, when in actuality, the person presents with a flat, expressionless affect. Conversely, clients with right hemisphere lesions tend to have a heightened state of euphoria that is often coupled with more severe impairments in insight, emotional maturity, and perceptual awareness.

CASE ILLUSTRATION: Brad—Behavioral Sequelae Following TBI

Brad is a 19-year-old male who sustained a traumatic brain injury (multiple injuries to his frontal, parietal, and temporal lobes) from an assault. He demonstrates a high level of agitation and is extremely restless. He frequently yells out profanities and is physically aggressive with staff. Brad is emotionally labile and very quickly escalates from laughing to crying and shouting out loud. Brad has also made several inappropriate sexual advances to female staff.

Discussion

Brad currently demonstrates many of the behavioral characteristics of a person recovering from brain injury at a Rancho Los Amigos Cognitive Level IV: Confused and Agitated. His behavior is not volitional or intentional. Brad is having difficulty processing all of the information from his environment. In order to maximize Brad's recovery in this stage, the occupational therapist can engage the client in gross motor activity (such as tossing a ball or taking a walk), vestibular stimulation activities such as riding around in a wheelchair, or simple one-step activities; minimize distractions; and establish trust by providing a safe and comfortable treatment environment.

The occupational therapist may interview family members to find out which activities have provided the greatest level of comfort for the client (e.g., eating, listening to music, etc.). Do not force the client to do something he does not want to do. Instead, listen to what he wants to do and follow his lead, within safety limits. Since the client is often distractible, restless, and agitated at this phase of recovery, remember to provide frequent breaks from activity and be prepared to change activities quickly. The occupational therapist can also modify the environment to increase the client's level of comfort by having family members bring in pictures and personal items from home.

PSYCHOSOCIAL SEQUELAE FOLLOWING BRAIN INJURY

Brain injury involves a sudden onset with little preparation for the impact of various changes, unlike persistent mental illness that can develop and be present over the course of a lifetime. One day, a person may be managing her or his own business or taking a family trip around the world, and the next day, the person may be paralyzed on one-half of the body, unable to communicate, remember, feel, or function.

While cognition and behavior can significantly and rapidly improve during the acute stages, brain injury can have a lifelong impact on the psychosocial adjustment of the individual. Thus, the psychosocial sequelae are sometimes the most devastating aspects of the disease for the affected individual and his or her family. Changes in overall mental health, personality, coping mechanisms, self-concept, social relationships, and the family dynamic can significantly alter the person's ability to adapt and master his or her environment.

Psychiatric Disorders

Due to the chemical changes in the brain following trauma and acquired events, the individual is often susceptible to mood disorders, anxiety disorders, and perceptual dysfunction that can contribute to hallucinations and paranoia. Premorbid mental illness, particularly personality disorders and alcohol and drug abuse, can significantly impact the recovery process and the severity of the psychosocial sequelae. For example, a person who suffered from depression and also had sociopathic behaviors prior to injury may have increased levels of depressed mood, agitation, and inappropriate social behaviors. Mood disorders, chemical dependency, delirium, psychotic disorders, aggressive disorders, and anxiety disorders are among the most common psychiatric disorders following brain injury (Yudofsky & Hales, 2002). In addition, approximately one-quarter of persons with brain injury also suffer from depression and other psychiatric illnesses post-TBI, which is affected by poor premorbid social functioning and previous psychiatric disorders pre-TBI (Fedoroff et al., 1992).

Changes in Personality and Impaired Social Pragmatics

Families often report that their loved one no longer has the same personality following brain injury. A variety of factors can contribute to an overall change in personality, such as cognitive and behavioral changes, changes in areas of the brain that contribute to personality, premorbid personality traits, and the severity of damage to the brain (Golden & Golden, 2003). An introverted person preinjury may suddenly become outgoing, and an outgoing person may become withdrawn and expressionless. Conversely, a person who "lived on the edge" may exhibit even more risky behaviors postinjury. Clients with TBI also tend to exhibit egocentric behaviors that interfere with their ability to participate in social activities that require turn-taking, sharing, reciprocal conversation, and other socially appropriate habits. These personality changes can have a devastating impact on the ability to maintain successful relationships with partners, friends, and family members, especially when the other person does not understand the course of recovery from brain injury. As time goes on postinjury, the person with brain injury often will find close friends and family members becoming less involved in her or his life. This can alter social roles immensely and lead to a feeling of isolation and abandonment. Even more difficult is building new relationships due to the lack of social pragmatic ability.

Impaired Coping Mechanisms

Due to impaired executive functions that inhibit problem-solving abilities and premorbid coping skills, clients with brain injury may have difficulty managing frustration, anger, and loss of function. Particularly in the later stages of recovery, the client with brain injury is required to deal with a tremendous amount of loss to his or her personality, social relationships, ability to engage in previously enjoyed occupations, and the ability to feel secure about the future. Compounding these issues are stressors regarding financial stability and sometimes legal issues postinjury. Ineffective coping strategies preinjury may also contribute to even more impairments with these abilities postinjury. The client is now required to manage greater amounts of stressors in his or her life, and may or may not have the ability to learn new strategies to cope with these stressors.

Altered Self-Concept

Self-concept is the internal image one has of self regarding body image; position in the family, peer group, and community; sexual and gender identity; and personal strengths and limitations. Brain injury can result in major disfigurement due to trauma, surgical craniotomies, and scars, which impacts a person's internalized self-image. Coupled with this change are reactions from society when the person enters the community for the first time postinjury. Individuals with brain injury are usually in adolescence or early adulthood when self-concept is still forming, which impacts their ability to deal effectively with the societal expectations for what is beautiful.

As individuals with brain injury recover, their long-term memory often will come back before their short-term memory. They often have a very good memory of who they were before the injury, and there is an internal conflict with having to let go of many of their goals, ambitions, and position in society. The individual is challenged to rebuild a postinjury self-concept that is meaningful and satisfying, which can lead to an identity crisis and deep depression due to the immense challenge of re-creating a life that has been lost (Ownsworth, 1998).

Impact of Brain Injury on Family Dynamics

Individuals with brain injury must cope with the loss of position within the family unit postinjury. The family members may also be resentful that their loved one may no longer be able to function as an effective partner, parent, or child. Coupled with this loss is the amount of dependence the individual will have postinjury. The client will often require close supervision and assistance from family members in daily activities. The lost ability to live independently in the community can further reinforce the individual's perceived loss of control or mastery over his or her environment. This can create strain in the relationship between the individual with brain injury and family members (Curtiss, Klemz, & Vanderploeg, 2000; Gosling & Oddy, 1999; Lanham, Weissenburger, Schwab, & Rosner, 2000). However, a study conducted by Perlesz, Kinsella, and Crowe (2000) concluded that "many families—despite their initial traumatic experience—eventually cope well, encouraging researchers and clinicians to focus future research efforts on those families who have made good adjustments to TBI" (p. 909).

> **CASE ILLUSTRATION: Tammy—Psychosocial Sequelae Following TBI**
>
> *Tammy is a 25-year-old who sustained a traumatic brain injury from a motor vehicle accident. She also suffered multiple facial trauma from the car accident, which has left her with permanent scarring. She was diagnosed three years ago with major depression. She is currently functioning at a Rancho Los Amigos Level VII: Automatic-Appropriate. While she has mild memory problems, her cognitive impairments are secondary to her psychosocial adjustment to disability. Tammy demonstrates a depressed mood, a flat affect, poor frustration tolerance, and poor self-concept. She avoids social situations and prefers to be alone. She states that she is embarrassed to be around her family and friends because of her disfigurement.*
>
> **Discussion**
>
> *Tammy demonstrates poor psychosocial adjustment to her disability. Her major depression is magnified by the recent brain injury, which has altered her mood, coping mechanisms, self-concept, and social pragmatics. In order to treat Tammy effectively, the treatment team will need to address the underlying psychiatric disorder and assist her in developing constructive coping mechanisms, opportunities for success in task performance, gradual group intervention to work on social skills, and community reentry activities to assist her in developing acceptance of her disability.*

INTERDISCIPLINARY ASSESSMENT AND TREATMENT

The **Rancho Los Amigos Levels of Cognitive Functioning** (Table 14-3) is a common rating scale used to assist the interdisciplinary team in determining the client's cognitive, behavioral, and functional status following brain injury (Hagen, Malkmus, & Stenderup-Bowman, 1973). The scale has established interrater reliability and validity (Dowling, 1985; Gouvier, Blanton, LaPorte, & Nepomuceno, 1987). The eight cognitive levels include a description of the common cognitive, behavioral, and psychosocial sequelae associated with recovery from brain

Table 14-3. Rancho Los Amigos Levels of Cognitive Functioning (2nd ed.)

Cognitive level	Behavioral characteristics	Interdisciplinary treatment approaches for managing cognitive, behavioral, and psychosocial sequelae
Level I: No Response	• Complete absence of observable change in behavior when presented with visual, auditory, tactile, proprioceptive, vestibular, or painful stimuli.	• Explain to the individual what you are about to do. For example, "I'm going to move your leg." • Talk in a normal tone of voice. • Keep comments and questions short and simple. For example, instead of "Can you turn your head towards me?", say, "Look at me." • Tell the person who you are, where he is, why he is in the hospital, and what day it is. • Limit the number of visitors to two to three people at a time. • Keep the room calm and quiet. • Bring in favorite belongings and pictures of family members and close friends. • Allow the person extra time to respond, but don't expect responses to be correct. Sometimes the person may not respond at all. • Give him rest periods. He will tire easily. • Engage him in familiar activities, such as listening to his favorite music, talking about family and friends, reading out loud to him, watching TV, combing his hair, putting on lotion, etc. • He may understand parts of what you are saying. Therefore, be careful what you say in front of the individual.
Level II: Generalized Response	• Demonstrates generalized reflex response to painful stimuli.	• Same approach as for Level I.

(continues)

Table 14-3. (continued)

Cognitive level	Behavioral characteristics	Interdisciplinary treatment approaches for managing cognitive, behavioral, and psychosocial sequelae
	• Responds to repeated auditory stimuli with increased or decreased activity. • Responds to external stimuli with physiological changes generalized, gross body movement, and/or not purposeful vocalization. • Responses noted above may be same regardless of type and location of stimulation. • Responses may be significantly delayed.	
Level III: Localized Response	• Demonstrates withdrawal or vocalization to painful stimuli. • Turns toward or away from auditory stimuli. • Blinks when strong light crosses visual field. • Follows moving object passed within visual field. • Responds to discomfort by pulling tubes or restraints. • Responds inconsistently to simple commands. • Responses directly related to type of stimulus. • May respond to some persons (especially family and friends), but not to others.	• Same approach as for Levels I and II
Level IV: Confused-Agitated	• Alert and in heightened state of activity. • Purposeful attempts to remove restraints or tubes or crawl out of bed. • May perform motor activities such as sitting, reaching, and walking, but without any apparent purpose or upon another's request. • Very brief and usually nonpurposeful moments of sustained alternatives and divided attention. • Absent short-term memory.	• Tell the person where he is and reassure him that he is safe. • Bring in family pictures and personal items from home, to make him feel more comfortable. • Allow him as much movement as is safe. • Take him for rides in his wheelchair, when this has been approved by the treating team. • Experiment to find familiar activities that are calming to him such as listening to music, eating, etc.

(continues)

Table 14-3. (continued)

Cognitive level	Behavioral characteristics	Interdisciplinary treatment approaches for managing cognitive, behavioral, and psychosocial sequelae
	• Absent goal-directed, problem-solving, self-monitoring behavior. • May cry out or scream out of proportion to stimulus even after its removal. • May exhibit aggressive or flight behavior. • Mood may swing from euphoric to hostile with no apparent relationship to environmental events. • Unable to cooperate with treatment efforts. • Verbalizations are frequently incoherent and/or inappropriate to activity or environment.	• Do not force him to do things. Instead, listen to what he wants to do and follow his lead, within safety limits. • Since he often becomes distracted, restless, or agitated, you may need to give him breaks and change activities frequently. • Keep the room quiet and calm. For example, turn off the TV and radio, don't talk too much and use a calm voice. • Limit the number of visitors to two to three people at a time.
Level V: Confused-Inappropriate-Non-Agitated	• Alert, not agitated, but may wander randomly or with a vague intention of going home. • May become agitated in response to external stimulation and/or lack of environmental structure. • Not oriented to person, place, or time. • Frequent brief periods of non-purposeful sustained attention. • Severely impaired recent memory, with confusion of past and present in reaction to ongoing activity. • Absent goal-directed, problem-solving, self-monitoring behavior. • Often demonstrates inappropriate use of objects without external direction. • May be able to perform previously learned tasks when structure and cues are provided. • Unable to learn new information.	• Repeat things as needed. Don't assume that he will remember what you tell him. • Tell him the day, date, name and location of the hospital, and why he is in the hospital when you first arrive and before you leave. • Keep comments and questions short and simple. • Help him organize and get started on an activity. • Have the family bring in pictures and personal items from home. • Limit the number of visitors to two to three at a time. • Give him frequent rest periods when he has problems paying attention.

(continues)

Table 14-3. (continued)

Cognitive level	Behavioral characteristics	Interdisciplinary treatment approaches for managing cognitive, behavioral, and psychosocial sequelae
	• Able to respond appropriately to simple commands fairly consistently with external structures and cues.	
	• Responses to simple commands without external structure are random and nonpurposeful in relation to the command.	
	• Able to converse on a social, automatic level for brief periods of time when provided external structure and cues.	
	• Verbalizations about present events become inappropriate and confabulatory when external structure and cues are not provided.	
Level VI: Confused-Appropriate	• Inconsistently oriented to person and place. • Able to attend to highly familiar tasks in nondistracting environment for 30 minutes with moderate redirection. • Remote memory has more depth and detail than recent memory. • Vague recognition of some staff. • Able to use assistive memory aid with maximal assistance. • Emerging awareness of appropriate response to self, family, and basic needs. • Emerging goal-directed behavior related to meeting basic personal needs. • Moderate assistance required to problem-solve barriers to task completion. • Supervised for old learning (e.g., self-care). • Shows carry-over for relearned familiar tasks (e.g., self-care). • Maximal assistance required for new learning with little or no carryover.	• You will need to repeat things. Discuss things that have happened during the day to help the individual remember recent events and activities. • He may need help starting and continuing activities. • Encourage the individual to participate in all therapies. He will not fully understand the extent of his problems and the benefits of therapy.

(continues)

Table 14-3. (continued)

Cognitive level	Behavioral characteristics	Interdisciplinary treatment approaches for managing cognitive, behavioral, and psychosocial sequelae
	• Unaware of impairments, disabilities, and safety risks. • Consistently follows simple directions. • Verbal expressions are appropriate in highly familiar and structured situations.	
Level VII: Automatic-Appropriate	• Consistently oriented to person and place, within highly familiar environments. Moderate assistance for orientation to time. • Able to attend to highly familiar tasks in a nondistracting environment for at least 30 minutes with minimal assistance to complete tasks. • Able to use assistive memory devices with minimal assistance. • Minimal supervision for new learning. • Demonstrates carryover of new learning. • Initiates and carries out steps to complete familiar personal and household routines, but has shallow recall of what he or she has been doing. • Able to monitor accuracy and completeness of each step in routine personal and household ADLs and modify plan with minimal assistance. • Superficial awareness of his or her condition, but unaware of specific impairments and disabilities and the limits they place on his or her ability to safely, accurately, and completely carry out his or her household, community, work, and leisure tasks. • Unrealistic planning for the future.	• Treat the person as an adult; show respect for his opinion when attempting to provide guidance and assistance in decision making. • Talk with the individual as an adult. There is no need to try to use simple words or sentences. • Because the individual may misunderstand joking, teasing, or slang language, be careful to check for understanding when using humor or other abstract language. • Encourage the individual to be as independent as is safe. Help him with activities when he shows problems with thinking, problem solving, and memory. Talk to him about these problems without criticizing. Reassure him that the problems are because of the brain injury. • Strongly encourage the individual to continue with therapy to increase his thinking, memory and physical abilities. He may feel he is completely normal. However, he is still making progress and may possibly benefit from continued treatment. • Be sure to check with the physician on the individual's restrictions concerning driving, working, and other activities. Do not rely on the brain-injured individual for information, since he may feel he is ready to go back to his previous lifestyle.

(continues)

Table 14-3. (continued)

Cognitive level	Behavioral characteristics	Interdisciplinary treatment approaches for managing cognitive, behavioral, and psychosocial sequelae
	• Unable to think about consequences of a decision or action. • Overestimates abilities. • Unaware of others' needs and feelings. • Oppositional/uncooperative. • Unable to recognize inappropriate social interaction behavior.	• Discourage him from drinking or using drugs. • Encourage him to use note taking as a way to help with memory problems. • Encourage him to carry out his self-care as independently as possible. • Discuss what kinds of situations make him angry and what he can do in these situations. • Talk with him about his feelings. • Learning to live with a brain injury is difficult and it may take a long time for the individual and family to adjust. The social worker and/or psychologist will provide family members and friends with information regarding counseling, resources, and support organizations.
Level VIII: Purposeful and Appropriate	• Consistently oriented to person, place, and time. • Independently attends to and completes familiar tasks for one hour in a distracting environment. • Able to recall and integrate past and recent events. • Uses assistive memory devices to recall daily schedule, "to do" lists, and record critical information for later use with standby assistance. • Initiates and carries out steps to complete familiar personal, household, community, work, and leisure routines with standby assistance, and can modify the plan when needed with minimal assistance. • Requires no assistance once new tasks/activities are learned.	• Same as Level VII.

(continues)

Table 14-3. (continued)

Cognitive level	Behavioral characteristics	Interdisciplinary treatment approaches for managing cognitive, behavioral, and psychosocial sequelae
	• Aware of and acknowledges impairments and disabilities when they interfere with task completion, but requires stand-by assistance to take appropriate corrective action.	
	• Thinks about consequences of a decision or action with minimal assistance.	
	• Overestimates or underestimates abilities.	
	• Acknowledges others' needs and feelings and responds appropriately with minimal assistance.	
	• Depressed.	
	• Irritable.	
	• Low frustration tolerance/easily angered.	
	• Argumentative.	
	• Self-centered.	
	• Uncharacteristically dependent/independent.	
	• Able to recognize and acknowledge inappropriate social interaction behavior while it is occurring and takes corrective action with minimal assistance.	

Source: Adapted with permission from Los Amigos Research and Educational Institute, Copyright 1975.

injury. However, because it is an ordinal scale, or a scale that ranks levels from low to high, differences between levels on the scale are not equivalent (Sachs et al., 1986). In other words, the differences between Levels I and II on the scale are not the same as the differences between Levels II and III. Moreover, some survivors of brain injury do not always proceed through each of the levels. Some clients skip many of the levels during the recovery process, and some individuals may progress only to a certain level and no farther (Corrigan & Mysiw, 1988; Rao, Jellinek, & Woolston, 1985). However, the Rancho Los Amigos Levels of Cognitive Functioning provides a useful tool for evaluating the cognitive and behavioral status of the client and also aids in the interdisciplinary treatment planning process. The Rancho levels can also serve as an effective family education tool by helping the caregiver to understand the progression of the recovery process and how to assist the client during recovery. Table 14-3 describes a variety of cognitive, behavioral, and psychosocial treatment strategies at each of the stages of recovery that can be implemented by the occupational therapist and the inter-disciplinary team.

Each person will progress differently, depending on the severity of brain dam-age, the length of time since the initial onset of injury, and the location of damage. Some individuals may progress through each of the eight cognitive levels, while others may progress only to a certain level and no farther. It is also important to remember that each person is an individual, and each person may fit some or all of the criteria under each level.

OCCUPATIONAL THERAPY INTERVENTIONS

In addition to interdisciplinary management, the occupational therapist plays a vital role on the interdisciplinary team in assisting the person with brain injury to resume previous life roles, assume new life roles post-TBI, effectively engage in occupations that are important to him or her, and assist the person with brain injury in adapting to home, community, school, and/or work environments. In the early stages of recovery, the occupational therapist may work on remediative or compensatory strategies for cognitive deficits, social skills retraining, and func-tional skills retraining. The task or environment may also be adapted to increase optimal functioning.

In the later stages of recovery, the occupational therapist uses a more client-centered approach to assist the person with brain injury to identify goals that are important to him or her and help him or her toward regaining occupational func-tioning in all areas of occupation, such as basic and instrumental activities of daily living, education, work, play, leisure, and social participation. A study conducted by Trombly, Radomski, and Davis (1998) concluded that "participants attending outpatient occupational therapy significantly improved and improvements were sustained after discharge, but no further improvement occurred spontaneously" (p. 810). Client-centered assessments, such as the Canadian Occupational Per-formance Measure, assist the occupational therapist in tailoring treatment goals to those activities that the client needs to do or wants to do in his or her environ-ment (Law et al., 1999). The unique contribution of the occupational therapist is to assist the client in managing and adapting to the cognitive, behavioral, and psy-chosocial impairments by engaging in productive, meaningful, and satisfying occupations that support role performance and social participation in the context of the person's unique environment.

Summary

Brain injury, which results from both traumatic and acquired events, is a public health concern that contributes to a high number of deaths and, for many who sur-vive, long-term disability. Brain injury presents with a complex clinical picture because of the effects of injury on the intricate neuronal networks throughout the brain that control cognition, behavior, perception, mobility, and vital life functions.

- Cognitive sequelae following brain injury include impairments in orientation, attention, memory, initiation and termination of activities, insight, judgment, safety awareness, information processing, executive functions, abstract reasoning, and new learning.
- Behavioral sequelae following brain injury include agitation, aggression, disinhibition, hypersexual behaviors, demotivational syndrome, and inappropriate emotional responses.
- Psychosocial sequelae following brain injury include psychiatric disorders, changes in personality, impaired social pragmatics, impaired coping mechanisms, changes in self-concept, and strains on the family dynamic.

The Rancho Los Amigos Levels of Cognitive Functioning assists the occupational therapist in describing the client's cognitive, behavioral, and psychosocial problem areas following brain injury and in planning appropriate interventions. The occupational therapist working with clients with brain injury are challenged to provide holistic, client-centered care that addresses the cognitive, behavioral, and psychosocial dimensions of the person's functioning to increase therapeutic effectiveness and to promote optimal recovery for the client.

Review Questions

1. Why is it important for the occupational therapist to consider an individual's premorbid psychosocial status prior to initiating treatment?
2. How do the Glasgow Coma Scale and the Rancho Los Amigos Levels of Cognitive Functioning help the occupational therapist to predict and plan the course of intervention for a person with brain injury?
3. How do the hierarchical levels of cognition influence the individual's ability to engage in occupation?
4. How can the occupational therapist capitalize on the client's current cognitive level to maximize task performance?
5. How do behavioral factors interfere with occupational performance?
6. How could the treatment environment be structured to decrease negative behaviors?
7. How does brain injury impact the individual's self-concept, social relationships, and internal drive to master her or his environment?

References

American Psychiatric Association. (2000). *Diagnostic and statistical manual of mental disorders* (4th ed.-Text Revision). Washington, DC: Author.

Brain Injury Association of America. (2001). *Types of brain injury.* Retrieved February 29, 2003, from www.biausa.org.

Bruns, J., & Hauser, W. A. (2003). The epidemiology of traumatic brain injury: A review. *Epilepsia, 44* (Supplement 10), 2–10.

Burgess, P. W., et al. (1998). Ecological validity of tests of executive function. *Journal of the International Neuropsychological Society, 4,* 547.

Bushnik, T., Hanks, R. A., Kreutzer, J., & Rosenthal, M. (2003). Etiology of traumatic brain injury: Characterization of differential outcomes up to 1 year postinjury. *Archives of Physical and Medical Rehabilitation, 84,* 255–262.

Centers for Disease Control (CDC). (2001). *Traumatic brain injury.* CDC.

Corrigan, J. D., & Mysiw, W. J. (1988). Agitation following traumatic head injury: Equivocal evidence for a discrete stage of cognitive recovery. *Archives of Physical and Medical Rehabilitation, 69,* 487–492.

Curtiss, G., Klemz, S., & Vanderploeg, R. D. (2000). Acute impact of severe traumatic brain injury on family structure and coping responses. *Journal of Head Trauma Rehabilitation, 15*(5), 1113–1122.

Dowling, G. A. (1985). Levels of cognitive functioning: Evaluation of interrater reliability. *Journal of Neurosurgical Nursing, 17*(2), 129–134.

Fann, J. R., Leonetti, A., Jaffe, K., Katon, W. J., Cummings, P., & Thompson, R. S. (2002). Psychiatric illness and subsequent traumatic brain injury: A case control study. *Journal of Neurology, Neurosurgery, and Psychiatry, 72*(5), 615–620.

Fedoroff, J. P., Starkstein, S. E., Forrester, A. W., Geisler, F. H., Jorge, R. E., Arndt, S. V., & Robinson, R. G. (1992). Depression in patients with acute traumatic brain injury. *American Journal of Psychiatry, 149*(7), 918–923.

Gelb, D. J. (2000). Introduction to clinical neurology (2nd ed.) St. Louis, MO: Elsevier Science.

Golden, Z., & Golden, C. J. (2003). Impact of brain injury severity on personality dysfunction. *International Journal of Neuroscience, 113*(5), 733–745.

Gosling, J., & Oddy, M. (1999). Rearranged marriages: Martial relationships after head injury. *Brain Injury, 13*(10), 785–796.

Gouvier, W. D., Blanton, P. D., LaPorte, K. K., & Nepomuceno, C. (1987). Reliability and validity of the Disability Rating Scale and Levels of Cognitive Functioning Scale in monitoring recovery from severe head injury. *Archives of Physical and Medical Rehabilitation, 68,* 94–97.

Gutman, S. A. (2001). Traumatic brain injury. In L. Pedretti & M. B. Early (Eds.), *Occupational therapy practice skills for physical dysfunction* (5th ed.). St. Louis, MO: Mosby.

Hagen, C., Malkmus, D., & Stenderup-Bowman, K. (1973). *The Rancho Levels of Cognitive Functioning* (2nd ed.). Downey, CA: Los Amigos Research and Educational Institute.

Hibbard, M. R., Uysal, S., Kepler, K., Bogdany, J., & Silver, J. (1998). Axis I psychopathology in individuals with traumatic brain injury. *Journal of Head Trauma Rehabilitation, 13*(4), 24–39.

Katz, N. (1998). *Cognition and occupational therapy in rehabilitation.* American Occupational Therapy Association.

Lanham, R. A., Weissenburger, J. E., Schwab, K. A., & Rosner, M. M. (2000). A longitudinal investigation of the concordance between individuals with traumatic brain injury and family or friend ratings on the Katz adjustment scale. *Journal of Head Trauma Rehabilitation, 15*(5), 1123–1138.

Law, M., Baptiste, S., McColl, M. A., Carswell, A., Polatajko, H., & Pollock, N. (1999). *Canadian Occupational Performance Measure* (3rd ed). Toronto: Canadian Association of Occupational Therapists.

Leahy, B. J., & Lam, C. S. (1998). Neuropsychological testing and functional outcome for individuals with traumatic brain injury. *Brain Injury, 12*(12), 1025–1035.

McGuire, L. M., Burright, R. G., Williams, R., & Donovick, P. J. (1998). Prevalence of traumatic brain injury in psychiatric and non-psychiatric subjects. *Brain Injury, 12*(3), 207–214.

Mooney, G., & Speed, J. (2001). The association between mild traumatic brain injury and psychiatric conditions. *Brain Injury, 15*(10), 865–877.

Occupational Therapy Practice Framework: Domain and Process. (2002). *American Journal of Occupational Therapy, 56,* 609–639.

Ownsworth, T. L. (1998). Depression after traumatic brain injury. *Brain Injury, 12,* 735–751.

Perlesz, A., Kinsella, G., & Crowe, S. (2000). Psychological distress and family satisfaction following traumatic brain injury: Injured individuals and their primary, secondary, and tertiary carers. *Journal of Head Trauma, 15*(3), 909–929.

Pulaski, K. H. (2003). Adult Neurological Dysfunction. In E. B. Crepeau, E. S. Cohen, & B. A. B. Shell (Eds.), *Willard and Spackman's occupational therapy* (10th ed.). Philadelphia: Lippincott Williams & Wilkins.

Radomski, M. V. (2002). Traumatic brain injury. In C. Trombly & M. V. Radomski (Eds.), *Occupational therapy for physical dysfunction* (5th ed.). Baltimore: Lippincott Williams & Wilkins.

Rao, N., Jellinek, H. M., & Woolston, D. C. (1985). Agitation in closed head injury: Haloperidol effects on rehabilitation outcome. *Archives of Physical and Medical Rehabilitation, 66,* 30–34.

Rothweiler, B., Temkin, N. R., & Dikmen, S. S. (1998). Aging effect on psychosocial outcome in traumatic brain injury. *Archives of Physical Medicine and Rehabilitation, 79*(8), 881–887.

Ruff, R. M., Camenzuli, L., & Mueller, J. (1996). Miserable minority: Emotional risk factors that influence the outcome of a mild traumatic brain injury. *Brain Injury, 10*(8), 551–565.

Sachs, P. R., Bell, E., Berger, M., Carroll, R. C., Davidson, K., Heavener, W., et al. (1986). A six-factor model for treatment planning and cognitive retraining of the traumatically head-injured adult. *Cognitive rehabilitation, 4,* 26–30.

Sadock, B. J., & Sadock, V. A. (2003). *Kaplan and Sadock's synopsis of psychiatry: Behavioral sciences, clinical psychiatry.* Lippincott Williams & Wilkins.

Tate, P. S., Freed, D. M., Bombardier, C. H., Harter, S. L., & Brinkman, S. (1999). Traumatic brain injury: Influence of blood alcohol level on post-acute cognitive function. *Brain Injury, 13*(10), 767–784.

Thurman, D. J., et al. (1999). *Traumatic brain injury in the United States: A report to Congress.* Washington, DC: U. S. Department of Health & Human Services, Centers for Disease Control, National Center for Injury Prevention and Control.

Trombly, C. A., Radomski, M. V., & Davis, E. S. (1998). Achievement of self-identified goals by adults with traumatic brain injury: Phase I. *American Journal of Occupational Therapy, 52*(10), 810–818.

Unsworth, C. (Ed.). (1999). Cognitive and perceptual dysfunction: A clinical reasoning approach to evaluation and intervention. Philadelphia: F. A. Davis.

Winkler, P. (2001). Traumatic brain injury. In D. Umphred (Ed.), *Neurological rehabilitation* (4th ed.). St. Louis, MO: Mosby.

World Health Organization. (2001). *International classification of functioning, disability, and health.* Geneva: World Health Organization.

Yudofsky, S. C., & Hales, R. E. (2002). *The American Psychiatric Publishing textbook of neuropsychiatry and clinical neurosciences* (4th ed.). Washington, DC: American Psychiatric Press.

Zafonte, R. D., Hammond, F. M., Mann, N. R., Wood, D. L., Black, K. L., & Millis, S. R. (1996). Relationship between Glasgow Coma Scale and functional outcome. *American Journal of Physical and Medical Rehabilitation, 75*(5), 364–369.

Suggested Reading

Angle, D. K., & Buxton, J. (1991). *Community living skills workbook for the life of the head injured adult.* Gaithersburg, MD: Aspen.

Bear, M. F., Connors, L. W., & Paradiso, M. A. (2001). *Neuroscience: Exploring the brain.* Philadelphia: Lippincott Williams & Wilkins.

Carney, N., Chesnut, R. M., Maynard, H., Mann, N. C., Patterson, P., & Helfand, M. (1999). Effect of cognitive rehabilitation on outcomes for persons with traumatic brain injury: A systematic review. *Journal of Head Trauma Rehabilitation, 14*(3), 277–307.

Crimmins, C. (2000). *Where is the mango princess?* New York: Random House.

Deboskey, D., Hecht, J., & Calub, C. (1991). *Educating families of the head injured: A guide to medical, cognitive, and social issues.* Gaithersburg, MD: Aspen.

Fraser, R. T., & Clemmons, D. C. (Eds.). (1999). *Traumatic brain injury rehabilitation: Practical, vocational, neuropsychological and psychotherapy interventions.* Boca Raton, FL: CRC.

Giles, G. M., & Clark-Wilson, J. (Eds.). (1999). *Rehabilitation of the severely brain-injured adult: A practical approach* (2nd ed.). London: Stanley Thornes.

Gutman, S. A. (2003). *Screening adult neurologic populations: A step-by-step instruction manual.* Bethesda, MD: American Occupational Therapy Association.

Yody, B. B., Schaub, C., Conway, J., Peters, S., Strauss, D., & Helsinger, S. (2000). Applied behavior management and acquired brain injury: Approaches and assessment. *Journal of Head Trauma Rehabilitation, 15*(4), 1041–1060.

CHAPTER 15

Psychosocial Aspects of Chronic Pain

Marti Southam, PhD, OTR/L, FAOTA

Key Terms

analgesics

chronic pain

conversion

neurobiological

opioids

Chapter Outline

Introduction

The American Chronic Pain Association (ACPA) (2003) reports that approximately 85 million Americans are afflicted with varying levels of disabling pain. This translates to a cost of about $90 billion annually to U.S. businesses and industry due to sick leave, lost productivity, and the high cost of medical benefits. Further, long-term analgesic users may suffer liver, stomach, or kidney damage, adding to their suffering and medical costs. About one-third of those on dialysis have a history of **analgesics** abuse (Frischenschlager & Pucher, 2002). In fact, pain has reached such a dimension that the U.S. Congress has designated the decade from 2001 to 2011 as "The Decade of Pain Control and Research" (Turk & Okifuji, 2002).

People in pain are not just suffering from a physical ailment. Psychosocial factors play important roles in pain perception, function in daily occupations, and response to treatments. "Ultimately, there is a psychogenic component to all chronic pain—if not as a primary cause, then as a result of the pain's duration and debilitating effects" (Edwards, 2000, p. 282). Because **chronic pain** may never completely disappear, teaching clients coping skills is crucial. A multidisciplinary treatment approach is recognized as the most effective way to help persons with chronic pain (ACPA, 2003). Professionals on a pain management team vary, but may include a physician, occupational therapist, physical therapist, psychologist, and case manager.

The International Association for the Study of Pain (1979) defines pain as "an unpleasant sensory and emotional experience associated with actual or potential tissue damage or described in terms of such a damage." This definition equalizes physical factors with emotional and cognitive factors and helps to provide an explanation for pain without an injury site, phantom limb pain, and pain relief from mind-body practices. It also allows for fear, depression, and life experiences to influence and perhaps modulate pain (Frischenschlager & Pucher, 2002).

Pain is a subjective experience, unique to each individual. Some people are able to withstand a great deal of pain while others are sensitive to the slightest injury. The health care professional must depend upon the ability of the client to communicate pain's severity through verbal and nonverbal expression. Acute pain is easier to address, as the cause is usually obvious (e.g., after a skiing accident, the ankle becomes swollen and is unable to bear weight). Medical personnel administer pain relief medication, dress the damaged part, and provide instructions on how to take care of the injury while it heals.

On the other hand, chronic pain may be more difficult to assess and diagnose. Often there is neither an apparent pathological indicator nor a physical cause for the pain. To the person's dismay, he or she may be turned away by health care professionals with comments like, "Sorry, we can't find any physical reason for your pain," or "It's all in your head." Feelings of anger may arise in the client when he or she finds that over and over again, help is not forthcoming. Helplessness and hopelessness may develop, which could lead the person to stop trying to manage the pain, and instead, to retreat from life's occupations (Frischenschlager & Pucher, 2002).

Chronic pain and its psychosocial aspects often have negative impacts on occupational performance within the individual's particular context (Birkholtz & Blair, 2001; Strong, 1996). Occupational therapists are uniquely situated by training to be able to offer skilled service to chronic pain sufferers that encompasses both the psychosocial and physical realms. This chapter focuses on ways for the occupational therapist to assess chronic pain; its impact on daily functioning and ways to assist adult clients in resuming a quality life through pain management. It is not within the scope of this chapter to address specific issues associated with pediatric and geriatric pain.

DIAGNOSTIC CRITERIA

In order to meet the criteria outlined in the *Diagnostic and Statistical Manual,* 4th edition, text-revised (*DSM-IV-TR*), the pain must be of sufficient severity to warrant clinical attention and cause significant distress or impairment of functioning (APA, 2000). The pain disorder may be specified as either acute or chronic and as being associated with psychological factors, with both psychological factors and a general medical condition, or with a general medical condition.

According to Lippe (2003), there are two categories of pain (Table 15-1). They can be distinguished by the amount of time the person reports the pain and whether the pain serves a useful purpose (i.e., alerting the person to bodily damage). Category I can be considered eudynia (good pain) and is acute. It serves a protective function by signaling tissue damage with an identifiable cause, such as being hit, burned, or cut. The site of injury is usually obvious and localized. As the pain threshold is reached, a neuronal signal is transmitted to the brain to warn the individual that damage to the body is occurring. Medication, either prescribed or over the counter, is the most common remedy for controlling acute pain. Category I pain goes away when the injury is healed and does not last more than six months.

Chronic pain is primarily Category II pain (i.e., maldynia or "bad" pain) because it is not related to acute injury and thus, serves no useful purpose (Lippe,

Table 15-1.	Categories of Pain
Category I	Eudynia ("good" pain) because it warns of bodily damage. Acute symptoms with an identifiable cause that do not last more than six months.
Category II	Maldynia ("bad" pain) because it serves no purpose. Chronic pain is primarily of this type and can last for months or years.

Source: Adapted from Lippe, 2003.

2003). Chronic pain is defined by the American Chronic Pain Association (2003) as pain that continues for a month or more after an initial injury has healed or pain that goes on over months or years sometimes without a discernible cause. It is considered a chronic illness, which may be continuous or intermittent, and is a long-term problem that will probably need lifelong attention. Types of chronic pain are described in Table 15-2.

Table 15-2.   Examples and Descriptions of Chronic Pain Types

Examples of Chronic Pain	Description
Back Pain	May be due to muscle spasms or vertebral disc damage or degeneration that leads to nerve irritation or impingement. Pain and/or numbness may extend down the legs to the toes (sciatica).
Fibromyalgia	Characterized by widespread soft tissue pain, sleep disorders, and fatigue. Must experience pain in at least 11 of 18 "tender points" throughout the body when pressed. No known cause.
Headache	Three common types: *Tension* headaches are caused by either muscular tension in the head, or neck and shoulders. *Migraine* headaches, characterized by pounding pain, nausea, sensitivity to light, and sometimes vomiting, may last for 12 to 72 hours. *Cluster* headaches are usually felt on one side of the head, behind one eye sometimes accompanied by tearing or facial swelling. Occur in groups during stressful times or a particular season.
Joint Pain	*Osteoarthritis:* Natural part of aging. Joint cartilage thins and dies; replacement rate slows with age. Bones rub together causing pain. *Inflammatory Arthritis:* Several types—rheumatoid arthritis, systemic lupus erythematosus, scleroderma, and ankylosing spondylitis. The immune system identifies the body's own connective tissue as foreign and triggers the inflammatory response. Over time, the immune cells destroy cartilage and joint lining and may go on to attack internal organs.
Myofascial Pain Syndrome	Begins with an injury as the surrounding muscles develop a holding pattern to protect the injured site. If muscles stay contracted for a long time, localized pain and spasm develop. "Auto-strangulation" occurs, depriving muscle cells of oxygen. Trigger point feels tender when pressed and pain radiates to another part of the body.
Neck Pain	Three common types: *Muscle tension* is caused by holding the head up for long periods (e.g., computer work, driving, cradling a telephone). *Whiplash* strains or sprains the neck's soft tissues. *Arthritis* or joint degeneration may occur in the cervical region. Any of these may cause pain in the neck, shoulders, and arms due to cervical nerve irritation.

(continues)

Table 15-2. (continued)

Examples of Chronic Pain	Description
Peripheral Neuropathies	Damage to a peripheral nerve that causes burning, shooting pain and/or numbness or dysesthesia. Commonly related to conditions such as diabetes, alcoholism, herpes zoster, and entrapped nerves.
Phantom Limb Pain	After an amputation, nerves spontaneously fire, transmitting pain messages in the absence of a stimulus. Burning in the fingers or other amputated parts may be reported.
Reflex Sympathetic Dystrophy (RSD)	May occur after a stroke (sometimes called shoulder-hand syndrome). Characterized by severe shoulder pain and a stiff, swollen, painful hand. Can lead to severely limited range of motion.
Repetitive Strain Injuries (RSI)	Soft tissue injury including carpal tunnel syndrome and tendonitis. Usually caused by repetitive motion, poor posture, and ergonomics.

Sources: Adapted from Dillard, 2002 and Hansen & Atchison, 2000.

NEUROBIOLOGICAL BASIS OF PAIN

As pain signals reach the brain, the messages are sorted and a response is generated. Multiple neurotransmitters and brain areas interact to modulate responses to pain and other stressors. Pain causes groups of brain cells to release chemicals called endogenous **opioids,** or as they are more commonly known, endorphins. These chemicals are the brain's natural painkillers and bind to mu-opioid receptors (Zubieta, Smith, Bueller, Xu, Kilbourne, Jewett, Meyer, Koeppe, & Stohler, 2001).

According to recent research from the University of Michigan, gender, hormone levels, and genetics are important to understanding individual differences in the release of endorphins and their ability to bind to mu-opioid receptors. Using positron emission tomography (PET), a mu-opioid radiotracer, and subjective pain scales, researchers were able to measure mu-opioid activation and a corresponding decrease in healthy volunteers' ratings of perceived pain (Zubieta et al., 2001).

Following up on this research, Zubieta et al. (2002) set up small, randomized, double-blind clinical trials to explore **neurobiological** sex differences in the suppression of pain. Data indicated that gender differences did exist when subjects were presented with intensity-controlled sustained deep tissue pain. The phase of the women's menstrual cycle appeared significant to the suppression of mu-opioid binding and to the women's perceived experience of pain. In the early follicular phase of the menstrual cycle, when estrogen and progesterone levels were low, women experienced significantly more pain than later in their cycles, when estrogen was higher. During the higher estrogen phase, women experienced levels of pain more similar to men. Studies with larger numbers of women to confirm these findings are underway. Zubieta, Heitzeg, Smith, Bueller, Xu, Xu, Koeppe, Stohler, and Goldman (2003) discovered that genetics may also play a role in individual responses to pain experience. Variations in a particular gene that interacts with dopamine seems to be important in a person's pain tolerance, regardless of gender.

Treatment that triggers release of natural opioids, endorphins, is helpful in an overall therapy regimen and may reduce the need for pharmaceuticals. Exercise has been shown to produce endorphin release, as has deep breathing. Rate and depth of breathing aid in the release of endorphins (Pert, 1997). Hearty laughter increases the heart rate and respiratory activity, causes blood pressure to drop, and releases endorphins. The result is a light, euphoric effect and a sense of pain relief that may last for 30 minutes to several hours. Muscle tension of the neck, face, and head, which often leads to headaches, may be relieved after laughter, which could decrease the need for medications (Black, 1984; Cousins, 1989; Fry, 1992). Helping a client use natural endorphin-releasing activities such as movement and laughter can reduce or eliminate dependence on pain medication and avoid the many serious associated health risks.

Pain is a complex phenomenon. Research supports subjective reporting of pain and emphasizes the importance of individual differences when trying to understand a person's description of pain, especially prolonged or sustained pain. The uniqueness of the pain experience may be related to the client's attitude toward pain and toward life and to the skills that the person possesses to handle daily challenges.

MENTAL ATTITUDE

Interfacing with the neurobiological factors associated with pain, an individual's mental attitude at a given time is critical to one's pain perception and the ability to endure it (Peolsson, Hyden, & Larsson, 2000). Because pain disrupts and disorganizes the person's daily occupations, it commands conscious attention (Craig, 1995). People react on a continuum from complaining about the pain and giving up, to mobilizing resources, support systems, and coping mechanisms.

CASE ILLUSTRATION: Michael and Bob— Chronic Pain, Different Attitudes

Michael, a 55-year-old manager, hurt his right dominant shoulder during a racquetball game with a colleague. Without medical advice, he iced it and put his arm in a sling for a couple of weeks. When out of the sling, he noticed his hand was swollen and blotchy and was extremely sensitive to light touch. He went to a physician who made the diagnosis of shoulder-hand syndrome or "frozen" shoulder. He received medical treatment, and occupational therapy was prescribed to improve function. Michael attended therapy inconsistently, tended to overprotect his hand, and declined most of the treatments that the OT recommended. He took all of his sick leave, stayed home, and became isolated from friends and family. Over the next year, Michael continued to suffer chronic pain in his right arm. He is currently out of work and on permanent disability.

Bob, a 56-year-old teacher, caused a cervical nerve to be pinched during an overly intense exercise session at his local gym. This resulted in pain and par-

tial loss of function in his left, nondominant upper extremity, which he tried to "work out" on his own. After a period of several months of chronic, recurring arm pain, weakness, and hand swelling, he finally decided to seek medical treatment. Cervical neck surgery was recommended to free the nerve and occupational therapy was prescribed to recover left arm and hand function. During his therapy, Bob enthusiastically discussed home program ideas with the OT, and he came up with the idea to make a Native American spear to decorate the cabin he owned. This creative, fun project involved planing and sanding a length of wood. Although this was a bilateral activity, the OT suggested doing most of the work with his left arm. The OT taught him to use good body mechanics, to pace the activity, and to practice relaxation and deep breathing if the pain increased. He was highly motivated to use his arm again and excited to complete the project. With gradual increase in use, the pain diminished and strength returned, allowing him to perform meaningful occupations at home and work.

Discussion

Bob and Michael are middle-age single men. They had similar injuries of the shoulders. Their stories illustrate how attitude makes a difference in compliance with treatment, healing, and returning to work.

Peolsson, Hyden, and Larsson (2000) argue that coping with pain is a "dynamic learning process" (p. 115). People who live with pain experience it as a companion that is always present, either in the background or in the foreground within the context of everyday occupations. They learn to sensitize themselves to the level of pain and what makes it increase or decrease. "The pain is, in a sense in command and thus requires continuous adaptation by the sufferer" (p. 118).

Everyone has good days and bad days. This is particularly true for those living with chronic pain. "In complex ways, physiologic stress responses interact with the sensory qualities of pain and with psychological coping" (Chapman, 1995, p. 298). One of the problems that people with chronic pain experience is poor pacing of activities. In other words, on a day when people feel good, they tend to do too much and then spend the next few days dealing with increased pain. Learning how to monitor activity levels and balancing activity and rest is key to pain management (Davis, 2002; Sasek, 2001). Depending upon what is happening in a person's life, shifts along the continuum occur, as illustrated in Figure 15-1.

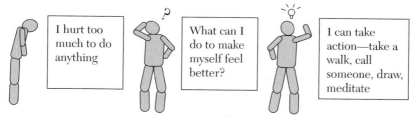

Figure 15-1. Pain Reaction Continuum

FACTORS IN CHRONIC PAIN

The way persons with chronic pain cope and respond to treatment is dependent upon a number of factors. Emotional states often vary with life's situations and can influence how well people deal with pain from day to day. Also, an individual's history may include underlying childhood or other traumas, which could surface as psychodynamic issues converted to pain that need to be recognized and treated. Sociocultural and personal values and beliefs (i.e., spirituality, optimism, and feelings of control) exert influences on perception of pain and coping abilities. The way in which these factors are manifested and handled by the client have an impact on pain management outcomes.

Emotions and Pain

Chronic pain is an emotional roller coaster ride. Often neither medical nor surgical treatments yield lasting results and the client vacillates between hope, fear, disappointment, further hope, and so on. After a period of time, helplessness and hopelessness could take root, and the person may become isolated and uninvolved in life's activities. Without meaningful occupations, the individual dwells on physical symptoms and may experience increased intensity of pain due to the attention paid to bodily sensations (Turk & Okifuji, 2002).

Symptoms of depression, including insomnia, are common in people with chronic pain. Pain management programs often combine analgesics and antidepressants along with psychological and physical protocols to help people cope with depression and lack of restful sleep (Diener, van Schayck & Kastrup, 1995). Learning to relax, which can be taught through cognitive-behavioral therapy, can be key in helping clients sleep. Progressive relaxation is one technique that is useful in redirecting attention from pain, releasing muscle tension, and diminishing emotional stress, thereby decreasing discomfort and aiding rest (Keefe, 1996).

> **CASE ILLUSTRATION: Janine—Chronic Back Pain Impairs Quality of Life**

Janine is a 32-year-old Caucasian female with a 4-year-old daughter. She has a college degree and worked throughout her 20s. During a one-year period, she experienced severe and incapacitating low back pain that occurred after three specific events: driving on a long road trip; falling down the stairs in her home; and helping to move a sofa. Following each of these episodes, Janine visited her physician, who prescribed pain relief medications and gave her a handout of stretches and exercises. However, her back never fully recovered, and now, one year later, she complains that the pain is always there. She expresses frustration that she cannot do the things she enjoys and needs to do, such as playing on the floor with her daughter or picking her up, shopping, home management tasks, and driving for more than one hour. She complains that she cannot get comfortable at night and rarely sleeps more than a few hours at a time. She also feels she cannot work, as she would not be a dependable employee, because she does

not know when her back pain will flare up and debilitate her to the point of hav-
ing to stay in bed for a few days. She reports feeling depressed because she has
to constantly self-monitor her activities. Fortunately, she has recently begun a
pain management program.

Discussion

Janine demonstrates emotional and behavioral aspects of chronic pain that can
restrict function and decrease engagement in occupations. Pain management
programs offer hope to many individuals and techniques to break the vicious
cycle of pain.

The ACPA (2003) recommends that people with chronic pain recognize, acknowledge, and deal with their emotions through various coping skills. Group support
can be valuable in encouraging people to express their feelings of pain and frustration to others who have had similar experiences and who understand pain. This validation can help reduce isolation and increase coping.

Psychodynamic Aspects in the Experience of Chronic Pain

Unconscious drives and emotional suppression in individuals with chronic pain
should be considered when developing a pain management program for clients
(Birkholtz & Blair, 2001). Psychodynamic themes that may be uncovered include
"early identification with ill or disabled family members; childhood sexual and physical abuse; . . . and pain as punishment (of self or others)" (Davis, 2002, p. 5). A predominant psychic mechanism is **conversion**, in which an unconscious fear, wish, or
conflict is transformed into physical pain, thereby providing an avenue for psychological release (Birkholtz & Blair, 2001; Frischenshlager & Pucher, 2002). In other
words, sometimes when people sustain a physical injury, they may hold onto the pain
or even extend it as a way to escape or avoid expressing an earlier psychological pain.

During expressive activities in an occupational therapy session, client responses
may arise that show deeper psychological levels of the experience of pain. Although
creative and artistic media are used by occupational therapists for a variety of reasons, from a psychodynamic perspective, the benefit is that "the therapist can elicit
feeling and meanings from their clients' painting and drawings, which might reflect
their [the clients'] inner lives" (Stein & Cutler, 2002, p. 541). This is especially helpful when clients have difficulty verbally explaining the impact of their pain. Very
often finding a way to express, name, and define the personal meaning of pain is the
first step in gaining control over it. Expressive media may bring up very powerful
images of one's past. These may be explored further during the occupational therapy session but should also be brought to the attention of the entire team.

Socio-Cultural Factors

Socio-cultural factors influence how people perceive and respond to pain as well
as how they communicate pain to other people. Pain perception is a private event

that only becomes public when the individual signals it, verbally or nonverbally, to others. Personal, cultural, and social factors influence how or if a person lets others know of her or his pain. Cultural groups have different perceptions of pain, depending on what they perceive as "normal" pain (Giger & Davidhizar, 1999; Helman, 2000). "Health care practitioners must investigate the meaning of pain to each person within a culturally explanatory framework to interpret diverse behavioral responses and provide culturally competent care" (Purnell & Paulanka, 1998, p. 44).

Societal expectations of different cultures may dictate how or if pain may be expressed according to gender. Men may be expected to bear pain and not show it, thus demonstrating strength and courage. For example, in the Anglo-Saxon tradition, men have been taught to "keep a stiff upper lip" or to "suck it up" when acute or chronic pain is encountered in sports or work (Helman, 2000). Women, too, demonstrate pain differently according to their culture. The symptoms of menopause that may extend for months or years (e.g., hot flashes, joint or muscle pain, vaginal or urinary burning, headache, etc.) are perceived according to social expectations. For example, Japanese women regard menopause, and its symptoms, as a normal life event, not a medical concern. Most never consult a physician. Women of the Papago Indian tribe of the Southwest seemingly ignore menopause, and in some cultures in India and South Asia, it is welcomed as freedom from fertility and menstruation (Papalia, Olds, & Feldman, 2001). However in dominant American culture, medical intervention, both allopathic and alternative, is common.

Spirituality and Chronic Pain

The Canadian Model of Occupational Performance (CMOP) and the Occupational Therapy Practice Framework (2002) recognize the relevance of spirituality in client-centered treatment of the whole person. Besides the feelings of hopelessness and helplessness that persons with chronic pain describe, clients may also discuss their courage, social support systems, and motivating factors that have helped them to endure. These strengths may be seen as spiritual aspects of the person that can be utilized in coping with chronic pain (Peloquin, 2003).

Christiansen (1997) describes "activities of the spirit" as those occupations that engage or reengage one with life's meaningful occupations. Through therapeutic use of self, the occupational therapist can empathetically view the client's world and can assist the person to live a life with quality that includes important spiritual and/or religious aspects. By being aware of a client's spiritual and/or religious beliefs, the occupational therapist may be able to identify persons, reading materials, audiotapes, and the like that may be helpful in coping with pain. A basic understanding of how different religions view pain is important to the therapeutic relationship and process. For example, in Buddhism, living includes suffering. The Dalai Lama said, "When you are aware of your pain and suffering, it helps you to develop your capacity for empathy . . . This enhances your capacity for compassion . . . So, as an aid in helping us connect with others, it can be seen as having value" (HH Dalai Lama & Cutler, 1998, p. 206). Likewise, Martin Luther King said, "What does not destroy me, makes me stronger." Occupational therapists who view the spiritual aspects of their clients as vitally important can engage them with an intervention plan that is meaningful on the deepest level.

Relationship between Cognition and Behaviors

Thoughts and actions are interdependent and learned, which leads one to the conclusion that they can be unlearned given the motivation of the client and the knowledge and skill of the therapist (Birkholtz & Blair, 2001). An individual's health beliefs predict compliance with treatment, and open the door for influencing clients' actions through education (Becker, Maiman, Kirscht, Haefner, Drachman, & Taylor, 1979).

In order to help adults with chronic pain, occupational therapists must recognize that clients have free will and make choices regarding their health and well-being. While this may seem obvious, it can be frustrating for the OT or the treatment team to put an intervention plan together only to have the client ignore it, change it, or try it without full commitment. Knowing the client's thoughts about committing to a behavioral change is paramount to therapeutic success.

Prochaska and DiClemente (1982) proposed a model to better understand the variables and processes involved in behavioral change. They performed a comparative analysis of 18 leading psychotherapy systems and identified four variables and five processes of change that people go through when choosing health behaviors. Their transtheoretical therapy model takes into account the subjective, verbal aspects as well as the objective, environmental elements of change. Research using this integrative model has involved clients with smoking, weight control, or alcohol abuse issues and seems applicable to working with people in chronic pain. The critical variables are described in Table 15-3.

Five stages for changing behaviors in the transtheoretical therapy model are shown in Figure 15-2. During precontemplation, the individual has no intention of changing, or has not acknowledged that he or she has a problem. The first real stage leading to change is contemplation. At this point, the person is thinking about making a change, but has not set goals or done anything specific. Readiness to enact a chronic pain self-management program can be assessed by discovering what the client's beliefs are regarding treatment. For example, those clients who believe that the only relief they will receive will come through medical channels (i.e., surgery, pain medications) may be less likely to apply a self-management approach. On the other hand, persons who have a belief that medical treatment has limitations may agree to try a self-management program (Turk & Okifuji, 2002).

Second, the person advances to the stage of determination and makes a serious commitment to make changes. He or she seeks information or a program to provide support in making a health behavior change. Interdisciplinary pain management programs have gained in popularity, but they are not universally available. However, "the responsibility of primary healthcare for treatment and

Table 15-3.	Variables in Choosing Health Behaviors
1. Preconditions for therapy	For optimal results, the client is motivated to change, has positive expectations about treatment, and will persevere with the treatment regimen. A good therapeutic relationship is also a key precondition.
2. Processes of change	Feedback and education are offered to the client to raise the individual's level of awareness. Through active listening, therapists can reflect and illuminate a client's thoughts and health beliefs. Using accurate information processing, the therapist can aid clients in making choices, "including the conscious creation of new alternatives for living" (p. 280). The environment is also a consideration in this integrative model, and changes in the client's context may also need to occur for a balanced intervention.
3. Content to be changed	Depending upon the client's history, current environment, and personality, therapeutic interventions will vary. Thus, the model is client-centered according to the content of the problem important to the client.
4. Therapeutic relationship	Progress depends upon the development of a caring, trusting relationship.

Source: Adapted from Prochaska & DiClemente, 1982.

rehabilitation of chronic pain patients has increased in the last decade" (Martensson, Marklund, & Fridlund, 1999, p. 157) and it is usually possible to find individual health care practitioners who are knowledgeable and skillful in treating chronic pain. In addition, there are several national and international organizations available to provide information and support to clients with chronic pain and related conditions. (See Appendix B for resources.)

In the third stage, the individual takes action and experiences a new lifestyle and ideally progresses to the fourth, or maintenance, stage in which she or he has successfully modified behavior for more than six months. This model should not be viewed as a strictly linear progression, as successful outcomes are not always achieved, especially in a first attempt to manage pain. People with chronic pain often relapse into previous pain-inducing behaviors. Therefore, the model includes a fifth or reentry stage, where the cycle of stages needs to be repeated if the individuals wish to pursue their health goals.

Knowledge of the variables and stages of the transtheoretical therapy model can benefit the therapist, because the stage that the client is in will help determine how successful a treatment program will be. In other words, if health education is introduced at the wrong stage, it is unlikely to be followed (Davis, 2002; Prochaska and Di Clemente, 1982; Nolan, 1995). As far as integrating therapy approaches, Prochaska and Di Clemente (1982) suggest that therapists use verbal approaches during the first three stages and behavior therapies during the last two stages. In this way, the therapist is matching the level and expectation for change that the client is experiencing.

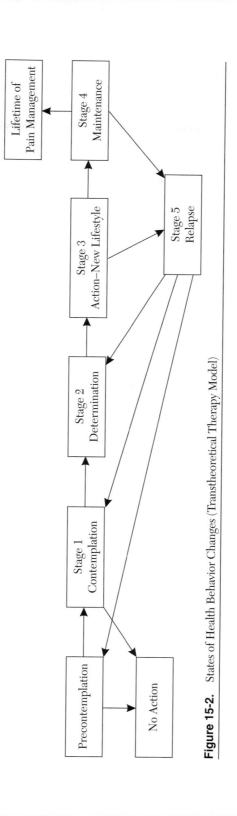

Figure 15-2. States of Health Behavior Changes (Transtheoretical Therapy Model)

Locus of Control

People have perceptions of whether events are under their control or not. Those with an internal locus of control operate from the belief that their actions and choices directly influence the outcomes of their experiences. Those with an external locus of control believe that events are caused by "fate, powerful others, or other factors out of their control" (Davis, 1998, p. 205). In terms of health education, persons with an internal locus of control seek out information when they have a health concern. In Arakelian's study (1980), clients with an internal locus of control were shown to have better health outcomes than matched subjects with an external locus of control.

In summary, it can be seen that clients' emotions, beliefs, values, and thought processes impact the therapeutic education that occupational therapists provide. The therapist needs to be aware of whether clients see a benefit to the treatment, how they perceive their own locus of control, and where they are in terms of making health behavior changes. This knowledge is necessary for the therapist to choose an educational approach that will engage and hold the learner's (i.e., the client's) attention so that information may be given in a comprehensible manner to guide the client toward mutually agreed upon goals.

MULTIDISCIPLINARY TREATMENT APPROACH

Due to the complexity of chronic pain, no single therapy is totally effective in its management (ACPA, 2003). Because chronic pain may continue for months or years, clients must learn to manage their own pain during daily occupations. Programs with the best results involve a multidisciplinary team that coordinates the knowledge and expertise of a variety of professionals. Overlap or redundancy is actually desirable to reinforce key concepts; however, each discipline will bring something unique to the treatment.

For a pain management program to have a positive outcome, clients must be evaluated by a pain management team and prescribed a treatment intervention that they follow regularly. Key team professionals often include a physician, an occupational therapist, a physical therapist, a psychologist, a social worker, and counselors (see Table 15-4 for examples of possible pain management team members).

Cognitive-Behavioral Therapy

Cognitive-behavioral therapy (CBT) is the overarching method that most chronic pain management programs use. The purpose is to help individuals understand the dynamics of chronic pain and to develop coping skills. Therapists teach people about the interrelationships between pain, thoughts, emotions, and physiology. CBT focuses on addressing chronic pain using multimodal strategies including stress management, relaxation, visualization, activity pacing, monitoring self-talk, assertiveness training, goal setting, and family training (Dillard, 2002; Keefe, 1996; Stewart, Law, Pollock, Letts, Bosch, Westmorland, & Everett, 2002; Turner & Romano, 1990).

Table 15-4.	Possible Members of a Multidisciplinary Team and Their Roles
Multidisciplinary Team Member	*Role*
Physician (MD) (neurologist, physiatrist, psychiatrist, or anesthesiologist with pain management expertise)	Makes the diagnosis, prescribes therapies and pharmaceuticals.
Occupational Therapist (OT)	Improves client's ability to perform daily occupations (activities of daily living, education, work, play or leisure, and social participation).
Physical Therapist (PT)	Improves client's flexibility, strength, and endurance.
Psychologist or Psychiatrist—the Commission on the Accreditation of Rehabilitation Facilities (CARF) requires a psychologist for a pain management program to be certified (Turk & Okifugi, 2002)	Through individual and group sessions, works with clients and families to resolve psychological issues, which may be contributing to pain. Psychologists may also lead or co-lead support groups and, along with the OT, strategize with clients to develop coping skills.
Registered Nurse (RN)	Nurse educators may be involved with workshop presentations, documenting client progress, and case management.
Biofeedback Therapist	Uses biofeedback equipment to help clients learn sensations of muscle tension and relaxation.
Family Counselor	Works with the family unit to promote understanding of client's pain, its impact on family dynamics, and ways to improve relationships.
Social Worker	Consults with family regarding economic and socio-cultural issues.
Vocational Counselor	Helps client to assess abilities to return to work or to change employment type.
Nutritionist	Works with client and family to adjust diet to incorporate foods and supplements that are helpful in reducing inflammation, increasing energy, and subduing pain.

Sources: Adapted from American Chronic Pain Association, 2003; Cayuga Medical Center at Ithaca, 2003; JFK Johnson Rehabilitation Institute, 2003.

CBT includes three important elements (Keefe, 1996). The first is education that teaches clients how their cognitions (thoughts) and behaviors impact pain perception and the ability to manage it. The second is description and rehearsal of coping skills to train clients in techniques so that they have choices of actions to take when pain strikes. Individuals are also taught options that help them avoid pain. The third aspect of CBT is the actual implementation and maintenance of learned coping skills by the client and family.

Most pain management programs use CBT with small groups for periods of four to eight weeks (Keefe, 1996; Sobel, Lorig, & Hobbs, 2002). There is debate in the literature over whether this is sufficient time to elicit permanent behavioral change. A study conducted by Soares and Grossie (2002) concluded that behavioral intervention produces several favorable outcomes for women with fibromyalgia, most notably an increased ability to control and decrease pain. However, with the exception of improvement in quality of sleep, these positive results disappeared within six months. Considering the possible lifelong course of chronic pain, it seems reasonable to assume that some form of maintenance therapy is essential.

Turner-Stokes, Erkeller-Yuksel, Miles, Pincus, Shipley, and Pearce (2003) concluded that there was no difference in effectiveness between delivering CBT in small groups or individually. Thus, the ability to reach more people in a cost-effective way was supported. A unique approach to group chronic pain management is a telemedicine program out of Warrawong, New South Wales, Australia. This interactive video program has been provided for many years and extends the hospital's group pain management program to remote areas. "Initial analysis indicates comparative outcomes between the two modes [in-hospital and remote] of service delivery" (Telemedicine Programs Database, 2003).

Groups provide support from others who experience and understand pain. Interactive problem solving between group members can help individuals develop self-efficacy in managing a variety of symptoms such as anger, depression, sleep issues, and pain. Other therapeutic aspects of groups include positive role modeling by peers, decreased isolation, increased confidence, and improved goal setting to perform daily occupations (Sobel, Lorig, & Hobbs, 2002).

Cognitive-Behavioral Treatment Methods in Occupational Therapy

The occupational therapist's presence on a pain management team is critical for clients to learn how to incorporate CBT into performing daily occupations. A study conducted by Engel (1994) using occupational therapy personnel and methods, including a "combination of a psychoeducational approach, and relaxation and attention diversion techniques, positive coping self-statements and homework assignment" resulted in "decreased pain complaints and improved mood . . . after completion of the program"(p. 82). Several CBT methods will be described in this section with an example of how they may be implemented in an occupational therapy pain management intervention program.

Stress management training is key to managing chronic pain successfully. A cycle between body and mind can develop, with pain causing stress and stress intensifying pain. Environmental stress such as being unable to perform meaningful occupations or having a fight with a family member can trigger an increase in pain. "No matter which comes first [stress or pain], the two are notorious for feeding each other" (Dillard, 2002, p. 14). Breaking this cycle is key to managing pain (Cayuga Medical Center, 2003; McCoy, 2002).

The first step is recognition that a stress reaction is taking place. Clients can be educated to sense bodily changes that indicate sympathetic nervous system activation such as increased heart rate and breathing, muscle tension, and perhaps digestive changes (e.g., upset stomach, diarrhea). In addition to these unpleasant physical symptoms, stress decreases immune function, an important fact for clients to be able to connect stress management with healing and overall health (Dillard, 2002).

Occupational therapists can utilize a variety of CBT methods to decrease stress and pain as clients perform daily occupations. Planning ahead, pacing during the activity, and relaxation techniques such as deep breathing, progressive relaxation, and positive/pleasant visualization help many people with chronic pain to participate more fully in life.

CASE ILLUSTRATION: Pain Management Group Activity

For their occupational therapy session, the pain management group chose to prepare a light meal as a way to resume cooking at home. Prior to the activity day, Brian, the pain management team occupational therapist, used information from the nutritionist to help the group plan to include foods that are helpful in reducing inflammation and pain. He also had the group rehearse the actions they would take to use good body mechanics, pace the activity, ask for assistance, and practice relaxation techniques if pain occurred during the cooking session. On the day of the meal preparation and before the cooking began, Brian asked the clients to find a comfortable spot and close their eyes. He recited a short relaxation visualization: "Take a deep breath for a count of four; hold it for four; release one, two, three, four; relax one, two, three, four [repeated two more times]. Now focus on relaxing your eyelids . . . feel the relaxation flow from your eyelids throughout your body, relaxing all of your muscles one by one. Let your attention move through your body to find points of pain or tension. Find an area of pain and give it a color. Now imagine a color that can wash the pain color out and pour rivers of that color on the pain. Feel the pain and tension drain away through your fingertips and toes. Take a deep, cleansing breath. Now imagine our pleasant cooking group. See yourself enjoying the activity, asking for assistance if you need it, and pacing yourself so that you only do what is comfortable and pain free." Brian continued to reinforce these images and then asked the group to slowly come back to full awareness and take part in the group session. During the cooking activity, Brian assisted the members in self-monitoring for stress and pain, asking for help, and pacing. The overwhelming comment at the end was that it had been a great experience. The OT requested that each member write down one goal for the week having to do with what they had learned and practiced that day, and to report back the following week.

Discussion

Incorporation and application of CBT techniques during an occupational therapy activity and receiving feedback throughout is a valuable way for clients to practice and learn its uses in everyday occupations.

SPECIFIC OCCUPATIONAL THERAPY ASSESSMENTS AND TREATMENT

The scope of occupational therapy practice includes areas of occupation, performance skills and patterns, activity demands, context, and client factors (Occupational Therapy Practice Domain, 2002). Therapists are trained to assess and treat the whole person. Due to their generalist education, occupational therapists are particularly well suited to work with persons with chronic pain because of the physical and psychological aspects of pain that impact daily occupations.

Occupational Therapy Assessments

Occupational therapists develop an occupational profile from the initial evaluation by assessing performance in areas of occupation: activities of daily living, instrumental activities of daily living, education, work, play, leisure, and social participation. For each of these areas, the therapist uses observation in combination with assessment tools to determine the client's performance skills and patterns. A client's abilities and deficits are viewed in relation to context, activity demands, and client factors. A list of possible assessments and a description of each may be seen in Table 15-5.

Occupational Therapy Treatment

Depending upon the results of the initial evaluation, an intervention plan is devised that meets the client's goals. CBT is the dominant therapeutic model to target emotional responses to stress and increase psychological coping to make chronic pain manageable in everyday occupations. Being generalist health care practitioners, occupational therapists can offer a wide variety of CBT techniques to alleviate problems for persons with chronic pain. Table 15-6 gives examples of specific CBT interventions that occupational therapists can use to help clients cope with pain.

Summary

Chronic pain is a complex phenomenon affecting millions of people and costing billions of dollars in lost productivity. Factors involved in the development, expression, and management of chronic pain include emotional status, socio-cultural attributes, spirituality, and learned cognitive and behavioral patterns. The most widely used and successful intervention for pain management is with an interdisciplinary team using an overarching cognitive-behavioral approach. Occupational roles, identity, and performance are disrupted with chronic pain, causing withdrawal from life's meaningful occupations. Successful intervention depends on a knowledgeable, compassionate, and dedicated pain management team that includes occupational therapy to address aspects of daily function.

Table 15-5.	Occupational Therapy Assessments and Descriptions	
Assessment	*Description*
Interview	Used to obtain demographic information; work, medical, and pain history; information about support systems. OT probes for beliefs about efficacy of pain treatments and ways of coping with pain that have been and have not been helpful.
Canadian Occupational Performance Measure, (Law, Baptiste, Carswell, McColl, Polatajko, & Pollack, 1999)	An interview to obtain information (pre- and post-treatment) about the client's abilities, difficulties, and satisfaction with performance in the areas of self-care, productivity, and leisure. Includes aspects of spirituality.
Role Checklist (Oakley, Kielhofner, Barris & Reichler, 1986)	Examines client's past, present, and future related to performance and value of occupational roles.
Neuro Psychiatric Institute (NPI) Interest Checklist (Matsusuyu, 1969)	Assesses client's interest levels (casual, strong, or no interest) in 80 activity items.
Numeric Pain Intensity Scale (Strong, 1996)	Self-report scale that measures client's perceived level of pain. On a scale from 0 to 10, clients rate how much the pain hurts, with 0 being no pain to 10 being the worst pain. This scale can be used during activities as well as at rest to help the therapist and client see the dynamic aspects of pain.
Daily Activity Log (Strong, 1996)	Clients record a log of the occupations that they engage in for a few days to a few weeks. This will give therapists and clients a better understanding of occupational patterns and activities that trigger a pain response.
Assessment of activities of daily living (ADL) and instrumental activities of daily living (IADL)	As the person performs routine ADL, (e.g., dressing, hygiene) and IADL (e.g., community mobility, shopping, caring for pets), the OT listens for complaints of pain and observes for unusual postures, holding patterns, grimacing, or other nonverbal signs of pain.
Physical measures of range of motion, strength, and sensation	Being sensitive to the client's verbal and nonverbal cues, the occupational therapist physically assesses baseline and progress.

Table 15-6. Occupational Therapy Cognitive-Behavioral Interventions for Pain Management

Intervention	Description	Rationale
Education in preparation for ADL, IADL, productive occupations, and leisure (Strong, 1996)	Assist clients in planning ways to participate in occupations so that pain will be minimized and reinjury will not occur. Teach body mechanics, pacing, range of motion and stretching, and use of adaptive equipment, if appropriate.	Movement is critical for one to engage in daily occupations and in occupational roles. By providing specific techniques that clients can use in planning and carrying out movement, participation in life will be improved.
Cognitive Restructuring	Teach clients to monitor negative self-talk and replace with appropriate thoughts; for example, replace "I can't live with this pain" with "I've had pain before and got through it. I can again. Right now, I'll practice deep breathing."	Thoughts about pain and its severity are destructive. By challenging and replacing negative thoughts with more realistic thoughts, a person can improve function in the present moment. Breathing focuses and calms the mind. Rate and depth of breathing aid in the release of endorphins, natural pain-killing chemicals (Pert, 1997).
Expressive Media	For play and leisure activities, use arts and crafts that clients find meaningful.	Arts and crafts engage clients in occupations that provide them with challenge and success. By focusing on a pleasurable self-expression, people can experience mastery and well-being (Strong, 1996).
Humor and Laughter	Encourage clients to socialize with friends who make them laugh; develop lists of favorite amusing books, television shows, and movies; clip cartoons; and gather funny greeting cards.	Laughter occurs more often in social groups. Laughter facilitates deep breathing, clears the respiratory system, and releases endorphins, natural pain-killing chemicals, and enhances the immune system functions (Berk, Tan, & Fry, 1993; Cousins, 1989).

Review Questions

1. Describe the differences between acute and chronic pain (definitions, treatment).
2. Explain the chronic pain reaction continuum. What is its significance to daily functioning?
3. How do socio-cultural factors impact pain perception?
4. What are some ways that occupational therapists use CBT?
5. Describe one assessment and one intervention for chronic pain.

References

American Chronic Pain Association. (2003, July). What is pain? [On-line]. Available: www.theacpa.org.

American Psychiatric Association. (2000). *Diagnostic and statistical manual* (4th ed., text-revised). Washington, DC: Author.

Arakelian, M. (1980). Assessment and nursing applications of the concept of locus of control. *Advances in Nursing Sciences, 3*(25), 25–42.

Becker, M. H., Maiman, L. A., Kirscht, J. P., Haefner, D. P., Drachman, R. H., & Taylor, D. W. (1979). Patient perceptions and compliance: Recent studies of the Health Belief Model. In R. B. Haynes, D. W. Taylor, & D. L. Sackett (Eds.), Compliance in health care. Baltimore: Johns Hopkins University Press.

Berk, L., Tan, S., & Fry, W. (1993). Eustress of humor associated laughter modulates specific immune system components. *Annals of Behavioral Medicine, 15,* 111.

Birkholtz, M., & Blair, S. E. E. (2001). Chronic pain—the need for an eclectic approach: 1. *British Journal of Therapy and Rehabilitation, 8*(2), 68–73.

Black, D. W. (1984). Laughter. *Journal of the American Medical Association,* 252(21), 2995–2998.

Cayuga Medical Center at Ithaca, Health Resource Library. (2003, July). Pain management: New research and treatments promise relief. [On-line.] *Health News: Medicine on the Horizon.* Available: http://12.31.13.113/healthnews/MedicineontheHorizon/MOTH42001.htm#diagnosis.

Chapman, C. R. (1995). The affective dimension of pain: A model. In B. Bromm & J. E. Desmedt (Eds.), *Pain and the brain: Nociception to cognition* (pp. 283–293). New York: Raven.

Christiansen, C. (1997). Acknowledging a spiritual dimension in occupational therapy practice. *American Journal of Occupational Therapy, 3,* 169–172.

Cousins, N. (1989). *Head first: The biology of hope.* New York: Penguin.

Craig, K. D. (1995). From nociception to pain: The role of emotion. In B. Bromm & J. E. Desmedt (Eds.), *Pain and the brain: Nociception to cognition* (pp. 303–316). New York: Raven.

Davis, C. M. (1998). *Patient practitioner interaction: An experiential manual for developing the art of health care* (3rd ed.). Thorofare, NJ: Slack.

Davis, P. (2002). *Pain management: Psychotherapeutic approaches.* Nashville, TN: Cross Country University.

Diener, H. C., van Schayck, R., & Kastrup, O. (1995). Pain and depression. In B. Bromm & J. E. Desmedt (Eds.), *Pain and the brain: Nociception to cognition* (pp. 345–354). New York: Raven.

Dillard, J. N. (2002). *The chronic pain solution: Your personal path to pain relief.* New York: Bantam.

Edwards, C. H. (2000). Chronic pain. In R. A. Hansen, & B. Atchison (Eds.), *Conditions in occupational therapy: Effect on occupational performance* (2nd ed.). Baltimore: Williams & Wilkins.

Engel, J. (1994). Cognitive-behavioral treatment of chronic recurrent pain. *Occupational Therapy International, 1*(2), 82–89.

Frischenschlager, O., & Pucher, I. (2002). Psychological management of pain. *Disability and Rehabilitation, 24*(8), 416–422.

Fry, W. F. (1992). The physiologic effects of humor, mirth, and laughter. *Journal of the American Medical Association,* 267(13), 1857–1858.

Giger, J. N., &. Davidhizar R. E. (1999). *Transcultural nursing* (3rd ed.). St. Louis, MO: Mosby.

HH Dalai Lama, & Cutler, H. C. (1998). *The art of happiness.* New York: Riverhead.

Hansen, R. A., & Atchison, B. (Eds.). (2000). *Conditions in occupational therapy: Effect on occupational performance* (2nd ed.). Baltimore: Williams & Wilkins.

Helman, C. G. (2000). *Culture, health and illness: An introduction for health professionals* (4th ed.). Oxford: Butterworth-Heinemann.

International Association for the Study of Pain. (1979). Pain terms: A list with definitions and notes on usage. *Pain, 6,* 249–252.

JFK Johnson Rehabilitation Institute, Adult Outpatient Programs and Services. (2003, July). *Pain management program.* [On-line]. Available: http://www.njrehab.org/painmgt.htm.

Keefe, F. J. (1996). Cognitive behavioral therapy for managing pain. *The Clinical Psychologist, 49*(3), 4–5.

Law, M., Baptiste, S., Carswell, A., McColl, M. A., Polatajko, H., & Pollack, N. (1999). *Canadian Occupational Performance Measure* (3rd ed.). Toronto: Canadian Association of Occupational Therapy.

Lippe, P. (2003, April). *History of pain and current legislation.* Paper presented at the annual meeting of the American Chronic Pain Association, Danville, CA. Synopsis available: http://www.acpa.org.

Martensson, L., Marklund, B., & Fridlund, B. (1999). Evaluation of a biopsychosocial rehabilitation programme in primary healthcare for chronic pain patients. *Scandinavian Journal of Occupational Therapy, 6*(4), 157–165.

Matsusuyu, J. (1969). The interest checklist. *American Journal of Occupational Therapy, 23,* 323–328.

McCoy, D. (2002). Fibromyalgia and cognitive behavioral therapy. Mental Health Information from PsychNet-UK [On-line]. Available: www.counseling.com/DrMcCoy/.

Nolan, R. P. (1995). How can we help patients to initiate change? *Canadian Journal of Cardiology, 11*(Supplement A), A16–A19.

Oakley, F., Kielhofner, G., Barris, R., & Reichler, R. (1986). The Role Checklist: Development and empirical assessment of reliability. *Occupational Therapy Journal of Research, 6,* 157–170.

Occupational Therapy Practice Framework: Domain and Process. (2002). *American Journal of Occupational Therapy, 56,* 609–639.

Papalia, D. E., Olds, S. W., & Feldman, R. D. (2001). *Human development* (8th ed.). New York: McGraw-Hill.

Peloquin, S. M. (2003). Spirituality: Meanings related to occupational therapy. In E. B. Crepeau, E. S. Cohn, & B. A. B. Schell (Eds.), *Willard & Spackman's occupational therapy* (10th ed., pp. 121–126). Philadelphia: Lippincott, Williams & Wilkins.

Peolsson, M., Hyden, L.-C., & Larsson, U. A. (2000). Living with chronic pain: A dynamic learning process. *Scandinavian Journal of Occupational Therapy, 7,* 114–125.

Pert, C. (1997). *Molecules of emotion: Why you feel the way you feel.* New York: Scribner.

Prochaska, J. O., & DiClemente, C. C. (1982). Transtheoretical therapy: Toward a more integrative model of change. *Psychotherapy Theory Research Practice, 19*(3), 176–288.

Purnell, L. D., & Paulanka, B. J. (1998). *Transcultural health care.* Philadelphia: F. A. Davis.

Sasek, H. (Ed.). (2001, September). *Managing chronic pain: Participant workbook.* Oakland, CA: Regional Health Education, Kaiser Permanente Northern California.

Soares, J. J. F., & Grosi, G. (2002). A randomized controlled comparison of educational and behavioral interventions for women with fibromyalgia. *Scandinavian Journal of Occupational Therapy, 9*(1), 35–45.

Sobel, D. S., Lorig, K. R., & Hobbs, M. (2002, Spring). Vohs award winner—multiple-region category: Chronic disease self-management program: From development to dissemination. [On-line]. *The Permanente Journal, 6*(2), 1–10. Available: http://www.kaiserpermanente.org/medicine/permjournal/spring02/selfmanage.html.

Stein, F., & Cutler, S. (2002). *Psychosocial occupational therapy: A holistic approach* (2nd ed.). Albany, NY: Delmar.

Stewart, D., Law, M., Pollock, N., Letts, L., Bosch, J., Westmorland, M., & Everett, A. (2002). The effectiveness of cognitive-behavioral interventions with people with chronic pain: An example of a critical review of the literature. In M. Law (Ed.), *Evidence-based rehabilitation: A guide to practice* (pp. 127–169). Thorofare, NJ: Slack.

Strong, J. (1996). *Chronic pain: The occupational therapist's perspective.* New York: Churchill Livingstone.

Telemedicine Programs Database, Group Chronic Pain Management by Telehealth (2003, July). [Online]. Available: http://tie.telemed.org/programs/ProgramListings.asp?ID=1422.

Turk, D. C., & Okifuji, A. (2002). Psychological factors in chronic pain: Evolution and revolution. *Journal of Counseling and Clinical Psychology, 70*(3), 678–690.

Turner, J. A., & Romano, J. M. (1990). Cognitive-behavioural therapy. In J. J. Bonica (Ed.), *The management of chronic pain* (Vol. 2, pp. 1711–1721). Philadelphia: Lea & Febiger.

Turner-Stokes, L., Erkeller-Yuksel, F., Miles, A., Pincus, T., Shipley, M., & Pearce, S. (2003, June). Outpatient cognitive behavioral pain management programs: A randomized comparison of a group-based multidisciplinary versus an individual therapy model. *Archives of Physical Medicine Rehabilitation, 84*(6), 781–788.

Zubieta, J. K., Heitzeg, M. M., Smith, Y. R., Bueller, J. A., Xu, K., Xu, Y., Koeppe, R. A., Stohler, C. S., & Goldman, D. (2003, February 21). COMT vall58met genotype affects mu-opioid neurotransmitter responses to a pain stressor. *Science, 299*(5610), 1230–1243.

Zubieta, J. K., Smith, Y. R., Bueller, J. A., Xu, Y, Kilbourne, M. R., Jewett, D. M., Meyer, C. R., Koeppe, R. A., & Stohler, C. S. (2001, July 13). Regional mu-opioid receptor regulation of sensory and affective dimensions of pain. *Science, 293*(5528), 311–315.

Zubieta, J. K., Smith, Y. R., Bueller, J. A., Xu, Y, Kilbourne, M. R., Jewett, D. M., Meyer, C. R., Koeppe, R. A., & Stohler, C. S. (2002, June 15). Mu-opioid receptor-mediated antinociceptive responses differ in men and women. *Journal of Neuroscience, 22*(12), 5100–5107.

Suggested Reading

Dobson, K. (2002). *Handbook of cognitive behavioral therapies* (2nd ed.). Guilford.

Carlsson, S. (2000). Coping with fibromyalgia: A qualitative study. *Scandinavian Journal of Caring Sciences, 14*(1), 29–36.

Gibson, L., & Strong, J. (1998). Assessment of psychosocial factors in functional capacity evaluation of clients with chronic back pain. *British Journal of Occupational Therapy, 61*(9), 399–404.

Leo, R. J. (2003). *Concise guide to pain management for psychiatrists.* Washington, DC: American Psychiatric Press.

Mcmanus, C. A. (2003). *Group wellness programs for chronic pain and disease management.* Philadelphia: Butterworth-Heinemann Medical.

CHAPTER 16

Occupational Therapy and Substance Use Disorders

Virginia C. Stoffel, MS, OTR/L

Penelope A. Moyers

Key Terms

decisional balance
FRAMES
harm reduction
lapses
occupational alienation
occupational deprivation
preferred defense structure

recovery
relapses
risk reduction
standard drink measure
tolerance
withdrawal

Chapter Outline

Introduction

Engagement in and performance of occupations deteriorate for persons who have substance use disorders, as the use becomes more frequent, is of longer duration, and involves greater quantities of the substance. Occupations involve generation of meaning in such a way that the individual forms a particular identity associated with the activity. Occupational therapists have a unique set of skills and perspectives that can contribute to promoting lifestyle changes needed to support recovery from substance use disorders.

Substance abuse and dependence may eventually impede engagement such that occupations are no longer meaningful and are no longer important to identity formation. These previously enjoyed occupations become a set of activities that one merely performs throughout the day. Dependency on a substance thus can lead to **occupational alienation**, which Wilcock (1998) describes as loss of meaning that was once associated with performance. Over time, if performance continues to deteriorate, one is deprived of those once important occupations necessary for a satisfying and meaningful life (called **occupational deprivation**) (Wilcock, 1998).

As a part of the occupational alienation/deprivation process, meaningful activities are gradually replaced with activities important for maintaining the addiction, such as: "a) raising money for the drugs, b) purchasing or making the deal to obtain the drug supply, c) protecting the supply from others, d) removing barriers to using, such as ignoring family members who object to the person's behavior, d) creating situations for using, e) seeking persons with whom to use, f) spending time using, g) recovering from the effects of using, and h) resuming the drug-using process all over again" (Moyers & Stoffel, 2001, 2001, p. 325). These "using activities" may have their own associated meaning, such as fulfilling the need to "escape, have fun, relax and sleep, avoid physical and emotional pain, gain confidence, increase sexuality, feel less inhibited and more creative, or increase energy and activity levels" (Moyers & Stoffel, 2001, p. 325). These using activities are structured into daily habit patterns that then preserve the using routine. Activities and occupations previously valued are avoided so that the using routines occur without disruption.

The process of **recovery** is much more than merely abstaining from the drug of choice (full cessation of drug use) or reducing drug use to the point where it is nonproblematic. Recovery involves a process of change in which the person assesses the need for lifestyle adjustments from drug use to healthy habits of daily living and meaningful occupations.

Recovery can occur within a very short or an extended period of time (as many as several years) and typically happens in nonlinear stages. The time spent in each stage of the process may be variable and may have an irregular course that intersperses progress with **lapses** (slips) and **relapses** (return to former drug-centered lifestyle). DiClemente and Velasquez (2002) have referred to this process as "recycling" through the stages of change (p. 213). The individual may have several lapses and relapses, but can still proceed toward recovery.

One example of recovery involving the return to full engagement in occupation to support participation is Ronaldo, a father who found meaning and pleasure in co-parenting with his wife and playing with his young children after successfully eliminating marijuana use from his daily habits. Another example is Harriet, an older woman who found that any alcohol intake interfered with the therapeutic effect of her antidepressant medications; she learned to change her former evening routine from isolating herself in her home while sipping on wine to attending the choir practice and music programs in her community center. An additional example may be Madeleine, a teenager, who after getting in trouble at school and home because of drug use, found a group of peers who supported her in staying chemically free, worked at getting the grades she needed to go to college, and enjoyed the peer support and exercise of being on the drill team at school. Occupational therapists are in the best position to influence these goals: regaining the motivation, confidence, and self-efficacy needed to support recovery. In this context, recovery reflects a change where a healthy mix of daily routines and engagement in meaningful occupations is incorporated into the person's lifestyle, replacing the destructive, habituated substance use patterns.

This chapter presents the *DSM-IV-TR* (APA, 2000) terminology of substance abuse and dependence and the prevalence rates associated with the use of a variety of drugs. Issues of co-occurring diagnoses are discussed as well. The impact of abuse and dependence on families and communities is described. Evidence-based evaluation and interventions important to resolving occupational alienation and deprivation are delineated particularly through the use of the transtheoretical model of behavior change. (See Chapter 15 for more information about this model.) As the client progresses through each of the stages of change, the transtheoretical model also guides the client's efforts to engage in different ways of thinking, planning, and doing, all actions important for the recovery process. Various intervention contexts are described to illustrate service delivery models within communities.

DIAGNOSTIC CRITERIA

The *DSM-IV-TR* (APA, 2000) defines various substance use disorders that are the primary focus of this chapter. Substance dependence and abuse involve ten classes of drugs, including alcohol, amphetamines, cannabis, cocaine, hallucinogens, inhalants, nicotine, opioids, phencyclidine (PCP), and sedatives. Caffeine is the only class of drug that does not have an associated abuse and dependence disorder, and instead is described as having only a substance-induced disorder related to intoxication. Therefore, a discussion of caffeine and nicotine falls outside the scope of this chapter.

Substance Dependence

The chief feature of substance dependence is "a maladaptive pattern of substance use, leading to clinically significant impairment or distress" (APA, 2000, p. 110). Maladaptive patterns typically include drinking or using the substance for a longer time period or in greater quantity than originally planned; having difficulty cutting down on use of the substance; organizing one's life around seeking the drug; obtaining and being under the influence of the substance; and giving up or reducing important social, occupational, or recreational activities. Despite having recurrent physical or psychological problems caused or exacerbated by the substance, the individual continues to use. Within a 12-month period, one's use may meet the criteria for dependence if there are at least three of the five types of maladaptive patterns.

If **tolerance** and **withdrawal** are present during the using experience, two of the three criteria needed for making the diagnosis of substance dependence exist. Tolerance occurs when increasing amounts of the substance are needed to achieve the desired effect, or when, with the same amount, there is less or little effect on the individual. Tolerance can lead to an overdose of the substance, which could present as a medical emergency.

CASE ILLUSTRATION: Jocanda—Developing Tolerance

Jocanda was on her way to work at the World Trade Center when she witnessed the destruction and devastation of the 9/11 attacks. She managed the difficult periods of moving to a new work site and attending many funerals for her work friends with regular counseling. However, she became alarmed when she realized that the beer or glass of wine she needed to sleep every night no longer helped her to sleep and she had started to need two or three drinks to sleep.

Withdrawal is "the development of a substance-specific syndrome due to the cessation of (or reduction in) substance use that has been heavy and prolonged" (APA, 2000, p. 116). To avoid withdrawal, the person with substance dependence might ingest more of the substance. Withdrawal can also lead to an emergency requiring medical monitoring and intervention, and may or may not be life-threatening.

Substance Abuse

Substance abuse is also a maladaptive pattern of substance use leading to clinically significant impairment or distress, but is differentiated from dependence by the absence of tolerance and withdrawal. In terms of maladaptive patterns, the person who experiences one of the following within a 12-month period would be classified as having substance abuse: (1) fails to fulfill major role obligations at work, school, or home; (2) takes physical risks, such as driving a car while under the influence of a substance; (3) incurs repeated legal problems related to substance use; or (4) displays social and interpersonal problems as a result of the effects of the substance. The person, though, must never have been diagnosed in the past with dependence in a particular class of substance as the one currently being abused (APA, 2000).

Classes of Substances and Their Prevalence

The varied classes of substances that are most commonly abused in the United States are outlined in Table 16-1 (SAMHSA, 2002). Information as to their "street" names, intended use, dosage, and prevalence should help the occupational therapy practitioner to recognize various terms that clients may use as they describe their use of substances, as well as to understand the possible effects that these substances might have on these individuals. The 2001 National Household Survey on Drug Abuse (NHSDA) (SAMHSA, 2002) presents national estimates for residents

Table 16-1. Classes and Substances of Abuse, Intended Effects, Risks, and Prevalence

Class of substances	Specific substances	Dosage, ingestion, intended effect	Prevalence
Alcohol	Beer, wine, vodka, whiskey, hard liquors, wine coolers, malt beers	Relaxing, release of inhibitions, social lubricant, heightened sexual effect *Standard drink* = 12 oz. beer; 1.5 oz. spirits; 6 oz. wine (Barry, 1999)	Of all Americans 12 or older, 48.3% were current drinkers, representing roughly 5 million more drinkers than in 2000. 20.5% of those older than 12 participated in binge drinking in the month prior to survey. Heavy drinking (5 or more drinks on 5 days in past 30 days) reported by 5.7% of the population 12 and older.
Amphetamine	Methamphetamine (crank, ice, speed), Desoxyn, Methedrine, Ritalin, Dexedrine, Tenuate	Stimulant, sense of energy and alertness	Incidence levels during the last decade around use of stimulants have not been seen since the mid-1970s. Number of new stimulant users reached 697,000 in 2000, peaking over the previous high of 646,000 new users in 1974.

(continues)

Table 16-1. (continued)

Class of substances	Specific substances	Dosage, ingestion, intended effect	Prevalence
Cannabis	Marijuana, Hash	Mellowing effect and escape reality	Average age of initiation in 2001 in the United States was 17.5 years old, with average age declining.
Cocaine	Crack, powder, free base, coca paste	Euphoria effect	Average age of initiation in 2001 in the United States was 20 years old.
Hallucinogen	LSD (acid), Ecstasy (MDMA), mescaline, peyote, psilocybin (mushrooms)	Altered sense of reality and escape into fantasy	Current use has risen nearly threefold since 1990, with 1.5 million new initiates in 2000. Ecstasy rates have risen, especially among 12- to 17-year-olds and 18- to 25-year-olds.
Inhalant	Amyl nitrite (poppers), correction fluid, gasoline, glue, shoe polish, ether, paint thinner, butane, nitrous oxide, spray paints, aerosol sprays	Quick rush	New inhalant users increased more than 50% between 1994 and 2000.
Opioid	Heroin, opium, non-medical use of pain relievers such as Morphine, Oxycontin, Methadone, Codeine, Vicodin, Dilaudid	Mood changes, drowsiness, and pain reduction effect	In 2000, there were 146,000 new heroin users per year, with heroin incidence rates rising.
Phencyclidine	PCP (angel dust)	Altered sense of reality with increased blood pressure and heart rate; paranoid thoughts and delusions effect	In 2000, there were almost 200,000 new users of PCP.
Sedative-Hyponotic- or Anxiolytic	Nonmedical use of sleeping pills, downers, Quaalude, Restoril, Halcion, Phinobarbital, Placidyl, Tuinal, Valium, Librium, Klonopin, Xanax, Ativan, Vistaril, Miltown	Relaxation and calming effect	Use by new nonmedical users of tranquilizers is higher than any point in time since 1965.

Source: Data from the 2001 National Household Survey on Drug Abuse, SAMHSA, 2002.

of the United States ages 12 and older that have been collected since 1971. The highest rate of illicit drug use among Americans peaked among 18- to 20-year-olds, was highest among American Indians/Alaska Natives, and was higher among unemployed persons despite the fact that most drug users were employed.

ASSESSMENT AND INTERVENTION FOR SUBSTANCE USE

The most common screening tool related to alcohol use is the CAGE (Ewing, 1984), an acronym standing for the four questions asked of the individual related to: needing to **C**ut down on drinking, feeling **A**nnoyed by others criticizing one's drinking, feeling **G**uilty about drinking, and needing an **E**ye opener, that is, a drink right after waking to avoid the symptoms of withdrawal. Two positive answers on the CAGE indicate a need to address the drinking problem (Ewing, 1984). These simple screening questions could be included within a broader health survey conducted as a part of the occupational profile, asking questions about sleeping habits, diet, and exercise, with additional questions related to quantity (how many drinks per occasion) and frequency (how many occasions per week) (American Society of Addiction Medicine, 1996). This part of the screening is positive for a man if consuming more than 14 drinks per week or greater than 4 drinks per occasion. For a woman, screening is positive if consuming more than 7 drinks per week or more than 3 drinks per occasion. (A **standard drink measure** is one 12-ounce can of beer, 1.5 ounces of spirits, or 6 ounces of wine.) When screening questions indicate the possibility of the person having alcohol- or drug-related problems, assessing readiness for change (abstinence or cutting down) can be conducted using a "readiness ruler" (Velasquez, Maurer, Crouch, & DiClemente, 2001). Here the clients are shown a scale of statements resembling a ruler where they select the term that most closely expresses their willingness to change their behavior, related to these four statements: "not at all ready, thinking about, preparing to, or actively working on or maintaining a change" (p. 30).

Stoffel and Moyers (1999) suggested that the Occupational Performance History Interview (Kielhofner, Henry, & Walens, 1989) be used to evaluate the impact of the person's alcohol or drug use on occupational performance. Other occupational therapy tools are also useful. The Role Checklist (Oakley, Keilhofner, Barris, & Reichler, 1986) can be used to consider the occupational roles affected by the use of substances. The Occupational Questionnaire (Smith, Kielhofner, & Watts, 1986) can be used to study the pattern of substance use during a typical week. It also can be a springboard for questions about substance use's influence on activity choice and performance. As a part of the goal-setting process, the Canadian Occupational Performance Measure (Law, Baptiste, Carswell, McColl, Polatajko, & Pollack, 1998) can be used to address the substance abuse issue as a part of the client's occupational therapy intervention. Coordination of care with other professionals such as specialized alcohol and drug counselors would be key to enhancing all rehabilitation outcomes.

Theoretical Models and General Treatment Strategies

In the past, occupational therapists who work with clients with substance use disorders have based their intervention decisions on theoretical propositions from models such as the cognitive-behavioral (Stoffel, 1992), 12-step (Moyers, 1997), and psychodynamic (Moyers, 1992). Current evidence-based practice strongly supports the transtheoretical model of behavior change (Prochaska & DiClemente, 1984; 1986). Key points of all of the models that have been shown to be effective are presented with an emphasis on the transtheoretical model of behavior change.

Cognitive-Behavioral Model. Principles from the cognitive-behavioral model indicate that substance use results from the interaction between social and interpersonal factors. The individual learns from social influences, such as peers, the media, and family members, who model and reinforce substance misuse behaviors (Beck, Wright, Newman, & Liese, 1993). The person's learning process regarding substance use is mediated through cognitions, attitudes, expectations, and personality. Thus, cognitive-behavioral interventions help the individual determine the environmental, interpersonal, and emotional situations linked to increased risk for using substances. Once these high-risk situations are identified, cognitive-behavioral strategies increase the individual's self-efficacy in utilizing improved and more varied coping skills in place of using substances. A cognitive-behavioral approach used by occupational therapists includes helping clients to use coping strategies in order to avoid relapse, and to routinize a healthy balance of nonusing occupations.

Twelve-Step Model. The 12-step model refers to those intervention programs that have adopted the principles of Alcoholics Anonymous (AA) grounded in the conception of alcoholism as a disease of the spirit, mind, and body (AA, 2001). Individuals are expected to attend AA meetings while participating in the intervention program and throughout life as a necessary part of long-term recovery. In addition to promoting the belief that AA affiliation is a central tenet for achieving sobriety, other principles include the importance of obtaining a sponsor, working through the 12 steps, and engaging in specific spiritual practices, such as developing a spiritual relationship with the higher power (Nowinski, Baker, & Carroll, 1995).

Psychodynamic Models. Psychodynamic models propose that psychological conflicts underlie the individual's propensity to misuse substances. These conflicts primarily involve unmet dependency needs that arise from early family problems. Over time, instead of mature interactions with others, the individual relies extensively on a **preferred defense structure** to ignore unmet needs as well as the problems related to substance abuse (Moyers, 1992). The preferred defense structure includes using such defense mechanisms (Freud, 1974/1936) as denial, rationalization, projection, minimization, obsession, and blame. Intervention is organized around helping the person mobilize this defense structure or individual defense mechanisms: helping the client to achieve abstinence as a first

Stage	Change
Table 16-2.	The Transtheoretical Model of Behavior Change Stages
Precontemplation	The individual is unaware of having problems with substance use; however, he or she may be able to recount some negative consequences related to a using incident.
Contemplation	The person is aware of pros and cons for using, but is ambivalent about change.
Preparation	The person has decided change is necessary and is considering and planning several alternatives for facilitating the change process.
Action	The person is learning new behaviors in place of substance use, though the new behaviors are somewhat fragile at this point.
Maintenance	The newly learned behaviors are incorporated into one's habits and routines on a long-term basis.

phase (e.g., encouraging the individual to replace the obsession with drinking with an obsession with sobriety); promoting the use of healthy coping strategies to replace the excessive reliance on defense mechanisms as a second phase (e.g., teaching the individual to use relapse prevention skills during high-risk drinking situations); and challenging the use of defense mechanisms in order to develop insight into one's own behavior as a third phase (e.g., helping the individual learn how to fulfill unmet needs in socially acceptable ways).

Transtheoretical Model of Behavior Change.   Moyers & Stoffel (1999) illustrate in a case report the application of the transtheoretical model of behavior change to occupational therapy. The transtheoretical model of behavior change is particularly useful because it may be used in any area of practice where the occupational therapist might come in contact with clients who are at high risk for drug and alcohol use. There are five stages of change representing the "process people go through when thinking about, beginning, and trying to maintain new behavior" (Barry, 1999, p. 14). Table 16-2 outlines the behavior expected in each stage. The therapist's role is to facilitate client movement from one stage to the next, realizing that the end result of therapy may be the client moving forward by only one step, such as from precontemplation to contemplation, rather than moving through all five steps. Different evaluations and interventions are targeted to facilitate movement, depending on the stage or readiness for change the client exhibits.

CASE ILLUSTRATION: Ronaldo—Using the Transtheoretical Model in Occupational Therapy

Ronaldo is a husband and father of two young children. He has smoked marijuana for over a decade, and his wife, Maria, has become increasingly concerned about the family's health due to his use in front of their children. Zwazzi, an occupational therapist, was seeing Ronaldo after he was involved in a fork-

lift accident where he failed the drug screen conducted at the worksite. As a part of the response team to any accident on the job, Zwazzi worked to determine how to eliminate all possible risks to the health and safety of the employees. After reviewing the drug screen and incident reports, she asked Ronaldo about his marijuana use. Ronaldo admitted that his marijuana use had become a dominating habit and a source of conflict with his wife, as she viewed him as isolating and being less engaged as a husband and father once he smokes. Zwazzi asked him to tell her how marijuana smoking has interfered with his roles. Ronaldo also disclosed that he has never been concerned about his daily marijuana use in the past, but that a part of him wonders if he should make a change since his 4-year-old asked about the funny smell in Maria and Ronaldo's bedroom. He also noted that his children are being screened for asthma, and he wonders if his smoking had anything to do with their symptoms of asthma. Zwazzi responded, "Would you be interested in knowing more about how marijuana may impact your family's health?" After positively accepting her suggestions about the impact of marijuana on his family's health, Zwazzi wondered what might be barriers to making changes in his drug use and what might facilitate his being more active in his valued occupations, particularly since he will be rehabilitating from his accident. Ronaldo considered other pros and cons of his drug use, such as "chilling out" versus being unsafe at his job. Finally, Zwazzi suggested that he take a vacation from his drug use for however long he thinks is reasonable. Ronaldo thought this vacation might be a good idea, and began to think of other occupational pursuits that he may enjoy with his family or soccer teammates.

Discussion

Ronaldo is moving from precontemplation ("I don't think I have any problems") toward contemplation (some ambivalence about change, not decided to change yet, but carefully considering it). His comments indicate a willingness to consider new information that might impact his decision to cut down or totally cut out his marijuana use. Strategies that have been found to be effective at the contemplation state of change (Velasquez, Maurer, Crouch, & DiClemente, 2001) include:

1. *Using motivational interviewing approaches ("Would you be interested in knowing more about how marijuana might be affecting your family's health?") to educate Ronaldo about the risks associated with smoking marijuana and its secondhand smoke.*
2. *Helping Ronaldo to self-evaluate what impact his marijuana use has on his daily occupational routines and valued roles as father, husband, worker, and athlete.*
3. *Having Ronaldo consider what might be a barrier in his various environments to making a change in his drug use and what might facilitate his being more active in his valued occupations.*
4. *Using **decisional balance** exercises to articulate the pros and cons of his current drug use and the pros and cons of cutting down.*

5. *Fostering his belief in his ability to change by suggesting he think about simply taking a vacation from his marijuana for a period of time that he sees as reasonable, and being prepared to replace his drug use with other meaningful occupational pursuits.*

The Occupational Perspective.   Although not a fully formed model, the *occupational perspective* provides a way of examining substance use as involving a set of activities, such as raising money for the drugs, purchasing or making the deal to obtain the drug supply, protecting the supply from others, and the like. These activities may eventually become of such central importance to the individual that they are actually occupations imbued with meaning, that is, they fulfill the need to escape, have fun, relax, and sleep (Moyers, 1992; 1997; Moyers & Stoffel, 2001). Furthermore, these occupations may eventually form the individual's identity, for example, of an addict or party person. We call these "using occupations" and they are often organized into specific habit patterns (e.g., having a drink in the morning to counteract effects of withdrawal) and routines (e.g., stopping off at the same bar every evening after work). As one becomes more involved in these substance-using occupations, performance in occupations and activities that do not incorporate substance use eventually deteriorates. Eventually the individual not only becomes more and more alienated from typical occupations but also is deprived of the occupations' healthy effects (Moyers & Stoffel, 2001).

According to this occupational perspective, occupational therapists are concerned with the way in which substance use impacts a person's engagement in valued occupational roles. They are also interested in how the therapeutic use of occupations and activities contributes to the prevention or recovery from problem drinking and substance use disorders.

In an evidence-based literature review conducted for the American Occupational Therapy Association, Stoffel and Moyers (2001) indicated that there was a dearth of research studies determining the effectiveness of occupational therapy interventions for persons with substance use disorders. Consequently, most of the research reviewed was from other fields, particularly psychology. Therefore, in reviewing the literature from other fields, research was selected related to interventions that had the potential for positively influencing the person's engagement in the occupations and activities necessary for role functioning, health, and quality of life. However, there was a lack of focus on the occupational areas of activities of daily living (ADL), instrumental activities of daily living (IADL), work, education, play, leisure, and social participation, all areas of occupations noted in the Occupational Therapy Practice Framework (2002). Therefore, the narrow focus on abstinence outcomes should be broadened to include an occupational perspective or outcomes focused on engagement in activity and participation within the community. The principles of these effective interventions, which were highlighted in the literature, should be considered when designing therapeutic activities and occupations for persons with substance abuse and dependence.

The AOTA evidence-based literature review focused on four main interventions, including brief intervention, cognitive-behavioral therapy, motivational strategies, and 12-step programs. Emerging evidence also supports the use of **harm reduction** strategies and the community reinforcement approach. These evidence-based interventions are presented here, but are also later woven throughout the section of the chapter that examines the timing, sequencing, and implementation of methods according to the readiness of the client to move forward toward abstinence and recovery. Table 16-3 describes literature that supports occupational therapy interventions.

Table 16-3. Evidence-Based Support for Occupational Therapy Interventions

Application of Evidence

Approach	Therapy Goals	Intervention Components	Resources
Brief Intervention	Curtail or reduce substance use	Screening for problematic substance use Providing feedback on amount of use Explaining risks of continued use Offering advice on reducing intake Setting use reduction goals	Barry, 1999 Moyers & Stoffel, 1999
Cognitive-Behavioral Therapy (CBT)	Develop coping skills needed to function within occupational areas Facilitate self-efficacy for making positive changes in substance use and in occupational performance Improve coping with situations that precipitate relapse	Functional analysis: identification of triggers, activating events, thoughts and beliefs, emotions, and actions and consequences Relapse prevention skill training Practice new coping and interpersonal skills Engagement in enjoyable and meaningful nonusing activities	Barry, 1999 Velasquez, Maurer, Crouch, & DiClemente, 2001 Stoffel, 1992
Motivational Strategies	Motivate to make changes in substance use Increase intervention participation rates/program retention	Collaborative partnership based on therapeutic style of open-ended questions, reflective listening, summarizing,	Valesquez, Maurer, Crouch, & DiClemente, 2001 Miller & Meyers, 1999

(continues)

Table 16-3.   (continued)

Approach	Therapy Goals	Intervention Components	Resources
	Reduce resistance during intervention	affirming self-efficacy, eliciting self-motivational statements	Miller, Zweben, DiClemente, & Rychtarik, 1995
		Emphasis on client values and strengths	Miller & Rollnick, 2002
		Focus is on motivation rather than challenging resistance/ambivalence	
Twelve-Step Programs	Foster acceptance of substance use as a disease that may be arrested but not cured	AA meetings and activities	Nowinski, Baker, & Carroll, 1995
	Develop commitment to attend AA meetings and to participate in fellowship activities of AA regularly	Twelve-steps of recovery	AA, 2001
		Sharing personal stories of substance use and recovery processes common to AA members	Moyers, 1997
	Develop a spiritually based recovery lifestyle	Helping others	
		Developing a spiritual relationship with the higher power	
Harm Reduction Programs	Consider alternative strategies that might lessen the potential negative impact of substance misuse.	Identify the potentially harmful consequences of behavior on self, family, and community	
		Adopt safer practices at both the societal and individual levels (i.e., needle distribution programs, designated driver programs, cutting down number of days drinking and eating food when drinking, alternate drinking alcohol with non-alcohol beverages	
Community Reinforcement Approach	Eliminate positive reinforcement for drinking/drug use	Increase motivation to stop drinking/using	Hunt & Azrin, 1973
	Enhance positive reinforcement for sobriety	Try a trial period of sobriety to explore	Meyers & Smith, 1997
		Do a functional analysis of drinking/using to	Meyers, Miller, Hill, & Tonigan, 1999

(continues)

Table 16-3. (continued)			
Approach	*Therapy Goals*	*Intervention Components*	*Resources*
	Be sure that abstinence is more rewarding than drinking/using!	determine the advantages of making a change	Miller, Meyers, & Tonigan, 2002
		Increase enjoyable activities with self and others in a chemically free environment	
		Train family in supporting sobriety and meet own needs for open communication and positive reinforcement for sobriety	

Brief Intervention Strategies.   Brief interventions may occur during a face-to-face visit with a therapist, via phone calls or e-mails, or through means other than therapist-client contact, such as a workbook or methods of independent learning (e.g., web site educational materials). Research does not clearly identify the way in which brief interventions are best administered, and is also unclear about whether outcomes are enhanced when multiple types of contacts are used (Poikolainen, 1999).

If involving a therapist, a brief intervention may just include one session, lasting from five minutes to one hour. However, very brief interventions of one session less than 20 minutes were not as effective in comparison to extended brief interventions of one hour over several sessions (Poikolainen, 1999). Brief interventions are not recommended as the main intervention for the client who has alcohol or drug dependence (Wilk, Jensen, & Havighurst, 1997). Brief interventions seem to have a more consistent benefit for women than for men (Poikolainen, 1999). Because brief intervention studies have primarily focused on reducing alcohol use and have not clearly discerned effectiveness in reducing other substances, more studies are being conducted related to amphetamine use (Baker, Boggs, & Lewin, 2001) and reducing alcohol use in persons who inject drugs (Stein, Charuvastra, Maksad, & Anderson, 2002).

Brief interventions usually incorporate principles from motivational strategies, the transtheoretical theory of behavior change, and cognitive-behavioral therapy. The focus of a brief intervention, depending upon the number of sessions involved, is initially for the occupational therapist to investigate with the client the potential substance use problem, or to help the client arrive at a conclusion about the health risk involved in using drugs or alcohol (Miller & Rollnick, 1991). In other words, the occupational therapist determines the client's readiness for change, and then motivates the client to move through successive stages of change to action and maintenance. Most often, the client is in the pre-contemplation or contemplation stage of change when coming into initial contact with a health professional. The goal is to increase awareness of the problem and to address the client's ambivalence for change in such a way that the balance of pros and cons for using is tipped in the direction favoring change.

To motivate the client, a variety of screening instruments are used. (See the previous section related to screening and assessment.) Because the goal in brief intervention is to motivate change, initially giving the client feedback from the screenings about his or her current situation is important. Then the occupational therapist provides the client with data about the pattern of drug or alcohol use the client typically follows within a day over a week-long period and how this pattern compares to those of others who do not have an addiction problem. The occupational therapist assists the person in evaluating the relationship between alcohol/drug consumption and any negative consequences in occupational performance that may result from drinking/using (Moyers & Stoffel, 1999). An occupational profile (AOTA, 2002) is an excellent method for determining how drinking and using has influenced engagement in occupations and activities. The professional also provides explanations of the physical and psychosocial risks associated with excessive alcohol or drug use. Discussions include the way in which using the substance less leads to improvements in physical and psychological health, as well as the way using less provides the opportunity to begin solving social problems arising from the excessive substance use.

Next, the occupational therapist motivates the person to do something about his or her substance abuse. The outcome of a brief intervention may be a natural, client-directed change, or the person seeks additional substance abuse treatment from a variety of alternative approaches, ranging from self-help groups to inpatient or outpatient substance abuse programs (Barry, 1999).

CASE ILLUSTRATION: Jackson—A Brief Intervention

Jackson was a sculptor whose hand injury prevented him from performing in his usual role of sculpting contemporary work for public spaces. The injury to his dominant hand also interfered with his self-care and hygiene. While conducting an occupational profile, Dante, a hand occupational therapist, discovered that his client's injury involved alcohol. Jackson had been working all night while he consumed three-quarters of a bottle of whiskey. Toward morning when he was very drunk, he had staggered against his worktable, knocked the sculpture off the table, and attempted to catch it. It had smashed his hand. Dante spent about 30 minutes questioning Jackson about his liquor intake and discussing its negative consequences, which Jackson readily admitted. He referred Jackson to a substance use program for artists.

Discussion

Although Dante did not work in a substance-related organization, he was able to discover substance abuse and use brief intervention strategies for Jackson, who was in a precontemplation state of change.

Cognitive-Behavioral Strategies. Cognitive-behavioral therapy (CBT) involves a combination of principles derived from behavioral and cognitive theories, with an emphasis on the cognitive aspects of behavior (Barry, 1999). To begin the change process, the individual in collaboration with the occupational therapist engages in a functional analysis. In a functional analysis the situations surrounding the client's substance abuse are probed to analyze what factors prompt substance use and the resulting consequences of using (Barry, 1999). The client is helped to understand the antecedents of a using incident, the underlying cognitions (beliefs, attitudes, and thoughts) that the individual has prior to the incident, and the resulting behavior and emotions from the cognitions. The main principle of CBT is to change the faulty cognitions from irrational thoughts into more rational thoughts. For example, one attempts to change the thought, "the problem at work is beyond my ability and the only way I can tolerate the stress is to drink" to "the problem can be solved if I break it down into manageable aspects and I am more likely to solve the problem if I don't drink." Actions and emotions subsequently change upon adjustment of thoughts. For example, an emotion may change from depression to self-efficacy, and an action may change from taking no action to implementing problem-solving steps.

When the client has not made the decision to change, CBT's success may be limited. In such cases, CBT may be more effective in combination with motivational and 12-step strategies (Project MATCH Research Group, 1997; 1998a, b). Also, considering cognitive capacity may be important because the functional analysis is dependent upon certain levels of insight and memory, and the use of coping skills requires cognitive flexibility and problem solving (Morgenstern & Bates, 1999; Roehrich & Goldman, 1993; Zinn, Bosworth, Edwards, Logue, & Swartzwelder, 2003).

The type of substance abused may also affect CBT outcomes. CBT might be more effective for persons with alcohol and polysubstance use than for persons who smoke tobacco or use cocaine (Barry, 1999; Irvin, Bowers, Dunn, & Wang, 1999). Additionally, CBT may not be effective when used as a primary prevention strategy for high-risk adolescents (Palinkas, Atkins, Miller, & Ferreira, 1996). CBT appears to be equally effective when delivered either in a group or in individual formats (Graham, Annis, Brett, & Venesoen, 1996), or when delivered in outpatient or inpatient settings (Irvin, Bowers, Dunn, & Wang, 1999).

CASE ILLUSTRATION: Susie—Cognitive-Behavioral Strategies

Susie had successfully graduated from a 30-day clinic, having readily admitted herself to deal with her long-time alcohol and marijuana use. After graduation, she regularly attended the hospital's outpatient program that consisted of various groups. While in an occupational therapy group she analyzed an incident. She called in sick to work on the two busiest nights for the restaurant where she worked as a sous chef, after which she had a slip. *She remembered that she had been particularly resentful of the master chef who had berated her for a slight mistake in front of many other kitchen workers. She remembered having obsessive thoughts about the evening. Subsequent to calling in sick, she ruminated that she was a poor worker who couldn't handle stress and maybe could never be any good. Donna, the OTR who led the group facilitated the other group members to problem-solve how Susie could have handled the incident and how else she could think about herself.*

Discussion

In a group focusing on maintaining one's vocational occupations, the therapist used cognitive-behavioral strategies of analyzing an antecedent event that led to drug use and facilitated group problem solving to change Susie's cognitions.

Motivational Strategies. Motivational strategies include motivational enhancement therapy (MET), motivational interviewing, and decisional balancing. The emphasis in all motivational strategies is to identify the person's readiness to change and enhance motivation to change, thereby influencing movement to the next stage as outlined in the transtheoretical model of behavior change (Barry, 1999). Motivational strategies are timed to correspond with the stages so that the strategies may be the primary intervention at the earlier stages and then in later stages may be used in combination with other interventions, such as CBT or 12-step programs (Project MATCH Research Group, 1997; 1998a, b). Motivational strategies have been shown to be effective for persons with alcohol and drug abuse (Project MATCH Research Group, 1997; 1998a, b; Saunders, Wilkinson, & Phillips, 1995).

MET is a stand-alone treatment aimed not only at getting the client to consider change, but strengthening the change process once the client has started to change (Project MATCH Research Group, 1997, 1998a). Therapeutic interventions involve five basic motivational principles, including expressing empathy, developing discrepancy, avoiding argumentation, rolling with resistance, and supporting self-efficacy (Miller, Zweben, DiClemente, & Rychtarik, 1995). These principles become clearer after reading about motivational interviewing and decisional balancing.

Motivational interviewing is client-centered and uses specific methods of communication that are highly empathic and nonconfrontational. **FRAMES** is the acronym that guides motivational interviewing, and includes feedback, responsibility, advice, a menu of alternate change options, empathy, and self-efficacy (Miller & Sanchez, 1994). The interviewer's role is to give feedback that is often based on the results of screenings about an individual's substance use and his or her health risk, to give advice about the need to change, and to emphasize the client's responsibility to make a change in these risk factors. A menu of a variety of change strategies are offered that may range from professional intervention in diverse settings to self-help groups.

The interviewer uses empathy and does not attempt to label the client as an alcoholic or addict, nor tries to break through denial, but recognizes how change could be difficult. Even though difficult, the interviewer stresses the client's ability to make change, thereby promoting self-efficacy. It is important when the client demonstrates resistance during the interview for the therapist to "roll with it" by not arguing for change, opposing resistance directly, or imposing new perspectives (Miller & Rollnick, 2002). Resistance is the client's signal that the therapist needs to act differently in responding to the client.

Exploring and resolving ambivalence toward change is a key aspect of motivational interviewing, where the therapist facilitates the client to eventually voice the arguments for change (Miller & Rollnick, 2002). Decisional balance exercises are used to explore the pros and cons of drinking or using drugs in order to help the client eventually come to the conclusion that it is in his or her best interest to abstain or cut down. Decisional balancing is thus a method for developing discrepancy based on the client's own arguments for change by noting the gap between one's personal goals and values and one's current using behavior (Miller & Rollnick, 2002). The therapist views the client as the primary resource in finding answers and solutions (Miller & Rollnick, 2002), and the client is invited to consider new perspectives.

Research indicates that motivational strategies may be more effective for those individuals who can tolerate more time in reaching a drinking reduction goal (Project MATCH Research Group, 1997; 1998a, b). Therefore, for those persons not in crisis, motivational strategies may be offered as a brief intervention (two to four sessions) or as a brief therapy (approximately four sessions over three months with telephone boosters) (Poikolainen, 1999).

Persons with serious mental illness (SMI) have a rate of dependence and abuse of alcohol that is three times higher than adults without SMI (SAMHSA, 2002). Another advantage of motivational strategies is that persons with schizophrenia are able to engage in decisional balancing-type intervention activities (Carey, Purnine, Maisto, Carey, & Barnes, 1999). Given that people with SMI have such a high rate of substance abuse and dependence, occupational therapists who work with the SMI population must actively monitor, provide feedback, support, and integrate services to the clients with these co-occurring disorders. Dealing with both the mental illness and the substance use disorder that are concurrent with one another, especially by attending to the daily routines associated with the person's optimal state of health, should guide the work of the occupational therapist and occupational therapy assistant.

CASE ILLUSTRATION: Jeb—Motivational Interviewing

Jeb had been living in an assisted independent living program in the community and working at a fast food restaurant one day a week for three hours. His case manager, Margaret, was an occupational therapist who visited him weekly. She noticed the smell of liquor on his breath during two of the visits and Jeb appeared to be drunk on the third. She confronted him about these times by asking him about his drinking quantity, habits, and possible interference with his daily life. Jeb seemed resistant to discussing these subjects, insisting that his drinking eventually helped him in his job because it was easier to be around people when he drank. Margaret empathized with his desire to feel less anxious at his job, and wondered aloud if his alcohol use helped him that much on his job. Jeb acknowledged that he often had a hangover while he worked and sometimes spent all of the money he earned on liquor. Margaret wondered out loud if it was worth it.

Discussion

Margaret used motivational interviewing techniques, empathy, rolling with it, and promoting decisional balancing to motivate Jeb to change his behavior.

Twelve-Step Strategies. Twelve-step strategies include treatment programs and 12-step facilitation methods that are consistent with the principles of 12-step self-help groups, such as Alcoholics Anonymous (AA) and Narcotics Anonymous (NA). Twelve-step strategies also include regular attendance and participation in self-help programming. However, there is lack of agreement about whether lay counselors with a personal history of substance use are key to successful 12-step programming or whether 12-step programming facilitated by professionals produces better outcomes (Project MATCH Research Group, 1998a).

The principles of 12-step self-help groups, such as AA and NA groups, involve the person identifying himself or herself as a recovering alcoholic or addict, seeking peer support and fellowship, incorporating spirituality into his or her daily life, and taking life "one day at a time." Key recovery-oriented behaviors involve the person attending 12-step groups and developing a connection to a person who can serve as a sponsor.

Twelve-step facilitation, 12-step treatment programs, and 12-step self-help groups all assist persons with substance abuse or dependence to (1) accept that they have a disease, (2) acknowledge that the only cure is abstinence, and (3) help them to surrender control over to a higher power (AA, 2001). Typically there are other objectives related to making cognitive, emotional, behavioral, social, and spiritual changes in one's daily life (Nowinski, Baker, & Carroll, 1995).

Cognitive changes involve the person understanding how his or her thinking has been affected by alcohol and may reflect denial of the problem and thus allowing continued drinking. Members of AA commonly refer to this type of thinking as "stinking thinking" (AA, 2001). Emotional states, such as feeling angry and lonely, also are thought to perpetuate drinking and therefore programs require the individual to incorporate AA strategies to change these states into more helpful and positive emotions. Behavioral changes involve replacing old drinking habits with habits and routines involving AA meeting attendance and volunteer work in helping others who are dependent upon alcohol. These meetings also contribute to the change in social relationships and activities so that the person no longer is tempted by being with others who use alcohol and drugs. The spiritual change involves recognizing that a higher power provides hope. In order to rectify the harm done to others, spirituality also involves acknowledging the immoral, unethical acts one may have committed while under the influence.

Although people who lack a support system often benefit from the network of support offered by AA (Project MATCH Research Group, 1997; 1998a), having a strong support network of relationships prior to receiving intervention seems to predict successful outcomes. However, if that social network includes a large number of persons who use alcohol, then research indicates that the more effective intervention is 12-step facilitation (Zywiak, Longabaugh, & Wirtz, 2002). Connection to AA thus seems important for replacing the person's social network that primarily included persons who also drank. There may be a minimal number of AA meetings one must initially attend in order to receive benefit, such as 90 meetings in 90 days (Ouimette, Moos, & Finney, 1998). Persons treated in 12-step programs are more likely to attend a greater number of 12-step meetings after completing treatment (Finney et al., 1998).

Persons with less severe forms of alcohol and drug abuse may not accept abstinence as the only goal of intervention or may not accept the disease concept of substance abuse (Project MATCH Research Group, 1998b). For these persons, programs based on CBT or MET might be more useful. In contrast, persons who are open to meaning seeking and its importance for one's life may respond better to a spiritual-based program than to programs that just offer CBT or MET (Project MATCH Research Group, 1997).

> ## CASE ILLUSTRATION: Harriet—Successful Use of 12-Step Programs

Harriet is a 72-year-old widow who, after discovering that her antidepressant medications were not working as effectively as they had in the past due to her drinking, asked for help from Mohini, an occupational therapist working in the community mental health center, to find ways to cut drinking out of her life. Mohini conducted an occupational profile to ascertain Harriet's daily occupational and health habits, and to understand the impact that drinking had on her other occupational choices. The occupational therapy intervention was to work with Harriet to develop a plan for her sobriety and to reengage her in occupations she had relinquished in the past. Mohini fostered Harriet's sense of self-efficacy by building on successful times without drinking and replacing her past isolated behavior at dinnertime by reengaging in a social meal plan at a nearby coffeeshop. Harriet was also able to identify people who would support her sobriety such as her minister, several friends in her congregation, and her next-door neighbor, who is a member of AA. In fact, she thought that she needed to bring back spirituality into her life and decided to attend AA meetings with her neighbor. While completing the Occupational Self-Assessment (Baron, Kielhofner, Iyenger, Goldhammer, & Wolenski, 2003), Harriet determined alternative occupations that she might like, such as attending choir practice and music programs in her community center and at church. Mohini also helped her to rid her home of all alcohol and supported her decision to talk with her grocery delivery service to let them know that she would like them to turn down any future requests to deliver wine. Mohini also assisted Harriet to identify possible obstacles to her follow through on the plan, and she developed and wrote down a strategy to remind herself of the costs associated with returning to drinking, such as saying to herself, "I don't want to feel so bad and be alone like I used to" and "I am happier than when I was drinking, and I want to stay with this change for my health." Harriet also planned to call Mohini with updates on her progress twice a week at first to taper off to e-mail contact every month.

Discussion

Harriet was at the preparation stage of change, so used strategies to facilitate her commitment to implement and act on her plan (Barry, 1999; Velasquez, Maurer, Crouch, & DiClemente, 2001). Once clients have made a reasonable set of plans that they feel they can enact, helping them move to the action stage of change by supporting new behaviors and encouraging new actions as needed becomes the way that the therapist matches her or his responses to a client's readiness to change. For many clients, putting the plans into action may include some trial-and-error learning, as well as feeling more comfortable and confident with their new behaviors. As time moves along, it is important for the client to find ways to establish habits and routines that can be maintained on a long-term basis.

Harm Reduction Strategies.   Harm reduction strategies, such as needle exchange programs, condoms for IV drug users, free cab rides for persons under the influence, and the "universal precautions" approach such as free bus rides for all on New Year's Eve, have been traditionally associated with public health initiatives to lessen the negative impact of substance-related behaviors. Typically, a harm reduction approach assumes a practical and nonjudgmental manner to lessening the negative consequences of behavior. As applied to persons with serious mental illness, harm reduction recognizes that abstinence is ideal, but accepts alternatives such as cutting down or using a less risky drug. Any step in the right direction is supported when it results in greater safety for both the individual and society overall. Marlatt (1998) contends that the therapist who adopts a harm reduction approach meets clients where they are, uses open-ended questions and reflective listening, provides choices, and is a guide, not an authoritarian. Occupational therapists in states like California have had to respond to state initiatives that mandate that harm reduction be integrated into public mental health programs (Stoffel, 2002). Although for some populations, any use of alcohol or drugs places them at significant health risk, the harm reduction model supports the step-wise process toward abstinence rather than demanding abstinence up front and risking losing the person who lacks the self-efficacy to lead a chemically free lifestyle.

Note that the term *harm reduction* should not be confused with **risk reduction**. Risk reduction programs are prevention programs where groups or individuals are identified as being at high risk for developing substance use disorders, such as children of alcoholics and addictions.

Community Reinforcement Strategies.   The community reinforcement approach (CRA), originally introduced by Hunt and Azrin in 1973, has as its underlying philosophy a positivistic approach to reinforcement for sobriety versus punishing continued drinking. Consistent with this approach, Babor and Higgins-Biddle (2001) advocate an awareness of good reasons for drinking less, which includes statements like "If I drink within low-risk limits I will live longer . . . sleep better . . . be happier . . . save a lot of money . . . stay younger for longer . . . be less likely to commit suicide . . . other people will respect me" (p. 41). Of particular interest to occupational therapists and occupational therapy assistants might be that the CRA approach explicitly involves the client in choosing enjoyable activities that do not involve drinking or using and using activity sampling if the client has a limited awareness of enjoyable alternatives. The importance of having clients select environments that reflect their personal interests and are chemically free are explicit components of the CRA (Miller & Meyers, 1999).

Family members play a role in the CRA approach by recognizing their opportunities to be engaged in positive communication and activities with their loved one, spending time with her or him when sober, and pulling back when drinking/using. Meyers and Smith (1997) also explored the use of CRA with family members whose loved one was not seeking help for the substance use disorder. With the same principles of supporting abstinence and removing inadvertent reinforcement for drinking, 64% of the family members who participated in CRA had family members who sought treatment (Miller, Meyers, & Tonigan, 2002). Similarly positive outcomes were also reported in a study funded by the National Institute on Drug Abuse, where family members successfully engaged two-thirds of previously unmotivated drug abusers into treatment (Meyers, Miller, Hill, & Tonigan, 1999).

Summary of Evidence-Based Intervention Strategies. Cognitive-behavioral, psychodynamic, 12-step, transtheoretical (stages of change), and occupational perspectives on substance use have guided the development of occupational therapy programs for persons with substance use disorders. These promising interventions developed from specific models of change, particularly the transtheoretical model of behavior change (Prochaska & DiClemente, 1984; 1986).

Impact of Substance Abuse on Families and Communities

Families and communities form the context of the life of a person who uses, misuses, abuses, and becomes dependent on substances. There are tremendous consequences of substance abuse and dependence that are experienced not only by persons with a substance use disorder, but also families and communities (work, school, churches, health care and civic arenas).

For some persons, the family may have a history of substance abuse and dependence, genetically predisposing them to suffer more serious consequences once they choose to drink or use substances. For others, the social consequences of being surrounded by family and friends who drink regularly might play a role in unknowingly making it more difficult for a family member pursuing change to cut down or abstain from substances. Occupational therapists must not only pay attention to the individuals with whom they intervene, but also to family, exploring the context of the community and social networks.

All family members may be affected by the substance disorder in the family, especially when the issues associated with substance abuse and dependence are considered. Issues of domestic violence, unemployment, crime, and accident-prone environments may be related to the kinds of disabling effects experienced by family members. Persons who use and abuse substances are likely to be involved in unintentional injuries such as car accidents, falls, drowning, burns, and unintended gunshot wounds (Hingson, Heeren, Jamanka, & Howland, 2000), with alcohol noted as the leading risk factor for such injuries. These factors are why many occupational therapists work, sometimes unknowingly, with persons affected by substance use disorders—because their client's presenting condition includes a head injury, or a gunshot to the spinal cord, or a near drowning, and, with full information from an occupational profile, the occupational therapist uncovers the dysfunctional impact related to a family member with a substance use disorder.

The impact of parental substance abuse on young children, from conception, and across their lifetime, has been studied. Young children from high-density alcoholism families have been shown to have different patterns of cognitive development when compared with children from families with no history of alcoholism (Corral, Holguin, & Cadaveira, 2003). In addition, mood disorders (with rates as high as 61%) are viewed as common among children who were prenatally exposed to alcohol (O'Connor, Shah, Whaley, Cronin, Gunderson, & Graham, 2002).

Providing Service in Natural Environments: Schools, Workplaces, Neighborhoods, and Families

Occupational therapists and occupational therapy assistants work in a variety of settings where the clients they serve are in need of support for changing their everyday routines away from destructive use of alcohol and other drugs to healthier occupational routines. As professionals who work in school settings and in the workplace, the opportunity to intervene in the lives of individuals and families whose lives are being harmed due to substance use disorders is readily available. Supporting the maintenance of a healthy balance of occupations and optimal occupational role performance is also a natural fit for occupational therapists who work in neighborhood community-based programs and programs directed at families. Advocating for community support of activities that are alcohol- and drug-free for adolescents and young adults might be one way that an occupational therapy practitioner could impact prevention and harm reduction options within their neighborhood. Raising awareness of family activities and the importance of parents being actively engaged in their children's lives would also fit what an occupational therapist might focus on to support a family at risk for substance use disorders.

CASE ILLUSTRATION: Madeleine—A Teenager Abusing Drugs

Madeleine, a teenage alcohol and drug abuser, was seen by Destiny, an occupational therapist in her school setting when she was in an alternative high school.

Although Madeleine had successfully completed an inpatient residential substance abuse treatment program, her return to school and her occupational roles of student and family member were rocky. Destiny taught Madeleine how to self-reward and give herself positive affirmations when she successfully stayed chemically free each day. Destiny also supported Madeleine's connections with others who were on the road to recovery so Madeleine found a number of peers who supported her active involvement in Narcotics Anonymous and her active involvement in the high school drill team. Destiny suggested that Madeleine serve as a sponsor to another teenager on her drill team who was struggling with drug use. As her self-efficacy as a chemically free person increased, Madeleine was able to establish routines that supported her academic performance, especially in studying and being ready for her classes each day. Destiny suggested that she reward herself for new occupational performance, such as getting a B or better or successful choreography of a drill team performance. Madeleine also found that Destiny was able to help her communicate more openly with her parents and sister, and use family members to support her when she felt vulnerable about certain social situations where alcohol or drugs might be and she was able to ask them for support to anticipate situations that might put her recovery at risk, such as going away to college and dealing with living in a dorm with peers who drink or use drugs.

Discussion

Destiny worked in a community setting where she was able to help a teenager redesign her lifestyle, reconnect with her family, and develop a plan for coping with future risky situations. (See Chapters 10 and 11 for more information on community-based and family interventions.)

Summary

This chapter emphasized the occupational nature of substance use, and how the destructive aspects of such use might lead a person to occupational alienation and deprivation. Intervention is best designed when it matches the client's readiness to change, and is supported in her or his natural environments, such as family, neighborhood, school, or workplace. A variety of strategies, such as brief interventions, cognitive-behavioral, motivational, 12-step, harm reduction, and community reinforcement, can be applied to occupational therapy practice situations. All interventions support healthier decision making, a variety of meaningful occupations, and engagement in occupation to support participation in context. Regardless of the practice area in which an occupational therapy practitioner works, problems associated with substance use disorders will likely be present. The occupational therapist's use of evidence-based strategies in all settings can be effective at preventing and lessening the negative effects of substance abuse. Regaining a healthy occupational lifestyle promotes well-being and reinforces the full participation of the individual in occupations in all pertinent contexts.

Review Questions

1. What are some questions about persons' substance use history and its impact on their occupational role performance and quality of life that can augment an occupational profile?
2. What is the most common general screening tool for alcohol or drug abuse? What occupational therapy assessments evaluate the impact of alcohol or drug use on occupational performance?
3. What is the transtheoretical model of behavior change and why is it important in occupational therapy?
4. How can you design occupational therapy interventions to address readiness to change related to a person's substance use disorder?
5. What are some ways to work with a client who has a family member with a substance use disorder to (a) develop meaningful occupational routines that support his or her own health, and (b) help him or her to cope with and assist the loved one to seek help for the substance use disorder?

References

Alcoholics Anonymous (AA). (1955). *Alcoholics Anonymous: The story of how many thousands of men and women have recovered from alcoholism* (rev. ed.). New York: Alcoholics Anonymous World Services.

Alcoholics Anonymous (AA). (2001). *Alcoholics Anonymous: The story of how many thousands of men and women have recovered from alcoholism* (4th ed.). New York: Alcoholics Anonymous World Services.

American Psychiatric Association (APA). (2000). *Desk reference to the diagnostic criteria for DSM-IV-TR* (text revision). Washington, DC: Author.

American Society of Addiction Medicine. (1996). *Patient placement criteria for the treatment of psychoactive substance use disorders* (2nd ed.). Washington, DC: Author.

Babor, T. F., & Higgins-Biddle, J. C. (2001). *Brief intervention for hazardous and harmful drinking.* Geneva: World Health Organization.

Baker, A., Boggs, T. G., & Lewin, T. J. (2001). Randomized controlled trial of brief cognitive-behavioral interventions among regular users of amphetamine. *Addiction, 96,* 1279–1287.

Baron, K., Kielhofner, G., Iyenger, A., Goldhammer, V., & Wolenski, J. (2003). *A user's manual for The Occupational Self Assessment*, Version 2.1. Chicago: University of Illinois at Chicago.

Barry, K. L. (1999). *Brief interventions and brief therapies for substance abuse.* Substance Abuse and Mental Health Services Administration, DHHS Publication No. (SMA) 99-3353.

Beck, A. T., Wright, F. D., Newman, L., & Liese, B. (1993). *Cognitive therapy of substance abuse.* New York: Guilford.

Carey, K. B., Purnine, D. M., Maisto, S. A., Carey, M. P., & Barnes, K. L. (1999). Decisional balance regarding substance use among persons with schizophrenia. *Community Mental Health Journal, 35,* 289–299.

Corral, M., Holguin, S. R., & Cadaveira, F. (2003). Neuropsychological characteristics of young children from high-density alcoholism families: A three-year follow-up. *Journal of Studies on Alcohol, 64,* 195–199.

DiClemente, C. C., & Velasquez, M. M. (2002). Motivational interviewing and the stages of change. In W. R. Miller and S. Rollnick (Eds.), *Motivational interviewing: Preparing people to change addictive behavior* (2nd ed.) (Chapter 15). New York: Guilford.

Dube, S. R., Anda, R. F., Felitti, V. J., Edwards, V. J., & Croft, J. B. (2002). Adverse childhood experiences and personal alcohol abuse as an adult. *Addictive Behaviors, 27,* 713–725.

Ewing, J. (1984). Detecting alcoholism: The CAGE questionnaire. *Journal of the American Medical Association, 252,* 1905–1907.

Finney, J. W., Noyes, C. A., Coutts, A. I., & Moos, R. H. (1998). Evaluating substance abuse treatment process models: I. Changes on proximal outcome variables during 12-step and cognitive-behavioral treatment. *Journal of Studies on Alcohol, 59,* 371–380.

Graham, K., Annis, H. M., Brett, P. J., & Venesoen, P. (1996). A controlled field trial of group versus individual cognitive-behavioral training for relapse prevention. *Addiction, 91,* 1127–1139.

Hingson, R. W., Heeren, T., Jamanka, A., & Howland, J. (2000). Age of drinking onset and unintentional injury involvement after drinking. *Journal of the American Medical Association, 284,* 1527–1533.

Hunt, G. M., & Azrin, N. H. (1973). A community-reinforcement approach to alcoholism. *Behavior Research and Therapy, 11,* 91–104.

Irvin, J. E., Bowers, C. A., Dunn, M. E., & Wang, M. C. (1999). Efficacy of relapse prevention: A meta-analytic review. *Journal of Consulting and Clinical Psychology, 67,* 563–570.

Kielhofner, G., Henry, A. D., & Walens, D. (1989). *A user's guide to the Occupational Performance History Interview.* Rockville, MD: American Occupational Therapy Association.

Law, M. (2002). *Evidence-based rehabilitation: A guide to practice.* Thorofare, NJ: Slack.

Law, M., Baptiste, S., Carswell, A., McColl, M. A., Polatajko, H., & Pollack, N. (1998). *Canadian Occupational Performance Measure* (3rd ed.). Toronto: Canadian Association of Occupational Therapists.

Lieberman, D., & Scheer, J. (2002). AOTA's evidence-based literature review project. *American Journal of Occupational Therapy, 56,* 344–349.

Marlatt, G. A. (1998). Basic principles and strategies of harm reduction. In G. A. Marlatt (Ed.), *Harm reduction—pragmatic strategies for managing high-risk behaviors* (pp. 49–66). New York: Guilford.

Meyers, R. J., Miller, W. R., Hill, D. E., & Tonigan, J. S. (1999). Community reinforcement and family training (CRAFT): Engaging unmotivated drug users in treatment. *Journal of Substance Abuse, 10*(3), 1–18.

Meyers, R. J., & Smith, J. E. (1997). Getting off the fence: Procedures to engage treatment-resistant drinkers. *Journal of Substance Abuse Treatment, 14,* 467–472.

Miller, W. R., & Meyers, R. J. (with Hiller-Sturmhofel, S.). (1999). The community-reinforcement approach. *Alcohol Research and Health, 23,* 116–120.

Miller, W. R., Meyers, R. J., & Tonigan, J. S. (2002). Engaging the unmotivated in treatment for alcohol problems: A comparison of three strategies for intervention through family members. *Journal of Consulting and Clinical Psychology, 70,* 1182–1185.

Miller, W. R., & Rollnick, S. (Eds.) (2002). *Motivational interviewing: Preparing people to change addictive behavior* (2nd ed.). New York: Guilford.

Miller, W. R., & Sanchez, V. C. (1994). Motivating young adults for treatment and lifestyle change. In G. Howard & P. E. Nathan (Eds.), *Alcohol use and misuse by young adults.* Notre Dame, IN: University of Notre Dame Press.

Miller, W. R., Zweben, A., DiClemente, C. C., & Rychtarik, R. G. (1995). *Motivational enhancement therapy manual: A clinical research guide for therapists treating individuals with alcohol abuse and dependence* (NIH Publication No. 94–3723). Rockville, MD: U.S. Department of Health and Human Services.

Morgenstern, J., & Bates, M. E. (1999). Effects of executive function impairment on change processes and substance use outcomes in 12-step treatment. *Journal of Studies on Alcohol, 60,* 846–855.

Moyers, P. A. (1992). *Substance abuse: A multi-dimensional assessment and treatment approach.* Thorofare, NJ: Slack.

Moyers, P. A. (1997). Occupational meanings and spirituality: The quest for sobriety. *American Journal of Occupational Therapy, 51,* 207–214.

Moyers, P. A., & Stoffel, V. C. (1999). Alcohol dependence in a client with a work-related injury. *American Journal of Occupational Therapy, 53,* 640–645.

Moyers, P. A., & Stoffel, V. C. (2001). Community-based approaches for substance use disorders. In M. Scaffa (Ed.), *Occupational therapy in community-based practice settings* (pp. 318–342). Philadelphia: F. A. Davis.

Nowinski, J., Baker, S., & Carroll, K. (1995). *Twelve-step facilitation therapy manual. A clinical research guide for therapists treating individuals with alcohol abuse and dependence* (NIH Publication No. 94–3722). Rockville, MD: U.S. Department of Health and Human Services.

Oakley, F., Keilhofner, G., Barris, R., & Reichler, R. (1986). The Role Checklist: Development and empirical assessment of reliability. *Occupational Therapy Journal of Research, 6,* 157–170.

Occupational therapy practice framework: Domain and process (2002). *American Journal of Occupational Therapy, 56,* 609–639.

O'Connor, M. J., Shah, B., Whaley, S., Cronin, P., Gunderson, B., & Graham, J. (2002). Psychiatric illness in a clinical sample of children with prenatal alcohol exposure. *American Journal of Drug and Alcohol Abuse, 28,* 743–754.

Ouimette, P. C., Moos, R. H., & Finney, J. W. (1998). Influence of outpatient treatment and 12-step group involvement on one-year substance abuse treatment outcomes. *Journal of Studies on Alcohol, 59,* 513–522.

Palinkas, L. A., Atkins, C. J., Miller, C., & Ferreira, D. (1996). Social skills training for drug prevention in high-risk female adolescents. *Preventive Medicine, 25,* 692–701.

Pierce, D. (2001). Untangling occupation and activity. *American Journal of Occupational Therapy, 55,* 138–146.

Poikolainen, K. (1999). Effectiveness of brief interventions to reduce alcohol intake in primary health care populations: A meta-analysis. *Preventive Medicine, 28,* 503–509.

Prochaska, J. O., & DiClemente, C. C. (1984). *The transtheoretical approach: Crossing the traditional boundaries of therapy.* Homewood, IL: Dorsey/Dow Jones-Irwin.

Prochaska, J. O., & DiClemente, C. C. (1986). Toward a comprehensive model of change. In W. R. Miller & N. Heather (Eds.), *Treating addictive behaviors: Processes of change* (pp. 3–27). New York: Plenum.

Project MATCH Research Group. (1997). Matching alcoholism treatments to client heterogeneity: Project MATCH posttreatment drinking outcomes. *Journal of Studies on Alcohol, 58,* 7–29.

Project MATCH Research Group. (1998a). Matching alcoholism treatments to client heterogeneity: Treatment main effects and matching effects on drinking during treatment. *Journal of Studies on Alcohol, 59,* 631–639.

Project MATCH Research Group. (1998b). Matching patients with alcohol disorders to treatments: Clinical implications from Project MATCH. *Journal of Mental Health, 7,* 589–603.

Roehrich, L., & Goldman, M. S. (1993). Experience-dependent neuropsychological recovery and the treatment of alcoholism, *Journal of Consulting and Clinical Psychology, 61,* 812–821.

Saunders, B., Wilkinson, C., & Phillips, M. (1995). The impact of a brief motivational intervention with opiate users attending a methadone programme. *Addiction, 90,* 415–424.

Smith, N. R., Kielhofner, G., & Watts, J. H. (1986). The relationship between volition, activity pattern and life satisfaction in the elderly. *American Journal of Occupational Therapy, 40,* 278–283.

Stein, M. D., Charuvastra, A., Maksad, J., & Anderson, B. J. (2002). A randomized trial of a brief alcohol intervention for needle exchangers (BRAINE). *Addiction, 97,* 691–700.

Stoffel, V. C. (1992). The American with Disabilities Act of 1990 as applied to an adult with alcohol dependence. *American Journal of Occupational Therapy, 46,* 640–644.

Stoffel, V. C. (2002, June). *Chemical dependency and the harm reduction models.* Paper presented at the Psychiatric Occupational Therapy Action Coalition of California, San Rafael, CA.

Stoffel, V., & Moyers, P. (1999). *Occupational therapy practice guidelines for substance use disorders.* Bethesda, MD: AOTA.

Stoffel, V. C., & Moyers, P. A. (2001). *AOTA evidence-based practice project: Treatment effectiveness as applied to substance use disorders in adolescents and adults.* Unpublished manuscript. Bethesda, MD: AOTA.

Substance Abuse and Mental Health Services Administration (SAMHSA). (2002). *Results from the 2001 National Household Survey on Drug Abuse: Volume I. Summary of National Findings* (Office of Applied Studies, NHSDA Series H-17, DHHS Publication No. SMA 02-3758). Rockville, MD.

Velasquez, M. M., Maurer, G. G., Crouch, C., & DiClemente, C. C. (2001). *Group treatment for substance abuse: A stages-of-change therapy manual.* New York: Guilford.

Wilcock, A. (1998). *An occupational perspective of health.* Thorofare, NJ: Slack.

Wilk, A. I., Jensen, N. M., & Havighurst, T. C. (1997). Meta-analysis of randomized controlled trials addressing brief interventions in heavy alcohol drinkers. *Journal of General Internal Medicine, 12,* 274–283.

Zinn, S., Bosworth, H. B., Edwards, C. L., Logue, P. E., & Swartzwelder, H. S. (2003). Performance of recently detoxified patients with alcoholism on a neuropsychological screening test. *Addictive Behaviors, 28,* 837–849.

Zywiak, W. H., Longabaugh, R., & Wirtz, P. W. (2002). Decomposing the relationships between pre-treatment social network characteristics and alcohol treatment outcome. *Journal of Studies on Alcohol, 63,* 114–121.

Suggested Reading

AOTA evidence briefs on substance use disorders found online at www.aota.org

Several Treatment Improvement Protocol (TIP) Series from the National Clearinghouse for Alcohol and Drug Information @ (800) 729-6686:

1) TIP 29 Substance Use Disorder Treatment for People with Physical and Cognitive Disabilities
2) TIP 34 Brief Interventions and Brief Therapies for Substance Abuse
3) TIP 35 Enhancing Motivation for Change in Substance Abuse Treatment

Occupational Therapy Intervention in Mental Health

The three chapters in Part VI focus on the process of intervention, that is, the assessments, methods, and approaches that practitioners use to understand and facilitate occupational engagement. The previous chapters detailed various psychosocial and developmental conditions and suggested clinical interventions specific to each condition, while these chapters suggest the broad individual and group processes used in every intervention.

The chapters on evaluation and assessment and methods and interpersonal approaches are new and reflect the unique perspectives of each author. Chapter 17 emphasizes occupational engagement, the impact of disorders on occupational engagement, the influence of stigma on recovery, and the nature of the recovery process. These ideas are the context or the background to a thorough evaluation using occupational therapy assessments. Chapter 18 focuses on personal approaches and techniques that are used in the context of the therapeutic relationship as well as the traditional occupational therapy processes of clinical reasoning and activity analysis used to deliver occupational therapy interventions. Both chapters follow and elucidate various sections of the Occupational Therapy Practice Framework (2002).

Chapter 19 has been updated to include information regarding group roles and tasks and case illustrations that reflect a group's process in a community psychosocial rehabilitation center based on a "clubhouse" model. Together the three chapters thoroughly cover the processes of evaluation and intervention from unique and innovative perspectives.

CHAPTER 17

Evaluation and Assessment

Deborah B. Pitts, MBA, OTR/L, CPRP

Key Terms

activity demands
analysis of occupational performance
assessment
client factors
comprehensive evaluation
contexts
evaluation
heterarchical

occupational profile
outcome evaluation
performance in areas
   of occupation
performance patterns
performance skills
reliability and validity
screening evaluation
validity

Chapter Outline

Introduction

In contemporary mental health practice, the **evaluation** process assists clients and occupational therapists to mutually determine the need for change in clients, their occupational performances, or their environments. The evaluation then guides collaborative interventions intended to facilitate that change. This chapter addresses the process by which occupational therapists perform such evaluations in mental health settings. It provides a select review of specific **assessment** methods and tools commonly used in those settings. In addition, the chapter also explains the process according to the Occupational Therapy Practice Framework (2002). This chapter provides a general review of the evaluation process and of assessments used in mental health practice. It is not a detailed study of assessments or psychometric properties of assessments.

THE EVALUATION PROCESS

Evaluation is a process that involves five steps: synthesizing, observing, selecting, interpreting, and developing. Synthesis involves gathering information about clients and then distilling it into essentials that are barriers to and strengths that support performance. Observation involves watching people's actions and listening to their words while they perform an activity. Selection involves choosing assessments that will further measure the essential areas of performance, whether context, activity, or client factors that influence skills and patterns. Interpretation involves determining the meaning of the assessment results, particularly as they affect meaningful and productive occupational engagement. Development involves detailing assumptions and refining hypotheses about the person's strength and weaknesses, **contexts**, and occupations that will guide interventions. Figure 17-1 briefly lists these steps.

There are two primary actions that organize the evaluation process. They are development of the **occupational profile** and **analysis of occupational per-**

1. *Synthesize* information from the occupational profile to focus on specific areas of occupation and their contexts that need to be addressed.
2. *Observe* the person's performance in desired occupations and activities, noting effectiveness of the performance skills and patterns.
3. *Select* assessments, as needed, to identify and measure more specifically context or contexts, **activity demands**, and **client factors** that may be influencing performance skills and patterns.
4. *Interpret* the assessment data to identify what supports or hinders performance.
5. *Develop* and refine hypotheses about the person's occupational performance strengths and weaknesses.

Figure 17-1.   Step-by-Step Evaluation Actions

formance (Occupational Therapy Practice Framework, 2002). The first two steps of the evaluation process will lead to an understanding of what the client wants and needs to do and what the barriers are to attaining desired goals. Ultimately this information will enable the occupational therapist to collaborate with clients in determining and developing interventions to accomplish the desired outcomes.

Synthesizing the Occupational Profile

The occupational profile (Occupational Therapy Practice Framework, 2002) is intended to provide an understanding of the client's occupational history and experiences, patterns of daily living, interests, values, and needs. In developing the profile, the occupational therapist collaborates with clients to identify problems and concerns about performing their occupations and daily life activities. The client's priorities are determined and these then serve as a focus for the next steps of the evaluation process. Typically the information for the profile is gathered through interviews and collecting the information may be based on various occupational therapy practice models. The therapist may use a specific interview format, such as the OPHI-II, or may let the interview unfold in each individual situation. Whichever format is used, the occupational profile will yield information that answers the questions listed in Figure 17-2.

Interviews. Interviews can be structured, semi-structured, or narrative. Structured interviews require occupational therapists to ask a specific set of questions

Who is the client (individual, caregiver, group, population)?

Why is the client seeking service, and what are the client's current concerns relative to engaging in occupations and in daily life activities?

What areas of occupation are successful, and what areas are causing problems or risks?

What contexts support engagement in desired occupations, and what contexts are inhibiting engagement?

What is the client's occupational history (i.e., life experiences, values, interests, previous patterns of engagement in occupations and in daily life activities, the meanings associated with them)?

What are the client's priorities and desired target outcomes?

- Improvement or enhancement of occupational performance
- Client satisfaction
- Role competence
- Adaptation
- Health and wellness
- Prevention
- Quality of life

Figure 17-2. Questions to Develop an Occupational Profile

Source: Adapted from the Occupational Therapy Practice Framework (2002, p. 616).

with no flexibility to modify the specific phrasing or order of the questions. However, structured interviews are not commonly used in occupational therapy and would more likely be used in the analysis of a specific aspect of occupational performance as opposed to the development of the person's occupational profile.

Semi-structured interviews are much more common in occupational therapy. In semi-structured interviews, an outline of performance domains that the interview is intended to target and a set of recommended questions are provided (Kielhofner, 2002). The interviewer is free to frame questions that are specifically matched to the unique individual being interviewed. Such flexibility allows for questions that have cultural relevance and sensitivity, as well as a sequence that flows out of the conversational nature common to clinical interviews.

Narrative interviews are a specific form of semi-structured interview and are the most open-ended of the three types of interviews (Kielhofner, Mallinson, Crawford, Nowak, Rigby, Henry, & Walens, 1997). In narrative interviewing, the therapist is encouraged to frame questions such that the people being interviewed tell a story about their occupations. The therapist uses verbal prompts that encourage the person to richly articulate the lived experience of occupational engagement. Clark's (1993) occupational storytelling and storymaking informed by phenomenology is an example of this approach. Clark argues that during the process of a narrative interview, the therapist and person must "build a communal horizon" of understanding to inform their work together. On the one hand, although less so in mental health settings, narrative approaches have been criticized as being too time-consuming, too costly and not reasonable and therefore not reimbursable given the demands of many health care settings (Duchek & Thessing, 1996). On the other hand, counter-arguments assert that the information derived from such approaches is more likely to optimize clinical outcomes and minimize costs associated with poorly planned interventions (Clark, Carlson, & Polkinghorne, 1997; Burke & Kern, 1996).

Occupational therapy practice in mental health has a long history of using interviews as a standard part of any evaluation process (Hemphill, 1982; 1988; 1999). Many of the interview-based assessments in use in modern occupational therapy practice were originally developed for use in psychiatric practice settings (Hemphill, 1999; Barris et al., 1988). One of the earliest of these, known as The Occupational History (Morehead, 1969), and its earliest revision, The Occupational Role History (ORH) along with the Environmental Questionnaire (Dunning, 1972), evolved out of efforts to further articulate what is known as the Occupational Behavior frame of reference developed by Mary Reilly in late 1960s as part of her effort to contribute to the development of theory to support occupational therapy practice. Other models of practice have incorporated the principles of the occupational behavior perspective (Barrett & Kielhofner, 2003). For a complete list of assessments mentioned in this chapter, refer to Table 17-1.

The Occupational Role History (ORH) (Morehead, 1969).   The ORH is a semi-structured or focused interview with the client as informant. It was developed as a preliminary device to identify critical information in two major areas: patterns of skills and achievement or dysfunction in past and current occupa-

Table 17-1. Assessments Used in Mental Health Practice

Assessment Type	Assessment	Acronym	Purpose	For	Time to Administer
Interview	Occupational Role History	**ORH**	Role status and balance of leisure and role activities	Adults	
	Environmental Questionnaire	**EQ**	Perspective about living environment	Adults	60 minutes
	Occupational Circumstances Assessment—Interview and Rating scale	**OCAIRS**	Extent and nature of occupational adaptation/functioning	Adolescents and adults	
	Occupational Performance History Interview-II	**OPHI-II**	Past and present adaptation, impact of environment, life history narrative		45–60 minutes
	Canadian Occupational Performance Measure	**COPM**	Perception of how well one performs and satisfaction with performance, prioritize problems and goals in occupational performance	Children to adult	40–60 minutes
Self-Report Checklists	Modified Interest Checklist	**Modified Interest Checklist**	Current interests, how interests have changed over time, desire to engage in interests in the future; unique pattern of interests that influence choices.	Adolescents and adults	
	Role Checklist	**Role Checklist**	Perception and value of roles	Adolescents and adults	
Self-Report Measures	Occupational Questionnaire	**OQ**	Record of daily activities for typical day, enjoyment, importance, how well they are performed	Adults	
	Adult Sensory Profile	**Sensory Profile**	Identifies response to sensations, how sensory processing patterns influence occupational performance	Adults	
Can be used as outcome measure	Occupational Self-Assessment	**OSA**	Perceptions of competence in occupations and impact of the environment on occupations. Personal values and identify desired changes	Adults	
Can be used as outcome measure	Child Occupational Self-Assessment	**COSA**	Perceptions of competence in occupations.	Children	

(continues)

Table 17-1.   (continued)

Assessment Type	Assessment	Acronym	Purpose	For	Time to Administer
Observation Tool for nonverbal reporters	Volitional Questionnaire	**VQ**	Observation of volitional behaviors in context	Adults	
Observation-based Performance Assessments	Assessment of Communication and Interaction Skills	**ACIS**	Social performance when engaged in daily occupations	Adults	20–60 minutes
	Kohlman Evaluation of Living Skills	**KELS**	Assesses ability to independently or with assistance complete self-care, safety and health, money management, transportation and telephone, and work and leisure.	Adults	30–45 minutes
Can be an outcome measure	Milwaukee Evaluation of Daily Living Skills	**MEDLS**	Basic daily living skills such as dressing, hair care, time awareness, etc.	Adults	
	Functional Needs Assessment	**FNA**	Criterion-referenced assessment of typical daily living tasks—perform an action by responding to instruction	Adults	
	Assessment of Motor and Process Skills	**AMPS**	Assesses daily living skills, motor and process skills used to complete daily living skills.	Adults, toddlers, children	30–60 minutes
	Allen Cognitive Level Test	**ACL**	Assesses person's ability to learn and need for environmental compensation according to person's performance on a task and placement on a cognitive level of functioning. Often used for quick screening.	Adults	15–60 minutes
	Allen Diagnostic Module	**ADM**	Twenty-four tasks that assess person's ability to learn and need for environmental compensation	Adults	15–60 minutes

tional roles; and the degree of balance or imbalance between leisure activities and those activities associated with occupational role. Information yielded from the ORH can be categorized according to two dimensions: role status (i.e., functional, temporarily impaired, dysfunctional) and balance. In determining the degree of balance or imbalance between leisure activities and those associated with occupational role, the criterion is whether individuals identified any interests, hobbies, and activities they did on a consistent basis separate from occupational role activities (Florey & Michelman, 1982).

The Environmental Questionnaire (EQ) (Dunning, 1972).   The EQ is a semi-structured interview designed to elicit the person's perspective about his or her living environment. An environmental grid that proposes relationships between space, people, and task is constructed through the use of the interview and serves to assist the practitioner in prioritizing interventions. Although there has been no further development of this instrument since, it serves as an early approach to assessing context (Dunning, 1972).

Since the 1980s, theoreticians and practitioners of the Model of Human Occupation have developed several interview-based instruments that have evolved from and expanded on Reilly's concepts regarding occupational behavior, including the Occupational Circumstances Assessment-Interview and Rating Scale (OCAIRS) (Haglund, Henriksson, Crisp, Freidheim, & Kielhofner, 2001) and the Occupational Performance History Interview-II (OPHI-II) (Kielhofner, Mallinson, Crawford, Nowak, Rigby, Henry, & Walens, 1997).

The Occupational Circumstances Assessment-Interview and Rating Scale (OCAIRS) (Haglund et al., 2001).   The OCAIRS is based on the Occupational Case Analysis Interview Rating Scale (Kaplan, 1984; Kaplan & Kielhofner, 1989) and provides a structure for gathering, analyzing, and reporting data on the extent and nature of the person's current occupational adaptation. Based on the Model of Human Occupation, it consists of a semi-structured interview that collects information on the person's occupational adaptation and participation, personal causation, values, goals, interests, roles, habits, skills, and the environment. Designed to be relevant to adolescent and adult clients with a wide range of backgrounds and impairments, it requires approximately 40 minutes to complete the interview and 15 minutes to complete the rating scale and comments. Studies about the Occupational Case Analysis Interview on which the OCAIRS is based that are cited in Kielhofner (2002) indicate good inter-rater **reliability**. Also, it discriminates between clients who have various severities of psychiatric illness.

The Occupational Performance History Interview (OPHI-II) (Kielhofner et al., 1997).   The OPHI-II, based on the Model of Human Occupation, is a three-part assessment intended to elicit information about the person's past and present occupational adaptation. It includes a semi-structured interview that explores the person's occupational life history; rating scales to identify the person's occupational identity, occupational competence, the impact of the person's occupational behavior settings; and a life history narrative that offers a qualitatively richer perspective of the person's occupational life history. Recommended questions for conducting the interview are provided and focus on five areas—activity/occupational choices, critical life events, daily routine, occupational roles, and occupational behavior settings. Administration of the interview takes approximately 45 to 60 minutes and the therapist then completes the three rating scales. Each item on the scale is scored with a 4-point rating indicating the person's level of occupational adaptation/environmental impact. The therapist then completes a written narrative of the person's occupational life history.

The Canadian Occupational Performance Measure (COPM) (Law, Baptiste, Carswell-Opzoomer, McColl, Polatajko, & Pollock, 1991).   The COPM, developed in Canada, is popular in the United States as well. (Evaluators are encouraged to review international journals, including the *Canadian Journal of*

Occupational Therapy, the *British Journal of Occupational Therapy,* the *Scandinavian Journal of Occupational Therapy,* the *Australian & New Zealand Journal of Occupational Therapy,* and others to become familiar with internationally developed instruments and research into the use of U.S.-developed instruments with international populations.)

The COPM is designed for use by occupational therapists to assess clients' perceptions of their occupational performance. Thus it is not an objective measure of occupational performance. The COPM identifies problem areas in occupational performance, assists in goal setting with regard to occupational performance, and measures changes in occupational performance over the course of occupational therapy. The COPM is designed for use among clients with a variety of disabilities and across all developmental stages.

Occupational performance is defined as consisting of three areas: (1) self-care—including personal care, functional mobility, and community management; (2) productivity—including paid or unpaid work, household management and school or play; and (3) leisure—including quiet recreation, active recreation, and socialization. Satisfactory performance in each of these areas is dependent upon the integration of physical, socio-cultural, mental-emotional, and spiritual performance components. Occupational performance must be defined for each individual according to the social roles he or she must fulfill, the environment he or she functions within, and his or her developmental stage. The individual being assessed defines performance in terms of how well he or she performs an activity and how satisfied he or she is with his or her performance.

The COPM is administered in the form of a semi-structured interview that includes five steps: problem definition, problem weighting, scoring, reassessment, and follow-up. Once the specific problems have been identified, they are prioritized. Then the person being evaluated is asked to rate the priority problems importance on a 10-point scale. For each problem area defined by the person being evaluated in the areas of self-care, productivity, and leisure, she or he is also asked if she or he can, does, and is satisfied with the way she or he performs that specific activity.

Other data collection methods that may be useful in completing the occupational profile are self-report checklists. These assessments give clients an additional method for communicating their needs and preferences for occupational engagement. They can be used to prompt discussion of important issues that may have not emerged in the interview.

Self-Report Checklists.   Instruments of this type include the Modified Interest Checklist (Matsutsuyu, 1969; Scaffa, 1981; Kielhofner & Neville, 1983), The Role Checklist (Oakley, Kielhofner, & Barris, 1985), and the Occupational Self-Assessment (Baron, Kielhofner, Iyenger, Goldhammer, & Wolenski, 2002).

The Modified Interest Checklist.   The Modified Interest Checklist, based on the Model of Human Occupation, is a revision of The Interest Checklist originally developed by Matsutsuyu (1969). The original instrument was part of the early theoretical development of the Occupational Behavior Frame of Reference. The original format of the assessment provided information about clients' interests in a select list of 68 activities, as well as a clustering of interests into categories (Rogers, 1988). The occupational therapist was also expected to provide a written summary. Revisions of the instrument were made by Scaffa (as cited in Kielhofner, 2002) and Kielhofner and Neville (as cited in Kielhofner, 2002) and expanded the response options to include what the person's current interests are, how interests have changed over time, and whether one currently engages or wishes to engage in the activity in the future. Useful for both adolescents and adults, the checklist primarily provides a perspective on the person's unique pattern of interests that affect his or her choices of activities. The checklist is quick to administer and easy to understand. Research studies did not support its use as a means for clustering or categorizing activities (Klyczek & Bauer-Yox, 1997; Rogers, Weinstein, Figone, cited in Kielhofner, 2002), but did show that the instrument can discriminate between people with disabilities and those without disabilities. Persons with disabilities exhibit fewer interests and less participation in valued interests (Eff, Coster, & Duncombe; Katz, Giladi, & Peretz, as cited in Kielhofner, 2002).

The Role Checklist.   The Role Checklist (Oakley, Kielhofner, & Barris, 1985), based on the Model of Human Occupation, is a self-report assessment and was developed to obtain information on clients' perceptions about their participation in occupational roles throughout their life and the value they place on those roles. The checklist can be used with adolescents or adults. The Role Checklist is interpreted by examining the pattern of responses, including loss of roles, lack of involvement in valued roles, and/or the desire for future role engagement. Content **validity** has been established and test-retest reliability indicated the checklist was stable over time with adolescents and adults (Oakley, Kielhofner, Barris, & Reichler; Pezzulli, as cited in Kielhofner, 2002).

The Occupational Self-Assessment (OSA).   The OSA (Baron, Kielhofner, Iyenger, Goldhammer, & Wolenski, 2002) is based on the Model of Human Occupation and is designed to facilitate understanding of the person's own perceptions of her or his occupational competence and the impact of aspects of the environment on occupational performance. Section I includes statements about occupational functioning, such as concentrating on tasks, and the client checks how well she or he does it on a 4-point scale that ranges from "I have lots of problems doing this" to "I do this extremely well." Then clients respond to the statements indicating the importance of each on a 4-point scale. Section II includes statements about their environment with responses on the same 4-point scale as in Section I. Then they list up to four things they would like to change in response to the same statements. This particular instrument has been designed to serve both as a intervention planning tool as well as an outcome measure, so it can be administered multiple times to identify change throughout treatment.

The OSA Studies (Iyenger; Kielhofner & Forsyth, as cited in Kielhofner, 2002), which examined the validity and reliability of the OSA, have found that the instrument is valid and reliable across cultural, language, and diagnostic differences.

There is also a form for children, the Child Occupational Self-Assessment (Federico & Kilehofner, as cited in Kielhofner, 2002), which is similar to the adult version except it does not include a section on the environment or listing changes, uses a simpler 3-point scale, and uses symbols for choosing responses that would appeal to children, such as happy faces or stars.

Although not a common approach to developing an occupational profile, observation tools may be necessary and useful when interviews or self-report measures are not likely to elicit the information needed. The Volitional Questionnaire (VQ) (de las Heras, Geist, Kielhofner, & Li, 2002) was developed to meet the need for an assessment tool that could elicit information about a person's values, interests, and goals when his or her ability to describe these verbally is limited.

The Volitional Questionnaire (VQ). The VQ (de las Heras, Geist, Kielhofner, & Li, 2002), based on the Model of Human Occupation, is an observational assessment of volition and is useful when self-report assessments are not able to be completed. It purports that people who have difficulty verbally articulating their goals, interests, and values communicate these through their active engagement in their environments. Therefore, it is composed of 14 items that describe behaviors reflecting values, interests, and personal causation. The rating focuses on clients' volitional behaviors in their environments rather than the environmental support needed to engage. Research (Chern, Kielhofner, de las Heras & Magalhaes, as cited in Kielhofner, 2002) shows that the items represent a continuum from less to more volition. The VQ is supported by a detailed manual (de las Heras et al., 2002) and content validity and inter-rater reliability studies (de las Heras, as cited in Kielhofner, 2002) have been completed.

There is also a version, The Pediatric Volitional Questionnaire, that is designed for children, 2 to 6 years old. However, it is often used for older children as well. The pediatric version can be used for children with significant developmental delays and other disabilities who are at significant risk for decreased volition. However, it also can be used with typically developing children (Kielhofner, 2002).

CASE ILLUSTRATION: Jackie—Evaluation in an Independent Living Situation

Jackie, an occupational therapist, was contacted by a local mental health agency that provides supervised and supported living environments for persons with psychiatric disabilities. She was recruited specifically to assist in the evaluation of potential tenants for the agency's new independent living apartment project that was still in the planning stage. In the development of a previous apartment program, the agency had had significant difficulty with tenants not being able to manage the demands of independent living with the level of support that had been provided. This new project would have the same level of support as the previous one and the agency wanted to ensure that they chose tenants who could successfully sustain their housing. Given the nature of the agency's request, Jackie considered the OCAIRS (Haglund et al., 2001) and the EQ (Dunning, 1972) interviews to develop a brief occupational profile to learn tenants' past and present functioning specifically in the activities of daily living area of occupation.

Discussion

Jackie considered interviews that would elicit information from clients about their living environments.

While the occupational profile develops an all-around picture of the client from her or his perspective, the observation of occupational performance focuses on behavior or what the client does.

Observing and Analyzing Occupational Performance Analysis

The second step of the evaluation process focuses on an analysis of occupational performance. Here the evaluator more specifically identifies the clients' strengths and available contextual supports, as well as barriers or potential challenges to engaging in their occupations. The occupational therapist orchestrates as much as possible observation of clients' actual performances in context so that the therapist can identify what supports or hinders performances. Various factors familiar to occupational therapists and within their domain of practice could support or hinder performance. Those factors identified by the Occupational Therapy Practice Framework (2002) are listed and defined in Table 17-2. Page numbers are listed

Table 17-2.	Factors That Support or Hinder Occupational Performance
Factor	*Definition*
Performance Skills	Skills are what one does, such as concentrate, not what one has, such as feelings, "related to observable elements of action that have implicit functional purposes," including motor, process, and communication skills (p. 621).
Performance Patterns	"Patterns of behavior related to daily life activities that are habitual or routine," including habits, routines, and roles (p. 623).
Context or Contexts	"Context (including cultural, physical, social, personal, spiritual, temporal, and virtual) refers to a variety of inter-related conditions within and surrounding the client that influence performance" (p. 623).
Activity Demands	"The aspects of an activity, which include the objects, space, social demands, sequencing or timing, required actions, and required underlying body functions and body structure needed to carry out the activity" (p. 624).
Client Factors	"Those factors that reside within the client and that may affect **performance in areas of occupation**. Client factors include body function and body structures" (p. 624). Body functions include psychological functions.

Source: Information from Occupational Therapy Practice Framework: Domain and Process. (2002). *American Journal of Occupational Therapy, 56,* 609–639.

so that the considerable additional information, explanations, and definitions can be easily accessed.

When considering these aspects in the evaluation process, they are best understood from a dynamic systems perspective as having a **heterarchical** relationship to each other. That is, no one aspect is considered to have more importance or to be at the core of successful and satisfactory performance in occupation. Each aspect may in a given occupation within a given context be identified as the constraining or supportive influence to engagement in that occupation. Therefore, all of these factors must be considered and understood in the evaluation process. However, though all factors may be considered, only selected aspects may be specifically assessed. Determining or prioritizing what specifically is assessed is determined by the findings from the occupational profile and by the client being served (Occupational Therapy Practice Framework, 2002). For example, members of a clubhouse program, Townehouse Creative Living Center, attend four days per week and are members of groups based on work in one of three vocational areas: clerical and computer, house and grounds, or food service. While attending and working in the vocational groups, staff are generally concerned with assessing activity demands so that the members can function in their work groups, and are generally aware of client factors, such as psychological or physical health that may influence members' abilities to function in the context of their community at Townehouse or where they live. However, when members express an interest in joining the transitional employment program, specific assessments are used. The assessments ascertain members' abilities to function safely, communicate in person and by phone, and travel to and from work. Specific observational assessments determine if they have the skills needed for particular job slots in the general community that are open to Townehouse members. Furthermore, the client can be a teacher, caregiver, spouse, parent, employer, family, or organization. For example, if a member from Townehouse was being evaluated for one of the transitional employment opportunities, ongoing consultation may be provided to the employer or supervisor at the job regarding the best way to communicate with the member, or the best way to use his or her particular skills. In addition, the member may express a desire to have his or her family be informed of the support that the member may need to maintain the job. In another example, an employer may request an analysis of the work environment in order to develop job slots for workers with mental illness.

Observation-Based Performance Assessments.   Observation-based performance assessments can be completed by the occupational therapist or another informant such as family member, teacher, or employer. These assessments are generally either contextual (Dunn, 1998) or noncontextual. Contextual observation-based assessments are designed for use in the actual contexts in which the person engages in the occupation. Like narrative interview approaches, contextual observation-based assessments are considered too costly and time intensive for many clinical settings. However, they are preferred over noncontextual observation-based assessments, which involve the use of simulated environments or assessment of a specific task performance that does not take into account environmental factors. If you choose to use noncontextual observation-based assessments they may be limited in predicting performance in the natural environment. Because many mental health interventions are now being provided in persons' natural environments such as homes, schools, or workplaces, contextual observation-based assessments are popular in mental health practice.

Occupational therapists working in mental health have more opportunities to observe people in their environment due to programs that emphasize community functioning, such as assertive community treatment (ACT), supported housing, supported employment, supported education approaches, and Medicare-reimbursed home health care. Instruments like the Assessment of Communication and Interaction Skills (ACIS) (Forsyth, Salamy, Simon, & Kielhofner, 1998) can be used in natural environments to measure social performance.

The Assessment of Communication and Interaction Skills (ACIS) (Forsyth et al., 1998). The ACIS, based on the Model of Human Occupation, is a formal observational assessment that measures a person's social performance when engaged in daily occupations. The ACIS observations should be made in those contexts that have meaning and relevance to the client. The ACIS has 20 items divided into three domains—physicality, information exchange, and relations. The items are rated on a 4-point scale and focus on the impact of skills on the progression of the social interaction, the impact on others with whom the client interacts, and the impact on the task being completed. The administration time for the ACIS can be 20 to 60 minutes, with the observation requiring between 15 and 45 minutes and the rating from 5 to 20 minutes.

When actual observation by the occupational therapist in context is not possible, simulated experiences will offer useful perspectives into how the person might perform that occupation in context. A noncontextual instrument such as the Kohlman Evaluation of Living Skills (KELS) (Kohlman-Thomson, 1992; McGourty, 1988) is an example of this type of assessment. Many of the simulated or noncontext observational assessments that have been developed by occupational therapists include the measurement of targeted client factors, such as impairments in attention, memory, or perception. These impairments can compromise a person's occupational performance in specific ways within certain contexts. Therefore, occupational therapy researchers have developed specific assessment tools designed to measure the impact of these cognitive impairments on the person's functioning. These assessments (other than the KELS) provide guidance for environmental modifications that will optimize the person's occupational performance within his or her preferred occupational contexts. Examples of this type of instrument include the Allen Cognitive Levels (ACL) (Allen, 1985), and the Allen Diagnostic Modules (ADM) (Allen, Earhart, & Blue, 1993).

When using simulated or noncontext-specific observations of occupational performance, it is useful to support this data with information from those involved with the client. Family members, teachers, employers, and others who have had extended and multiple opportunities to interact and observe the person performing occupations can be interviewed or can complete checklists that describe the person's performance. This information from other informants is particularly helpful when evaluating children and/or adults who are nonresponsive to interview questions or who are unwilling or unable to complete self-report checklists. The following sections discuss noncontextual observation-based assessments.

The Kohlman Evaluation of Living Skills (KELS) (Kohlman-Thomson, 1992). The KELS is an assessment of basic living skills that combines interview and task performance techniques. It is intended to be administered and scored within 30 to 45 minutes. It assesses 18 living skills grouped within five major categories of self-care, safety and health, money management, transportation and telephone, and work and leisure. Scoring criteria have been formulated to indicate the minimum standards required for living independently within the community. Items scored as "needs assistance" are given a score of one point except those in the work/leisure category, which are assessed one-half point. Items scored Independent are given a score of zero. Therefore, higher scores indicate more dependent functioning. Studies cited in the manual indicate that the KELS has good inter-rater reliability and that the scale was able to correctly differentiate persons living in a sheltered setting versus those living independently with an accuracy of 90%.

The Milwaukee Evaluation of Daily Living Skills (MEDLS) (Leonardelli, 1988b). The MEDLS is an assessment of basic daily living skills and was developed out of a desire to provide a standard procedure for measuring the behavioral performance of daily living skills for persons with psychiatric disabilities. It consists of 20 subtests such as dressing, hair care, and time awareness. Specific subtests are selected for use according to the expressed goals and needs of each person. MEDLS can provide baseline data for beginning intervention and can also be used to provide a quantifiable measure of change. Screening and Reporting Forms provide quick, easy-to-read information for the entire interdisciplinary treatment team.

The Functional Needs Assessment (FNA) (Dombrowski, 1990). The FNA provides an integrated, systematic method for assessment, treatment planning, clinical program designing, and progress monitoring. The program is comprehensive and does not require an extensive amount of time to administer. It was designed as a criterion-referenced assessment, that is, one in which the client's performance is measured against specific criteria for each skill (Crist, 1998; Duncan, 1998). The component skill areas were chosen to reflect common or typical tasks in daily living and the developmental process of identification, recognition, generalization, and integration of performance. The assessment is a "show me" assessment, which requires clients to demonstrate their ability to understand by performing a specific action or by responding to an instruction. The functional components in the program are neurologically based and developmentally sequenced and address several areas of daily functioning. Each component is developmentally sequenced into five skill levels. The objective at each skill level assumes integration of lower skill levels.

The Assessment of Motor and Performance Skills (AMPS) (Fisher, 1999). The AMPS conceptual model was based on the Model of Human Occupation (and led later to a revision of MOHO) (A. Fisher, personal communication, January 30, 2004) and gathers information on skills by observing the person doing certain activities of daily living, including instrumental activities of daily living, in her or his own environment. Therefore, it is a contextual test of occupational performance. The AMPS has been designed in such a way that cross-culturally standardized tasks can be used to measure occupational performance, of those 3 years old and above, because it has been standardized, on 46,886 participants (Fisher, 2003). When administering the AMPS, information on performance skills, that is, motor skills (i.e., observable goal-directed actions done to move oneself or task objects) and process skills (i.e., observable actions that are enacted to logically sequence actions, select and appropriately use tools and materials, and adapt to problems) are observed and collected simultaneously. In addition, the design of AMPS allows the therapist to consider the level of difficulty of the task the person is performing and for the severity/leniency of the rater. Occupational therapists choosing to use the AMPS as part of their evaluation portfolio must be trained and calibrated for their severity/leniency scoring tendencies. Many studies cited in the AMPS manual (Fisher, 2003) and in Kielhofner (2002) support the validity, reliability, internal consistency of the scales, stability of the measures over time, and ability of the measures to remain stable when the AMPS is scored by different raters. Administration and scoring of the AMPS takes 30 to 60 minutes and includes a brief interview and observation of the person performing at least two preferred standardized tasks from 83 standardized ADL tasks. Sixteen motor (effort) and 20 process (efficiency) skill items are rated on a scale of 1 (deficit) to 4 (competent). Scores for the AMPS are then computer generated.

The Routine Task Inventory (RTI) (Allen, Earhart, & Blue, 1992; 1996; Heimann, Allen, & Yerxa, 1989). The RTI, developed within the Cognitive Disabilities Model, is an observational guide. It consists of 14 tasks that describe behavioral actions consistent with six, hierarchical, cognitive levels for understanding how cognitive impairments impact a person's occupational performance. The RTI, although it describes how a person can be expected to function according to each level, is a description of the functional severity of a disability; it is a here-and-now assessment of the impact of a disease. The 14 routine tasks of the RTI are divided into two scales, the physical scale and the instrumental scale. The six tasks on the physical scale are grooming, dressing, bathing, walking, feeding, and toileting. The eight tasks on the instrumental scale are housekeeping, preparing food, spending money, taking medication, doing laundry, traveling, shopping, and telephoning. Under each of the 14 tasks, behavioral descriptions are written in connection with each cognitive level. Administration of the interview requires the identification of an informant who is well acquainted with the individual's performance and willing to provide information. The informant and the occupational therapist review the inventory together and the behavioral descriptions that match the individual's routine task performance are noted. Estimated time needed to administer the RTI is about one hour.

The Allen Cognitive Levels Test (ACL) (Allen, 1985; Allen, Earhart, & Blue, 1992; 1996). The ACL is based on the Cognitive Disabilities Model (Allen, 1985) and is designed to obtain a baseline measure of a person's capacity to learn and the need for environmental compensations. As noted previously, the cognitive levels represent a six-level hierarchical model that describes what behaviors a person is capable of doing, and for understanding how cognitive impairments impact a person's occupational performance. This performance test is usually administered at the end of the initial interview. Therapists use the score as a guideline for the treatment goals that are achievable at the present time. The ACL is a leather-lacing task that provides an estimate of a person's ability to learn to do other sensoriomotor tasks. Reliability and validity studies have found the instrument to be a dependable measure of cognitive levels consistent with the model (Allen, 1985; 1990; Katz & Heimann, 1990).

The Allen Diagnostic Module (ADM) (Allen, Earhart, & Blue 1993).   The ADM provides standardized activities for the evaluation and treatment of people with a cognitive disability. Twenty-four craft projects have been analyzed according to their cognitive complexity based on the six levels described by the Cognitive Disabilities Model. The ADM is designed to be used as a bridge between the Allen Cognitive Level (ACL) (1985) test and the Routine Task Inventory (RTI) (Allen, Earhart, & Blue, 1992; 1996). Projects in the ADM have been pilot tested though no empirical investigation has been conducted to see how strongly the ADM correlates with the ACL or the RTI. Training in using the ADM and assistance in setting up descriptive, prospective studies are offered by Allen, Earhart, and Blue (1992).

Self-Report Measures.   Self-report measures are also used in the analysis of occupational performance and may be particularly helpful in trying to understand the difference between the person's perspective of her or his performance and the perception of others in the environment, particularly parents and employers. As noted earlier, occupational therapy researchers have developed assessment tools that measure specific client factors, performance in particular areas of occupation, and particular performance skills or patterns. Self-report measures like the Routine Task Inventory-Self Report Version (Allen, 1985) measure performance in activities of daily living (area of occupation); the Occupational Questionnaire (Smith, Kielhofner, & Watts, 1986) measures performance patterns; and the Adult/Adolescent Sensory Profile (Brown & Dunn, 2002) targets the specific sensory functions.

The Occupational Questionnaire (OQ) (Smith, Kielhofner, & Watts, 1986). The OQ asks clients to record daily activities for a typical day in half-hour increments. For each activity they are then asked to identify the activity as work, leisure, daily living task, or rest; how much it is enjoyed; how important it is; and how well it is performed. The instrument is understood to elicit information about volition states, habit patterns, and occupational participation. In addition to being used as self-report measure, it can be used as part of an interview as well. Often the person is asked to identify a typical weekday and a weekend day separately. Scores can also be computed for each activity in order to give the person an alternative view of his or her lived experiences. Research has found that the OQ has adequate test-retest reliability and concurrent validity (Riopel, cited in Kielhofner, 2002).

The Adult/Adolescent Sensory Profile (Dunn, 1999; Brown, Tollefson, Dunn, Cromwell, & Filion, 2001).   The Adult/Adolescent Sensory Profile is a self-report measure designed to identify sensory processing patterns and effects on occupational performance following Dunn's Model of Sensory Processing (Dunn, 2001). The instrument can be used to develop a person's awareness of sensory processing needs and strategies to optimize the desired sensory environment (Brown et al., 2001). The person answers questions regarding how he or she generally responds to sensations. Based on the intersection of two dimensions (neurological threshold and behavioral response/self-regulation), Dunn's model describes quadrants identified as Low Registration, Sensation Seeking, Sensory Sensitivity, and Sensation Avoiding. Each quadrant has its own score. It is possible for an individual to have any combination of scores and some patterns that seem to be mutually exclusive (e.g., sensation seeking and sensation avoiding) may be present in the same individual. There are a total of 60 items with 15 items for each quadrant. These quadrants cover the sensory processing categories of Taste/Smell, Movement, Visual, Touch, Activity Level, and Auditory. Psychometric evidence supports the claim that scores from the profile can provide reliable and valid inferences about an individual's sensory processing patterns. Sensory Profiles (Dunn, 1999) are also designed for children and infants. For these measures the caregiver provides information and completes the items.

CASE ILLUSTRATION: Jackie—Thinking about Observation-Based Performance Assessments

After selecting interviews to develop the occupational profile, Jackie, the occupational therapist working for the agency mentioned in the previous case illustration, also wanted to know whether clients experienced any cognitive limitations that might impact their ability to perform routine tasks safely. Therefore, she selected a screening, noncontextual assessment, the Allen Cognitive Levels Assessment (Allen, Earhart, & Blue, 1992), which would predict functioning in activities of daily living (area of occupation).

Discussion

Jackie integrates her understanding of the psychiatric disabilities literature that has found cognitive functioning (client factor) to be an indicator of community functioning (Allen, Earhart, & Blue, 1992). This noncontextual assessment predicts functioning in one's environment based on cognitive abilities. Because of the specific purpose of the evaluation, to assess ability to manage the present level of support in the apartments that are not yet built, she chose this noncontextual assessment.

CRITERIA FOR SELECTING TOOLS

To choose the correct assessment, several factors can guide selection of instruments. They are relevance, feasibility, utility, reliability, and validity of the instruments (Hinojosa & Kramer, 1998). In addition, the role and purpose of occupational therapy in context, the setting in which you work, the model of practice that you may follow, the type of clients that you treat, and the performance areas pertinent to occupational therapy may dictate information that you will want to gather. These factors are listed in Table 17-3.

You may have a specific role and purpose in occupational therapy depending on the setting you work in. For example, when an occupation therapist worked in an inpatient hospital exclusively for women, a large part of the treatment was directed towards women with eating disorders. However, she treated those with eating disorders in general groups and did not specify occupational therapy indi-

Table 17-3.   Criteria for Selecting Instruments

Relevance	Does the instrument generate information that fits your needs? Does the assessment elicit information that addresses the overall purpose of the evaluation? Is this the right assessment for this person, in this context, at this time?
Feasibility	Can the assessment be done with available resources? Do you have the competency, time, materials, support, and the like to perform the assessment? Certain assessments are time-intensive to learn how to use as well as to administer; some may only be administered by a practitioner with particular credentials; or they may require specific equipment and materials that are costly, technical, or nonportable.
Utility	Who benefits and how do they benefit? Many assessments are time-intensive and therefore costly to the clients being served and to the organization that serves them. Therefore, the information should have value—it should be meaningful to the client served or result in critical information that will improve the likelihood that the intervention plan will be successful. Although some assessments in other areas of practice may include equipment and may be costly, many assessments in mental health are not expensive. Also, because they have been researched and developed over time, and have proven reliable and valid, they are often more cost-effective (Kielhofner & Forsyth, 2002)—they enable therapists to gather the most important information in the most efficient way so you will not waste time gathering information that is not needed.
Reliability	How accurately do scores reflect a true performance of the individual?
Validity	Does the instrument measure what it proposes to measure?
Role of Occupational Therapy	Are there other professionals that have specific roles? What is the purpose of occupational therapy–generalist or specialist?
Setting	Brief or long-term? Community or inpatient? Home or hospital?
Model of Practice	Occupation-based or skill-based? What are the assessments developed by the model?
Age	Developmental and chronological age dictates the specific focus of assessments.
Diagnosis	Acute or residual? Positive or negative symptoms that interfere? Primary issues?

vidually for them because a psychologist and nutritionist were on staff who designed programs for those with eating disorders. Because of the occupational therapists role in that specific setting, she did not design treatment specifically for eating disorders, but included women with that disorder in general occupational therapy groups that addressed self-efficacy, roles, habits, and coping and communication skills. Because of her role and the purpose of occupational therapy in addressing women with various issues and diagnoses, the occupational therapist did not specifically use assessments designed to elicit information about eating habits and behavior, but used general assessments of overall performance areas and narrative self-report assessments.

The setting you are in may dictate what information is pertinent. For example, inpatient treatment may be very brief where the goal is to stabilize someone, so you may want to evaluate when a person is stable and able to be discharged. For example, in a large inpatient hospital with acute treatment, clients could have a brief treatment stay of three days. In this case, observation with the Allen Diagnostic Module (1996) indicates when the clients are stable enough to be discharged, and also predicts the environment that they will function best in when discharged. In contrast to inpatient treatment, clients may attend a day treatment or psychosocial rehabilitation organization for a year or more. The organization may become the clients' communities where they go to work every day, or participate in community functions and holidays with friends. In this case they may not be considered clients but be club members. You may not know a past psychiatric history, but may only be concerned with how clients function in the present, and how they may enhance or learn new skills for living in the community. In such a setting, evaluation might be concerned simply with which vocational group they might be interested in, or which skills they would like to learn.

The model of practice you follow or your workplace follows may dictate the type of evaluation and assessments that you use. For example, if you follow the model of cognitive disabilities you will most likely be interested in a person's cognitive functioning and being able to place a person according to the levels of functioning that are explained by the model (Allen, 1985). Assessments used to assess cognitive functioning are typically crafts or routine activities of daily living. However, if you follow other models that are broader, such as the model of human occupation (Kielhofner, 2002), occupational adaptation (Schultz & Schkade, 2003), or person-environment-occupation (Stewart, et al., 2003) based in the context of occupations, you may engage in a longer evaluation process that uses assessments that measure broad areas of occupation, adaptation, or motivation as well as assessments that measure specific occupational performance skills.

The age of clients may dictate the evaluation process and assessments that you use. For example, the process for infants and toddlers will necessarily involve caregivers and may involve observation and task assessments of sensory, motor, and perceptual performance skills as well as assessing the occupational area of play. Assessing children may involve verbal, task, and observation assessments of sensory, motor and perceptual, process and communication/interaction skills, performance patterns and the occupational areas of activities of daily living, instrumental activities of daily living, education and play. The process for adolescents and adults will involve assessments that are verbal, task, and observational of all performance skills and patterns, in all contexts. For adolescents, assessments may focus on volitional processes and self-identity and occupational areas of education, and work, whereas for adults they may focus on volitional processes and occupational areas of leisure and work. For the older adult, assessments may focus on activities of daily living, instrumental activities of daily living, leisure and social participation in the context of maintaining skills, and retirement. Obviously, for all ages in mental health, including the infant in the context of caregivers and family, psychological factors will be in the forefront of the evaluation process and assessments.

Diagnosis may dictate the evaluation process and assessments you use. For example, for those with schizophrenia in the acute stages, it may be difficult to elicit information in an assessment that is client-centered, such as the COPM or the OSA, and demands broad and abstract thinking that may be impaired by positive symptoms such as hallucinations and delusions. In this case, more structured assessments, with specific simple questions that elicit information or task assessments may be in order.

For those with major depression, motivation and pleasure are most likely major issues that demand attention, so the evaluation process or assessments may focus on volition and performance patterns and their influence on activities of daily living. Those with personality disorders may respond best to narratives of occupational engagement and to broad assessments of ability to function in occupational performance areas, primarily work and social participation. In addition, assessments that focus on roles, process and communication skills, and client factors of regulating emotions would be useful.

There are other considerations in addition to selecting the best instruments. For example, one should have the appropriate level of training to administer the assessment according to its standard protocol. One should always elicit the person's cooperation and "best performance" by ensuring the proper assessment environment. Cultural differences should be considered. The examiner should be aware if the assessment has been developed primarily with a white, middle-class population. Also, the examiner should consider that people may not have experience with tests; they may not understand the importance of tests, or tests may not be meaningful to them. Additionally, language differences may be obvious barriers; tests that have to be translated may lose much of their dependability or reliability. (See Chapter 2 for more information regarding environments.) Subject privacy and confidentiality should also be taken into account; that is, the client has a right to privacy and to be thoroughly informed of the assessment and its purpose, and of the intended use of the assessment (Richardson, 2001). Assessments should not be used in isolation, that is, there should be a broad spectrum of information that gives an in-depth view of the client.

Often in mental health contexts, occupational therapists complain of not having enough time to administer assessments. However, "the amount of effort each assessment takes is proportionate to the kind of information one gathers" (Kielhofner & Forsyth, 2002, p. 282). Indeed, it seems short-sighted not to use the assessment tools that have been developed for occupational therapy practice. Assessments are developed so that therapists can be sure that they will be consistent and measure what they want them to measure. Assessments have been researched so that therapists can compare the performance of their clients with average performances of other clients. They have been designed so that therapists can be assured of obtaining the information needed in the quickest possible time without obtaining useless information. Assessments also define therapists' practice domain and in most cases are designed so that they can be used in research that further illuminates practice and improves treatment interventions.

Assessments can also be used creatively so that they become a part of treatment (Kielhofner & Forsyth, 2002). For example, they can be given in groups (particularly a craft assessment), or they can be given as an intervention (such as completing a narrative lifeline of important and significant positive and negative events in one's life), or they can be given to clients to fill out in their own time (such as an interest or role checklist).

Therapists in mental health practice sometimes complain of the time-consuming process of having to learn the assessment administration and scoring. However, it seems equally short-sighted not to read a manual and practice an assessment that then can become "second nature" and another tool of the trade. Therapists are licensed to practice and so must follow legal and ethical guidelines. One of those guidelines is to be competent and to continue to remain up-to-date with developments in the field that influence treatment. Learning to administer, score, and use assessments in treatment planning is a part of therapists' job as professionals, just as it is a part of any professional's job on a mental health treatment team.

In addition, emphasizing the time and effort it takes to use assessments or refusing to use them because you think that you already gather that information may be a way of fostering a negative stereotype about mental health practice. For example, occupational therapists who work in areas other than mental health may feel that the people who work in mental health are "not together" themselves, or somehow those who work in mental health really do not do much of anything that is productive or worthwhile. Another stereotype is that those who have mental illness may not do anything that is productive and may not change, so therefore time-consuming assessments may not be particularly useful. Refusing to use well-researched, valid, and reliable assessments that serve to develop more information about the individual, and determine interventions as well as define valuable work in mental health and demonstrate the need and outcomes of occupational therapy, may perpetuate those stereotypes.

Limits of Data

While assessments are important tools for eliciting information to guide interventions, assessment data has its limits, particularly the ability to predict how a person is likely to perform in a given context. Occupational therapists in mental health practice as well as other health care professionals may be asked to use their evaluations to contribute to decisions regarding a person's eligibility for rehabilitative and support services from the Department of Rehabilitation Services, for disability funding determinations such as social security disability income, supplemental security income, or worker's compensation, and/or for legal competency determinations. Decisions are based on the expectation that occupational therapists can use their findings to predict the person's ability to perform specific occupations within particular contexts, the person's potential response to particular interventions, or the likelihood that a person's recovery will progress to a particular level of functioning.

There is evidence that personal causation and other volitional factors may mediate the impact of psychiatric symptoms on occupational performance (Anthony, 2001). Occupational therapy researchers and instrument developers as well have argued that the impact of cognitive impairments on occupational functioning can be specifically identified and used in determining the level of functioning that is likely given a particular context's safety risks (Allen, Earhart, & Blue, 1992; Fisher, 1992a; 1992b). However, occupational therapists who are asked to participate in predictions of future performance should be thoughtful about the impact of such decisions on the lives of the persons they serve and keep in mind a dynamic systems perspective on occupational performance. Such a perspective emphasizes the complex, nonlinear and emergent nature of development and change in occupational performance (McLauglin-Gray, Kennedy, & Zemke, 1996). That is, occupational performance may change over time and be dependent on each specific context or situation.

COMMUNICATING EVALUATION FINDINGS AND INTERVENTION RECOMMENDATIONS

An important part of any evaluation process is the responsibility to communicate findings and recommendations to the person, members of his or her support system, other professionals, or payer sources. Communicating findings is a professional competency that often influences the overall impression and perception that those therapists collaborate with have about occupational therapy. In some instances, as when occupational therapists have been asked to consult only, the communication of the findings may be the final contact that they have with the person and those involved with her or his care.

As was noted previously in this chapter, occupational therapy assessment findings in mental health settings may be used to determine eligibility for services or funding, as well as make competency decisions, but they can also be used to instill hope of recovery and to engage the person that you are serving in a sustained commitment to efforts needed to accomplish that recovery (Davidson, 2003; Davidson & Strauss, 1992). Therefore, a helpful perspective is to consider the reporting process and format as a rhetorical tool meant to persuade the recipient of the report—whoever that may be—to a particular way of understanding the person and his or her circumstances. With this perspective and ethic in mind, the occupational therapist can more effectively determine the format and content of the assessment report method.

Written reporting methods include checklists, graphs, or narrative reports. The selection of a written method is influenced by several factors, including the time available to collect and analyze the data and to complete the report; reimbursement or payment sources for conducting the assessment and preparing the report; the credentialing and skill level of the practitioner conducting the assessment; and the characteristics of the recipient of the assessment information. In most mental health settings reporting these formats are standardized and significantly influenced by the requirements of the payer sources and other regulatory processes.

In addition to written documentation, the oral communication of assessment findings is made during meetings with the person and her or his support system, as well as in meetings with other professionals. Communicating evaluation findings to the person and her or his support system should be done in a manner that is meaningful and understandable, and is likely to be considerably different in style and language than oral communications with other professionals. Findings should be communicated with a warm, objective, and positive attitude so that information can truly be shared and collaborative decisions made. It is important that the occupational therapist be committed to the use of person-first, nonstigmatizing language in all written and oral communications.

OTHER CONSIDERATIONS IN EVALUATION: ASSESSMENT, SCREENING, AND OUTCOME EVALUATION

A distinction has been made in occupational therapy practice between assessment and evaluation. Depending on your practice area this distinction may vary. For example, in education-based practice settings, *assessment* is the term that has been used to describe the overall process and *evaluation* is the term that has been used to describe the actual instruments that practitioners use in the assessment process. In rehabilitation-based practice settings, *evaluation* is used to describe the overall process and *assessment* to describe the instruments used during the evaluation process.

The Occupational Therapy Practice Framework (2002) adopts the rehabilitation perspective for distinguishing between evaluation and assessment. However, it is important to understand how the terms are used in individual practice settings so that occupational therapists can collaborate effectively with other professionals.

Occupational therapists also distinguish between **screening and comprehensive evaluations** (Crist, 1998). Screening evaluations are intended to provide an initial indication of the person's need for services. Assessments used in screening evaluations often identify global levels of disability or expressed desire for change. Given that they identify global levels of disability, screening assessments may be less useful in determining the specific change that is needed to assist the person. They may not require a context-based observation of occupational performance and may identify a need for change that upon a more comprehensive evaluation is not indicated.

Screening evaluations are often used to triage persons toward particular programs or settings where a more comprehensive evaluation will identify the specific targets of intervention. It is important to understand whether a screening or comprehensive evaluation will be needed to meet the needs of the program or setting in which you are working for various reasons. In some mental health settings, the number of referrals may be greater than the occupational therapist can serve. In these instances, screening instruments can be very helpful to identify who would most benefit from occupational therapy services. For example, an inpatient chemical dependency unit of a large hospital had a waiting list of many potential clients. When openings became available the hospital screened those who were waiting for admittance for cognitive deficits because the treatment unit tended to require abstract thinking and ability to be reflective. The hospital staff used the ACL (1985; Allen, Earhart, & Blue, 1996) to determine level of functioning and those who placed below 4.6 of the six-level hierarchy, indicating difficulty with exploratory learning, were referred elsewhere.

In addition, in some mental health settings occupational therapists may serve as gatekeepers for multidisciplinary psychiatric rehabilitation teams. That is, the use of a screening instrument facilitates linking clients with practitioners that will best meet their needs. (See the first case illustration, where Jackie used a screening evaluation to quickly measure tenants' abilities to live independently.)

Unlike screening assessments, comprehensive evaluations are designed to gather a complete contextually specific understanding of the client's occupational performance strengths, needs, abilities, and preferences. Assessments used in comprehensive evaluations are most often context-based observations and include contact with members of the person's support system. Comprehensive evaluations may also be consultative in nature. In those instances, the occupational therapist may not actually provide direct service, but the evaluations may give guidance to clients and their caregivers on how to optimize client success and satisfaction in their occupations of choice.

CASE ILLUSTRATION: Oksana—Comprehensive Evaluation

Oksana, an adolescent who had been hospitalized for the first time for a manic episode, quickly improved. However, the plan was to transfer her to a day treatment program for teenagers to assure aggressive intervention that would prevent another episode. Therefore, when she was admitted to the day program, a comprehensive occupational therapy evaluation included the OCAIRS and the MEDLS. The OCAIRS determined her strengths and weaknesses, environmental supports or constraints, social environments that fit with her level of interest and skills, roles and habits that she desired to maintain or develop, how effective she believed herself to be, what aspects of personal identity needed to be developed, and motivation to participate in treatment based on her short- and long-term goals. The MEDLS determined her ability to complete basic activities of daily living and could also be used to determine functioning in ADLs at admission and discharge, and perhaps be useful halfway between admission and discharge.

Discussion

Because the adolescent day program was a longer-term comprehensive treat-ment program in which Oksana would most likely spend about six months and would serve as a school and social community, the OCAIRS was chosen to pro-vide comprehensive information from her point of view. In addition to serving as an outcome measure, the MEDLS served as a performance-based measure that could be used in Oksana's home and treatment environment.

Another important distinction in the evaluation process is the difference between the use of assessments for **outcome evaluation** and evaluation for intervention planning. In contemporary health care practice, outcome evalua-tion is a necessary aspect of program evaluation and is required by most ac-crediting organizations and in some instances by funding or payment sources. Outcome evaluation refers to the process of tracking the specific changes that the program, service, or intervention makes in the lives of the people it serves. In mental health practice, outcomes evaluation has focused on three factors that impact the lives of people with psychiatric disabilities: psychiatric symptomatol-ogy, level of function, and quality of life. The Occupational Therapy Practice Framework (2002) recognizes the last two outcomes as legitimate occupational therapy outcomes. The process of outcome evaluation involves measuring each of these factors at a minimum of three points in time: prior to the start of an inter-vention (often referred to as the "baseline"), at the close of the intervention (either at discharge or transition from one level of care to another), and at some reasonable time period after the intervention has been concluded. For example, an assessment such as the OSA (Baron, Kielhofner, Iyenger, Goldhammer, & Wolenski, 2002) may be used when a client first enters an acute hospital, later when discharged to community care, and after six months of treatment in com-munity care. Assuming continuity of occupational therapy treatment, the assess-ment will show if clients' satisfaction and ideas about their performance have improved, thus demonstrating quality of life changes, or if they have made the changes that they indicated were important to them in specific performance areas, patterns, and skills.

The important point for this chapter is that the assessment tools that are used in outcome evaluation in mental health practice tend not to be useful for plan-ning the specific and discrete details of occupational therapy interventions and changes that these interventions are intended to make. Occupational therapy assessment tools may contribute to the outcome data collection process, but the rich and detailed information needed for planning intervention is not usually met by the outcome evaluation tools commonly used in mental health practice.

Role of Theory

Conceptual models provide the practitioner with a framework for thinking through how the various aspects of the domains of occupational therapy interact and influence each other and facilitate prioritizing occupational therapy interven-tions. For occupational therapists practicing in mental health settings, theoretical perspectives regarding occupation, the nature of psychiatric disorders, and recovery from those disorders assist in analysis and interpretation of evaluation and assessment findings. Theoretical perspectives are useful because they bring unique and meaningful professional knowledge about occupations to clients. There is a growing body of work from occupational science regarding the lived experience of occupation that can particularly contribute to the occupational therapist's development and framing of the person's occupational profile (Zemke & Clark, 1996).

Research and theoretical perspectives regarding the etiology and nature of psychiatric disorders must be taken into account as well, particularly research that investigates the functional aspects of these disorders, like the research on cognition noted above. Knowledge of psychiatric disorders is important because symptoms influence occupational performance.

Research and theoretical developments in our understandings of recovery are also critical. For example, first-person narratives regarding the recovery experience provide rich examples of the role of occupation in the recovery process. In addition, these stories remind us of the predictive limits of data, and can motivate change because many writers of these accounts recall being told emphatically by professionals that they would never be able to work, go to school, or live on their own (Deegan, 1988; 1993; 1996; Leete, 1989). A final case illustration describes how to integrate information from an evaluation process.

CASE ILLUSTRATION: Brandon—Occupational Profile and Analysis of Occupational Performance

Jackie's findings and recommendations from the initial occupational therapy evaluation assisted the agency in identifying the supports that each tenant would need to successfully maintain her or his apartment. An example of Brandon's evaluation follows.

Brandon's occupational profile obtained from an interview using the OPHI-II, indicated that he was excited about being considered for the new apartment complex. He wanted to "get his life back." He had been living in a group supported living setting for the last year or so and wanted very much to have his own apartment. He especially wanted the freedom and privacy of having his own place, and was particularly interested in these apartments both because they were affordable and he would have understanding neighbors since the other tenants would have similar problems. He knew some of the other potential tenants from previous supported group living situations and experienced them as supportive. He was also aware that there would be support staff available at the apartment if he needed assistance and this too was important. He reported having previously lived on his own for a short time when he first left home when he was 23. He had an apartment and two roommates and had been able to manage the apartment without any problems. However, since first experiencing (about five years ago) his psychiatric symptoms, which included hypomania, paranoid/suspicious thoughts, and auditory hallucinations, he had resided in mental health treatment environments or other special residences. He reported having had no problems with his home maintenance responsibilities while in these group living settings. Although his self-report indicated no problems with home maintenance, he agreed with Jackie that an assessment of his ADL skills when he was actually living in the apartment would help them know exactly how well he performed. They both agreed to an ADL assessment using the AMPS. He also expressed a desire to go back to work, as he had stopped working at the onset of his psychiatric symptoms. He described his family as very important to him and experienced them as very supportive. He visited them regularly at their home and hoped to have them visit him when he moved into the apartment. His family expressed excitement and pleasure in the possibility of him being able to have his own apartment and planned to continue to assist him in the ways that they had been.

Brandon's occupational performance analysis indicated that he would be successful in maintaining his apartment with the level of support that was available from his family and that was expected to be available at the apartment (i.e., one to two hours per day for help with problem solving, and supportive counseling). It was noted that he would likely need assistance with money management and self-monitoring of symptom level with particular attention to its impact on his tenant-to-tenant relationships. Given the functional impact of his periodic hypomania, his father was currently serving as social security payee and gave him an "allowance" each week to purchase the items he needed. It was expected that this would continue, at least initially, upon move-in until Brandon and his father were satisfied that he could manage his own funds without risking his financial stability. Most likely Jackie would consider using the KELS to assess his ability to manage everyday basic skills with money. Given the functional impact of his periodic paranoid and suspicious ideation, he would occasionally experience his former roommates as "threatening" and get into arguments with them. He thought that access to direct feedback and support for reality testing from apartment support staff would help to mediate this problem. In discussing what made him suspicious, Jackie was alerted to possible sensory processing issues. She considered giving Brandon the sensory profile.

Summary

Evaluation is a planned and ongoing process that requires the occupational therapist to have a thorough understanding of occupation, both as a life activity and as a therapeutic measure. Through the thoughtful and skilled selection and use of assessment tools, evaluation findings guide the development of interventions that will promote occupational engagement. Ethical considerations influence all aspects of the evaluation process from the beginning question of accepting the referral to the manner in which the evaluation findings are communicated to the person served and her or his support network. This chapter highlights the evaluation process and specific assessments that are used to develop occupational profiles and measure occupational performance. However, other assessments mentioned throughout this text may be used according to specific occupational therapy practice models and target performance skills and patterns, client factors, activity demands, or contexts.

Review Questions

1. How do you differentiate evaluation from assessment? Screening from comprehensive evaluation and assessments? Assessments used in outcomes evaluation from those used for intervention planning?
2. Describe the focus of AOTA's Occupational Therapy Practice Framework occupational profile and analysis of occupational performance as they relate to evaluation and assessment in occupational therapy.
3. What should you take into consideration when determining specific assessments you will use in any given evaluation process?
4. Which assessments would be most useful for your practice when determining occupational performance barriers?
5. What influences the manner in which you communicate and report the findings from your evaluation?

References

Anthony, W. (2001). Assessing readiness for change among persons with severe mental illness. *Community Mental Health Journal, 37*(2), 97–112.

Allen, C. K. (1985). *Occupational therapy for psychiatric diseases: Measurement and management of cognitive disabilities.* Boston: Little, Brown.

Allen, C. K., Earhart, C. A., & Blue, T. (1992). *Occupational therapy treatment goals for the physically and cognitively disabled.* American Occupational Therapy Association.

Allen, C. K., Earhart, C. A., & Blue, T. (1993). *Allen Diagnostic Module: Instruction manual.* Colchester, CT: S & S Worldwide.

Allen, C. K., Earhart, C. A., & Blue, T. (1996). *Understanding cognitive performance modes.* Colchester, CT: S & S Worldwide.

Baron, K., Kielhofner, G., Iyenger, A., Goldhammer, V., & Wolenski, J. (2002). *The Occupational Self Assessment (OSA) (Version 2.0).* Chicago: Model of Human Occupation Clearinghouse, Department of Occupational Therapy, College of Applied Health Sciences, University of Illinois at Chicago.

Barrett, L., & Kielhofner, G. (2003). An overview of occupational behavior. In E. B. Crepeau, E. S. Cohn, & B. A. B. Schell (Eds.), *Willard and Spackman's occupational therapy* (10th ed., pp. 209–212). Philadelphia: Lippincott Williams & Wilkins.

Barris, R., Kielhofner, G., et al. (1988). *Occupational therapy in psychosocial practice.* Thorofare, NJ: Slack.

Brown, C. (2001). What is the best environment for me? A sensory processing perspective. *Occupational Therapy in Mental Health, 17*(3/4), 115–125.

Brown, C. E., & Dunn, W. (2002). *Adolescent/Adult sensory profile.* San Antonio, TX: The Psychological Corporation.

Brown, C., Tollefson, N., Dunn, W., Cromwell, R., & Filion, D. (2001). The adult sensory profile: Measuring patterns of sensory processing. *American Journal of Occupational Therapy, 55,* 75–82.

Burke, J. P., & Kern, S. B. (1996). Is the use of life history and narrative in clinical practice reimbursable? Is it occupational therapy? *American Journal of Occupational Therapy, 50*(5), 389–392.

Clark, F. (1993). Occupation embedded in a real life: Interweaving occupational science and occupational therapy. *American Journal of Occupational Therapy, 47*(12), 1067–1068.

Clark, F., Carlson, M., & Polkinghorne, D. (1997). The legitimacy of life history and narrative approaches in the study of occupation. *American Journal of Occupational Therapy, 51*(4), 313–317.

Crist, P. (1998). *Standardized assessments: Psychometric measurement and testing procedures.* In J. Hinojosa & P. Kramer (Eds.), *Evaluation: Obtaining and interpreting data* (pp. 77–106). Bethesda, MD: American Occupational Therapy Association.

Davidson, L. (2003). *Living outside mental illness: Qualitative studies of recovery in schizophrenia.* New York: New York University Press.

Davidson, L., & Strauss, J. S. (1992). Sense of self in recovery from severe mental illness. *British Journal of Medical Psychology, 63,* 131–145.

Deegan, P. (1988). Recovery: The lived experience of rehabilitation. *Psychosocial Rehabilitation Journal, 11*(4), 11–19.

Deegan, P. (1993). Recovering our sense of value after being labeled. *Journal of Psychosocial Nursing, 31*(4), 7–11, 33–34.

Deegan, P. (1996). Recovery as a journey of the heart. *Psychiatric Rehabilitation Journal, 19*(3), 91–97.

de las Heras, C. G., Geist, R., Kilehofner, G., & Li, Y. (2002). *The Volitional Questionnaire (VQ) (Version 4.0).* Chicago: Model of Human Occupation Clearinghouse, Department of Occupational Therapy, College of Applied Health Sciences, University of Illinois at Chicago.

Dombrowski, L. B. (1990). *Functional needs assessment: Program for chronic psychiatric patients.* Tucson, AZ: Therapy Skill Builders.

Duchek, J. M., & Thessing, V. (1996). Is the use of life history and narrative in clinical practice fundable as research? *American Journal of Occupational Therapy, 50*(5), 393–396.

Duncan, M. (1998). Interpretation and application. In J. Hinojosa & P. Kramer (Eds.), *Evaluation: Obtaining and interpreting data* (pp. 47–76). Bethesda, MD: American Occupational Therapy Association.

Dunn, W. (1998). Person-centered and contextually relevant evaluation. In J. Hinojosa & P. Kramer (Eds.), *Evaluation: Obtaining and interpreting data* (pp. 47–76). Bethesda, MD: American Occupational Therapy Association.

Dunn, W. (1999). The Sensory Profile. San Antonio, TX: The Psychological Corporation.

Dunn, W. (2001). The sensations of everyday life: Empirical, theoretical, and pragmatic considerations. *American Journal of Occupational Therapy, 55,* 608–620.

Dunn, W., Brown, C., & McGuigan, A. (1994). The ecology of human performance: A framework for considering the effect of context. *American Journal of Occupational Therapy, 48,* 595–607.

Dunning, H. (1972). Environmental occupational therapy. *American Journal of Occupational Therapy, 26*(6), 292–298.

Fisher, A. G. (1992a). Functional measures, Part 1: What is function, what should be measured, and how should we measure it? *American Journal of Occupational Therapy, 46,* 183–185.

Fisher, A. G. (1992b). Functional measures, Part 2: Selecting the right test, minimizing the limitations. *American Journal of Occupational Therapy, 46,* 278–281.

Fisher, A. G. (2003). *Assessment of motor and process skills:* Volume I: *Development, standardization, and administration manual* (5th ed.). Ft. Collins, CO: Three Star.

Florey, L., & Michelman, S. (1982). Occupational Role History: A screening tool for psychiatric occupational therapy. *American Journal of Occupational Therapy, 36,* 5.

Forsyth, K. Salamy, M., Simon, S., & Kielhofner, G. (1998). *The Assessment of Communication and Interaction Skills (Version 4.0).* Chicago: Department of Occupational Therapy, University of Illinois at Chicago.

Haglund, L., Henriksson, C., Crisp, M., Freidheim, L., & Kielhofner, G. (2001). *The Occupational Circumstances Assessment-Interview and Rating Scale (OCAIRS) (Version 2.0).* Chicago: Model of Human Occupation Clearinghouse, Department of Occupational Therapy, College of Applied Health Sciences, University of Illinois at Chicago.

Heimann, N. E., Allen, C. K., & Yerxa, E. J. (1989). The routine task inventory: A tool for describing the functional behavior of the cognitively disabled. *Occupational Therapy Practice, 1,* 67–74.

Hemphill, B. J. (Ed.). (1982). *The evaluative process in psychiatric occupational therapy.* Thorofare, NJ: Slack.

Hemphill, B. J. (Ed).(1988). *Mental health assessment in occupational therapy*. Thorofare, NJ: Slack.

Hemphill, B. J. (Ed.). (1999). *Assessments in occupational therapy mental health: An integrative approach*. Thorofare, NJ: Slack.

Hinojosa, J., & Kramer, P. (Eds). (1998). *Occupational therapy evaluation: Obtaining and interpreting data*. Bethesda, MD: American Occupational Therapy Association.

Kaplan, K. (1984). Short-term assessment: The need and a response. *Occupational Therapy in Mental Health, 4*(3), 29–45.

Kaplan, K., & Kielhofner, G. (1989). *The Occupational Case Analysis Interview and Rating Scale*. Thorofare, NJ: Slack.

Katz, N., & Heimann, N. (1990). Review of research conducted in Israel on cognitive disability instrumentation. *Occupational Therapy in Mental Health, 10*, 1–15.

Kielhofner, G., & Neville, A. T*he modified interest check list*. Unpublished manuscript. University of Illinois at Chicago.

Kielhofner, G., Mallinson, T., Crawford, C., Nowak, M., Rigby, M., Henry, A., & Walens, D. (1997). *A user's guide to the Occupational Performance History Interview-II (OPHI-II) (Version 2.0)*. Chicago: Model of Human Occupation Clearinghouse, Department of Occupational Therapy, College of Applied Health Sciences, University of Illinois at Chicago.

Kielhofner, G., & Forsyth, K. (2001). Development of a client self-report for treatment planning and documenting occupational therapy outcomes. *Scandanavian Journal of Occupational Therapy, 8*(3), 131–139.

Kielhofner, G., & Forsyth, K. (2002). How to know the client best: Choosing and using structured assessments and unstructured means of gathering information. In G. Kielhofner, *Model of human occupation* (3rd ed.), pp. 280–295. St. Louis, MO: Mosby.

Klyczek, J.P., Bauer-Yox, N., et al. (1997). The interest checklist: A factor analysis. *American Journal of Occupatinal Therapy, 51*, 815–823.

Kohlman-Thomson, L. (1992). *The Kohlman Evaluation of Living Skills, Third Edition*. Bethesda: MD: American Occupational Therapy Association.

Law, M., Baptiste, S., Carswell-Opzoomer, A., McColl, M., Polatajko, H., & Pollock, N. (1991). *Canadian Occupational Performance Measure* (COPM). Toronto: Canadian Association of Occupational Therapist Publications.

Leete, E. (1989). How I perceived and manage my illness. *Schizophrenia Bulletin, 15*(2), 197–200.

Leonardelli, C. (1988a). The Milwaukee Evaluation of Daily Living Skills: Evaluation in long-term psychiatric care. In B. J. Hemphill, *Mental health assessment in occupational therapy: An integrative approach to the evaluative process* (pp. 151–162). Thorofare, NJ: Slack.

Leonardelli, C. (1988b). *The Milwaukee Evaluation of Daily Living Skills* (MEDLS). Thorofare, NJ: Slack.

Leonardelli, C. A. (1989). Specification of daily living skills for persons with chronic mental illness. *Occupational Therapy Journal of Research, 6*, 323–333.

Matsutsuyu, J. (1969). The Interest Checklist. *American Journal of Occupational Therapy, 23*, 368–373.

McGourty, L. K. (1988). Kohlman Evaluation of Living Skills (KELS). In B. J. Hemphill (Ed.), *Mental health assessment in occupational therapy: An integrative approach to the evaluative process* (pp. 133–146). Thorofare, NJ: Slack.

McLaughlin Gray, J., Kennedy, B. L., & Zemke, R. (1996). Application of dynamic systems theory to occupation. In Zemke & Clark (Eds.), *Occupational science: The evolving discipline*. Philadelphia: F. A. Davis.

Morehead, L. (1969). The occupational history. *American Journal of Occupational Therapy, 23*(4), 329–334.

Oakley, R., Kielhofner, G., & Barris, R. (1985). An occupational therapy approach to assessing psychiatric patient's adaptive functioning. *American Journal of Occupational Therapy, 39*, 147–154.

Occupational Therapy Practice Framework: Domain and Process. (2002). *American Journal of Occupational Therapy, 56*, 609–639.

Richardson, P. (2001). Use of standardized tests in pediatric practice. In J. Case-Smith (Ed.), *Occupational therapy for children* (pp. 217–245). St. Louis, MO: Mosby.

Rogers, J. C. (1988). The NPI Interest Checklist. In B. J. Hemphill (Ed.), *Mental health assessment in occupational therapy: An integrative approach to the evaluative process* (pp. 93–114). Thorofare, NJ: Slack.

Scaffa, M. E. (1981). *Temporal adaptation and alcoholism.* Unpublished master's project, Virginia Commonwealth University, Richmond.

Schultz, S., & Schkade, J. (2003). Occupational adaptation. In E. B. Crepeau, E. S. Cohn, & B. A. B. Schell (Eds.), *Willard and Spackman's occupational therapy* (10th ed., pp. 220–223). Philadelphia: Lippincott Williams & Wilkins.

Smith, N. R., Kielhofner, G., & Watts, J. (1986). The relationship between volition, activity pattern, and life satisfaction in the elderly. *American Journal of Occupational Therapy, 40,* 278–283.

Stewart, D., Letts, L., Law, M., Cooper, B. A., Strong, S., & Rigby, P. J. (2003). The person-environment-occupation model. In E. B. Crepeau, E. S. Cohn, & B. A. B. Schell (Eds.), *Willard and Spackman's occupational therapy* (10th ed., pp. 227–231). Philadelphia: Lippincott Williams & Wilkins.

Zemke, R., & Clark, F. (1996). *Occupational science: The evolving discipline.* Philadelphia: F. A. Davis.

Suggested Reading

Asher, I. E. (1996). *Occupational therapy assessment tools: An annotated index* (2nd ed.). Bethesda, MD: American Occupational Therapy Association.

Barham, P., & Hayward, R. (1995). *Relocating madness: From the mental patient to the person.* London: Free Association Books.

Carpinello, S. E., Knight, E. L., Markowitz, F. E., & Pease, E. A. (2000). The development of the mental health confidence scale: A measure of self-efficacy in individuals diagnosed with mental disorders. *Psychiatric Rehabilitation Journal, 23*(3), 236–243.

Clark, E. N., & Peters, M. (1984). *Scorable self-care evaluation.* Thorofare, NJ: Slack.

Estroff, S. E. (1989). Self, identity, and subjective experiences of schizophrenia: In search of the subject. *Schizophrenia Bulletin, 15,* 189–196.

Mann, W. C., & Klyczek, J. P. (1991). Standard scores for the bay area functional performance evaluation task oriented assessment. *Occupational Therapy Journal in Mental Health, 11,* 13–24.

Nippert-Eng, C. E. (1995). *Home and work: Negotiating boundaries through everyday life.* Chicago: University of Chicago Press.

Scheid, T. L., & Anderson, C. (1995). Living with chronic mental illness: Understanding the role of work. *Community Mental Health Journal, 31,* 163–176.

Stainsby, J. (1992). Schizophrenia: Some issues. *Schizophrenia Bulletin, 18,* 543–546.

Van Dongen, C. J. (1996). Quality of life and self-esteem in working and nonworking persons with mental illness. *Community Mental Health Journal, 32,* 535–548.

Weingarten, R. (1989). How I've managed chronic mental illness. *Schizophrenia Bulletin, 15,* 635–640.

Methods and Interpersonal Strategies

Elizabeth Cara, PhD, OTR/L, MFT

Key Terms

clinical reasoning
intersubjective process

strategies
techniques

Chapter Outline

Introduction

To some occupational therapists, learning about methods and interpersonal strategies may seem dry and technical. However, knowing how to use these methods and strategies often makes the difference in motivating or not motivating clients to engage in treatment. Also, how an individual therapist incorporates interpersonal strategies to match his or her individual style and specific therapeutic situation is what makes working fun! Although therapists understand methods and general interpersonal strategies, they are uniquely applied to each client, setting, and situation that occurs in practice. Deciding which strategies to use and specifically how to deliver them in each encounter is what may motivate clients and is what makes clinical practice successful as well as interesting and rewarding. Creative ways of applying methods in interpersonal strategies in mental health practice are embedded throughout this text, but this chapter introduces and explains them so that you can understand and artistically use them in your specific clinical practice.

This chapter discusses universal and specific strategies used primarily in mental health but they can also be used in physical rehabilitation, pediatric, and other practices. This chapter also discusses the Occupational Therapy Practice Framework (2002) when applicable, particularly those methods that are unique to this domain of practice and make up the process of practice.

This focus on interpersonal strategies is particularly important because the therapeutic relationship assumes primacy in mental health practice. Also, in mental health practice there are not typically tangible disorders to work with and, therefore, abstract techniques assume prime importance. This chapter uses the terms *techniques* and *strategies* interchangeably according to the following definitions. **Strategies** or **techniques** include the tangible tools that are often readily identified or observed in practice. However, particularly in mental health treatment, strategies and techniques also include abstract abilities the person uses to fulfill the plan, or apply the methods, such as the style, finesse, capacity, craftsmanship, virtuosity, or resourcefulness of the therapist. A tangible example of an occupational therapy strategy is grading an activity according to the cognitive functioning of an individual or providing just enough tools in a group so that members have to interact with each other around sharing their use. An abstract technique may include clinical reasoning about the client, which intervention may work best, and how to apply the intervention in context.

This chapter focuses on the interpersonal dimensions of strategies, such as how the occupational therapist conveys, communicates, makes contact with, relates to, proposes, and presents techniques. An example of an interpersonal emphasis may be the specific and unique way an occupational therapist discusses an activity with a client, including tone of voice, physicality, and gestures of the therapist, the timing of the discussion, and how the therapist conveys the words (in a serious or humorous manner).

INTERPERSONAL STRATEGIES

Various strategies have been identified in different ways in occupational therapy. Some are based in a model of practice (Kielhofner, 2002) while others are listed in chapters on the therapeutic use of self (Hagedorn, 2000; Peloquin, 2003). Some are explained in relationship to interactive clinical reasoning (Swartzberg, 2002) or client-centered practice (Fearing & Clark, 2000). Whichever means have been used to explain strategies in occupational therapy, they are universal strategies used by most health professionals.

Perhaps the most important information that can be added to explanations of strategies is that they should be individualized or used on a case-specific basis. As stated above, all interpersonal strategies that one chooses should be based on each individual client and the specific situation in which the client and therapist interact from moment to moment. Also important is the fact that personal techniques should be congruent with the occupational therapist's personality. Although interpersonal strategies can be learned and practiced, and usually will deepen with clinical experience, it is nevertheless critical to be authentic and genuine. Clients in the mental health system are very attuned to therapists' personalities and styles (even though they may not show) and can recognize when someone is not being genuine. For example, if you tend to be matter of fact and less demonstrative, it will not benefit most clients in most situations for you to falsely show enthusiasm for a minor daily accomplishment, such as attending a daily group. The broad and universal interpersonal techniques are explained briefly and then illuminated with examples or case illustrations.

Validation

Validating is conveying respect for a client's experience or perspective, acknowledging one's understanding of a client's experience (Kielhofner & Forsyth, 2002), conveying that you value the individual (Hagedorn, 2000), and demonstrating that the client's concern is accepted (Schwartzberg, 2002). Clients in mental health care are often cast in a deviant role, certainly in a role that is devalued by most of society. Often due to their psychiatric symptoms they are feared, if not disregarded. Therefore, it is essential that their therapist convey an understanding and acceptance of their experiences. Validation could be verbal, such as greeting a person and saying you are glad to see him or her, or acknowledging her distress about talking to herself around others, or it could be nonverbal, such as sitting with and listening to a person although he or she may seem to make little sense.

Setting Limits

Setting limits and personal boundaries is identifying behavior that you are unwilling to tolerate. Setting limits is a common clinical strategy in mental health, but not often explained. It is sometimes elusive to novice clinicians because it takes practice, assertiveness, knowing yourself, knowing what the client needs in that specific situation, and understanding the goals of mental health practice. Also, students sometimes mistake setting limits for not caring. However, establishing behavior that you are unwilling to tolerate or accept actually conveys much caring because often the client behavior that one "sets limits on" is the very behavior that is a barrier to satisfying occupational performance, roles, habits, or successful relationships.

CASE ILLUSTRATION: Athena—Setting Limits

Athena attended a psychosocial treatment program based on a clubhouse model. Although she was very smart and clever, residual behaviors from her co-occurring bipolar and addictive disorders were barriers to successful occupational performance. Specifically her barbs and vicious comments directed to others often resulted in her being asked to leave jobs or in others terminating friendships. She had difficulty recognizing her responsibility or role in these "messy" work or relationship situations.

When she arrived at a daily group that discussed the agenda for the day, many members greeted her warmly. Having never experienced unconditional caring and believing herself unworthy, she was embarrassed and made a sarcastic remark, denigrating their warmth. The occupational therapist, who was aware of Athena's problems, immediately commented on Athena's comment by saying, "That was a pretty hurtful comment" and indicated that this was not an acceptable way to interact with peers. She asked the other clients to tell Athena how it made them feel. Although two clients said they were no problem, two others were able to say that her sarcastic comments were somewhat hurtful.

The occupational therapist pointed out to Athena that these were the very type of comments that led to her problems with work and relationships.

Discussion

The occupational therapist understood Athena's problems and treatment needs and was able to set limits on destructive behavior, and hopefully provide some reality testing for Athena. Reality testing meant that through acknowledgment of this situation, Athena might begin to recognize and work on behaviors that were barriers to productive living and her quality of life.

Encouragement

Encouraging is providing emotional support (Kielhofner & Forsyth, 2002) and assurance for clients' actions, behaviors, or choices. In a mental health setting, encouragement is often needed for clients to engage in activities, try out new occupations or new situations, or move to the next level of treatment. In fact, it seems that encouragement is the most consistent strategy that occurs with clients in mental health. Perhaps encouragement implies that the therapist holds that somewhat elusive attitude of hope (Fearing & Clark, 2000; Schwartzberg, 2002) and conveys that hope through his or her encouraging. Although it seems simple and a commonsense technique, it also has to be timed and specific to individual situations and clients so as not to seem that the occupational therapist is a "Pollyanna" or cheerleader. Sometimes, therapists mistake encouragement for validation, or give encouragement when validation is required. The case illustration of Jocelyn provides an example of validation and encouragement.

CASE ILLUSTRATION: Jocelyn—Encouragement and Validation

Jocelyn experienced depression and anxiety and attended an outpatient writing group to help alleviate her sadness and anxiety about being alone. However, she did not attend her writing group one week. The occupational therapist called her as the group started but was unable to reach her. Later, the occupational therapist e-mailed her saying that she had been missed. Jocelyn did not answer the e-mail, so the occupational therapist called her again with the same message. She reached Jocelyn on the last call and Jocelyn spoke about her distress due to a conflict she had had earlier with her only friend. The therapist listened to her story and validated that such conflicts were very difficult to handle, and must be very distressing because Jocelyn was already anxious about being alone and isolated. The therapist also stated that this conflict might have confirmed for Jocelyn that she was not lovable. After a long conversation, she encouraged the client to come to the group, suggesting that writing about it might alleviate the distress and that the group would be helpful for suggestions on how to proceed with her friend. She also mentioned that the group members and she missed her. Jocelyn agreed to attend the next group and felt less alone.

Discussion

The occupational therapist was persistent in reaching Jocelyn and both validating Jocelyn's concerns and encouraging her to come back to the group. In this case, relying on a case-specific strategy, the therapist decided to interact with Jocelyn because she believed that Jocelyn wanted this specific response from the therapist. In other situations, she may have encouraged the group members to contact her.

Advice

Advising is recommending a course of action or choice. Occupational therapists advise clients when they set goals and share desired outcomes with the client and recommend how the client can reach goals and desired outcomes. Advice is also given regularly during treatment when clients seek help to accomplish their intervention program. Advice also may be offered when the therapist wants to discourage action that is not in the client's best interest. Naturally, advice is offered judiciously and not overbearingly. For example, in practice, occupational therapists often discuss plans with their clients beginning with the phrase, "You need . . ." This phrase indicates that the therapist would like to control the situation or that clients are not capable of knowing their own needs. Care must be taken to assure that advice is given in a manner that conveys respect.

Coaching

Coaching implies all the things that a therapist does when she or he instructs clients during an activity. Coaching includes demonstrating, guiding, or prompting when necessary for clients to accomplish tasks. Coaching can also be a motivating factor because it redirects clients to performance aspects that may be satisfying or validating of their skills or habits (Kielhofner & Forsyth, 2002).

Confrontation

Confronting is to oppose or bring together for examination or comparison, or present for acknowledgment or contradiction. Occupational therapists may have face-to-face conversations with clients that are frank discussions of clients' behaviors, actions, skills, or performances that may be harmful or destructive. For example, an occupational therapist may confront a client who has not followed through with plans to look for a job, or may confront a client who has made denigrating remarks about other group members, and therefore has alienated herself from the group members. For example, in the case illustration of Athena, the occupational therapist set limits by confronting her behavior.

Confrontation is not carried out when the therapist is angry, but with honesty and directness, often with an appraisal of the client's actions or behavior. In a way confrontation provides or sets limits because it is letting the client know that his or her behavior or actions are unacceptable. Confronting also conveys caring, that the therapist cares enough about the client to notice and attempt to intervene when the client may be harming himself or herself.

Reframing

Reframing is providing alternative interpretations of behaviors, actions, performance patterns, or skills. Very often in mental health settings clients are unsure of their strengths and very knowledgeable about their weaknesses. Sometimes it is much easier for clients to see what they themselves cannot do, or what they lack, than it is to see what they themselves can do or what skills they have intact. This useful cognitive therapy technique highlights other aspects of clients' behaviors, actions, skills, or patterns when clients can only see usually negative aspects. The therapist is able to accentuate or acknowledge the "other side of the coin" when clients only focus on one side. For example, when a client working on the computer entering a menu for the catering group complained about being too slow in typing when the therapist seemed so much quicker, the occupational therapist noted that it was particularly important to have accurate menus and that the client seemed to be taking care to be accurate. In another instance an addict in a chemical dependency program lamented how he had "messed up his life." After validating his thoughts, the OTR suggested that at least he had recognized it and could now begin to change.

Interpretation

Interpreting conveys the therapist's understandings of the client's motivations, usually understood concurrently or intersubjectively by observation of the client's actions and verbalizations and self-observation of the therapist's own thoughts and feelings about clients. Although interpretation is usually thought of in connection with psychotherapy or psychoanalysis, occupational therapists may interpret clients' motivations or the meaning of activities or occupations. Usually, an interpretation is offered in a timely manner and when the therapist is absolutely sure that the interpretation will further the therapy process or performance.

CASE ILLUSTRATION: Denny Mike—Interpretation

During an assessment, Brian, the occupational therapist, noticed that Denny Mike was seemingly interested in all activities with equal enthusiasm. As the assessment continued, Brian began to feel anxious and began to think that maybe Denny Mike was being sarcastic at best or dishonest at worst; however, Denny Mike also seemed polite and interested in the process. Brian thought that perhaps his anxiety mirrored that of the client, and perhaps Denny Mike's anxiety was driving the apparent self-report of enthusiasm for all activities. Brian offered an interpretation that maybe the client was nervous about performing well, and really did not know what he wanted, in addition to believing that to be cooperative, Denny Mike had to like everything Brian offered. Brian further stated that while he appreciated his cooperation and his courtesy, the best use of the assessment was really to find out what activities were important to him, and it was okay not to know exactly because in the process of occupational therapy he would clarify his likes and dislikes, values, and interests. Denny Mike appeared relieved and started to mention that he really did not value some interests that he had checked.

Discussion

Brian used the intersubjective experience to understand Denny Mike. Brian then was able to offer an interpretation that seemed correct because Denny Mike was visibly relieved. Also, the interpretation motivated Denny Mike to act more congruently with his desires and values and to use the assessment reliably.

Metaphors

In the language of metaphors there is a transfer of meaning (Jones, cited in Schwartzberg, 2002) and a way of quickly grasping a concept without having to explain it in lengthy words. Using metaphors in conversations may not be a natural way of talking but can be learned and practiced (Bandler & Grinder, 1975;

1976; Lakoff & Johnson, 1980; 1993). Using metaphors in occupational therapy is a skill that comes with clinical experience.

CASE ILLUSTRATION: Olivia—Use of Metaphors

After three years of practice, Tenaya, the occupational therapist, had attended many communication workshops and read many books about metaphors. When a group member, Olivia, who had many more skills that she could still learn and was not yet ready for discharge, announced that she was cured and ready to go, Tenaya used a metaphor to convey that she was not yet ready to leave. She stated that Olivia was like an ice cube that is partially on its way to being but not yet frozen. It may look like it is frozen and ready to be used, but when you put it into water, it will immediately crackle and melt. However, if you wait until the ice is completely frozen, when it is put into water, it will change the temperature of the water while it will remain intact for a long time. After listening to Tenaya, Olivia thought that she might still need to learn some skills.

Discussion

Olivia implicitly understood her own needs and changed her mind about leaving prematurely when Tenaya used a metaphor of ice cubes that conveyed her need to stay in treatment.

Reality Testing

Reality testing is offering an explanation of a situation that occurs in reality to counter obvious distortions or denials that clients may use. The understanding of what is actually happening is offered in such a way that the therapist encourages the client to think about and reflectively examine a situation. For example, in the previous case of Athena, the occupational therapist set limits around a situation that had just occurred by asking others to describe how Athena's comments had made them feel. In this situation Athena could not as easily deny the implications of her sarcastic behavior.

In addition to these universally used interpersonal strategies, the Occupational Therapy Practice Framework (2002) delineates methods that are unique to occupational therapy.

OCCUPATIONAL THERAPY METHODS

Broad strategies as well as methods of interventions and outcomes are specified in the Occupational Therapy Practice Framework (2002). The outcome of engagement in occupation to support participation in contexts is emphasized, but specific outcomes are also listed. This rendition of intervention makes it easier to set specific goals and to assess their outcomes. Because the practice framework defines broad strategies and methods of intervention, it also makes it easier to assess the outcomes of those strategies that you may use in practice.

Methods are: (1) to create and promote health, called health promotion; (2) to establish or restore health, called remediation or restoration; (3) to maintain health; (4) to modify, called compensation or adaptation; and (5) to prevent, called disability prevention. These broad methods are delivered through four interventions:

- Therapeutic use of self
- Therapeutic use of occupations
- Consultation
- Education

Application—Clinical Reasoning and Motivating

Perhaps because of the assumption that occupational therapists will use the Occupational Therapy Practice Framework (2002) in thinking and in documentation, the framework implies a clinical reasoning process. In fact, the practice framework mentions clinical reasoning: "During the intervention process, information from the evaluation step is integrated with theory, frames of reference, and evidence and is coupled with clinical reasoning to develop a plan and carry it out" (p. 617). Thus, the forms of clinical reasoning always guide methods and interpersonal strategies used in practice in collaboration with the client. The **clinical reasoning** process (Mattingly & Fleming, 1994) forms the guide for how the therapist will think about the client, plan step-by-step procedures (procedural reasoning), empathize with what is meaningful for the client (interactive reasoning), envision a past and a new future for the client (conditional reasoning), and perhaps engage in storytelling or storymaking with the client and with oneself (narrative reasoning) as a technique of facilitating the therapeutic relationship and change.

The plan is directed by the client's priorities and the interaction of the client's performance skills, patterns, contexts, activity demands, and client factors. The process of intervention is dynamic and unpredictable and really depends moment to moment on clients' skills and patterns as they influence or are influenced by particular contexts, activities, or internal attributes. For example, clients in a psychosocial rehabilitation program may be the most skilled workers when it comes to clerical work; however, their skills may seem to deteriorate if they are required to perform the same skills in a different work environment (context), or if they have a different supervisor for the day (context), or if they are asked to complete a job with which they are not familiar (demands of the activity), or if they begin to hear voices (client factors). The context, the demands of the activity, or client factors may interfere with their ability to complete the task. Therefore, occupational therapists will use specific methods directed toward the contexts, the demands of the activity, or the client factors, and they will design specific interpersonal approaches that address the client, and most likely these approaches will motivate the client to change.

In suggesting a way of addressing motivational deficits that often accompany mental illness, Wu, Chen, and Grossman (2000) provide another useful way of thinking about the context, demands of the activity, or client factors in mental health. Essentially, they propose that a social context in which individuals' basic psychological needs are satisfied promotes intrinsic motivation. Basic psychological needs are the need for autonomy or to determine one's own behavior; competence, or the need to experience productivity and to control outcome; and relatedness, the need to care for others. Thus an environment (context) in which a client will experience motivation will be one in which basic psychological needs (client factors) are met. Such needs can be met, and therefore intrinsic motivation can be facilitated by a combination of autonomy support, structure in activities (activity demands), and significant people being involved in therapy.

Depending on what motivates a given client, an occupational therapist may provide support, structure, and involvement in the following ways. Autonomy support can be generated by the therapist valuing and *validating* the client's goals and interests, *encouraging* participation, providing the client with choices and abilities to make decisions, encouraging the client to act on one's own expectations rather than those of others, helping the client to take responsibility for changes rather than attribute change to the therapist, and *empathizing* with experiences of frustration due to gaps between present performance and future goals. Structure can be provided by including some challenge to clients' abilities, communicating clear expectations, providing clear feedback regarding performance, assisting clients to understand consequences of behavior (*reality testing and setting limits*), the relationship of goals and occupational therapy services, and the nature of personal gratification with one's interests versus performing for approval. Involvement may include educating, supporting, or consulting clients' significant others in the therapy process, encouraging clients' participation in group and social or community functions, or providing an empathic therapeutic relationship (Wu, Chen, & Grossman, 2000). The therapeutic relationship and therapeutic use of self will be discussed in more detail because they are methods discussed in occupational therapy's domain of practice. However, more important, they will also be discussed in a way that suggests an expanded understanding of the ideas.

No matter how a therapist chooses to address context, activity demands, or the client implementation of an occupational therapy plan is carried out by types of interventions broadly stated as therapeutic use of self, or therapeutic use of activities and occupations. Other types of interventions are consultation and education, but since these are self-explanatory, they will not be discussed in this chapter.

Interventions

Occupational therapy interventions are guided by the Occupational Therapy Practice Framework's (2002) broad methods of therapeutic use of activity and occupations and therapeutic use of self. Under those broad categories are the techniques and methods unique to occupational therapy—activity and occupational analysis and gradation—and those techniques and methods that are borrowed or common to other practices—therapeutic use of self.

Therapeutic Use of Self in Relationship—Empathy

Therapeutic use of self is defined in the practice framework (2002, p.628) as "a practitioner's planned use of his or her personality, insights, perceptions, and judgments as part of the therapeutic process." The planned use of personality, insights, perceptions, and judgments can be thought of as personal approaches that a practitioner adopts in the interpersonal interaction with the client or clients. Occupational therapy literature has more specifically defined those traits of a professional and approaches that a practitioner adopts with a client (Borg & Bruce, 1997; Crepeau, Cohn, & Schell, 2003; Fearing & Clark, 2000; Hagedorn, 1995; 2000; Kielhofner, 2002; Schwartzberg, 2002). Professional traits and approaches are meant to be used in service of a client-centered practice where the meaning and subjective experience of the client is to be taken into account at all times in a collaborative process.

To effect a client-centered approach, the occupational therapy literature has focused on two important skills that must be apparent in the therapeutic relationship: empathy and trust. However, in discussing the therapeutic relationship or alliance that should engender empathy and trust, empathy is considered at times as part of a therapeutic relationship and a means of establishing trust and a climate of caring, or recognizing the uniqueness of clients and clients' needs (Peloquin, 2003). At other times it is considered a quality of the therapist in the therapeutic use of self (Hagedorn, 2000; Kielhofner, 2002; Schwartzberg, 2002). Empathy is a professional skill that can be developed, and thus is necessary to the therapeutic relationship, and in fact is one ingredient of the therapeutic relationship that effects change (based on the beliefs and theories of self-psychology, and its founder, Heinz Kohut [1971, 1977, 1985; 1987; Siegel, 1997] and his followers [Elson, 1986; Grief, 2000; Kohut & Wolfe, 1978; Lee, 1991; Rowe, 1989; Shane, 1997]).

Contextual and Case-Specific Empathy. Empathy can be further distinguished as contextual empathy and case-specific empathy. Contextual empathy conveys caring, putting oneself in another's shoes, and the spirituality (or what Peloquin calls covenant) of "holding" a relationship sacred. An implicit aspect of each encounter in mental health is the empathic attitude that the client is valued and understood.

Case-specific empathy is used in clinical situations or therapeutic relationships by the therapist to formulate an accurate response to an individual client in a specific context. If the therapist's responses convey empathy, then the client in turn will feel understood (Babiss, 2002) and *be more motivated to continue treatment*. So just as occupations and activities are considered the prime motivator of change in occupational therapy intervention, in mental health, the therapeutic relationship is equally important in motivating change in occupational therapy. This last statement is supported by research that finds the therapeutic relationship has proven to be important to the effectiveness of therapy (Krupnik et al., cited in Hagedorn, 2000) and is the most important aspect of psychotherapy regardless of which theory or type of therapy a therapist espouses (Roth & Fonagy, 1996). An empathic response not only conveys caring, but also may be a response to a client's specific needs. Therefore, a case-specific response may be confronting or limit setting. It may be coaching or offering validation or reality testing. In that specific moment the therapist's response may not seem caring or appear to be caring although it ultimately is because the response is exactly what is needed for the client in that specific situation. This understanding of empathy, contextual or case-specific, also demonstrates more than the therapeutic use of self.

Intersubjectivity. The use of empathy as a contextual attitude and as a case-specific response conveys that there is more than only the therapeutic use of self that occurs in a therapeutic relationship; there is also therapeutic use of the other and the other-in-relationship to the therapist. For example, empathy, empathic responses, and client progress imply that the client also has an influence on the relationship and on the therapist. Although occupational therapy emphasizes the therapeutic use of self for the therapist and understanding the meaning of the client's world through clinical reasoning, there is less emphasis on the fact that the client also influences the therapist's world, and that the therapist's reactions and responses take the subjectivity of the client into account. Thus, particularly in a mental health setting the **intersubjective process** (Crepeau, 1991; Stolorow, 1994; Stolorow & Atwood, 1992), rather than only the therapeutic use of self, must be emphasized.

Emphasizing the intersubjective process means that the occupational therapist is more reflective and self-aware, or insightful (Hagedorn, 2000), in the therapeutic alliance, always reflecting on herself or himself in a self-analytical process (Stolorow, 1994). With this analytical vantage point the therapist uses his or her thoughts and feelings to give clues about or recognize the thoughts and feelings that may be implicit with the client. The analytical vantage point and understanding of the intersubjective nature of any therapeutic interaction or alliance then guides the occupational therapist in choosing and using various techniques or strategies on a case-specific basis. That is, the occupational therapist will choose strategies and techniques according to the subjective needs of each client in context. Obviously occupational therapists analyze client factors, contexts, and activities on a case-specific basis, but understanding the client's needs emerges out of awareness of the intersubjective nature of therapeutic encounters. The intersubjective nature of therapeutic encounters takes both the clients' and therapists' factors or subjective meanings into account.

Therapeutic Use of Activity

Although the practice framework finally defined therapeutic use of activity and occupations as the domain of occupational therapy, activities and occupations have been recognized throughout the history of occupational therapy as the core process of the profession. (See Chapter 3 for a detailed historical discussion of activities and occupations.)

There are many ways to think about and discuss activities and occupations, and there is much information regarding activity and occupational analysis in occupational therapy (Crepeau, 2003; Fidler & Velde, 1999; Hagedorn, 2000; Levine & Brayley, 1991). The practice framework (AOTA, 2002) specifically includes activity demands, and *Willard and Spackman's* 10th edition (2003) includes an occupation-based activity analysis format based on the information in the practice framework. Thus, this broad activity analysis includes categories of:

- Objects and their properties
- Space and social demands, thus attending to physical, social, and cultural contexts
- Required actions
- Required body functions and structures

However, within these broad categories, it is often difficult to ferret out which aspects of the activity demands are most useful for psychosocial purposes. Fidler and Velde (1999) note that there is still little information "regarding the inherent characteristics of activities, those elements that make up and define the nature of a given activity" (p. 1) and that "the social, cultural, and personal meanings and metaphors inherent in an activity are an essential aspect of understanding purposeful activity" (p. 3).

In addition to a perspective on activities that attends to their inherent characteristics and social, cultural, and personal meanings and metaphors, Fidler and Velde (1999) espouse another important emphasis (in Chapter 2 of her book that is written by Susan Fine) that is pertinent to mental health practice: an acknowledgment of a person's inner life. By inner life they mean mental processes that deal with thoughts and feelings and influence our behavior and that are influenced by activity and occupational performance. An apt quote captures a societal attitude that sometimes seems to be adopted by occupational therapists but that explains the significance of attending to unconscious elements of activity demands.

> Acknowledging the unconscious inner life in the context of today's dynamic biopsychosocial dialectic does not commit one to the couch. It simply, and profoundly, opens the door to *a fuller understanding of how human activities at one level influence processes at another.* Exploring it is well worth the risk! (p. 13)

Because the practice framework provides essentially a broad overview of activity analysis, but lacks a focus on psychosocial demands, symbolic and metaphorical meanings, or unconscious aspects that are provoked or inherent in activities, this chapter's information is based primarily on Fidler's view of activities and activity analysis. In addition, this chapter introduces another view of activity analysis that focuses on explicit and implicit methods in psychosocial activities (Eklund, 2002) because sometimes the goal in psychosocial occupational therapy is not so obvious.

Activity Analysis

The basic elements of an activity analysis are: (1) form and structure, (2) properties, (3) action processes, (4) outcome, and (5) realistic and symbolic meaning. Each of these categories is explained in more detail in the following paragraphs.

Form and Structure.   Form and structure provide the rules and procedures, time to complete, and sequences that ensure predictable products or outcomes. Form and structure tell us how extensive and explicit the rules are, if the rules can be changed without significantly changing the activity, what the sequences in the activity are, and how long the activity will take to complete. A comparison of two crafts, forming a hand-built ceramic pot or constructing a wooden birdhouse, gives different structure due to the inherent pliable (clay) and nonpliable (wood) nature of the materials. Likewise, a self-grooming activity compared with completing a meal following a specific menu will provide more creativity and flexibility (self-grooming) or less creativity and flexibility (following a specific menu). The previous case illustration of Denny Mike indicated that he had difficulty expressing his unique opinions and attempted to please the therapist without thinking of his own interests. Therefore, if Denny Mike engaged in a concrete craft, it would most likely be more beneficial to give him one whose form is more pliable, so that he can experiment with fashioning his own unique design instead of following one in which he has no unique options.

Properties.   Properties of an activity are the objects, materials, space, setting, equipment, and number of people required for an activity. These requirements dictate the nature of the activity and how it will impact the client. The properties of the activity form its "character" (Fidler & Velde, 1999, p. 51). For example, projects that can be accomplished by hand or with the aid of tools may convey different meanings. How might the project have different meanings depending on if it is crafted by hand or by power tool? A knitting project that is done by hand usually claims more respect (and more money) in our society than a knitting project that uses a knitting tool. Another example may be a work project that is completed in assembly line fashion. How might the project have different meanings for each of the clients that are required for the activity? How might the number of people required influence the interaction of those involved? In the case illustration of Athena, who required some limit setting due to her sarcastic comments subsequent to having difficulty accepting caring, it might be useful to engage her in a group project such as an outreach group in which members actively contact other members, or in a gardening project in which members work with each other in caring for plants.

Action Processes.   Action processes identify the sensorimotor, cognitive, psychological, and interpersonal functions that the activity may demand. For example, a sports game such as flag football involves more sensorimotor processes than does watching sports, but watching sports may involve more cognitive processes than a sports game. Using the same example, the game of flag football may involve more psychological processes such as competition and aggression than cognitive processes of watching the game. Finally, the sports game may involve more interpersonal processes than watching sports if one watches a sport alone. However, if in playing the game a person only attends to his or her position and if being a spectator is a group activity, the sports viewing may include more interpersonal processes than playing the game (and many reports of superstars in baseball, such as Barry Bonds; football, such as Randy Moss; or basketball, such as Kobe Bryant, attest to isolation even while playing a game).

Outcome.   The end product of activities may be a tangible product, such as a cake, or an abstract outcome, such as a decision made or a problem solved. Also, the end product may convey socio-cultural meanings or meanings concerning individual values. For example, a cake might convey a cultural transition, such as in a cake celebrating graduation or a birthday, or may simply be a pleasing food item. A decision to discontinue a community vocational skills group may mean movement to the next level of work in the community or recognition that work is not important at this time in one's life or illness process.

Realistic and Symbolic Meaning.   Activities and their elements have an actual, literal meaning and also have significance symbolically in personal associations or societal beliefs and cultural values. For example, maintaining a community garden may mean growing vegetables that may sustain an individual's family or psychosocial rehabilitation community by providing organic foods. Symbolically, it may mean the ability to nurture and sustain living things and to contribute in some positive way to one's community or to solving the problem of global warming. In the example of a gardening project suggested for Athena, when considering the properties of an activity, the symbolic nature of nurturing and sustaining living things and contributing to one's community may give her a way of accepting that she has the ability to nurture and care for plants, and that others may extend that same nurturing to her.

Activity Categorization

Fidler & Velde (1999) also classify activities into broad categories that can influence which activities one will use in practice according to each specific individual and context. Based on others' research (Moore & Anderson, cited in Fidler, 1999), socialization could be explained as developing from certain experiences with games and activities. Although this idea of how one develops through games and activities is readily acceptable when thinking of children, it is somehow lost when thinking of adults. However, it is no less true when thinking about adults in mental health settings, let alone adults in other settings. So this manner of categorizing activities according to the characteristic of games that contribute a socializing factor in people's lives is particularly important for individuals with mental illness whose overarching problems keep them functioning as best they can in society. These categories are listed in Table 18-1.

CASE ILLUSTRATION: Sylvia—Characteristics of Activities

Sylvia had been hospitalized twice in her 20s because of suicide attempts after the termination of relationships that she thought were the "loves of her life." While hospitalized she had been diagnosed with major depression and borderline personality disorder. During the hospitalizations it was discovered that she also had post-traumatic stress disorder because of her mother's periodic loss of control and physical abuse, and because she often had been placed in various foster homes prior to being adopted when she was 12. While hospitalized she was unable to sustain her denial of her abusive past and to maintain the picture of her mother as someone treated unfairly by "the system."

Table 18-1. Categories of Activities

Activity Category	Examples	Characteristics
Puzzles	Knitting, weaving, orienteering, survivor programs Learning computer software Negotiating the Internet	Contain much form and structure, predictable outcomes, clear sequences and procedures. Performer can control and predict the outcome.
Chance	Card games—poker or solitaire Board games—Scrabble or Sequence Watching sports	Contain little form and structure, unpredictable outcomes, few rules and procedures. Performer has little control or prediction of outcomes.
Games of Strategy	Card games—bridge, hearts Board games—chess, checkers Sports participation—tennis, basketball, soccer, softball, running track	Contain some form and structure, sequences and procedures, but they depend on the other person playing—anticipation of the other's plan in conjunction with one's own plan—and are constantly and dynamically changing. Performer has some control but less prediction of outcomes.
Aesthetic	Attending concerts, museums, plays and critiquing music, art, or drama Obtaining antiques or "collectibles" Refereeing sports Performing music, art or drama for an audience.	Less defined external form and structure and rules and procedures determined by the person. Contains an evaluative element. Performer can control the process through element of making evaluative judgments or through performance. Actual performance is subject to less control of other's evaluative judgments.

While hospitalized and working with these issues that caused considerable stress, Sylvia worked on activities that could be categorized as puzzles. In occupational therapy, she particularly enjoyed weaving scarves on a hand-loom and finding information about Native American textiles on the Internet. She also enjoyed the occupational therapy groups in which she could discuss her feelings but in an intellectual way about various issues of daily life, including how to save money, how to have casual relationships, how to get along at work, and ways to access personal resources and develop a self-identity (see Cara, 1992 for further discussion of these ideas).

After discharge Sylvia had been able to function for 10 years without rehospitalization, during which time she attended individual and group therapy.

During those 10 years she had continued to have various chaotic and unhappy love relationships, most of which ended unhappily and often caused her to request extra therapy time. At these times her psychiatrist would suggest that she attend an ongoing community mental health occupational therapy group so that she could identify and pursue some new interests. Sylvia also was able to renew her interest in weaving that she had learned in the hospital, and that interest sustained her during periods of turmoil.

Now as she entered her 40s, Sylvia realized that maybe her life was satisfying without a long-term, significant relationship. She had two cats that she took care of, and she also grew plants and vegetables that she used in cooking. She had learned to cook with these natural ingredients. She had become increasingly active in a tennis league and had purchased season tickets to the ballet. In addition to supporting the ballet in a volunteer role, she also was active in Amnesty International, and felt gratified that she was able to support political prisoners.

Discussion

During acute periods of her illness and during times when she was particularly vulnerable, Sylvia engaged in activities, such as weaving, that provided much form and structure and predictable outcomes. She satisfied her nurturing desires by taking care of plants and animals, and by her volunteer roles. She also used her strength of intelligence and thought about how she felt about various instrumental activities of daily living. She began to sort out her values and interests and acquire new roles as she formed a personal identity. When she became more able to regulate her emotions, Sylvia realized that perhaps she could enjoy life although she was not attached to a man. She broadened her interests into games that included some form and structure but also some change and interactions with another person. She also broadened her interests into aesthetic activities in which each performance was less predictable and offered an element of surprise and in which she could satisfy her inquiring mind by evaluating.

Implicit and Explicit Methods

Another broad way of analyzing psychosocial interventions is placing the intervention on a continuum of explicit or implicit methods (Eklund, 2002). Although thinking in terms of explicit or implicit methods is most useful in explaining occupational therapy to those unfamiliar with it, thinking in these terms can help organize how one will deliver services. On the one hand, in an explicit method the relationship between the purpose of the activity and the end goal is clear and direct and the skill being learned is obviously necessary in an occupational performance. For example, a transportation group may be carried out because a client needs to learn how to travel to a job independently. On the other hand, in an implicit method, the purpose of the activity and the end goal are less clear and more indirect and the skill being learned is not as obviously necessary for performing a given occupation. For example, a transportation group may be carried out because a client needs to learn how to handle change, read signs, make appropriate small talk with strangers, or learn how to maintain concentration.

There are differences in various dimensions of activities that are important when thinking of using either method (Eklund, 2002). Those dimensions are: short-term goals, activities used, time required, and position in the profession. In explicit methods, the short-term goal is typically better skills in occupational performance; activities used are ADL, work, or leisure skills directly related to the goal; time required is the time it takes to master the current activity; and the methods constitute the core of occupational therapy—therapeutic use of activity. In implicit methods, the short-term goal is typically better functioning in performance components or patterns; the time required is the time it takes to master the current activity and the underlying components; and the methods are not as linked to the core of occupational therapy, but are inherent in all occupational performance.

The case of Brandon and his occupational therapist, Jackie, in the previous chapter demonstrates the interpersonal strategies discussed in this chapter. Refer to Chapter 17 to review Brandon's occupational profile and barriers or supports to his occupational performance before reading about the interpersonal strategies that Jackie used with Brandon.

CASE ILLUSTRATION: Brandon—Jackie's Interpersonal Strategies

Jackie's use of strategies began with evaluation although she did not know at the time that she would be working with Brandon after the evaluation. She had been hired by the agency for occupational therapy intervention after the apartments were built and after she had completed her first contract.

During the evaluation process, Jackie provided empathic responses *to Brandon's frustrations about having mental illness, not being independent, and wanting very much to live on his own. Through the interactive clinical reasoning process she was able to gain an understanding of Brandon, his hopes, fears, dreams, and frustrations. Through* conditional reasoning *she was able to form an image of Brandon that included his past and what he might become or where he might be in the future. She encouraged Brandon to share his own personal story and* validated *his statements about himself and his situation, about his feelings toward his family, staff, and other tenants, about his frustrations when he experienced hypomania, paranoid thoughts, or hallucinations.*

During the intervention process Jackie continued to provide encouragement, validation, and empathic responses. However, empathic responses did not always mean some positive statement about Brandon's behavior, choices, or feelings. For example, at times, Brandon believed that he was doing so well that he probably did not really have mental illness but was just "stressed sometimes." At those times, Jackie provided an empathic response concerning how hard it might be to accept mental illness, particularly when one seemed to be functioning so well, but that indeed she along with many others observed that he did have a mental illness and the symptoms did interfere with his life.

Because Jackie was often working in Brandon's apartment, she often encoun-tered situations that called for limit setting, confrontation, *and interpretation. For example, during an intervention in which the objective was making tea for a guest as the rudimentary step to having his family for dinner, Brandon stated that having her for tea really was like a date, and since she was not married and they got along so well, that maybe they should extend their "friendship" into something more serious. Jackie stated that she thought working in someone's home made it very difficult to always be aware that this work was a professional encounter. Furthermore, the type of interventions, like meal planning and hosting a dinner party that they worked on, further blurred the reality that this was a professional encounter. Nevertheless, she thought that Brandon's idea was somewhat grandiose and his grandiosity was most likely influencing him to read more into her actions and behavior than was actually there. This symptom was one of the very reasons he attended his group and for which he requested* reality testing *and she would not be doing her job if she did not let him know about it. Brandon became angry and initial-ly accused Jackie of encouraging his romantic feelings toward her. However, Jackie accepted his expression of anger and continued to confront his denial, grandiosity, and hurt feelings. Eventually, she stated an* interpretation *that she understood that he liked, respected, and appreciated her, and perhaps it was difficult to express his feelings without "sexualizing" them. After this very difficult situation, Brandon and Jackie were able to work within professional boundaries.*

At times Jackie coached Brandon, particularly when they attended the enti-tlement workshops, implemented the intervention plan in the supermarket, or when carrying out an objective in his plan by having tea. She often used metaphors *and* reframing *during these times and also when Brandon reported his problems back to her after having friends or his brother and sister for break-fast (another objective in the intervention plan). After the first time he had a friend for breakfast, he reported his discouragement that he could not get everything ready at the same time. Jackie stated that this was one of the hard-est, intangible aspects of cooking meals that often doesn't show up until you cook a large meal, and that he was most fortunate that it came up so early so that he could get this intangible aspect correct for the family dinner. Additionally, putting a meal together and having everything ready at the same time is like a dress rehearsal, and you want things to go wrong at the dress rehearsal not at the final performance. Brandon responded humorously that, indeed, maybe this was an example of a situation where you wished that you were a little manic!*

Discussion

During evaluation and treatment Jackie used interpersonal strategies that kept the plan on track and further motivated Brandon to continue his efforts to achieve his goals.

Summary

The Occupational Therapy Practice Framework (2002) specifies the domain and the process of occupational therapy. The occupational therapy domain is use of occupations and activities for intervention. The occupational therapy process involves clinical reasoning and interpersonal techniques and strategies to apply occupations or activities. Activity and occupational analysis and gradation are unique to occupational therapy and ways of thinking about activities in psychosocial practice (Eklund, 2002; Fidler & Velde, 1999; Wu, Chen, & Grossman, 2000) were suggested. Although interpersonal strategies are common in other fields, they are efficacious when used in occupational therapy, particularly for motivating clients to engage in treatment. An overall interpersonal approach is client-centered and grounded in empathy and trust while useful interpersonal strategies are validation, setting limits, encouragement, advice, coaching, confrontation, setting limits, reframing, use of metaphors, and reality testing.

Review Questions

1. Why are limit setting and interpretation useful strategies in mental health care?
2. What is case-specific empathy and how is it carried out in occupational therapy? How is it different from contextual empathy?
3. What is an important perspective regarding activities in a mental health practice?
4. What is intersubjectivity and why is it discussed apart from therapeutic use of self in this chapter?
5. What are the categories of activity and how do these categories define activities?

References

Babiss, F. (2002). Treatment experiences: Helpful and not helpful. *Occupational Therapy in Mental Health, 18*(3/4), 39–62.

Bandler, R., & Grinder, J. (1975). *The structure of magic: A book about language and therapy* (Vol. 1). Palo Alto, CA: Science & Behavior Books.

Bandler, R., & Grinder, J. (1976). *The structure of magic, II* (Vol. 2). Palo Alto, CA: Science & Behavior Books.

Borg, B., & Bruce, M. A. (1997). *Occupational therapy stories: Psychosocial interaction in practice.* Thorofare, NJ: Slack.

Cara, E. (1992). Neutralizing the narcissistic style: Narcissism, self-psychology, and occupational therapy. In S. C. Merrill (Ed.), *Occupational therapy and psychosocial dysfunction,* (pp. 135–156). New York: Haworth.

Crepeau, E. B. (1991). Achieving intersubjective understanding: Examples from an occupational therapy treatment session. *American Journal of Occupational Therapy, 45*(11), 1016–1025.

Crepeau, E. B. (2003). Analyzing occupation and activity: A way of thinking about occupational performance. In E. B. Crepeau, E. S. Cohn, &. B. A. B. Schell (Eds.), *Willard and Spackman's occupational therapy* (10th ed., pp. 189–198). Philadelphia: Lippincott Williams & Wilkins.

Crepeau, E. B., Cohn, E. S., & Schell, B. A. B. (Eds.). (2003). *Willard and Spackman's occupational therapy* (10th ed.). Philadelphia: Lippincott Williams & Wilkins.

Eklund, M. (2002). Explicit and implicit methods in psychosocial occupational therapy. *Occupational Therapy in Mental Health, 18*(2), 3–15.

Elson, M. (1986). *Self-psychology in clinical social work.* New York: Norton.

Fearing, V. G., & Clark, J. (Eds.). (2000). *Individuals in context: A practical guide to client-centered practice.* Thorofare, NJ: Slack.

Fidler, G. S., & Velde, B. P. (1999). *Activities: reality and symbol.* Thorofare, NJ: Slack.

Grief, G. (2000). *The tragedy of the self: Individual and social disintegration viewed through the self-psychology of Heinz Kohut.* Lanham, MD: University Press.

Hagedorn, R. (1995). *Occupational therapy: Perspectives and processes.* New York: Churchill Livingstone.

Hagedorn, R. (2000). *Tools for practice in occupational therapy: A structured approach to core skills and processes.* Edinburgh: Churchill Livingstone.

Kielhofner, G. (2002). *Model of human occupation: Theory and application.* Baltimore: Lippencott Williams and Wilkins.

Kielhofner, G., & Forsyth, K. (2002). Therapeutic strategies for enabling change. In G. Kielhofner (Ed.), *Model of human occupation: Theory and application* (3rd ed., pp. 309–324). Philadelphia: Lippincott Williams & Wilkins.

Kohut, H. (1971). *The analysis of the self.* New York: International University Press.

Kohut, H. (1977). *The restoration of the self.* New York: International University Press.

Kohut, H. (Ed.). (1985). *How does analysis cure?* Chicago: University of Chicago Press.

Kohut, H., & Wolfe, E. (1978). The disorders of the self and their treatment: An outline. *International Journal of Psycho-Analysis, 59,* 413.

Lakoff, G. (1993). The contemporary theory of metaphor. In A. Ortony (Ed.), *Metaphor and thought* (pp. 202–251). Cambridge: Cambridge University Press.

Lakoff, G., & Johnson, M. (1980). *Metaphors we live by.* Chicago: University of Chicago Press.

Lee, R. (1991). *Psychotherapy after Kohut: A textbook of psychotherapy.* Hillsdale, NJ: Analytic.

Levine, R. E., & Brayley, C. R. (1991). Occupation as a therapeutic medium: A contextual approach to performance interventions. In C. Christiansen & C. Baum (Eds.), *Occupational therapy: Overcoming human performance deficits.* Thorofare, NJ: Slack.

Mattingly, C., &. Fleming, M. H. (1994). *Clinical reasoning: Forms of inquiry in a therapeutic practice.* Philadelphia: F. A. Davis.

Occupational Therapy Practice Framework: Domain and Process. (2002). *American Journal of Occupational Therapy, 56,* 609–639.

Peloquin, S. (2003). The therapeutic relationship: Manifestations and challenges in occupational therapy. In E. B. Crepeau, E. S. Cohn, & B. A. B. Schell (Eds.), *Willard and Spackman's occupational therapy* (10th ed., pp. 157–184). Philadelphia: Lippincott Williams & Wilkins.

Roth, A. R., & Fonagy, P. (1996). *What works for whom?: A critical review of psychotherapy research.* New York: Guilford.

Rowe, C. E. (1989). *Empathic attunement: The "technique" of psychoanalytic self-psychology.* Northvale, NJ: Jason Aronson.

Schwartzberg, S. (2002). *Interactive reasoning in the practice of occupational therapy.* Upper Saddle River, NJ: Prentice-Hall.

Shane, M. (1997). *Intimate attachments: Toward a new self-psychology.* New York: Guilford.

Siegal, C. (1997). *Heinz Kohut and the psychology of the self: The makers of modern psychotherapy.* New York: Routledge.

Stolorow, R. (1994). The intersubjective context of intrapsychic experience. In R. Stolorow, G. Atwood, & B. Brandchaft (Eds.), *The intersubjective perspective.* Northvale, NJ: Jason Aronson.

Stolorow, R., & Atwood, G. (1992). *Contexts of being: The intersubjective foundations of psychological life.* Hillsdale, NJ: Analytic.

Wu, C., Chen, S., & Grossman, J. (2000). Facilitating intrinsic motivation in clients with mental illness. *Occupational Therapy in Mental Health, 16*(1), 1–14.

Groups

Elizabeth Cara, PhD, OTR/L, MFT

Key Terms

activity group
group
group content
group dynamics
group norms
group process

group protocol
group structure
personhood skills
psychodynamic
psychoeducational

Chapter Outline

Documentation and Outcome
Summary

Introduction

Occupational therapists in the psychosocial arena conduct much, if not most, of treatment in **group** settings. Group treatment can be incredibly exciting, stimulating, and interesting. It is exciting to implement or to "lead" groups, and it is stimulating to develop or "create" them. Developing and implementing groups includes both artistic and scientific elements. The science is involved in developing the **group structure**, organizing a **group protocol**, recognizing the needs of the setting and the population with whom one works, applying a knowledge of occupations and occupational skills, and utilizing good communication and interpersonal skills. The art lies in being aware of the **group process**, using oneself in a therapeutic way, and knowing, and responding to, the here-and-now needs of the individual group participants and to the participants as a group—simultaneously. Both the art and the science can be learned through acquiring knowledge and practicing experientially. This chapter discusses groups in general and how to think about occupational therapy groups so that they can be developed and implemented creatively and competently, in any setting, and with any participants.

Specifically, this chapter explains how to develop, conduct, and lead groups. It also distinguishes occupational therapy groups from other types, notably psychotherapy groups, which are conducted by other professionals.

What Makes a Group a Group?

There are various definitions of groups, all of which include a situation in which three or more people come together and think of themselves as a group. A group can be thought of as an intentional coming together to produce change for the members (Borg & Bruce, 1991; Hagedorn, 2000; Howe & Schwartzberg, 2001) and also as a microcosm of society, in which participants can learn about themselves and their relationships (Corey & Corey, 2002). There are common properties that characterize almost any group. These include:

- A background, history, and purpose
- A structure imposed by the group leader, which usually consists of preparations, expectations, a composition, and arrangements
- An interaction pattern, for example, member-to-member or member-to-leader
- Communication or action taking place, whether verbal or nonverbal
- Usually, a cohesion, or a "we" feeling
- Standards or rules of acceptable behavior

The **group norms** or standards of a group usually contribute to cohesion and a feeling of safety and trust. Norms can be explicit or implicit, verbalized or unstated, developed initially by the leader or based on the group interaction (Cole,

1998). Norms are often set and monitored by how the group leader models expected behavior and handles unwanted behavior. In addition to the leader, the environment—both physical space and how people react in and to it—and goals of the group also are responsible for the development of norms (Borg & Bruce, 1991). For example, a norm of talking to other group members and not to the leader is developed when the leader does not answer every question directed to him or her, but instead asks the group in general to answer the question. A norm of talking to, not about, each other is established when the leader asks an individual who is talking about another person in the group to direct his or her comments to the person about whom he or she is speaking. A norm of the members' acceptance and importance in the group is set when the group meets at a regular time, is held in a comfortable, distraction-free place that accommodates everyone and is identified as the space where occupational therapy happens, and supplies are made readily available. In addition, the therapist should greet participants warmly, start the group on time, and always begin and end the meeting in a similar manner. When the group leader states the clear goals of the group and the purpose for the group to each new member—or asks participants to do so—a norm is established concerning how new members will enter the group and what individuals should learn in the group is made explicit.

Common norms necessary in any group are confidentiality, a here-and-now focus, respect for each individual, and participation—though each member has a right to choose how to interact, what to disclose, and what to do in the group (Corey & Corey, 2002).

Advantages and Limitations of Groups

Practically speaking, group treatment in mental health is time- and cost-effective. It costs less to treat people in groups than it does to treat them on an individual basis, and they allow more people to be seen in a shorter amount of time. Group treatment facilitates personal growth by virtue of providing more people with whom to interact. Participants can learn about themselves through identifying with others; observing, and being able to compare and contrast, their own experience with those of others; experiencing closeness and caring; and having opportunities to be around others in a safe or trusting context. Groups support experimentation and trying of new behavior, with a variety of feedback provided by different people (Corey & Corey, 2002). More specifically, occupational therapy groups facilitate learning new skills from others. Groups are like mini-laboratories in which one can practice skills for living in a simulated experience.

Of course, there are some limitations to group treatment. Not everyone is suited for groups. For example, an individual may be too disoriented, confused, or suspicious of others to be able to tolerate a group. A group may be too distracting or require too high a degree of abstract ability. Some clients may require individual treatment; for example, if they are inpatients in an acute care hospital, they may not be able to leave their room or setting due to precautions or illness. Last, some people may simply need the concentrated effort of individual treatment. The following section discusses some of the properties, norms, stages, and themes of groups.

OVERVIEW OF GROUP THERAPY

"Since humans have inhabited the earth, we have joined and been influenced by groups" (Barlow, Burlingame, & Fuhriman, 2000, p. 115). However, the history of groups has been written mostly in the beginning of the last century, and group psychotherapy has been practiced in one form or another since the early 1900s (Scheidlinger, 1994). While group therapy may bring to mind a psychoanalyst silently treating a group of adults, group therapy has been conducted by various professionals for problems ranging from psychopathology to problems in living. It has been brief to long-term and occurs in many settings. Because various disciplines have contributed to its application and theory, the history of group therapy is complex, nonlinear, and distinguished by somewhat disparate research.

A Short History

Although Europe contributes to the history, group therapy is generally thought to be an American phenomenon resulting from the energy of this open culture in the twentieth century (Barlow, Burlingame, & Fuhriman, 2000). "The professionally guided helping group is an American invention" (Scheidlinger, 1994, p. 197). Although early pioneers included Freud and Adler in Europe, it was Pratt in the United States who first conducted groups for individuals with tuberculosis in 1905. Shortly after Pratt, in 1909, Marsh, a minister who became a psychiatrist, gave his psychiatric clients inspirational group lectures (Scheidlinger, 1994). In the 1920s milieu therapy and the psychoeducational method was introduced for "mental" clients. Principles of using members' influence, maintaining a here-and-now focus, and analyzing the group emerged from the group treatment of the mentally ill. Also in the first two decades of the twentieth century, Jacob Moreno founded psychodrama and began to use group action methods called sociodrama. Techniques of psychodrama that later became mainstream practice included role playing and role reversal. In the 1930s groups re-created the family, the method was introduced for children, and group leaders established credentials for leadership. These diverse applications were based on diverse theories, for example, classical psychoanalysis, existentialism, and behaviorism.

In the mid-1940s, the understanding of group process became popular as a result of World War II, which caused numerous psychiatric casualties at a time when there was a shortage of psychiatrists. Therefore, therapy in groups became a necessity. Also in the 1940s, researchers attempted to confirm the efficacy of groups and to categorize them. However, the groups were too diverse to catalogue adequately. An explosion of group practice models and outpatient groups continued throughout the 1950s. With the opening of community mental health centers in the 1960s, innovative group therapy models were developed (Scheidlinger, 1994). During the same decade research methods became more rigorous, and researchers were better able to describe diverse variables or factors in group therapy. Diverse aspects of groups such as therapeutic factors (hope, altruism, identification, etc.), interventions (feedback, reality-testing, role flexibility, etc.), and leader traits (directive, warm, active, etc.) were researched throughout the 1990s. Regardless of which aspects of groups have been studied, the outcomes suggest that "groups do appear to work" (Barlow, et. al., 2000, p. 117).

Currently, managed care and the emphasis of biology in treatment point to certain future trends. Most likely, short-term groups with one leader will proliferate, as well as large-group treatments and psychoeducational and medical self-help groups; also, groups will be tailored to specific client populations.

Models of Group Therapy

The increasing use of group therapy techniques has paralleled the rise in popularity of different psychological models. For example, from the concept's inception through the 1950s, groups were based on a psychoanalytic model, which was popular in the United States during this period. Today, self-help groups and brief cognitive and behaviorally oriented groups are popular because of the growth of behavioral and cognitive models and a community self-help movement.

Different concepts, techniques, and leadership roles will be assumed depending on which model a group is grounded. A brief explanation of various psychological models of group therapy is presented in Table 19-1. Although one may pattern a group specifically on one model, in actuality many groups are implemented utilizing various principles. Each group developer and leader will generally blend what they feel to be the most effective concepts and techniques to create a unique group (Corey & Corey, 2002).

Group Content and Structure

The **group content** is the activity that is planned and carried out in the group (Denton, 1987) or what is said in the group (Cole, 1998; Howe & Schwartzberg, 2001). It can be either verbal or nonverbal. The way in which the activity is presented; the directions, procedures, techniques, and time arrangements; and the way in which membership is organized comprise the group structure. The content and structure of a group will naturally flow from its purpose and the style of the leader. Group content and structures have been combined in various ways to produce many types of occupational therapy groups.

Group Dynamics and Process

Group dynamics are the forces that influence the relationships of members and the group outcome (Cole, 1998). Some important dynamics of a group are the process and stages of groups, leadership styles and leader behaviors, roles that members assume, norms and expected standards of behavior, the behavior and interaction of the group members, the group structure, and the environment in which it is held.

The group process refers to how the work of the group is carried out (Howe & Schwartzberg, 2001), including how participants relate to each other, who talks to whom, how tasks are accomplished, and how decisions are made. Group process involves two tiers (Yalom, 1995). On the first tier, it includes the here-and-now experience of the group members, who focus their attention on their feelings

Table 19-1. Models of Group Therapy

	Psychoanalytic	Humanistic	Behavioral	Cognitive-Behavioral
Philosophy	Childhood experiences	Self-actualization	Changing behavior	Changing thoughts or schemas
Emphasis	Make the unconscious conscious	Self-awareness	Learning effective, eliminating maladaptive, behavior	Learning more adaptive thinking, eliminating maladaptive thinking
Key Concepts	Work through resistance and transference	Understanding values and discovering meaning	Increasing effective, decreasing ineffective, behavior	Change cognitions, thoughts, or schemas
Goal	Insight	Maximize climate of growth and awareness	Change behavior	Change thinking to influence behavior
Role of Leader	Interpret	Keep focus in the present; model authenticity	Organize, direct, teach new skills	Organize, direct, teach new skills
Techniques	Interpret and analyze	Understanding modeling, confronting, clarifying; coaching, role modeling	Learning principles: delineating, reinforcing, extinguishing	Various principles: clarifying, changing or eliminating thoughts, learning schemas that influence behavior

toward other group members, the therapist, and the group as a whole. The immediate events in the meeting take precedence. The second tier involves the group's focus on recognizing and understanding its own process. The group becomes self-reflective in looking at the here-and-now behavior that has just occurred. This two-tiered process is what facilitates learning and generalization as the group becomes a microcosm for the participants' outside lives. It becomes a personal laboratory in which to discover, study, and change one's life experience. In psychotherapy groups, "processing" about the group experience may occur during the meeting, whereby individuals may become reflective and analytical, which allows them to understand, integrate, and generalize their behavior from the group experience to their everyday life. Continual processing about the group does not usually occur as an **activity group** experience, although members may reflect and analyze their experience through the activity of the group or as it pertains to activities generally (Fidler, 1969); moreover, group leaders may—and, in fact, should—analyze and reflect on each group meeting after its completion.

CASE ILLUSTRATION: One Group's Process

Townehouse Creative Living Center was a clubhouse following the model of Fountainhouse in New York. Members who lived in board and care homes and who usually were severely and chronically mentally ill attended five days per week. All members attended groups depending on which work the group carried out. For example, the house and grounds group cleaned houses and apartments, did recycling and car washes, and conducted gardening and landscaping. The nutrition group cooked lunch daily for the members and accepted catering jobs in the community. The clerical group took on work such as stuffing envelopes, compiling and sending out mailings, and making notecards. The transitional employment program (TEP) had volunteer and paid jobs in the community that members could work at for six months at a time to gain work experience. The group also required attendance once per week at a work support group where members discussed any issues or questions that concerned work.

One of the weekly TEP groups had started and Lucius was talking about his new job at the local fast food place as the lot and lobby person. He was excited after his first day, explaining that this was the first time he had worked in 10 years. As he was talking, LaBrea came in late, dressed much fancier than usual and sexier and inappropriate for her role as a member of the day program. She said nothing and sat down. The members did not acknowledge LaBrea but all stared at her and Lucius stopped talking in mid-sentence. After a short silence of about 45 seconds, Thomas began to talk about a date that he hoped he could make when he got paid for his job on Friday. Dante began to talk boastfully about his car and how he had a girlfriend. Enrique began to talk rapidly and incoherently and Keiko then talked about a job she had had years ago making pretty dresses. When Gus, the group leader, asked Lucius if he was finished, Lucius said yes and sat sulkily while LaBrea interrupted to talk about her desire for a job as a hostess in a fast food restaurant.

The content of the group started out as a discussion group where members could share their thoughts and feelings about work. Lucius verbalized his thoughts and feelings about his new job. After LaBrea arrived what was said in the group changed to discussions about dates and jobs a long time ago. The non-verbal content of the group indicated that LaBrea was dressed inappropriately and that after she arrived late, Lucius became silent and sulked, Dante became boastful, Enrique became incoherent, and Keiko talked about work that was not meaningful to the group.

Discussion

Some hypothetical ideas about the process of the group might be:

LaBrea *needed attention and achieved it by her clothes and late entrance to the group. Perhaps she was romantically interested in one of the group members and dressed and arrived late so she would be noticed. Alternatively, she may have wished to have a job as a hostess and believed that if she dressed as she thought a hostess should dress she might somehow get such a job.*

Lucius *was excited about his first job in a long time and was doing the work of the group by telling other members how he thought and felt about it. When interrupted by LaBrea he was hurt or angry but was unable to acknowledge that when given the opportunity by Gus.*

The *other members were influenced by LaBrea's appearance and her late entry. Thomas and Dante made associations to LaBrea's appearance and associated it with dating. Alternatively, perhaps Thomas and Dante became anxious by the interruption and LaBrea's inappropriate appearance and/or the 45-second silence but were unable to keep on track with the purpose of the group. Enrique and Keiko perhaps also became anxious and made loose associations that did not make sense for the group. Alternatively, this may be their current state and the way they participate in the group.*

Group Stages and Patterns

The stages and patterns of a group can be considered as happening over a length of time in different sessions or, with the advent of shorter treatment, within one session. Stages have been described primarily with traditional psychotherapy groups in mind; however, these stages and themes can be recognized in all types of groups, including activity groups. In fact, it appears that activity groups are often nonthreatening, causing stages to occur more rapidly. Although stages are written about as if they were linear, in fact, different stages can overlap. The group process consists of the patterns or stages that groups usually go through; these are characterized by recognizable feelings and behaviors that are usually unspoken or not made explicit (Corey & Corey, 2002). Group stages have been characterized in different ways according to certain themes that arise in each stage (cited in Borg & Bruce, 1991; Cole, 1998). The themes have been described as "forming, storming, norming, and performing"; "inclusion, control, and affection"; "flight, fight, unite, and orientation"; and "conflict, harmony, and maturity." The general themes describe or explain the participants' own thoughts and feelings about the group and the other group members, including the leader. They connote the process of coming together with unknown others and involve an unknown future process: (1) wondering if one will be accepted and liked, (2) deciding on standards for the group, (3) agonizing about the degree to which one wants to be in the group and whether one can follow the norms, (4) a cohesive stage of acceptance of the self and others and investment in using the group for the work that needs to be done, and (5) an ending and consolidation of growth and learning.

Initial. In the initial stage, participants generally learn the norms and expectations, get acquainted, and attempt to determine whether they will be included or excluded. Members will decide whom they can trust and will like, how much they will be involved, and how deeply they wish to disclose. Some tasks of the group member are to begin to behave in a way that will establish trust, learn how to express feelings (especially fears, concerns, and hopes for the group), being involved in the creation of the group norms, and establishing goals for themselves. The leader functions are usually to role-model active participation, develop the rules, assist members to establish a trusting atmosphere and establish goals, and structure the group so that it will have the right balance, discouraging both excessive dependence and excessive floundering. Possible problems involving group members are the failure to participate, an unwillingness to reveal themselves, and the refusal to accept a role of advice giver or problem solver.

Transition. In the transition stage there tend to be more feelings of anxiety on the part of group members. Participants may be concerned about being accepted, how safe the group is, and the leader's competence. They may struggle with ambivalence between choosing risk taking or compliance and, possibly, control or conflict and confrontation. Tasks may include recognizing and expressing negative feelings, learning how to deal with one's own personal resistances, and overcoming conflict with others. The leader functions so as to support the group through the transition so that members will accept and resolve conflict and personal resistances. The leader provides a model of tact and directness, assists members to recognize their personal resistances and interpersonal conflicts, and encourages them to "stay with" expressing reactions that pertain to the here-and-now happenings in the group. Problems may arise if members are categorized as problem types and scapegoated, refuse to express feelings or engage in handling conflicts, or form subgroups to discuss negative reactions outside of the group but not in the presence of the group as a whole.

Working. The working stage is characterized by a high level of trust and cohesion. Members tend to communicate openly in a responsible way, the group shares leadership functions, there is a willingness to take risks, conflict is recognized and handled constructively, and participants generally feel energized to change their behavior outside the group. There is a general tone of high energy and hope. Members function as independent initiators, bringing topics that they are willing to express openly to the group, offering and accepting constructive feedback, and striving to be both more challenging and more supportive of each other. The leader functions as a role model who provides a balance of support and confrontation, interprets the meaning of behavior patterns so that members can engage in a deeper level of self-exploration, explores common themes to link the work of the individual members, and encourages members to practice new skills. Possible problems include members' tendency to challenge each other, the possibility of gaining insufficient insight in the group but to understand the necessity of behavior change on the outside of the group, and the risk of becoming more anxious because of the intensity of group meetings.

Final. In the final stage group members may feel sadness and fear over the group's eventual ending, hopes and concerns for each other may be expressed, members generally ready themselves for dealing with the reality of the world outside the group, and there may be an evaluation of the group experience. Members' tasks are to deal with their feelings regarding separation, offer feedback to others, complete any unfinished business concerning others in the group, discuss changes still to be made and how to make them, and attempt to generalize what they have learned to everyday life. The leader assists the members in dealing with their feelings regarding termination, reinforces changes, and assists members to consolidate what they have learned in the group and understand how it might be applied to everyday life. Possible problems concern members' avoidance of reviewing their experience or putting it into a framework that enables generalization and the danger they may distance themselves from the other group members, thus limiting the possibility of expressing and consolidating feelings. Table 19-2 reviews group properties, norms, stages, and themes.

With the advent of shorter treatment duration, fewer groups will have the luxury of smoothly moving through the various stages to completion. Instead, groups may remain at one stage and fail to progress to the next. However, the various themes that characterize each stage may still become apparent. For example, in a short-term evaluation group, the theme of wanting to be accepted may be expressed by a group member refusing to participate in the assessment or, in a

Table 19-2. Group Properties, Norms, Stages, and Themes

Properties	*Norms*
Background, history, purpose	Confidentiality
Structure	Here-and-now focus
Interaction pattern	Manner of participation
Communication	Activities
Cohesion	Individual respect
Rules and standards	

Stages	*Themes*
Initial	Learning expectations
	Getting acquainted
	Wondering about inclusion/exclusion; disclosure/involvement, trust
Transition	Wondering about acceptance/rejection; safety; leader competency
	Struggle with compliance verses risky behavior
Working	Trust and cohesion
	Responsible communication
	Constructive resolve
	Sharing of responsibility
Final	Evaluation of experience
	Feelings of ending/separation
	Completion of unfinished business
	Continuing change

daily movement group, a member may only participate by watching from the sidelines. A theme of deciding how to be in a group may be expressed by a member attempting to take care of other group members or attempting to assume responsibility like the group leader. Harmony or affection may be achieved in a daily group that runs for a week, yet at the end some members may fail to show up for the last meeting or demean their accomplishments in the group.

The Group Roles

In addition to stages characterized by certain themes, group members may also assume certain roles that can be characterized by the group tasks that they undertake in their roles. Some roles are helpful for accomplishing the group's task while other roles help the group maintain the status quo or keep the group functioning. For example, some participants may take on a helper role, while others may seem to do the work of the group and therefore act in accordance with the purpose or goals of the group. Table 19-3 lists some roles that have been universally identified by many theorists (Cole, 1998).

By recognizing these group roles the therapist can help members take on the roles, particularly in a task group. A successful group can be defined as one in which participants take on a variety of the roles because learning takes place as each participant experiences these roles. Also, a healthy group is usually one in which there is a balance of all of the roles. Often, participants will naturally assume these universal group roles. However, a therapist in a more structured group can explicitly assign the roles to the participants.

CASE ILLUSTRATION: Group Roles

Due to the economy, Townehouse Creative Living Center experienced a reduction in funds from the county that necessitated a cutback in the program. The staff of the clubhouse met and came to the consensus that the best way to deal with the reduction in funds was to eliminate the drop-in program that was held every day for people who did not attend regularly or consistently, but because the program was a clubhouse, members were generally not turned away. The staff presented this option to the clubhouse governing board members who had been elected president, vice-president, secretary, and treasurer. The governing board agreed that eliminating the drop-in program was the best option. They also recognized that some of the drop-in members could form another vocational group based on doing clerical work. Furthermore, they thought that the drop-in members should decide among themselves who should become everyday members and who would be referred elsewhere for services. The staff followed the dictates of the governing board and planned a series of groups facilitated by a staff person for the members to form the clerical section.

At the beginning of the week, the staff facilitator, Song, informed the drop-in group of the cut-back in funds and what had been recommended by both the staff and governing board. She posed a problem for the drop-in members to solve in the next few days of group. The problem was how to decide who would

Table 19-3. Group Roles and Functions

Roles That Further Group Tasks	Function of the Roles
Initiator	Often the first to suggest solutions or ideas and sometimes literally the first person who responds to the leader's suggestions or inquiries.
Elaborator	Usually expands upon suggestions or inquiries but usually does not initiate.
Information or opinion seeker	Asks for clarification of facts or of participants' or the group's attitudes, values, and thoughts.
Information or opinion giver	Offers generalizations or facts automatically without being solicited or offers facts or opinions instead of feelings.
Coordinator	Discusses the relationship of various ideas that may organize the ideas for other participants.
Orienter	Will keep the group on track by defining how the group is keeping to or straying from the goals of the group.
Critic	Critiques the group's accomplishments or functioning as a group.
Energizer	Facilitates some action or decision making by the group.
Operator	Does things for the group following the procedures, such as putting chairs around a table or getting supplies that help move it toward its goal but the things are not necessarily recognized because they are procedural.
Recorder	Writes down suggestions or decisions or what happens in the group.

Roles That Maintain Group Functions	Function of the Roles
Encourager	Praises or generally accepts the contributions of the participants.
Harmonizer	Moderates any differences among group members; usually actions are directed toward "keeping the peace."
Compromiser	Consistently changes own opinion in order to keep group harmony.
Standard setter or follower	Expresses the ideals to which the participants can aspire or goes along with the other group participants.
Group observer or commentator	Observes and comments on the group process.

Source: Adapted from Cole, 1998.

remain as members of a clerical section and who would be asked to seek other ser-
vices. Starting the next day and for the next four days and maybe the next week
she told the members that they were all welcome to join in this decision-making
group. She informed the group that there were two roles that should be assigned
each day, the procedural role and the recorder role, and she explained each role.

Mingus volunteered for the procedural role for the next day's group, and Aki
volunteered for the recorder role for the remainder of the groups. Song thanked
Aki for volunteering but wondered aloud if perhaps other members might like to
share that role. Khalil spoke up and said he would like to function as the recorder,
too. Dorothy agreed with Khalil and further suggested that after tomorrow mem-
bers could volunteer for each role and the group would vote for the volunteers if
there were more than one. Lilly followed up Dorothy's suggestion with a request
that the group vote for either Aki or Khalil to be the recorder today.

After the group voted for Aki for the day's recorder the group sat in silence.
Then Newton began to talk about the coffee he was drinking. Amy offered that
she and Newton had gone to Peete's instead of 7-11 for their coffee in the morn-
ing and that Peete's coffee was much stronger and tasted much better. Khalil
said he would be interested in going to Peete's tomorrow and asked where it was
located. Silvio said that he had been to Peete's but he liked the 7-11 better
because they sold donuts and had larger coffee cups.

After another silence, the leader, Song, wondered aloud if the group would
like to discuss how the group members would be selected for the clerical group.
Khalil suggested that they vote today on who would become the members of the
clerical group. Dorothy suggested that maybe the members had different ideas
and perhaps they should talk about them. Lilly agreed with Dorothy and stat-
ed that she thought the members should each have a chance to state their opin-
ions. Rosetta stated that she, too, wanted to go to Peete's in the morning and
Amy said that she would go with Rosetta. Newton stated that he would meet
them there and Silvio said that he was still going to the 7-11. Etta wondered if
the clubhouse would be having coffee with lunch and the group discussed if they
should have coffee with lunch. The leader, Song, wondered aloud if perhaps the
group was having a hard time keeping to the task because they were afraid of
hurting someone's feelings.

After a silence, Khalil stated that he was afraid of being voted out of the
group. Silvio thought that was not a bad idea and stated that he would vote
Khalil out of the group. Khalil became angry and raised his voice as he stated
that he knew Silvio did not like him since he (Khalil) had started to date
LaBrea, who had been Silvio's girlfriend for a while. As both Silvio and Khalil
started to argue, Newton told both Silvio and Khalil to calm down and the
group members were tired of them arguing. Dorothy suggested that they make
some rules about acceptable and unacceptable group behavior. Lilly agreed and
stated that arguing was not acceptable. Dorothy wondered if group members
should be thrown out if they argued. Newton thought that there should be a rule
against arguing, but that Silvio and Khalil should have another chance. Doro-
thy agreed that maybe they should have another chance, and Lilly suggested

that members vote on that rule. At this point Aki wondered if she should be writing "all of this down."

The leader, Song, observed that the group seemed to have a hard time discussing how to select members of the clerical group, and wondered if Aki should be writing about everything that happened or should be writing down the rules that the group decided on. Khalil apologized for fighting and thought that Aki should be writing everything down. Dorothy wondered what they needed all of the information for, and Lilly thought that they would want all of the information because she would want to know what had happened just in case she missed a group. Dorothy changed her mind and thought that Lilly had a good idea. Newton thought that if they wrote everything down it would also include the rules so why not write everything to make sure that those who only came once or twice knew what happened. The leader, Song, suggested that perhaps what was to be recorded should be voted on by the group and the group proceeded to vote.

After the vote Song noted that it was time to stop and wondered aloud if there were any other comments or business that needed to be done. Khalil thought that they should elect a procedures person for the next day, since the chairs needed to be arranged. Dorothy suggested that the group make their own coffee in the morning and that the procedures person could be the one to make it. Lilly agreed and suggested that they vote. Newton thought that they should ask Mingus if he wanted to make the coffee and Mingus stated that he would make the coffee for the group the next day. The leader, Song, asked if Mingus needed some instructions about making coffee, but he mentioned that he had assumed that role in another group. Mingus asked if he should set up the chairs again tomorrow, and Aki then asked if she was the recorder tomorrow. No one answered but the members looked at the leader, Song.

Song wondered aloud if the group remembered that they had voted to have a person volunteer each day for the recorder. Khalil stated that he did remember voting that a person should volunteer to be the recorder each day if more than one person volunteered. Dorothy seconded Khalil, and thought that they should vote again tomorrow. Lilly wondered if anyone else wanted to be the recorder, but no one else spoke. The leader, Song, suggested that maybe they should complete the task of choosing the recorder in the beginning of tomorrow's group and the group members agreed to do that. Amy, Newton, and Khalil stated that since Mingus was making coffee tomorrow, they would meet at Townehouse and go to Peetes another time.

Discussion

The various participants and the leader assumed different roles during the group. In this session, each of the group's participants functioned primarily in the same role throughout the group, for example, Khalil consistently initiated, Dorothy consistently elaborated, and Lilly consistently energized the group, while Newton became the harmonizer. Some of these members assumed more than one role, for example, Dorothy also became a compromiser. The leader,

Song, assigned two roles to the members throughout the group, and she herself assumed the roles of information seeker, energizer, and group commentator. Song chose her roles strategically to further the group process.

Problems in Groups

In addition to the roles that further the group process or maintain the group's function, theorists have also identified individuals' roles. Often the individual roles become a detriment or interfere with the movement of the group and there is a temptation to label certain people as the source of problems in groups (such as the storyteller, the avoider, the monopolizer) instead of simply labeling their behavior (Cole, 1998; Corey & Corey, 2002). It seems very human to attribute a person's behavior in a particular situation to an enduring character trait. However, this can be a danger in groups (as it is in the practice of psychiatry) due to the tendency to then consistently characterize the person by a single instance of behavior, which in reality may not occur again or may be inconsistent and only happen in certain situations. In particular, a group situation should allow for testing of behavior, and often, participants are unaware that their behavior is considered a problem. With this caveat in mind, we will now review behaviors that may interfere with the normal development of groups if allowed to persist, and that may be addressed by the group leader in fundamental ways.

Although in some instances, problematic behavior may have to do with the participant's thoughts and feelings about the group leader, in general, "problem" behavior is not usually personally directed to the leader. Often, it is mostly unconscious and unintentional. (This is a basic assumption of psychiatry.) Generally, the best procedure to use in handling "problem" behavior is to (1) attempt to understand the meaning of the behavior for that specific time, group, and group members; (2) accept the behavior in a nondefensive way and address it in a manner appropriate to the situation, the functioning of the person, and the level of disruption (disruption either in the behavior itself or to the group); and (3) allow the person to "save face" and avoid power struggles whenever possible.

Nonparticipation. A group member's nonparticipation, silence, or withdrawal is not an overt problem, but it will influence the other group members if it continues and is usually not helpful for the individual participant. Natural silences do occur in individual or group treatment, and often they may define a therapeutic moment or positive transition point. Naturally occurring silence can be distinguished from silence that is more defiant or defensive. The latter, which will be discussed here, is ongoing and noticeable as a behavior pattern, and it is not necessarily spontaneous. It may occur because the individual is not cognitively competent to handle the demands of the group or because symptoms, such as hallucinations, may be a barrier to participation. The individual may fear looking foolish or being rejected, feel unlovable and vulnerable, be paranoid or uncertain about how the group works, or not trust or want to be in the group. The leader should invite participation in the group, direct comments to the person, or make contact in some way, and if possible, he or she should directly explore what makes the person behave in that way. In an activity group, this is less problematic because clients usually will become involved. For example, a task can be adapted (e.g., graded to make the steps more simple) or the individual who does not want to participate can be asked to at least remain with the group. An extreme of non-participation is leaving a group before its completion. Again, the leader should consider whether the client may have been cognitively incompetent or too distracted for that specific group. Contact should be made with nonparticipants to assure their safety and let them know that their presence is valued. If appropriate, the leader should explore the reasons for departure. Sometimes clients are unable to consciously recognize or discuss their behavior. If that is the case, then the leader should either just make contact or provide a choice of reasons that they may agree to or at least think about.

Monopolizing. Monopolizing behavior is at the opposite end of the spectrum, with storytelling, questioning, advice giving, and intellectualizing somewhere in between. A person's symptoms, such as symptoms of mania, may interrupt the group or the individual may be driven by the same fears and concerns that lead to unnatural silences. Monopolistic behavior can be more problematic than silence because it demands to be addressed and will eventually cause the other members to resent the person. If the behavior is part of a person's symptoms, the leader should continually address it by interrupting the person and redirecting him or her. The behavior can be confronted by gently describing the situation, stating, for example, "I don't know if you realize that you are taking up all the group's time. Your thoughts and feelings are important, but I think other group members would also like to participate." Alternately, the leader may attempt to deepen the person's self-understanding, as appropriate to the person and the situation, by saying, for example, "You seem to want a lot of attention, but I sense that the way you are asking for it is turning people off, which is not really what you want."

Hostility. Hostile behavior can be direct or indirect. Indirect hostility may come subtly in the form of sarcasm, jokes, seeming bored and detached, or arriving late. The individual may fear looking foolish, fear rejection, feel unlovable, be uncertain about how the group works, or not trust or want to be in the group. The person may be expressing himself or herself in a learned manner and may not recognize that this is distancing. The person may be disappointed and hurt, or he or she may be feeling angry and expressing it in an indirect way. A special case occurs often with activity groups and occupational therapists, whereby clients will denigrate an activity—or the occupational therapist who suggests it—as being too simple, childish, or totally unrelated to treatment or change. For some people, this may mean that the activity is too challenging and, perhaps, cognitively overwhelming. In that case, acknowledging the right to decline participation or changing the activity may take care of the situation. If the level of difficulty is not the apparent problem, gentle confrontation may be enough to change the behavior, such as by saying, "You seem upset today—is that so?" or "I don't know if you realize that your comment sounds somewhat angry—is that how you are feeling?" In the case of denigration of the activity, there may be different ways to approach the situation. A serious explanation of the rationale for the activity and how it may be helpful to the person will often defuse the situation. Alternately, an acceptance of the person's feelings and explanation that although the activity may appear overly simple it has additional benefits may defuse the hostility. Sometimes an exploration of how the person felt when engaged in the activity helps to shift or reframe the situation. In all instances of problem behavior, the leader's response will depend on the situation, the person's level of functioning, and the leader's understanding of the behavior's meaning.

CASE ILLUSTRATION: Handling Problem Behaviors in a Group

In a life skills group for young adults that met daily, participants at times discussed how to use cognitive techniques to quiet their minds and avoid distractions when asked to do group projects together with other students in their classes. They acknowledged that their anxiety, as demonstrated by obsessive and negative thoughts about themselves as individuals, often prevented them from even starting the projects. They were then labeled "lazy," ostracized from the class, and more than likely denied a grade indicative of their knowledge. After the first week of the group, Maria, the OTR, was feeling increasingly uneasy about the sessions. For the most part, the group was functioning, but two members often interfered with the process. The first, John, declined to comment when asked to share some pertinent cognitive problem or solution and often physically separated himself from the others. Most of his comments were aimed at interpreting other people's problems or offering solutions for others in the group. Another member, Louise, participated in group exercises and made comments but also often directed comments with subtle sexual innuendos to the therapist.

After careful consideration in supervision of each member's difficulties and circumstances, Maria decided to handle the two individuals in two different ways. Knowing John and observing him in other groups, she believed that he felt less intelligent than the others and feared they would find this out if he acknowledged his perceived shortcomings. Maria raised this fear as a group issue, not mentioning John but rather questioning whether others worried about rejection and acknowledging how difficult it is to reveal perceived weaknesses that have seemed hopelessly intractable. The group members, including John, were able to discuss their fears of seeming inadequate and thus to identify with, and support, each other.

Knowing Louise, the leader judged her comments to reveal a more personal issue—that Louise either liked the group leader and was expressing it in this indirect, almost unconscious, way or, perhaps, was expressing a fear about the leader's competency. She decided to discuss this with Louise personally and inquire whether Louise was aware of the nature of her comments. In fact, Louise was surprised and embarrassed to realize that she had made such comments; however, she also acknowledged her affection for Maria, who represented a healthy, strong model that Louise wished to emulate.

Discussion

Each instance of "problem behavior" meant something different for the individual participant and the group and was, therefore, handled differently. In each case, however, the therapist's reaction was congruent with her assessment of the group process, the meaning of the comment, and each person's individual process.

In addition to considering the individual's behavior as a personal problem, it is useful to consider whether one's own leadership style and manner of interacting or the group structure or content may be contributing (Howe & Schwartzberg, 2001). For example, is the activity matched with the person's ability? Is the person able to meet the demands of the group? Is the reason for the activity clear? Has the leader successfully created norms of safety and trust and interacted in a respectful and genuine manner? Has the leader assumed too much responsibility for the process of the group? Perhaps neither the leader, the interaction, nor the person is a cause of problem behavior and instead, some outside influence has affected the group or its members. For example, was there an incident on an inpatient unit, such as a suicide attempt or theft, or was the person just notified of a workplace review by his boss or social security audit? Perhaps visitors have just left. Indeed, there are many potential outside influences.

The Group Leader

The role of the group leader may change somewhat according to the type of group, but there are also general leadership aspects that define the role, communication skills that can be utilized in the role, and general **personhood skills** (which translate into leadership skills) (Corey & Corey, 2002). Every group has properties and norms and goes through stages characterized by certain themes. Table 19-4 lists ideal roles, communication skills, and personhood traits of group leaders.

Roles and style of leadership.   Overall, the leader is the organizer of the group. He or she initiates action and interaction, directs the activities of the group, and establishes an atmosphere of trust and openness. The leader can be thought of as the "holder" of the group by virtue of his or her development, implementation, and overall investment (Yalom, 1995). Group leaders must remain aware that ongoing careful attention to the structure and content of the group through their interactions and directions continually establishes its tone and influences its success and the degree of member participation.

By establishing the norms and boundaries of a group through organization and attention, a group leader can assist members in feeling comfortable and motivated to participate. The group leader should strive to establish an "ambiance of safety." More specific aspects of the leader's role are:

- Demonstrating by example
- Setting rules and limits, such as confidentiality, not interacting in subsets, not interrupting
- Providing orientation
- Being tuned in to the mood of the group

Table 19-4. The Group Leader

Roles

Organizer	Sets and maintains norms, boundaries, and rules Establishes a tone, or ambiance, of safety and participation
Role Model	Demonstrates by example Provides orientation
Facilitator	Determines and directs or enables the group activity and participant interactions

Communication Skills

Active Listening	Absorbing the content, noting a person's gestures and changes in expression, sensing underlying messages (what a person is not saying) while simultaneously remaining fully present and concentrated in the moment for each interaction
Reflecting	Communicating back to a person the essence of what she or he has communicated to you
Clarifying	Recounting what a person has communicated
Blocking	Prohibiting, either directly or by your interpretation, types of communication that are destructive to the group process or members. Examples of destructive communication are gossiping, breaking another's confidence, and invading another's privacy
Facilitating	Inviting others to participate, that is, to express thoughts or feelings or to work on the activity of the group; to work or interact with other members or to make comments concerning other members' statements or products
Empathizing	Providing a response to indicate you understand a person and what he or she has wished to communicate; that you can "put yourself in another person's shoes"

Personhood Skills

Courage	The ability to admit mistakes, express fears, or act on hunches; to be direct and honest with members; to be genuine and not defensive in the face of criticism; to do what the leader expects others to do in that group situation
Willingness	To model or exhibit behaviors that one expects of group members
Being Present	Fully experiencing the group's activity or interactions and not being distracted from the purpose of the group
Belief in the Group	Believing in the value of what is being done or is happening in the group
Ability to Cope Nondefensively	Not personalizing, retaliating, or withdrawing from comments or actions that you perceive as critical of you or your performance
Self-Awareness	Awareness of personal goals, identity, motivations, needs, strengths and limitations, values and feelings
Sense of Humor	The ability to laugh at yourself and to see and understand the frailty of the human condition
Inventiveness	The capacity to be spontaneous and creative, often combined with the ability to learn from every experience in life

Source: Adapted Corey & Corey, 2002.

Basically, as group leader, you are a role model. Through your behavior and attitude, you model the norms you would like to create in the group (Corey & Corey, 2002; Howe & Schwartzberg, 2001; Kaplan, 1988). *This is true for all groups* whether the members only work in the presence of others or interact with each other, the content is activity-based or psychodynamic, and the structure is verbal or nonverbal. This is true even though you may perceive your role as being simply an organizer or resource guide.

Your natural style of leadership may be broadly considered as active and directive in your involvement or as more facilitative and supportive. As a directive leader, you actively control or direct the group, usually choose the activity and direct the process, and actively direct interactions to motivate clients. A facilitative leader will remain more in the background, perhaps supporting the members as they make their own decisions and interact among themselves. Often the structure of a group may dictate the leadership style; for example, the leader may be introducing a new or novel activity, the group members cognitively may require direction, or the goal of the group may be to increase motivation or interpersonal skills. In these cases, a directive and active leadership style is required. Another example is a group whose goal is to determine community resources that support finding a job. In this task, members should be more independent and can benefit from interacting with, and supporting, each other, skills that will be required in a job. In this case, the leadership style must necessarily be facilitative. See the group roles case illustration for an example of a facilitative group leadership style and notice that the leader, Song, assumes the roles of organizer and role model. Notice the communication skills that Song uses in the group, and imagine the personhood skills that she must possess to be an astute and successful group leader.

Communication Skills.   There are many communication skills that can be learned and become part of a group leader's repertoire of skills. Although there are many skills, some of the most important are active listening, reflecting, clarifying, blocking, facilitating, and empathizing. (These skills are explained more fully in Table 19-4.)

Personhood Skills.   Other skills sometimes are more difficult to explain or acquire because they often have to do with an individual's personality, or personal traits, temperament, and experience. These can be called personality traits, but the term *personhood skills* (Corey & Corey, 2002) better conveys that these are particular traits that positively influence how one person relates to another. In occupational therapy the concept that comes closest to "personhood skills" is therapeutic use of self, defined in the Occupational Therapy Practice Framework (2002) as "planned use of . . . personality, insights, perceptions, and judgments as part of the therapeutic process" (p. 628). (See Chapter 18 for further discussion of these ideas.) Therapeutic use of self or personhood skills can sometimes be learned by observing the behavior of someone who has the traits and noting how he or she practices the skills in everyday life. (The personhood skills are listed and explained in Table 19-4.)

OCCUPATIONAL THERAPY GROUPS

Occupational therapy groups have much in common with groups based on other models. Often they borrow techniques, such as assertiveness training or role playing, that originated according to other psychological models. Such a blending of methods and techniques is not uncommon in the field of mental health. However, occupational therapy groups tend to be unique in two ways. They are unique in their *focus on the activity*, which is the aspect that produces change. They are also unique in their *emphasis on occupations*, which involves changing areas of occupation and performance skills and patterns. This broad purpose can be incorporated in any occupational therapy model. Although people often erroneously assume that every group's purpose is interaction, broad categories of activity groups show that the purpose of occupational therapy groups extends far beyond simply social interaction.

Definitions of Groups in Occupational Therapy

Activity.   Activity groups have been defined in different ways in occupational therapy. A variety of activity groups are defined and practiced by occupational therapists and modeled after occupational therapy frames of reference, but no consensus has yet been reached on an inclusive, unique definition of the type of activity group employed exclusively by occupational therapists. Groups have been developed according to occupational therapy models (Kaplan, 1988; King, 1974); they generally follow the principles of other systems, especially the psychoanalytic and developmental approaches (Borg & Bruce, 1991; Fidler, 1969; Mosey, 1970; 1981), and they may delineate a specific structure (Cole, 1998; Howe & Schwartzberg, 2001; Kaplan, 1988). What they all have in common is that the content focuses on activity, emphasizes occupation, and addresses areas of occupation performance skills and patterns to aid in adaptation, improve or enhance occupational performance and quality of life, promote role competence, client satisfaction, health and wellness, or prevent unhealthy lifestyles. All groups also share a common structure, which deemphasizes reflecting on the group process throughout the duration of the whole group.

Activity groups have been considered to have the properties of both psychotherapy groups and task groups (Borg & Bruce, 1991; Denton, 1987). A psychotherapy group usually emphasizes group process with a goal of resolving inter- or intrapersonal issues, whereas a task group usually emphasizes an outcome or product, which can be tangible, such as an art project, or intangible, such as a decision or recommendation and the goal of the task group is to accomplish a group task. An activity group falls somewhere in between the two types of groups. It may emphasize a group goal, yet the interaction concerning the group goal may be considered as important as the goal. Alternately, the interaction may occur through a medium of activity.

Activity groups have been defined (Howe & Schwartzberg, 2001) as those in which members are engaged in a common task directed toward occupational performance. The group focuses on function and replicates living in the community or family. The activity focuses the group's attention, and the group members learn from direct experience. The task provides form and organization and serves the needs of members in different ways, including utilizing purposeful activity in developing skills. A functional group has been proposed based on adaptation and occupation. According to this approach, groups enhance the use of occupations to help people adapt to the environment or vice versa, and groups utilize purposeful activities and active involvement (doing) so that members can maintain or develop skills in areas of occupation.

The goal of the activity group is to enable change in the areas of occupation, whether activities of daily living, instrumental activities of daily living, work, play, or education; in performance skills, whether motor, process, or communication and interaction; and performance habits, whether focusing on habits, routines, or roles. Groups in mental health settings may also focus on various contexts, whether cultural, physical, social, personal, spiritual, or virtual. Cole (1998) suggested a seven-step format for activity groups, involving introduction, the activity, sharing one's own product or experience, processing or reflecting and making sense of the experience, generalizing or summing up the responses to the activity, applying what was learned to everyday life, and summarizing the group experience. The steps can be adapted to maximize learning for any population according to the purpose of the group and the overall level of functioning of the group members.

Task. In the classic task-oriented group (Fidler, 1969), a task was defined as either an end product or a service, though task accomplishment was not the purpose of the group. Instead, the task provided a shared experience whereby the participants could reflect on the relationship between behavior, thinking, and feeling and explore their impact on others. What is demonstrated in the process of participating in the task and encountering problems in doing or interacting can be observed and thus become the focus of group problem solving and trying out alternative patterns. In this way the group becomes engaged in processing behavior and then trying out more adaptive modes.

Developmental. Group interaction skills have been described as a developmental sequence necessary for adaptation (Mosey, 1970; 1981; 1986). Five types of groups, from least to most developed, are (1) parallel, where tasks are done side-by-side and interaction is not required; (2) project, emphasizing task accomplishment and some interaction; (3) egocentric-cooperative, requiring more interaction and responsibility; (4) cooperative, requiring much interaction and taking care of others' needs; and (5) mature groups where the members take on all necessary leadership roles to facilitate task accomplishment and caring for others' needs. In the hierarchy, initially task accomplishment is emphasized while interaction and meeting each other's needs are deemphasized. At each successive level, interaction becomes more important and the role of the therapist or leader becomes less primary. At the highest level, task accomplishment is emphasized equally with meeting the needs of other group members.

Directive. The directive group (Kaplan, 1986; 1988)—and also the focus group (Yalom, 1983), which was modeled on the directive group—meets the needs of the most severely and acutely mentally ill and most minimally functioning patients, representing a wide range of diagnoses, ages, and problems. The environment is actively structured in form, organization, and leadership to assure maximum participation. The directive group format is a consistent one involving orientation, introduction, a warm-up, selected activities, and a wrap-up, while the focus group format is orientation, warm-up, structured exercises, and review. The formats enable group goals of participation, interaction, attention, and initiation; within this broad range, goals can be individualized.

Neurodevelopmental. Neurodevelopmental groups (King, 1974; Levy, 1974; and Ross, 1987, cited in Cole, 1998) utilize movement activities often based on sensory integration theory and techniques. The movements are usually imitative, gross motor movements and involve tactile, kinesthetic, and proprioceptive input. The groups are designed for persons with chronic schizophrenia who have been in the mental health system for a long time.

Other. Although activity groups' goals are to enable change in areas of occupation, performance skills, or habits with respect to different contexts, the content of some groups may also be described by areas of occupation, performance skills, or habits with respect to different contexts. For example, some groups may be described as an activity of daily living group, a communication group, a habit-change group, or a cultural or computer group. In these cases the activity makes up some of the content of the group and the goals of the group are really explained by the activity.

There are also other types of groups that are explained by their content and activity, but are not specific to occupational therapy, but may forward goals of occupational therapy that were mentioned previously. For example, a thematic group (Mosey, 1981; cited in Denton, 1987) is organized around a topic or theme. The aim is to help the participants change or examine attitudes or acquire knowledge and skills in certain areas. Examples of thematic group titles are "Grieving and Loss," "What Do You Say after You Say Hello?" "On Depression," "On Anger," "On Guilt," and "Recognizing Feelings."

An expressive/projective group (Denton, 1987) uses creative media to facilitate the recognition, acknowledgment, or expression of feelings and ideas. Examples of expressive groups are art or craft groups, play groups, and recreation or sport activity groups.

A sensory group is one in which the activity increases the awareness of bodily sensations and responses or facilitates bodily relaxation. Examples include training in progressive relaxation, shiatsu, yoga, karate, or other Eastern forms of movement.

The **psychoeducational** group has a clear objective: to teach specific information or techniques to clients and their families, thus supporting clients and their families' well-being (Ruiz-Sancho, Ivanoff, & Linehan, 2001). It is typically time limited and utilizes cognitive-behavioral and social learning theory (Alonso & Swiller, 1993). For example, a group for people with eating disorders may provide facts on nutrition and the social correlates and medical consequences of eating disorders and the group may be open to those who have eating disorders and to their families or significant others. Due to the shorter duration of mental health treatment and the dictates of managed care, many professionals utilize the techniques of psychoeducation.

In all these categories, the structure of the group, pattern of interaction, leader's role and methods, and techniques utilized in the group are dictated by the group developer or implementer. In one sensory group the leader may demonstrate how to stretch and have the participants practice the technique. The only verbalization may be the leader's. In another sensory group, participants may share knowledge and demonstrate their own relaxation techniques. The leader's role may be simply as facilitator or the sessions may contain both elements.

In one expressive group participants may simply sit silently together in a room, working on their own, individual crafts. The role of the leader will be to help each person initiate and follow through. Alternately, in another expressive group participants may draw themselves in a certain setting and then discuss the emotions and thoughts that the drawing evoked. In this case, the role of the group leader is more active, that is, to help members interact with each other or make connections between their drawings and their thoughts and feelings.

In a thematic group, the group leader may provide education about a topic, such as, "How Thoughts Get in Our Way." Then participants might individually write down negative things they say to themselves and when they do so. Participants may then engage in an interactive discussion facilitated by the leader.

An *ADL* group in an acute psychiatric unit may consist of learning skills for showering, personal hygiene, and grooming. The group leader may provide supplies and demonstrate the skills, while the group participants will practice skills for themselves or will help others when appropriate.

An *IADL* group on community outreach may consist of the group participants deciding who or what institution they would like to visit, discussing transportation and setting time schedules, and deciding who will use the phone book and phone to make the necessary arrangements. The group leader may facilitate by making resources available or giving advice when asked.

A *vocational* group may involve working on a clerical task on an assembly line. The role of the leader will be to set up the project, decide who will perform which roles, and monitor the work and the end products. Participants may interact and help each other or they may work only on their task.

An *education* group may include a group of residents of a board and care home identifying topics that they might be interested in and how they might obtain the information. The group together reads through adult-education brochures and pamphlets, and visits the local library and community college. The group leader obtains the pamphlets, helps the clients decide what questions they might ask, finds out from the clients if they can take public transportation or may need a van, and accompanies the clients to the institutions.

A *leisure* group in the day treatment program decides that they would like to meet other singles. They decide that they will have a dance. The group leader helps them to explore community facilities to find a low-fee rental hall. They plan the dance, including who can be invited, how they will advertise, how they will assure safety, and what food they can have. They decide to sponsor a monthly dance.

A house and grounds section of a clubhouse spends a week learning *how to organize space and objects* for cleaning vacant apartments. The group leader is directive, bringing in tools, explaining processes, and inviting apartment managers to talk about their needs.

In preparation to attend the monthly dances, the *communication* group learns the ways people communicate with their bodies. They practice asking someone to dance and "making small talk," the rules of personal space, how to maintain gaze, and how to assume a posture that indicates warmth, openness, and interest. The group leader assigns role-plays and helps the group members to evaluate the role-plays and analyze the group process.

A 12-step group for addictive behaviors meets weekly to discuss useful *habits* that members would like to cultivate and dominating habits that they would like to eliminate. The group leader functions as a consultant, advising the group when they have questions.

A combined *spiritual/physical contexts* group of retired older people from the same community who call themselves "the transcendentalists" meet twice weekly. At the beginning of the week they discuss a physical environment, often a natural one such as the mountains or the oceans, but sometimes a man-made environment, such as a historical monument, that they wish to explore. Once they determine the environment, they plan how they will explore it. During the second meeting they explore the environment, discussing how the place affects their well-being, and general sense of efficacy and comparing the places that they have visited. The group leader functions as a consultant, advising the group when they have questions or discussing the power of environments to influence people.

Starting a Group

There are basic steps involved in starting a group (Rerek, 1966). At each step there are questions to ask to clarify your thinking and make the group development a smooth process. If you know the steps and questions, you will know how to think about groups, and consequently, you will be able to develop and utilize groups in any setting and with any population. You will be able to work alone as a group leader, effectively and successfully, to provide meaningful treatment. Table 19-5 reviews the steps to starting a group.

The first step is to survey the client population. The questions to ask yourself are, "Who are the clients and what are their needs?" An inpatient acute setting where people of all ages stay for three days to be stabilized on medication will dictate a group setting that addresses here-and-now functioning or cognitive reorganization. An outpatient setting that provides service primarily to women who may be depressed would dictate a group for women that provides opportunities for success and mastery and addresses longer-term occupational areas or daily functioning. A setting in which intense, **psychodynamic** work is the daily focus would dictate a group that provides relaxation/restoration or recreation.

Table 19-5.   Starting a Group: Tasks and Critical Questions

Therapist Task	Critical Questions
1. Survey of client population	Who are they? What are their needs?
2. Setting	Short- or long-term? Inpatient or outpatient? Specific disorder or special services? Roles for other health professionals? Your job description?
3. Purpose	Why is this group necessary? What do you and the participants want to accomplish? What are the types of outcomes that are expected?
4. Selection criteria	How will you select participants? Who will and will not benefit? Why? Are evaluation and screening based on issues, problems, diagnosis, cognitive level, interests, gender, age?
5. Specific activities	Concrete or abstract? Simple or complex? Short or long duration? Based on a model? Easy to transport?
6. Your skills and knowledge	Are your skills adequate? Is a consultant, supervisor, or mentor available? Are you interested in this group? Is it a good fit for you?
7. Structure and logistics	Minimum and maximum allowable participants? Voluntary or required? Open or closed? When? How often? How long? Where? One or more leaders?
8. Outcome measure	How will you determine success, whether goals and purpose are being achieved?

Source: Adapted from Rerek, 1966.

The second step is to consider the constraints of your setting. Is your setting a short-term, acute unit where people who function differently are treated together? Is it a long-term setting where people live in the community and attend four days a week? Does the setting provide treatment for a specific disorder, such as addiction, or does it provide special treatment, such as vocational services? Does the setting include many other health professionals, such as psychologists, nutritionists, social workers, recreational therapists, or movement therapists, with specific roles? Are you the only health professional with a more generalized role? Is your job description specific or are you allowed some freedom?

An important step is to establish the purpose of the group. What do you want to accomplish? What do you want the participants to accomplish? What do the participants wish to accomplish? Why is this group necessary? These questions often translate into group goals. In some groups the purpose is not to change one's life forever but rather to increase one's recognition of the internal resources needed for a transition from the structured setting or a return home. Some groups may allow people to be creative and explore the meaning of their lives, while others may help people reorganize their thinking and decrease confusion. Another type of group may be designed to improve members' personal appearance and therefore will address grooming and self-care. The purpose of a group in a day treatment setting may be to provide a sense of belonging to a community, whereas the same group in an acute care center may be intended to provide a sense of community safety and comfort.

Another step is to consider selection criteria. How will you select participants? Who will benefit from this group and who might not? Some groups will evaluate and screen participants, while others will be open to anyone who wishes to attend. Some groups may require an ability to think abstractly and will therefore screen out individuals who are actively psychotic. Some may address retirement issues and therefore will not benefit adolescents.

A step that is often dictated by the purpose and goals of the group and the nature of its membership is the consideration of what activities to use. What will be the specific activities featured? Will they be tangible or abstract? Will they be short- or long-term? Will they vary? Will they be easy to use and transport? Stress management groups may use meditation, movement, and music or writing; activities of daily living groups may use discussion and demonstration; and craft groups may use specific modalities, such as clay, jewelry, or leather. Some groups may be nonverbal, while others may involve a great deal of talking.

A step that has been implied in discussing group development and implementation is for the leader to consider his or her skills and knowledge. Are your skills and knowledge adequate for this group? Is there someone who can consult or mentor you? Are you excited about this group? Is it a good fit for you (does it match your personality and strengths)? Although it is important to be aware of the members' needs, which should be paramount, some of the best groups are those that interest their leaders. In fact, if you are not excited or interested in some way by a group, you should not lead it.

The structural details of the group should be well thought out. How large will the group be? Will it be voluntary, or is it required in the program? Will it be open (that is, members may enter and leave at any time) or closed (that is, membership remains stable for a time period)? For how long should the group meet? When and how often will it meet? Where will it meet? Will it be led by the same person or persons? Who has primary responsibility for the group? How will participants be kept informed? Often, such structural details about the group are written down in a group protocol.

A final consideration is to determine a measure of effectiveness for the group. How will you determine if this group is successful and achieves its purpose and goals? Often therapists develop and implement groups and informally assess success, usually as based on attendance or comments of the group members. If at all possible, however, a more formal evaluation of the group's success—an outcome measure—should be established. This is not a requisite in most institutions and in many fields. However, outcome measures document the usefulness and utility of your group and the profession. An ongoing formal evaluation also gives feedback about what does and does not work. It guides the therapist in providing the most useful treatment.

Formal evaluation does not have to be complicated, perplexing, or time-consuming. It could simply involve consistently taking attendance and comparing it with your institution's census to learn the percentage of patients who attend. It could involve a questionnaire about the group to be filled out by the members at various times after their attendance. It could involve questions posed before, during, and after the group experience. It could mean posing the same questions about the group after trying out different activities or techniques. A professional who engages in research (your occupational therapy professor or consultant or a psychologist on staff) will usually assist you.

The Group Protocol

The group content and structure are often written in a protocol. Protocols vary in form but usually include similar content. They often include the group's name, purpose, goals, content or methods, structure and logistics, method of entry, requirements, and referral criteria. They also generally cover who would and would not benefit, contraindications for membership, and name of the group leader. They often also include a short description or narrative about the group. Two examples of protocols are presented in Table 19-6. Protocols can be more extensive (Borg & Bruce, 1991; Cole, 1998; Howe & Schwartzberg, 2001) and include a more detailed description of the client population, a rationale, a frame of reference, an outline of treatment sessions, and a listing of outcome criteria.

Writing a group protocol is a way of organizing your thinking about a group. In a narrow sense, it is an aid for yourself, while in a broader sense, it is an aid for others with whom you work. It provides them with a brief, useful description of the group and helps them in referring people to your group and knowing what type of treatment clients are receiving. In these different ways, the group protocol contributes to the functioning of the organization for which you work, in that it also aids the institution to describe its services to prospective clients. Sometimes, the group protocol serves to demystify psychological treatment.

You may also share your protocols with your clients or members of the group, particularly on entry, as a way of explaining the group. Providing this information can relieve the fears and satisfy the curiosity of new members. Often it favorably disposes the new member to the group and aids in the rapid cohesion and integration. Group members may share protocols with their families, often giving relief to worried or curious family members and providing a basis of discussion regarding the client's difficulties and experiences, or prompting family members to join the psychoeducation groups offered for clients and families.

Documentation and Outcome

It is becoming increasingly important to document outcomes, and group outcomes can indeed be documented. In addition to suggesting group goals or activities, the Occupational Therapy Practice Framework (2002) defines types of outcomes that can measure group success, such as improvement or enhancement in occupational

Table 19-6. Group Protocols

Occupational Therapy MAC Group: Mastery and Accomplishment through Crafts

Purpose: Provide opportunities for participants to master concrete activities in a parallel group setting that is not threatening or demanding.

Goals: Long-term—Increase sense of effectiveness as demonstrated by participant self-report.

Short-term—Improve concentration and attention span and ability to plan sequentially, as demonstrated by daily assessment.

Group Content: Concrete activities (craft).

Group Structure: Therapist will present participants with crafts. Often all will be working on the same type of craft though each will have his or her own project. Crafts will be structured and graded according to Allen's Cognitive Levels (see attached). Therapist will prepare projects and client decision making will be minimal. Interaction will not be required or encouraged, although it often occurs.

Logistics:

Place:	CCB 209
Number of Patients:	Maximum of 8
Meeting Schedule:	Daily, Mondy–Friday, 9:00–10:00 A.M.
Group Facilitator:	James Lopez, OTR

Occupational Therapy—Life Skills

Who: • Those who identify areas of daily life that are problematic or that they would like to change.

• Those who use few coping mechanisms or one for all situations

Goal: • Provide opportunities to learn a range of coping mechanisms or ways of adapting

• Provide opportunities to practice old skills of managing in new ways that are more satisfying

• Provide opportunities to clarify values and ways of being in the world, ultimately expanding choices.

Method: Occupational therapist will provide a theme or topic for each session that occurs twice a week from 7 to 9 in Room A of the community center, and will provide specific experiential exercises for the group to follow.

Contraindications: Those who are presently or those who have difficulty thinking abstractly, or are easily distracted, for example, those with psychotic or hypermanic symptoms.

Group Leader: Ahmad Wallace, OTR

---

performance, client satisfaction, or quality of life, role competence, adaptation, health and wellness, prevention, or promoting healthy lifestyles. A simple measurement of outcomes is self-report (Howe & Schwartzberg, 2001), whereby members are asked to evaluate a group either at the end of each session or at the end of a series of meetings. The form can be structured, providing forced choices such as "always," "sometimes," "rarely," or "never," or it can be unstructured, perhaps asking participants open-ended questions regarding their experiences.

Members can be asked to monitor their progress by filling out a behavioral assessment regarding their own behavior in the group. A behavioral observation form (Kaplan, 1988) can also be filled out by the group leaders. Assessment and observation should always tie in to the goals and the purpose of the group as a whole and the individuals in the group. This implies that an initial assessment has been performed to ascertain baseline functioning and that assumptions regarding the group and the frame of reference in which it is grounded will be explicit.

An ideal method of evaluating a group or the individual participants is goal attainment scaling (Ottenbacher & Cusick, 1990). This method employs operational goals and outcomes and explicit time sequences that are determined by the therapist, individuals, and others involved in treatment. It also includes a quantitative measurement of treatment effectiveness. It can be used both for the evaluation of group efficacy and for the evaluation of treatment efficacy for group members.

Documentation may cover the group process and content or discuss each individual in the group. It is generally written in the form of a narrative note; a more structured, problem-oriented or behavioral outcome format; or a list (Acquaviva, 1992; Borg & Bruce, 1991; Denton, 1987; Kaplan, 1988). Generally, a note regarding the group will contain a description of the activity and clients in attendance and a summary of the group experience, or what has occurred. This includes what has been accomplished, any changes since the previous group session, and any unusual occurrences. It may restate the purpose and goals of the group and whether the goals were accomplished. It may include the plan for the subsequent group meeting. A note regarding each individual in the group generally will include descriptions of the person's behavior in the group, how the person interacted and responded to interaction, how the individual participated in the activity, and changes in performance from previous group sessions. Goals may be reiterated, or the plan for an individual in the next group meeting may be stated. As with the group narrative, a baseline assessment and explicit grounding in a frame of reference are required.

CASE ILLUSTRATION: Developing a Group, Protocol, and Plan

Janice Nyugen is an OTR in a large psychiatric hospital that treats people of all ages and diagnoses. One of her roles is as evaluator of incoming clients. After six months of evaluating six to eight clients per week, she noticed that 70 percent had a diagnosis of depression. Of this group, 90 percent were female, 60 percent were between the ages of 25 and 40, and about 15 percent had accompanying problems, such as eating disorders or addictions, for which they were attending other groups or self-help programs based on the 12 steps of Alcoholics Anonymous.

At the hospital, no groups specifically targeted people with the diagnosis of depression. Janice had been interested in this topic in school and so welcomed the opportunity to learn more. She read about depression and spoke with her supervisor about her ideas for a group. She attended case consultations and interviews and spoke with her colleagues concerning how a group for people who were depressed might fit into the program. She attended communication workshops to supplement what she learned in her occupational therapy classes and observed other people whose traits and skills of group leadership she admired. She then developed a group protocol and an explanation of the group that she had designed. Table 19-7 shows the protocol she wrote for the group. Table 19-8 delineates the group leadership, activity, process, and desired outcomes of the group.

Discussion

Janice demonstrated the correct way to go about developing a group; that is, she noticed a need and a population that were not served in her organization, she sought consultation and more knowledge, she observed other leaders' styles, she developed a logical group plan and description, and she determined how she would measure types of outcomes the group sought.

Table 19-7. Protocol for a Group Dealing with Depression

Name: Making Friends with Your Demons: Dealing with Depression

Purpose: Increase opportunities for mastery and success, improve participants' strategies and tools to cope with depression, and educate participants regarding the warning signs of depression.

Goals: Given participation in the group daily for two weeks, the participants will be able to accomplish two concrete activities successfully, report improved mood as measured by the Beck Depression Inventory, state three strategies for coping with depressed mood, and state three warning signs of impending depressed mood.

Group Content: The group will include simple craft activities that can be worked on independently and finished successfully in one session, identification of thoughts and feelings relating to depressed moods, and identification of coping strategies and signs of impending depressed mood through written exercises, exploration, and discussions.

Group Structure: The leader will provide opportunities for engagement with concrete activities and assist members to complete them. The leader will actively direct written exercises and discussion and provide education regarding coping strategies and recognizing signs of impending depression. The sequence of the group is such that initially there will be little demand on the participants as they successfully complete activities, and then gradually demands will increase as exploration and discussion are introduced. However, participants do not have to initiate in this group, and interaction is initially mostly between the leader and individuals, gradually giving way to group discussion with other members, facilitated by the leader.

Who Would Benefit: This group would primarily benefit women between the ages of 25 and 40 with depressed mood who also are dealing with issues of addiction. They must be able to think abstractly and should demonstrate some capacity for self-reflection.

Who Would Not Benefit: Those who are unable to think abstractly or have psychotic thinking; those who are unable to attend to a group for at least one hour or concentrate on abstract concepts; those who are presently in a manic state.

Logistics: Monday–Friday, 9–10 A.M., 2/1–2/12.
The Rose Room, #200
Group Leader: Janice Nyugen, OTR

Table 19-8. Making Friends with Your Demons: Dealing with Depression (Two-Week Process)

Day	Group Leadership	Group Activity	Group Process	Desired Outcome/Rationale
1	Explains the group to the participants, giving them the group protocol and discussing it. Gives them self-report questionnaires to fill out concerning improvements that they seek in occupational performance, satisfaction, occupational roles, customary ways of adapting to daily situations, self-assessment of their current state of physical and mental health, and current quality of life. Solicits questions and concerns.	Reading and discussing thoughts and feelings regarding the group protocol; stating desired personal outcomes. Filling out the Beck Depression Inventory, a list of strategies each individual uses to cope with depression, and a list of behavioral and cognitive warning signs of impending depression.	The leader introduces herself or himself and members introduce themselves to each other. Most interaction is between the leader and the members.	Introduction to each other. Developing rapport with leader and members. Beginning comfort among members. Completion of evaluative measures.
2–4	Provides categories of craft activities: ceramics, jewelry, or leather. Assists members in their projects.	Craft projects.	Members work independently and individually on their chosen craft projects, with assistance from the leader when necessary. They speak casually with each other, though this is not required. They display their finished projects on the last day.	Developing rapport and comfort in the group and with each other. Increased sense of ability and mastery and therefore awareness of self-effectiveness. Beginning group participation in a nondemanding way.
5	Provides a written handout, "On Depression," that describes the symptoms of depression and theories of its cause. Directs an active discussion by asking each participant to comment on various aspects.	Group discussion with a handout about various aspects of depression.	Members read and listen to the leader's thoughts and depression. Members are asked to comment by the leader. The interaction is primarily leader-to-participant.	Beginning interaction. Education about depression. Beginning ability to identify specific, personal aspects of depression.

(continues)

Table 19-8. (continued)			
Day	Group Leadership	Group Activity	Group Process	Desired Outcome/Rationale

Day	Group Leadership	Group Activity	Group Process	Desired Outcome/Rationale
6	Provides written exercise, "Stressful Events." Directs participants how to do the activity. Directs a discussion of how everyday events cause more stress than one is likely to realize. Asks members to share their stress test and validates thoughts and feelings. Points out similarities with other participants.	From a list of stressful events weighted from most stressful to least stressful, chooses those that have occurred in the last year and adds up the stress score. Discusses thoughts and feelings regarding the scores and the events.	Members complete the activity individually, and share their comments, at first with the leader, then with the other members.	Recognition of stressful events. Realization of how each event may cause stress. Validation of thoughts and feelings. Decrease of isolation and guilt.
7	Provides written exercise, "Chalk Talk." Directs participants how to do the activity. Directs a discussion of how automatic negative thoughts contribute to depression. Asks each member to share their "chalk talk," validates, and points out similarities with other members. Ends with a symbolic erasure or throwing away of the negative "chalk talk," while carefully saving the positive "chalk talk."	Introduces the concept that automatic, usually negative, thoughts contribute to depression. Introduces the concept of the "chalk talk," that is, that individuals are constantly coaching themselves as they go about daily life. Members choose an event from the previous day that causes moderate stress, then list the thoughts that usually occur before, during, and after that event.	Members write their "chalk talk" individually and share their comments, at first with the leaders and then with the other members. Members begin to validate and initiate with each other.	Participants become aware of the effect of their internal, usually negative, thoughts. Participants become aware of how their thoughts interfere with behavior and occur with depression. Participants learn strategies for coping with the negative thoughts.
8	Provides written activity, "Practice." Directs participants how to do the activity. Directs a discussion of how automatic behavior contributes to depression. Asks members to share their prac-	Introduces the concept that automatic behavior often contributes to depression. Introduces the concept of automatic practice routines that need to be changed. Members choose	Members individually write their "practice routine." Members share their routine with others and validate others' comments.	Participants become aware of how their actions are automatic and can lead to depression. Participants learn new strategies to practice different behavior.

(continues)

Table 19-8. (continued)

Day	Group Leadership	Group Activity	Group Process	Desired Outcome/Rationale
	tice routines. Validates and points out similarities with other members. Asks members to work with each other in dyads to create a new practice routine.	the same stressful event from the previous day and list their behavior before, during, and after the event.		
9	Provides written activity, "Creating Positive Chalk Talk and New Practice Routines." Directs members how to do the activity. Asks members to share their thoughts and feelings. Facilitates the group working together to help each other create new talk and new routines.	Written exercises, the "Next Chalk Talk" and "Creating New Practice Routines." Leader introduces the concept of anticipating events that lead to depression. Members choose one situation/event that will evoke depression in their environment. Members create new talk and new behavior to prevent depressed mood.	Members individually choose and share the anticipated event and their automatic thoughts and behavior. Members work together designing new practice routines and chalk talks.	Members anticipate events connected to depressed mood and create prevention strategies. Members cooperate with each other, decrease isolation, and learn how to accept help.
10	Group leader asks members to fill out the Beck Depression Scale and a self-report of the types of outcomes concerning improvements that they sought, written during the first session, in occupational performance, satisfaction, occupational roles, customary ways of adapting to daily situations, self-assessment of their current state of physical and mental health, and current quality of life. Group leader guides the wrap-up, in which each member says good-bye and expresses a message directly to every other member.	Each member individually fills out evaluative measures and comments on them. Each member directly interacts with the other members.	Each member has a chance to express any ending thoughts or feelings about the group, each other, and what she or he had anticipated, thereby having a chance to realize a positive sense of completion.	To have comparative outcome measures so that members may recognize personal change and progress. To have comparative outcome measures regarding group goals to evaluate the efficacy of the group.

Summary

Much treatment in the psychiatric arena is provided in groups. Groups are cost-effective, facilitate personal growth, and provide feedback by more than one person (though not everyone is suited for group treatment). The content, the structure, and leadership contribute to the process of the group.

Occupational therapy groups often combine principles and techniques of psychological models, but they are unique in their emphases on activity and on areas of occupation performance skills and patterns with respect to contexts. Various types and models of activity groups have been proposed for occupational therapy. A theory of activity groups is evolving; currently, occupational therapy groups can be fit into broad categories based on content.

Certain steps can be followed to successfully start a group. Starting a group involves planning and writing a group protocol. A successful group combines following the appropriate steps while assuming leadership and modeling communication skills. Group outcomes can be subsequently evaluated.

Review Questions

1. What are the differences between group process and group content? How do you define each?
2. What are the stages of a group? What are the questions that group participants might have in each stage?
3. How can a leader handle monopolizing behavior in a group? Why is it important to do so?
4. What are some questions you might reflect on as you develop a group?
5. How would you describe the group process in the case illustration of group roles?

References

Acquaviva, J. (Ed.). (1992). *Effective documentation for occupational therapy*. Rockville, MD: American Occupational Therapy Association.

Alonso, A., & Swiller, H. (Eds.). (1993). *Group therapy in clinical practice*. Washington, DC: American Psychiatric Press.

Barlow, S. H., Burlingame, G. M., & Fuhriman, A. (2000). Therapeutic application of groups: From Pratt's "Thought control classes" to modern group psychotherapy. *Group Dynamics: Theory, Research and Practice, 4*(1), 115–134.

Borg, B., & Bruce, M. A. (1991). *The group system: The therapeutic activity group in occupational therapy*. Thorofare, NJ: Slack.

Cole, M. B. (1998). *Group dynamics in occupational therapy.*(2nd ed.) Thorofare, NJ: Slack.

Corey, G. (1991). *Theory and practice of counseling and psychotherapy* (5th ed.). Pacific Grove, CA: Brooks/Cole-Thomson Learning.

Corey, M. S., & Corey, G. (2002). *Groups: Process and practice* (6th ed.). Monterey, CA: Brooks/Cole-Thomson Learning.

Denton, P. L. (1987). *Psychiatric occupational therapy: A workbook of practical skills*. Boston: Little, Brown.

Fidler, G. S. (1969). The task-oriented group as a context for treatment. *American Journal of Occupational Therapy, 23,* 43.

Hagedorn, R. (2000). *Tools for practice in occupational therapy: a structural approach to core skills and processes.* Edinburgh: Churchill Livingstone.

Howe, M., & Schwartzberg, S. L. (2001). *A functional approach to group work in occupational therapy* (3rd ed.). Philadelphia: Lippincott Williams & Wilkins.

Kaplan, H., & Sadock, B. (1991). *Synopsis of psychiatry: Behavioral sciences: Clinical psychology* (6th ed.). Baltimore: Williams & Wilkins.

Kaplan, K. L. (1986). The directive group: Short term treatment for psychiatric patients with a minimal level of functioning. *American Journal of Occupational Therapy, 40,* 474–481.

Kaplan, K. L. (1988). *Directive group therapy: Innovative mental health treatment.* Thorofare, NJ: Slack.

King, L. J. (1974). A sensory integrative approach to schizophrenia. *American Journal of Occupational Therapy, 28*(9), 529–536.

Levy, L. L. (1974). Movement therapy for psychiatric patients. *American Journal of Occupational therapy, 28*(6), 354–357.

Mosey, A. C. (1970). The concept and use of developmental groups. *American Journal of Occupational Therapy, 24,* 272.

Mosey, A. C. (1981). *Occupational therapy: Configuration of a profession.* New York: Raven.

Mosey, A. C. (1986). *Components of psychosocial occupational therapy.* New York: Raven.

Occupational Therapy Practice Framework: Domain and Process (2002). *American Journal of Occupational Therapy, 56,* 609–639.

Ottenbacher, K. J., & Cusick, A. (1990). Goal attainment scaling as a method of clinical service evaluation. *American Journal of Occupational Therapy, 44* (6), 519–526.

Rerek, M. (1966). *The use of groups in occupational therapy.* Unpublished manuscript.

Ruiz-Sancho, A. M., Ivanoff, A. M., & Linehan, M. (2001). Psychoeducational approaches. In W. J. Livesley (Ed.), *Handbook of personality disorders: Theory, research and treatment* (pp. 460–475). New York: Guilford.

Sadock, B., & Kaplan, H. (2000). *Comprehensive textbook of psychiatry* (7th ed.). Baltimore: Williams & Wilkins.

Scheidlinger, S. (1994). An overview of nine decades of group psychotherapy. *Hospital and Community Psychiatry, 45*(3), 197–225.

Yalom, I. (1983). *Inpatient group psychotherapy.* New York: Basic.

Yalom, I. (1995). *The theory and practice of group psychotherapy* (4th ed.). New York: Basic.

Suggested Reading

Bion, W. (1961). *Experiences in groups and other papers.* New York: Basic.

Kaplan, H., & Sadock, B. J. (1993). *Comprehensive group psychotherapy* (3rd ed.). Baltimore: Williams & Wilkins.

Expanded Roles for Occupational Therapy in Mental Health

Just as occupational therapists treat psychiatric conditions, lifespan issues, and psychosocial consequences of physical disorders, they also intervene with psychiatric conditions within various systems and through systematic treatment approaches. Part VII considers psychosocial occupational therapy for those with mental disabilities who are incarcerated, need vocational programs to assist with work, or need a manager to coordinate their services. These broad interventions have been part of occupational services for many decades though perhaps they have been known more readily in practice but less through the literature.

In Chapter 20 occupational therapy is discussed in different settings in the criminal justice system covering the city prison as well as the federal penitentiary. In Chapter 21 vocational programming is discussed as a broad intervention not limited to one program but as an intervention that can be adapted in all settings. In Chapter 22 case management is discussed from the same viewpoint as vocational intervention, not limited to one county, city, or facility, but able to be adapted in all settings. The chapters are filled with creative and innovative programming ideas for these broad interventions.

CHAPTER 20

Occupational Therapy in the Criminal Justice System

Fred Snively, OTR/L

Jane Dressler, OTR, JD

Key Terms

adjudication   incarceration
commitment   jails
forensics   prisons

Chapter Outline

Introduction

An understanding of the criminal justice system is mandatory for all occupational therapists working in mental health. The mental health and criminal justice systems overlap, and the boundaries between the two systems have become more blurred in the last 10 years. The number of people with mental illness in America's **jails** and **prisons** is significant and rising. The estimated prevalence of mental illness in jails and prisons is as follows (Beck & Maruschak, 2001):

- 13%, or one in eight state prisoners were receiving some mental health therapy or counseling service.
- 10% were receiving psychotropic medications.
- 20% of the inmates in five states (Maine, Montana, Nebraska, Hawaii, and Oregon) were receiving psychotropic medication.
- There were 155 state facilities specializing in psychiatric confinement, but two-thirds of all inmates receiving therapy/counseling or medication were housed in facilities that did not specialize in providing mental health services.

Conversely, many people receiving mental health treatment in traditional, non-criminal justice settings have a history of contact with the criminal justice system. At any point in their **incarceration**, individuals from criminal justice institutions may be referred to traditional mental health settings for special services. The blurring of these systems will surely continue as trends such as rising unemployment, homelessness, cuts in community based mental health services, hospital closures, and legislation that favors stiffer criminal sentences persist. Criminal justice institutions will continue to be faced with growing mental health needs.

The role of the occupational therapist in the criminal justice system is as varied as in other mental health settings. Occupational therapy facilities, referral procedures, the institution's physical settings, frames of reference, modalities used, and goals of programs differ widely across the country. Occupational therapists may work in an administrative and consultation role or offer a range of services directly, including evaluation, group and individual treatment, program development, case management, and student supervision. A therapist may work with patients in high-security correctional facilities such as jails, prisons, and forensic state hospitals, as well as with outpatients in the community.

Occupational therapy evaluation and treatment procedures in the criminal justice system rely on the same principles and procedures that are applied in traditional, noncriminal justice settings. Occupational therapists work as part of an interdisciplinary team, evaluate functional abilities, and use structured, graded therapeutic activities with individuals and groups to achieve specific goals. They facilitate skill development in order to help patients function at their maximum potential within their current institutional environment and be more productive and successful when they reintegrate into the community.

CRIMINAL JUSTICE SETTINGS

There are several different criminal justice settings, each of which has potentially different populations and treatment issues. For the purposes of this chapter, the discussion will focus on jails, prisons, forensic state hospitals, and community programs. The term *inmate* is used to identify a member of the prison population at large, while the term *patient* identifies an individual in need of or receiving mental health services.

Jails

As depicted in Figure 20-1, jails are the entry points of the criminal justice system. They are city- or county-funded and operated, and serve as holding facilities for arrested individuals awaiting arraignment, trial, or transfer to another facility. They also function as the institution in which people found guilty of a crime and given a sentence of under one year serve out their time.

The **adjudication** process is often complicated, filled with delays, and misunderstood by the accused. The jail environment is stressful. In large population

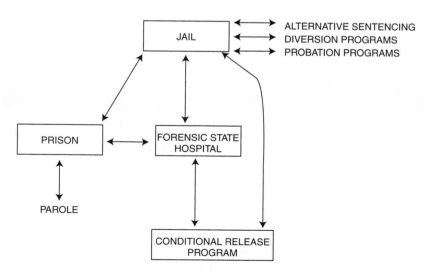

Figure 20-1. Jail Is the Entry Point of the Criminal Justice System

areas the jail facilities tend to be cramped, overcrowded, noisy, and chaotic. The accused have lost their freedom, they are separated from their support network, the ability to make life choices has been removed, and individual privacy is gone. Most American jails have minimal outdoor recreational opportunities and limited rehabilitation programs of any type (NAMI & PCHRG, 1992).

Adjusting to jail is difficult. Depression, suicidal ideation, confusion, and a sense of total loss of life control are frequent reactions among newly arrested individuals. People with a history of a major psychiatric disorder are vulnerable to decompensation in jail. Decompensation typically includes an increase in symptoms such as suicidal ideation, mutilation attempts, assaultive or violent behavior, auditory and visual hallucinations, delusional beliefs, loss of appetite, change in sleep patterns, and change in grooming and hygiene.

The availability of high-quality, comprehensive psychiatric treatment in jails varies widely across the country. All jails are required to have an operational plan that includes psychiatric screening and evaluation, crisis intervention, treatment, and discharge and transfer planning (American Psychiatric Association Task Force, 2000); however, the extent of these services may be limited to the on-call availability of a single mental health professional. The most effective and complete programs offer an array of services that include separate housing for people with mental illness with seven days per week clinical coverage, day treatment programs, training in community living skills, and an acute hospital unit for emergencies.

Occupational therapists are most likely to be found as part of the acute hospital program, which may be located at the jail or at a nearby hospital. The length of stay at these facilities is usually under two weeks. A wide variety of diagnoses are seen, but a majority of the hospitalized inmates have a chronic history of mental illness, and frequently their crimes are a manifestation of this condition (NAMI & PCHRG, 1992). Some typical arrest scenarios are described in Table 20-1. The occupational therapist in the acute hospital setting focuses on functional assessment, stabilization, treatment, and discharge planning. Treatment programs are designed to create a safe, nonthreatening environment that emphasizes patient

---

Table 20-1. Typical Arrest Scenarios

- A woman with schizoaffective disorder is arrested for assault after she entered a department store and began rearranging the shelves because of a delusion that she worked there. When asked to leave, she struck a store manager.
- A man with schizophrenia who was behaving in a bizarre manner on the street is arrested for assault after striking a teenager who was making fun of him.
- A man with bipolar disorder–manic is arrested for theft after he impulsively stole a yacht at a dock and then drove it around until it ran out of gas.
- A homeless man with chronic schizophrenia and a substance abuse problem is arrested for defrauding an innkeeper after running out without paying at the end of a meal because he was very hungry and had no money.
- A woman with schizophrenia is arrested for trespassing after she refused to leave a building due to having the delusional belief that she owned it.

strengths and engages the patients in activities at the appropriate cognitive level to allow for success. Initially, self-care and social skills training are a main focus. Discharge planning involves assessing when the patient is stable enough to return to jail or choosing the right community placement based on his or her skill level. Stability to return to jail usually involves the patient being able to eat and perform basic hygiene routines independently, to safely tolerate and/or cooperate with others, and to adequately control self-injurious behavior.

The occupational therapist working in a jail setting may have a limited amount of time in which to devise and implement a meaningful treatment plan, and security restrictions may substantially limit patient access to traditional occupational therapy materials such as wood, leather crafts, or even cooking utensils. Jails do, however, offer a fast-paced environment with a varied caseload and the opportunity to provide a positive, supportive therapeutic program for individuals experiencing multiple problems.

San Francisco General Hospital, a public hospital in California, utilizes occupational therapy on its 12-bed, acute, inpatient psychiatric jail unit. Patients are referred to the unit by jail psychiatric workers if they meet the criteria for involuntary psychiatric hospitalization (danger to self, danger to others, or grave disability). Typical admission scenarios involve patients assaulting cell mates; attempting to cut or hang themselves; not eating, sleeping, washing, or being totally unable to communicate with others due to psychosis.

Most patients have a psychiatric and/or substance abuse history that predates their legal problems. A full range of diagnoses are seen, but the most common are schizophrenia, bipolar disorder–manic, major depression, schizoaffective disorder, cognitive disorders, delusional disorder, and (jail) adjustment disorder. Legal charges vary from minor offenses like trespassing to more serious charges, including murder. The typical length of stay is five days, but occasionally a patient stays as long as two weeks.

The occupational therapist works as part of an interdisciplinary team consisting of nurses, psychiatrists, psychologists, and social workers. Deputy sheriffs guard the unit and attend selected patient treatment–planning sessions. When first admitted, patients are often agitated, physically aggressive, and verbally abusive, and they may require seclusion and/or physical restraints. Patients are carefully evaluated for behavioral control and only begin to attend programming after they can reliably agree, as assessed by the treatment team, not to hurt themselves or others. Once exerting behavioral self-control, all patients attend community meetings, discussion groups, and two occupational therapy groups a day.

Patients are evaluated by the occupational therapist with the Allen Cognitive Level Test (a screening tool that detects the presence of cognitive disability) (Allen, 1985), a brief interview, and observation in groups. The Kohlman Evaluation of Living Skills Assessment (interview and task observation of living skills) (Kohlman Thomson, 1992) may be used to further assess functional level. These assessments provide unique and vital information regarding patients' current and baseline functioning, specific assets and limitations when coping in the jail environment, and readiness to return to jail or another facility.

The overall goal of treatment is the stabilization of acute symptoms and an improvement in jail-coping skills. Groups are planned daily according to the patients' needs and abilities. Patients are generally appreciative of the opportunity for productive therapeutic activity and a respite from the jail environment, and patient cooperation with treatment activities tends to be high. Task skills groups, including crafts, light work, and gardening, are very effective for increasing organizational skills, problem solving, and the ability to concentrate. For safety reasons, no sharp tools are allowed and patients are not allowed to keep projects of any type. Consequently, all work is donated to other parts of the hospital or to charity. Games and physical activities are used for stress management, the productive channeling of excessive or aggressive energy, and improving basic social and communication skills. Focus and art expression groups create a sense of a safe, cohesive community and provide an opportunity for patients to express themselves. Focus groups typically explore subjects such as frustration, respect, and living in close quarters. Cooking provides an opportunity to explore the knowledge of basic nutrition and issues surrounding caring for oneself. Psychoeducational groups on goal setting, anger management, leisure time management, stress management, and journal writing are used in higher-functioning groups.

Prisons

After the adjudication process and having been found guilty of a felony, a crime that carries a sentence greater than one year, the felon is transferred to a prison. A prison is a state or federally operated facility where the environment tends to be more stable than that of a county jail. However, in the highly controlled, but unpredictable, prison environment there are many stresses due to the potential for violence, victimization, or being cited and reprimanded for infractions of prison rules. Inmates frequently describe their experience as a daily "struggle for survival." As high as two-thirds of prison inmates are in need of some form of psychiatric care at one time or another during their incarceration (Jemelka et al., 1989).

Like jails, prisons have mandated requirements for providing psychiatric services. Mental health services can be provided by either the state mental health system, the state correctional system, or a combination of the two. The services provided vary widely from state to state and may include prison-based, acute, inpatient hospital units; prison-based, day treatment programs; "outpatient" (in prison, but out of the acute hospital phase) programs; and special, mental health program prisons (MacKain & Streveler, 1990).

Improving task and interactional skills is an important focus for prison-based occupational therapy programs. Many patients lack the basic skills to complete a task, such as the needed attention span, memory, cognitive skills, concentration, problem-solving and sequencing abilities, the ability to follow instructions and to work with others, and frustration tolerance. Occupational therapy programs focus on these task skills as well as interpersonal and intrapersonal skills such as assertiveness, stress management, coping skills, and basic social skills. In order to function effectively and safely in prison, inmates must be hyper-alert to the environment and very cautious about how they present themselves to other individuals. Role-playing, videotaping, and structured communication exercises can be very helpful in developing necessary social skills.

Prison settings are challenging environments for the occupational therapist. Antisocial behavior and institutional restrictions to program planning are prevalent, but the opportunity to help patients make real changes in their lives and develop new skills is genuine. In the prison setting, therapists can form positive, long-term professional therapeutic relationships with their clients. The unique projects created in occupational therapy clinics seem to have increased significance to prison inmates, perhaps because so little else in their life is individualized. Figure 20-2 displays actual projects completed in a prison-based occupational therapy clinic.

The California Medical Facility in Vacaville, California, utilizes occupational therapy. This is a 3,000-man prison housing physical medicine, psychiatric, and general population inmates. The occupational therapists assigned to mental health services provide treatment to 600 plus psychiatric inmates with a Global Assessment of Functioning (GAF) below 50. This facility is the inmates' community, and the role of occupational therapy is to work with the pathology that restricts the inmates' productivity within their community.

Many of the patients have been socially and culturally deprived. By focusing on the patients' abilities and capabilities, the occupational therapist helps individuals use their strengths for growth and stability through such modalities as an intake assessment (structured questionnaire and interview), structured activities, individual counseling, and task-oriented activities. The treatment objectives are to explore the performance ability and capability of each patient; to maintain or improve reality awareness, concentration, self-esteem, self-image, social skills, and problem-solving abilities; and to develop tolerance and respect for individual needs and differences.

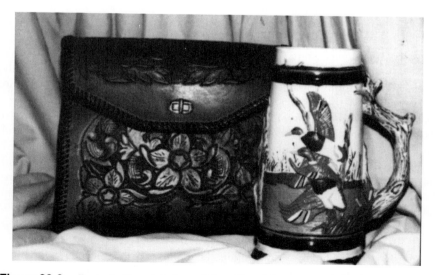

Figure 20-2. Projects Completed in a Prison-Based Occupational Therapy Clinic

Occupational therapy services are provided in a central location for the various program units. Interdisciplinary treatment teams comprised of a psychiatrist, psychologist, social worker, and psychiatric technician provide referrals to occupational therapy services for reasons such as withdrawn or unfocused behavior, lethargy, poor motivation, anxiety, depression, inability to relate to others or express emotional needs, and acting-out behaviors that violate departmental rules and regulations.

Occupational therapists treat a multitude of psychiatric disorders. Based on statistical information about inmates treated in occupational therapy at California Medical Facility, Vacaville, California, for the year 2001 approximately 83% of the patients treated in occupational therapy have a dual or multi-axis I diagnosis of schizophrenia, schizoaffective disorder, major depressive disorder, polysubstance abuse/dependence, psychiatric disorder not otherwise specified, and/or bipolar disorder. Sixty-seven percent of the patient population also have an axis II diagnosis of antisocial personality disorder, borderline intelligence, personality disorder not otherwise specified, and/or borderline personality disorder. Due to the lifestyles affecting the patients' health, 35% of those treated also have an axis III diagnosis that may include a history of head injury, seizure disorder, hepatitis B or C, visual impairments, diabetes, or HIV.

Patients are initially interviewed by the occupational therapy staff to obtain a personal history of the individual; assess cognitive function, memory, and treatment needs; and set treatment goals. The observation of mood and body language is vital to this process, and these observations are often more valuable than the patient's direct statements. The interviewer must acquire the trust and confidence of the patient so as to reduce defensive behavior in an effort to obtain accurate, unguarded responses. The nonthreatening atmosphere of the occupational therapy clinic, which has arts and crafts projects displayed and music playing in the background, helps the patient to relax defensive barriers and talk freely.

Occupational therapy provides a highly structured program, with the average length of treatment being 2.5 months. Average patients have had a life of negative environments, negative behavior, and no positive reinforcement. They usually make poor decisions and choices, feeling they are the victims of society with no power to change their lives. Using the Allen Cognitive Levels frame of reference, patients are matched with activities suited to their level of functioning in order to facilitate success. This process provides patients with positive feedback and increases self-esteem and sense of personal accomplishment. Learning that they can be successful builds confidence, and patients will explore new directions and face challenges that they previously considered stumbling blocks. Mistakes are reframed, not as failures, as was their experience in the past, but as lessons in learning, growth, problem solving, and decision making.

Forensic State Hospitals

Forensic state hospitals are maximum security psychiatric hospitals, administered by state mental health systems, that serve jails and prisons. The laws vary from state to state, but generally, three categories of patients are treated at forensic state hospitals, consisting of individuals who are considered to be one of the following:

1. incompetent to stand trial
2. not guilty by reason of insanity/not criminally responsible
3. competent, criminally responsible, adjudicated, guilty, but mentally ill

Incompetent to stand trial.   The word *incompetent* has a specific legal meaning, which differs from the ordinary understanding of the word. *Incompetent to stand trial* means that:

> a person, as the result of a mental disorder or mental retardation is unable to consult with a defense lawyer with a reasonable degree of rational understanding and otherwise assist in his or her own defense and/or does not have a rational, as well as factual, understanding of the criminal proceedings being conducted against him or her. (American Bar Association, 1989, pp. 167–168).

This means that an individual does not understand the criminal court proceedings. For example, he or she may not understand the role of the judge, jury, or attorneys or may not be able to communicate effectively or cooperate with a lawyer.

Individuals who are ruled incompetent to stand trial undergo **commitment** to a forensic state hospital for the specific intent of restoring them, through psychiatric treatment, to a sufficiently healthy mental state to permit an understanding of the nature of the criminal proceedings. Once this objective has been achieved, the individual is considered to have been returned to competence. The time frame for such restoration varies widely from case to case. The law then mandates that the competent person be returned to court for a reinstatement of the criminal proceedings (Donovan, 1991). The individual will then be returned to jail in the county in which the alleged crime was committed and the adjudication process will continue.

Not guilty because of insanity/not legally responsible.   People who are considered not guilty because of insanity/not criminally responsible comprise another category of patients treated at forensic state hospitals. The terminology and criteria vary from state to state, but the key issue is

> whether or not, a defendant, due to mental disease, disorder or defect at the time of the commission of an offense, was incapable of appreciating the criminality of his/her conduct and incapable of conforming that conduct to the requirements of the law. (American Bar Association, 1989, p. 294).

People may be found not guilty because of insanity/not criminally responsible if they are incapable of distinguishing right from wrong (Donovan, 1991). When individuals are found to be not guilty because of insanity/not criminally responsible, they are committed to a state forensic hospital.

Those evaluated as incompetent to stand trial or not guilty by reason of insanity will remain hospitalized and under close supervision until their illness is deemed to be in remission by a team of psychiatrists. When or if a patient is released back into the community, it will be under close court-ordered supervision.

Competent, criminally responsible, guilty, but mentally ill.   The third category of patients treated at forensic state hospitals is made up of individuals who are considered competent, criminally responsible, guilty, but mentally ill. These individuals are transferred from other criminal justice institutions because they are in need of mental health treatment. Some patients are acutely ill and are transferred to the forensic state hospital under emergency conditions; others may be more stable or chronic and are transferred for a specific type of treatment or training. Some patients are transferred specifically for preparation and training before being released into the community.

Forensic state hospital treatment programs and occupational therapy programs vary widely depending on patient and security needs and the state's resources. Some hospitals allow patients to wear their own street clothes, while others require uniforms. Some programs are sparse, while others are quite rich with services and opportunities. Some even provide outings (usually requiring court notification of approval), both on and off hospital grounds.

The forensic state hospitals with sufficient resources may have large occupational therapy departments that offer comprehensive, specialized programming to meet the specific needs of the patient. Sensorimotor activities, living skills training, cooking, task groups, prevocational programming, and expressive arts are all typical of the offerings. These settings offer the advantage of the availability of a wide variety of modalities and have a clear institutional mission for treatment. A special challenge in this setting is combatting institutional dependence and motivating the more chronic patient.

A role for the occupational therapist that is unique to the forensic state hospital setting is leading a pretrial competency group for patients identified as incompetent to stand trial. This group uses role-playing and paper-and-pencil tasks to increase patients' understanding and appreciation of their current legal charges, their own social interaction styles, and the roles and procedures of a courtroom. The overall goal of the group is to facilitate the patient's return to competency. Specific group goals include increasing the abilities to verbally express charges, verbally express what charges mean, verbally identify the participants in a courtroom, verbally identify a range of possible criminal penalties, cooperate with others, and express both positive and negative feelings appropriately.

Community Programs

In the community, occupational therapists work with newly released individuals. There are a number of ways in which people can be released from custody while remaining under court-ordered supervision. Some states are experimenting with alternative sentencing for mentally ill individuals, which includes referrals to traditional, non–criminal justice, mental health programs and intensive case management. Individuals may also be placed in diversion programs, be put on probation or parole, or be referred to a conditional release program. Diversion programs typically mandate services such as structured, supervised living situations; volunteer community service time; mental health treatment; drug counseling; and participation in educational activities, work, and other meaningful daytime activity. Individuals released on probation in lieu of jail time and inmates paroled from prison are subject to legal guidelines that require monitoring by either a probation or parole officer. If a condition of release is violated, the individual will be returned to custody. Common conditions of probation and parole include required community service, testing for controlled substances, warrantless search conditions, restraints on certain types of employment, restraints on associations and activities, abstinence from the use of alcohol and drugs, involvement in educational activities, and mental health or substance abuse treatment (Mental Health and Forensic Task Force, 1989).

Newly released individuals may also be court-ordered to participate in formal conditional release programs, which are comprehensive psychiatric programs providing services such as individual therapy, case management, group therapy, skills training, family therapy, home visits, and screening for drug and alcohol use (California Department of Mental Health, 1991).

At the community level, occupational therapists working in a criminal justice setting have a vital role in providing living and job skills training and activities that focus on self-confidence, accomplishment, goal setting, taking responsibility, and problem solving. They also have the very important function of focusing on skill development to facilitate compliance with release requirements and court-ordered conditions. For example, they may help individuals develop the transportation or telephone skills needed to contact their probation officer or facilitate the development of appropriate communication skills needed for court appearances. Occupational therapists also evaluate patients' level of function, information that may be used to help determine how long a patient will need to remain under close supervision.

Community programs offer the occupational therapist the advantage of working with a stable, motivated group of patients for whom medication compliance may be a condition for release. The potential exists in this community for drug and alcohol abuse, and therapists must be aware of this possibility and be skilled in substance abuse treatment methods and resources.

Riverside and San Bernadino Counties in California have a conditional release program that utilizes occupational therapy. The overall goal of the program is to prevent relapse and/or reoffense while stabilizing the patient in the community. Close observation, support, and immediate response to potential problems are provided. Supervision and support are then gradually reduced while promoting the patient's ability to function in the community. Skill building, symptom recognition, acceptance of mental illness, substance abuse prevention, social skills training, stress management, and building a sense of self-determination are all critical.

Before they are admitted to the program, patients sign a contract in which they agree to follow the rules, participate in treatment, take prescribed medication, and remain drug and alcohol free. Abiding by the contract is a condition of their court-ordered release into the community, and patients may be reincarcerated if they violate it. Most patients, at least initially, attend a highly structured day treatment program, although some participate in a less-structured program of outpatient visits.

Patients represent a wide range of ethnic and socioeconomic backgrounds. Many report a poor educational history and have been in the forensic state hospital for several years before release. The primary diagnoses cover a wide spectrum, but the most common are schizophrenia, bipolar disorder, and alcohol- or substance-induced psychosis. About half the patients carry a diagnosis of personality disorder. The average length of treatment is 2.5 years. Discharge from the program is primarily dependent on an evaluation of the person's potential for relapse or reoffense.

The occupational therapist works with an interdisciplinary treatment team consisting of several clinicians (social workers, psychologists, or marriage, family, and child counselors), a program manager, and a psychiatrist. The occupational therapist screens new patients for day treatment using an interview and questionnaire adapted from the Occupational History (an interview protocol focusing on educational and occupational history and living skills). Once in day treatment, patients are evaluated by observation in a wide variety of groups as well as with specific evaluations, including the Kohlman Evaluation of Living Skills (Kohlman Thomson, 1992) as well as various educational and vocational assessment tools.

The occupational therapist addresses work skills, independent living skills, and the development of social supports. Work skills are addressed on two levels, with role-play and psychoeducational groups for the higher-functioning patients and a token economy for the lower-functioning group. Acting as a liaison for the patient, the occupational therapist will provide, as necessary, in-depth prevocational evaluations and, if appropriate, make referrals on behalf of the patient to the state Department of Vocational Rehabilitation. Training in independent living skills is approached through cooking groups, shopping groups, problem-solving groups, and discussion groups. When needed, the occupational therapist can provide more intensive, one-on-one training in independent living skills, perhaps even working in the patient's own home. The occupational therapist addresses developing a support system within the community through engaging in altruistic activities, humor, crafts, games, expressive art, and community outings.

CLINICAL COMPETENCIES IN A CRIMINAL JUSTICE SETTING

Criminal justice settings provide a unique set of challenges requiring occupational therapists to refine their competency in a number of areas. They must be able to understand and adapt institutional environments, redefine the concept of independence in a confined setting, blend therapeutic practice with safety and security issues, and be creative problem solvers when they encounter difficult patients and institutional blocks to good treatment. These skills are required in all mental health settings, but they must be well developed to function effectively within the criminal justice system, particularly within the locked environments of jails, prisons, and forensic state hospitals.

Analyzing the Environment

Performance is greatly affected by environmental influences and how the patient interprets them (Spencer, 1978). Correctional facility environments vary between states, between facilities within states, and between housing units within facilities, but all have demanding and unique environments. Therapists in the criminal justice system must understand the specific demands of the various environments in which their patients function. They must also understand the difference between the institutional environment and the community (Michael, 1986).

Jails and prisons are closed societies, with their own rules and culture. They are, essentially, small cities providing all the services of a city while maintaining a high degree of security. Although there are a variety of positive roles that inmates may assume within these institutions (church member, volunteer, student, worker), many factors in the jail and prison environment reinforce maladaptive behavior. Victimization is common, and inmates may learn how to protect themselves by fighting or gathering support by joining a gang. While rigid institutional structures attempt to control inmate access to legal and illegal goods, underground economies controlled by the inmates themselves often flourish. Complicated systems develop for the distribution of extra food and the "good" work and housing assignments, as well as for contraband such as cigarettes, drugs, alcohol, and weapons. Inside the facility, inmates may learn ways of meeting their needs that foster continued criminal behavior. Occupational therapists are faced with the challenge of creating programs to improve individuals' coping skills, decision-making ability, and self-esteem and counseling inmates on how to develop alternative strategies for controlling and eliminating criminal behavior.

Forensic state hospital environments offer another set of demands. These hospitals tend to be highly structured and organized. Compliance and conformity to external controls are emphasized, which can foster dependence, passivity, and social withdrawal on the part of the patients. The structured environment of the hospital is in sharp contrast to the lack of structure encountered in the community. Occupational therapy programs in forensic state hospitals focus on increasing patients' sense of competency, autonomy, and productivity in an effort to combat the institution's tendency to create passivity and dependency.

All programming must keep the patients' current and future environments in mind. Therapists may be called on to help patients make the transition from mental health housing to mainstream prison housing, from prison to a forensic hospital, from prison or a forensic hospital to the community—and there are many other possibilities. Each of these environments is different and requires a different adaptive performance in order for patients to be successful.

Effective social skills, ways of expressing feelings, and communication skills may greatly differ from one criminal justice unit to another, one institution to another, and, certainly, from inside to outside this system of institutions. In jail, for example, it would be considered adaptive to develop a quiet interpersonal style whereby one keeps to oneself, does not initiate conversation or does not openly express emotion, and remains detached from other people's problems. In many community mental health programs, however, quite the opposite is considered adaptive. People are encouraged to form close personal relationships, make inquiries regarding each other's lives, openly express their feelings, and assist each other when needed. It is also considered adaptive in jail to develop a tolerance for long stretches of inactivity and engage in quiet, solitary interests like solitaire, journal writing, and reading, whereas most community settings expect tolerance for a more active, social, and productive schedule. Moreover, how one projects one's self-image is very different inside and outside of jail. On the outside, it is frequently considered good to have a realistic sense of one's assets and limitations, and be open about one's frailties, and be proud of one's accomplishments and material assets. In jail, however, adaptive functioning involves presenting a low-key, but confident, persona, with little said about personal assets (for fear of angering someone) or personal weaknesses (for fear of victimization). Thus, each area of patient functioning must be evaluated within the context of the particular environmental demands and norms.

Maintaining Safety and Security

Safety and security are the primary mission of all criminal justice settings. Correctional facilities usually have a number of security levels or classifications, ranging from light to moderate and, finally, to close custody status. Policies and procedures are outlined for each security level and must be adhered to without deviation. Automatically locking doors, increased awareness of danger, the presence of custody staff, clear emergency plans, high staffing ratios, security cameras, buzzer systems, emergency alarms, and restrictions on materials are vital to the security of an institution.

To maintain safety, occupational therapists must maintain close, continual communication with other staff members and avoid situations where they may be isolated or lack immediate staff support. Patients must be carefully assessed, especially those with a high violence potential or a history of impulsive or explosive behavior. All clinical staff must be observant, sensitive to subtle changes in a patient's behavior and affect, and constantly alert to the surroundings. Treatment planning in these settings starts with the highest degree of structure and control, which lessen only as a patient demonstrates reliability and predictability.

Occupational therapists must be cognizant of tools and supplies since quite a few of these items are considered contraband. They must also be aware of alternative, and potentially dangerous, uses of common materials, such as using chewing gum to jam locks or sharpening plastic and wooden items into weapons. Some glues are very flammable; some paints can be "sniffed" for an intoxicating effect. Because of the potential of misusing occupational therapy supplies and equipment, body searches and metal detectors are common in this system. Figure 20-3 reflects the policy and procedures for tool safety and security for one prison-based occupational therapy clinic; the photograph in Figure 20-4 illustrates this application.

General
- The OT tool room will be locked at all times and out of bounds to all inmates unless under the direct supervision of staff.
- All OT tools will be painted using assigned department color code and engraved "OT Clinic" to denote origin.
- Periodic, unscheduled searches of the entire OT clinic will be made for safety and security.

Tool Accountability
- Tools are stored in locked rooms, secured inside cabinets and on shadow boards.
- Each morning tools are inventoried.
- Tools are accounted for at the end of each group before inmates are released to their housing areas. No one is allowed to leave until all tools are accounted for.
- All inmates will be given a clothed body search for contraband before leaving the OT clinic.

Use of Tools
- Inmates and OT staff are assigned a number with five corresponding numbered tags for checking out tools. For each tool used by an individual one tag assigned to that person is placed where the tool is stored. No one will be allowed to use more than five tools at a time.
- Large floor power tools will only be used under the direct supervision of an OTR.

Figure 20-3. Policy and Procedures for Tool Safety and Security in a Prison-Based Occupational Therapy Clinic

---

Strict adherence to infection control policies is mandatory, as tuberculosis, HIV infection, and hepatitis are common in correctional institutions. Groups, such as cooking and grooming, that involve eating communal food or close physical contact require adherence to standard precautions.

Professional and modest clothing for the occupational therapist is mandated. While most inmates' crimes are not of a sexual nature, incarceration deprives individuals of privacy and inhibits normal sexual outlets, creating a heightened degree of sexual tension. Therapists will be more effective when their clothing does not act as a disruption or distraction to the therapeutic process. Fashionable clothing is quite acceptable, but short skirts, low-cut blouses, exposed midriffs, and tight-fitting clothing, for example, are not.

Overcoming Obstacles

The safety and security policies for any given correctional facility may drastically alter the modalities and scope of occupational therapy that is provided. There may be policies to avoid "overfamiliarity" with patients that discourage one-on-one contacts or place restrictions on the types of materials patients can take out of the occupational therapy clinic. For example, sharp tools may be prohibited altogether. The occupational therapist must model positive problem-solving strategies. Each obstacle can serve as a creative opportunity for problem solving. For example, if sharp tools are not permitted, the occupational therapist can explore alternative, and perhaps more creative, novel, and meaningful,

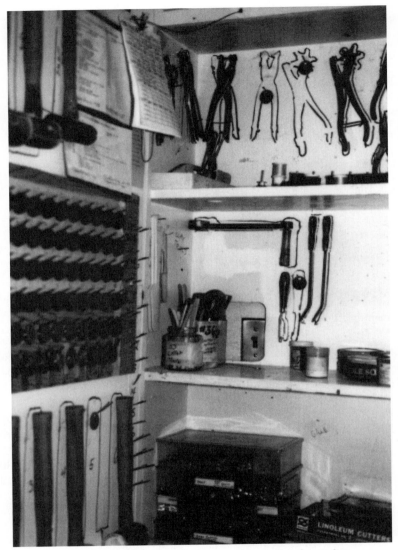

Figure 20-4.   A Tool Closet Arranged as Required by Tool Safety Policies

activities. Similarly, if patients cannot take finished projects out of the occupational therapy clinic, they can be encouraged to donate their work to charity or make a gift of it.

Developing Team Relationships

In any criminal justice setting, the occupational therapist will interface with the non–mental health, criminal justice staff, such as deputy sheriffs, prison or security

- Increases safety by providing productive, creative outlets for aggression.
- Increases safety by building cooperation and a sense of cohesiveness among inmates.
- Increases safety by reducing individuals' feelings of tension and stress.
- Provides unique evaluation material and a new view of inmates' abilities, deficits, and capabilities and how they best learn.
- Provides inmates with new skills that ultimately will help with productive integration into their community and decrease the possibility of reoffense.

Figure 20-5. Benefits of Occupational Therapy in Criminal Justice Settings

guards, parole officers, and correctional case managers. These staff may be unfamiliar with mental health treatment philosophy and benefits and concerned instead with public safety and compliance with institutional rules. Some correctional staff may feel that patients should be punished because of past criminal behavior and do not understand the value of providing any form of therapy to the population. In other words, there is potential for conflict between mental health and criminal justice staff due to philosophical differences.

Occupational therapists can build alliances with all staff by clearly articulating the benefits of occupational therapy for the patient and the institution. Some of these "selling points" are listed in Figure 20-5. The occupational therapist must also try to understand the other staffs' perspective. Relationships can be developed by including other disciplines in decisions, program planning, and in-service training. Clear lines of communication, well-defined staff roles, and an attitude that promotes sharing ideas is beneficial for all staff. It is always recommended to use humor when appropriate, to be persistent, and, above all, to be flexible in meeting conflicts and working toward resolution.

Building Therapeutic Alliances

One challenge when working in the criminal justice system involves developing and maintaining relationships with patients who are impaired in their ability to trust and cooperate with others, find it difficult to express their thoughts and feelings, and are unable to interact in a socially acceptable manner. The general atmosphere of mistrust and suspicion typical of correctional facilities increases the difficulty of fostering therapeutic relationships.

Personality disorders, and antisocial personality disorder in particular, are quite common within the criminal justice setting (Jemelka et al., 1989). People with personality disorders typically exhibit difficulty with conflict resolution, delaying gratification, repressing impulses, and forming stable relationships. Internal feelings are often transformed into social or somatic complaints or are projected onto another person. These patients often have difficulty assuming responsibility for their actions. They frequently try to bend and break rules, divide the staff, and undermine authority. People with personality disorders tend to view themselves as tough, smart, entitled, and victimized by the legal system and may view the therapist as foolish and weak, ineffective, and easily manipulated. Such patients are likely to view situations with concrete thinking, with their ultimate goal a self-centered, self-serving one. They view conflicts in terms of right or wrong, seeing things in black and white rather than in shades of gray, and are unable to comprehend others' emotions.

Knowing this information about personality disorders, the therapist can be better prepared and avoid taking conflicts personally. Patients seem to respond to a genuine show of respect and concern. This population can be very enjoyable and satisfying, and these problematic traits described are found in patients in traditional mental health settings as well. Guidelines for building effective therapeutic alliances include being assertive and honest while maintaining a healthy degree of suspicion, as the patient's word may not always be reliable. Occasionally, it is necessary to give firm, direct orders and set clear limits. Above all the therapist should only focus on current, relevant factors to communicate to patients exactly what is expected of them. Unacceptable patient behavior is best handled through immediate limit setting. Occupational therapists are most effective when they are fair and consistent and when they use rational limits that apply to everyone, without deviation.

Recognizing Malingering

Malingering is defined as the conscious, planned simulation of an illness for the sake of gain or the pretense of a slow recuperation from a disease once suffered; in either case, the intent is to receive benefits (Rogers, 1988). There are several reasons why patients within correctional institutions may want to feign or exaggerate psychiatric symptoms.

Malingerers may believe that being diagnosed with a mental illness will make them appear more sympathetic to a judge or a jury. Some individuals prefer mental health programs to mainstream jail or prison, as these programs are often associated with fewer restrictions and work expectations. Some patients may also be "medication seeking," trying to obtain prescription drugs to "get high," alter consciousness, or ease the frustration and boredom associated with incarceration rather than for the intended purpose of reducing specific psychiatric symptoms.

Clinicians within the system need to share observations with other team members and carefully document suspicious or unlikely symptoms. The occupational therapist is often the first person to observe or confirm malingering as patients tend to relax and let their guard down in occupational therapy. Malingerers become fully absorbed in their tasks during treatment sessions and forget to "act sick," thus revealing the inconsistencies in their functioning.

Documenting Accurately

Documentation must be clear, accurate, concise, and in accordance with professional guidelines. The focus, as in other mental health settings, is on functional ability, progress toward goals, and treatment plans for future intervention. The occupational therapist's observations and documentation regarding cognitive and functional abilities can be instrumental in the treatment team's decisions regarding a patient's transfer and discharge and therefore are taken very seriously. In preadjudication settings, documenting specific information regarding an individual's charges, the circumstances resulting in arrest, and the patient's beliefs regarding his or her innocence or guilt should be avoided. It is not the occupational therapist's responsibility to investigate a case or pass judgment regarding a crime.

Although the issue is becoming controversial, medical records tend to be more accessible to patients and their lawyers in the criminal justice system than in the traditional mental health system. In some prison systems, patients are allowed to review their charts by simply asking to see them. Criminal justice medical records are frequently subpoenaed, either in reference to an individual's criminal case or medical treatment or as part of a class action lawsuit concerning jail or prison conditions. Such class action lawsuits are not uncommon in these settings. Every therapist is ethically and legally obligated to inform patients of confidentiality guidelines within this system in order to maintain a therapeutic, trusting relationship.

Knowing the Criminal Justice Language

Having a knowledge of the basic terminology used in criminal law will increase the occupational therapist's credibility with staff and patients, who will frequently make reference to the adjudication process. The occupational therapist must understand this process to understand the stressors, demands, and decisions facing patients. Jail and prison slang words are also commonly used. Table 20-2 defines some of the basic legal terminology, and Table 20-3 describes slang vocabulary commonly used in this system.

Summary

An understanding of the criminal justice system is mandatory for all occupational therapists working in mental health, as it impacts many patients. The mental health and correctional systems overlap and will continue to blend in line with current trends of economic hardship, hospital closures, and the general decrease in mental health resources.

Occupational therapists in the criminal justice system may work in jails, where the treatment program focuses on evaluation, crisis intervention, and symptom stabilization; in longer-term prisons and forensic state hospitals, where the focus is on improving task skills, interactional skills, and the opportunities for choices and decision making; or in the community where the focus is living skills and vocational skills training. All programs must take the institutional environments and legal process into account.

To function effectively in the criminal justice system an occupational therapist must develop expertise in several areas. These include a thorough knowledge of **forensics**, the ability to understand and adapt to institutional environments, the ability to blend therapeutic practice with safety and security issues, the ability to think flexibly and creatively to overcome obstacles, the ability to form strong team relationships with mental health and correctional staff alike, the ability to

Table 20-2. Basic Criminal Law Vocabulary

Term	Description
Arraignment	An initial step in the criminal process wherein the defendant is formally charged with an offense.
Bail	A monetary or other security given to ensure the appearance of the defendant at every stage of the criminal proceedings.
Defendant	The accused.
District Attorney	The prosecuting attorney.
Felony	A class of criminal offenses that are considered more serious than misdemeanors and are usually punishable by imprisonment for more than a year (possibly death).
Misdemeanor	A class of criminal offenses that consists of offenses less serious than felonies, which are sanctioned by less severe penalties, usually including fines, community service, probation, or a sentence of under one year in jail.
Parole	A conditional release from imprisonment that entitles the person receiving parole to serve the remainder of the term outside the prison provided he or she satisfactorily complies with all the terms and conditions of the release and remains under the supervision of a parole officer.
Plea Bargaining	The process whereby the accused and the prosecutor negotiate a mutually satisfactory disposition of a case, thus avoiding a complete trial.
Probation	A procedure whereby a defendant found guilty of a crime upon verdict or pleas of guilty is released by the court to the community without imprisonment, subject to conditions imposed by the court, under the supervision of a probation officer.
Prosecute	To bring legal action against the accused.
Public Defender	A lawyer whose duty it is to defend accused persons who are unable to pay for legal assistance.
Revocation	To recall a power of authority previously conferred, as in revoking probation or parole if a condition of release is not met and requiring a return to jail or prison.
Sentence	The punishment ordered by the court to be inflicted on a person convicted of a crime.
Trial	An examination involving the offering of testimony before a judge and/or jury.

form therapeutic alliances with difficult patients, the ability to recognize malingering behavior, the ability to document occurrences in an unbiased manner, and a basic understanding of the legal system.

Occupational therapy provides professional diversity to the criminal justice environment. The profession's understanding of one's ability to adapt in different environments, its emphasis on problem-solving strategies, and its commitment to treating people with dignity makes occupational therapy an asset to the criminal

Table 20-3. Jail and Prison Slang

Term	Description
Beef	A written action against an inmate.
Behind the wall	Inside the prison.
Bunkie/cellie	Someone who sleeps above or below an inmate (in a bunk bed).
"Burn rubber"	"Get lost, leave, you're not wanted."
Canteen	A version of a store in which inmates are allowed to purchase needed and wanted items, based on how much money is available in their trust account.
Chrono	Information written about an inmate that is either negative or positive and becomes part of the inmate's "central" (permanent) record.
Clean time	Period of time for which an inmate has been infraction free.
Date	Prison release date.
Down	Amount of time in prison.
Gooner	A correctional officer on the prison's security and investigation task force.
Hang	Staying with someone to the end, no matter how tough the situation gets.
Hog	Tough guy, leader.
"Homes"	General greeting, refers to "homeboy" or someone from your hometown.
In the car	Refers to being in the in-group.
Jacket	Inmate's central file or record.
Mainline	Areas of prison accessible to inmates.
On the leg	Describes inmates who spend time with the staff to cultivate influence.
PC	Protective custody, where inmates are housed for their own safety when they need to be locked away from others.
Pruno	Prison-made alcohol.
Punk	Young, defenseless inmate who is forced into homosexual activity.
Road dog	Friend who can be trusted for life.
Rolled up	To be locked up in a security housing unit.
Schooled	Inmate who has earned respect; someone who knows how to survive in prison.
Shakedown	What officers do when they search the work or living areas of the prison.
Take care of business	To do what is necessary for day-to-day living or to protect oneself.
To the house	Home, getting out on parole.
Yard	Outside space for recreational activity.

justice setting. Although personal observation and anecdotal reports show the success of occupational therapy in criminal justice settings, there is an urgent need for outcome research and the development of strong evidence-based practice for these settings.

It is time to demystify some of the myths related to the criminal justice system and to encourage increased involvement in it. There is currently a paucity of occupational therapists in the criminal justice system and a growing need. The population is compelling and opportunities are rewarding: The work is fascinating and satisfying.

Review Questions

1. Name and define the four criminal justice settings where an occupational therapist might work.
2. Define "incompetent to stand trial."
3. Why could the accused be committed to a state forensic hospital?
4. What limitations would be placed on a therapeutic modality or intervention in a jail, prison, or forensic hospital?

References

Allen, C. (1985). *Measurement and management of cognitive disabilities*. Boston: Little, Brown.

American Bar Association. (1989). *Criminal justice mental health standards*. Washington, DC: Author.

American Psychiatric Association Task Force. (2000). *Psychiatric services in jails and prisons* (2nd ed.). Washington, DC: American Psychiatric Association.

Beck, A., & Maruschak, L. (2001, July). *Mental health treatment in state prisons 2000*. Bureau of Justice Statistics Special Report. U.S. Department of Justice, Washington, DC. http://oip.usdoj.gov/bis/

California Department of Mental Health. Forensic Services Branch. Office of Forensic Services. (1991). *The Forensic Conditional Release Program: An orientation guide*. Sacramento, CA: Author.

Donovan, J. (1991). *Forensic Conditional Release Program: An overview of laws pertaining to Conrep*. Unpublished paper.

Jemelka, R. P., Trupin, E. W., & Chiles, J. A. (1989). The mentally ill and the prisons: A review. *Hospital and Community Psychiatry, 40*, 481–489.

Hodgins, S. Muller-Isberner, R. (2000). *Violence, crime and mentally disordered offenders: Concepts and methods for effective treatment and prevention*. West Sussex: Wiley.

Kielhofner, G. (1995). *A model of human occupation: Theory and application* (2nd ed.). Baltimore: Williams & Wilkins.

Kohlman Thomson, L. (1992). *The Kohlman evaluation of living skills*. Bethesda, MD: American Occupational Therapy Association.

Livesley, J. (2001). *Handbook of personality disorders*. New York: Guilford.

MacKain, S. J., & Streveler, A. (1990). Social and independent living skills for psychiatric patients in a prison setting. *Behavior Modification, 14*, 490–518.

Mental Health and Forensic Task Force (California). (1989). *Violence and treatment*. Unpublished paper.

National Alliance for the Mentally Ill (NAMI) and Public Citizen's Health Research Group (PCHRG). (1992). *Criminalizing the seriously mentally ill*. Arlington, VA: Author.

Rogers, R. (1988). *Clinical assessment of malingering and deception*. New York: Guilford.

Spencer, E. A. (1978). *Willard and Spackman's occupational therapy* (5th ed.) Philadelphia: Lippincott.

Suggested Reading

Chiles, J. A., Von Cleve, E., Jemelka, R. P., & Trupin, E. W. (1990). Substance abuse and psychiatric disorders in prison inmates. *Hospital and Community Psychiatry, 41*, 1132–1134.

Curran, W. J., McCarry, A. L., & Shah, S. A. (1988). *Forensic psychiatry and psychology.* Philadelphia: F. A. Davis.

Fansworth, L., Morgan, S., & Fernando, B. (1987). Prison based occupation therapy. *Australian Journal of Occupational Therapy, 34*, 40–46.

Farnsworth, L. (2000). Time use and leisure occupational of young offenders. *American Journal of Occupational Therapy, 54*(3), 315–325.

Fowles, G. P. (1988). Neuropsychologically impaired offenders: Considerations for assessment and treatment. *Psychiatric Annals, 18*, 692–697.

Freeman, M. (1982). Forensic psychiatry and related topics. *British Journal of Occupational Therapy, 45*, 191–194.

Green, N. S. (1984). OT Education Bulletin: Utilizing inmate populations in training occupational therapy assistants. *Occupational Therapy News, 38*(10), 9.

Halleck, L. S. (1986). *The mentally disordered offender.* Rockville, MD: National Institute for Mental Health.

Hamm, M. S., & Schrink, J. L. (1989). The conditions of effective implantation: A guide to accomplishing rehabilitative objectives in corrections. *Criminal Justice and Behavior, 16*, 166–182.

Idzinga, R. (1997). Occupational therapy, forensics and the care and treatment of addicts. *World Federation of Occupational Therapists (WFOT) Bulletin, 36*, 16–20.

Jones, E. J., & McColl, M. A. (1991). Development and evaluation of an interactional life skills group for offenders. *Occupational Therapy Journal of Research, 11*, 80–92.

Lloyd, C. (1983). Forensic psychiatry and occupational therapy. *British Journal of Occupational Therapy, 46*, 348–350.

Lloyd, C. (1985). Evaluation and forensic psychiatric occupational therapy. *British Journal of Occupational Therapy, 48*, 137–140.

Lloyd, C. (1987a). The role of occupational therapy in the treatment of the forensic psychiatric patient. *Australian Journal of Occupational Therapy, 34*, 20–25.

Lloyd, C. (1987b). Working with the female offender. *British Journal of Occupational Therapy, 50*, 44–46.

Lloyd, C. (1988). Discharge preparation for the forensic psychiatric patient: A proposed model. *Journal of the New Zealand Association of Occupational Therapists, 39*, 12–14.

Lloyd, C. (1995). Trends in forensic psychiatry. *British Journal of Occupational Therapy, 58*(5), 209–213.

Lloyd, C., & Guerra, F. (1988). A vocational rehabilitation programme in forensic psychiatry. *British Journal of Occupational Therapy, 4*, 123–126.

Maier, G. J., & Miller, R. D. (1987). Models of mental health service delivery to correctional institutions. *Journal of Forensic Sciences, 32*, 225–232.

Michael, P. S. (1991). Occupational therapy in a prison? You must be kidding! *Mental Health Special Interest Section Newsletter, 14*(2), 3–4.

Miller, R. K., Maier, G. J., Van Rybroek, G. J., & Widermann, J. A. (1989). Treating patients "doing time": A forensic perspective. *Hospital and Community Psychiatry, 40*, 960–962.

Morrison, E. F. (1991). Victimization in prison: Implications for mental health professionals. *Archives of Psychiatric Nursing, 5*(1), 17–24.

National Alliance for the Mentally Ill. (n.d.). *A guide to mental illness and the criminal justice system: A systems guide for families and consumers.* Arlington, VA: Author.

Nelson, S. H., & Berger, V. F. (1988). Current issues in state mental health forensic programs. *Bulletin of the American Academy of Psychiatry and the Law, 16*, 67–75.

Penner, D. A. (1978). Correctional institutions: An overview. *American Journal of Occupational Therapy, 32*, 517–524.

Platt, N. P. (1977). Level I field placement at a federal correctional institution. *American Journal of Occupational Therapy, 31*, 385–387.

Police Executive Research Forum. (1986). *Special care: Improving the police response to the mentally disabled*. New York: Author.

Reed, K. L. (1991). *Quick reference to occupational therapy*. Gaithersburg, MD: Aspen.

Rogowski, A. (1997). Forensic psychiatry. In J. Creek (Ed.), *Occupational therapy and mental health*. Edinburgh: Churchill Livingstone.

Sadler, C. (1989). Held without help . . . Mentally ill offenders. *Nursing Times*, 85(4), 16–17.

Samarneh, G. (1993). Taking treatment behind bars. *OT Week*, 7(47), 20–22.

Samson, S. T. (1990). Occupational therapy in a forensic psychiatric unit. *Journal of the New Zealand Association of Occupational Therapists*, 41, 18–22.

Seek, N. (1989). The New Zealand prison system: The potential role of occupational therapy. *Journal of the New Zealand Association of Occupational Therapists*, 40, 16–19.

Simon, R., & Aaronson, D. (1988). *The insanity defense: A critical assessment of law and policy in the post-Hinkley era*. New York: Praeger.

Smith, J. A., & Faubert, M. (1990). Programming and process in prisoner rehabilitation: A pison mental health center. *Journal of Offender Counseling Services and Rehabilitation*, 15, 131–153.

Stein, F., & Cutler, S. (2002). *Psychosocial occupational therapy: A holistic approach* (2nd ed.). Albany, NY: Delmar.

Sturm, H. V. (1988). OT gives new outlook to inmates of a Texas prison. *OT Week*, 2(22), 16–17.

Taylor, E. (1997). Forensic practice for the occupational therapist—The Alberta experience. *World Federation of Occupational Therapists (WFOT) Bulletin*, 36, 6–10.

Wittman, P. (2001, October 15). Occupational therapy behind bars. *OT Practice*, 11–15.

Vocational Programming

Eileen S. Auerbach, MS, OTR/L
Glenda Jeong, PhD, OTR/L

Key Terms

Americans with Disabilities
Act (1990)
assertive community treatment
(ACT)
community support team
Individual Placement and Support
(IPS) model
job coach
prevocational services

psychiatric or psychosocial
rehabilitation
Role Acquisition Frame
of Reference
seriously and persistently
mentally ill (SMI)
supported employment (SE)
work programming

Chapter Outline

Introduction

A primary goal of occupational therapists working in community mental health is to support independent living. Assisting someone to enter or reenter the workforce provides a real and meaningful context in which both the occupational therapist and the client can address issues of daily living. The work arena becomes the backdrop for occupational therapy interventions aimed at assisting an individual to reestablish his or her age-appropriate balance in work, play, and leisure.

Providing occupational therapy within a community context requires the recognition that one is truly operating in an open, dynamic system with many players. Maintaining sensitivity to the community context ensures that the activities pursued are both personally and socially meaningful. Figure 21-1 depicts the multiple levels of collaboration necessary when operating in a dynamic community context and shows how the vocational approach is the most useful and meaningful model for clients and therapists.

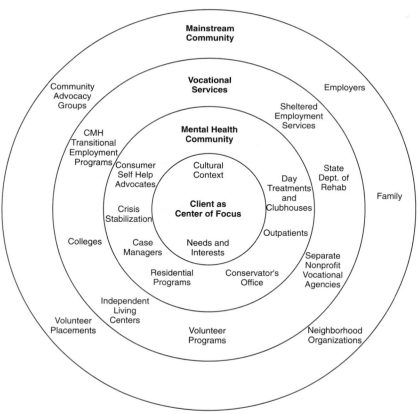

Figure 21-1. Levels of Collaboration

HISTORY OF WORK PROGRAMMING IN OCCUPATIONAL THERAPY

Occupation involves engaging with clear intent in activity that nourishes and sustains one's relationship to oneself (body, mind, and spirit) and one's relationship to the community. The value of work—that is, productive activity—has always been key to the philosophical basis of the profession. The roots of occupational therapy come from moral treatment, an approach that was used in the early 1900s for humane treatment of the mentally ill. During World War I, occupational therapy assisted disabled soldiers to regain their self-discipline, build their morale, and obtain training for reentering the civilian workforce. Operating from a holistic perspective, occupational therapy continued to be actively involved in the work adjustment of soldiers through the early 1900s during the immediate post–World War I period. During that same period, the Vocational Rehabilitation Act (Smith-Fess Act, Public Law 66-236) of 1920 established rehabilitation as a necessary service benefit for disabled individuals to enable them to return to remunerative employment (Flexor & Solomon, 1993). Occupational therapists actively developed **prevocational services** through the 1930s, and in 1943, with the passage of the Vocational Rehabilitation Amendment (Barder-La Follete Act/Public Law 78-113), people with psychiatric and developmental disabilities became eligible for such benefits. During this time, occupational therapists, including those in mental health, were actively involved with work adjustment programming.

In spite of the clear need and opportunity for occupational therapists to continue and expand their roles within work programming during the post–World War II era, there was a decline in professional interest during the 1950s. However, during the 1960s the profession saw a resurgence in this area with the emergence of evaluation practices in industrial therapy.

Only from the 1980s to the present has **work programming** begun to progress beyond being seen as a specialty within community mental health practice and have occupational therapists begun to practice work-related interventions as part of their expected role. If occupational therapy began as a forerunner in this arena in clear alignment with rehabilitation, what contributed to the shifting paradigm? With respect to work programming, some noteworthy occurrences during the 1950s and 1960s had a significant impact in shaping the direction of mental health occupational therapy and the changes it is making today.

A phenomenon that was most prevalent in the 1950s was the adoption of the medical model of diagnosis and treatment that prevailed in all arenas of health care, including psychiatry. Occupational therapy was no exception. Embracing the medical model, occupational therapy shifted away from its holistic perspectives and adopted the more popular scientific, reductionist perspectives (Lang, 1991). This philosophical perspective viewed human behavior as purely a result of biological and physiological, mechanical function. Like a machine, the human could be dismantled and reduced and then understood by examining its structural parts. Hence, humans were considered separate from nature and the mind considered separate from the body. This perspective manifested itself in medicine as specialties in practice emerged. Emphasis was placed on developing expertise in specific modalities and techniques. While occupational therapists in physical disabilities became experts at adaptive equipment, occupational therapists in mental health became experts at craft modalities and projective techniques for supporting the psychoanalytic process.

Although the 1960s was also the era of deinstitutionalization, it was marked by greater focus on occupational therapy practice to assist the individual to "process" feelings through activity. The therapeutic focus was limited to a part of the client—the psyche—without a visibly meaningful link to the whole client as a center of focus for community function. That is not to say occupational therapy did not address function, but within the medical model, function had a biomechanical meaning. For instance, occupational therapeutic interventions were aimed at structuring medication management, with the end goal being to alleviate symptoms. Given the prevailing viewpoint of the era—that people with mental illness could never improve—achieving maintenance and stability of the condition was considered achieving function.

Ironically, while the medical model took precedence, the 1950s also saw the emergence of the psychosocial rehabilitation programs in community mental health. Hallmark agencies such as Fountainhouse and Thresholds were established throughout the country with the mission of improving the lives of people with mental illness by providing a supportive environment for learning skills and encouraging mastery through community membership and activity. The goal of the **psychosocial or psychiatric rehabilitation** model is to assure that the person with a psychiatric disability can perform those physical, emotional, social, and intellectual skills needed to live, learn, and work in the community with the least amount of professional support necessary (Anthony & Liberman, 1992). The specific professional grounding of psychiatric rehabilitation was in vocational rehabilitation, and, although the concept of psychiatric rehabilitation has more recently expanded to include domains of social and community functioning, the area of work remains its primary focus. Its two main intervention strategies are client skill development and environmental resource development. As in occupational therapy's Role Acquisition Frame of Reference, the conceptual framework of this model relies upon skill development in expected social roles in the expected environment.

It was not until the late 1960s that the occupational therapy profession expressed concern over the paucity of work programming in mental health, and it was not until the late 1970s and early 1980s that occupational therapy began to increase its involvement with work programming for people with psychiatric disabilities.

Occupational therapists began to recognize that the psychosocial rehabilitation perspective was similar philosophically to the perspective held by the profession of occupational therapy. Indeed, the following principles are common to both:

- There can be no health without meaningful occupation.
- People can change themselves by their own efforts, and they have the choice—and responsibility—to do so.

- To effect change requires enlisting client choice and engaging in activities that promote skill building, exploration, education, and community role development.

The two fields share common interests, philosophies, and modes of treatment. Although it is possible to regard the two areas as competitive, many consider occupational therapists to be full practitioners of psychiatric rehabilitation, albeit with their own developed practice framework.

An example is occupational therapy's **Role Acquisition Frame of Reference**, which is concerned with the learning of social roles required of the individual in an expected environment (Mosey, 1996). Decisions about areas of focus in treatment are determined in the context of the individual's society and cultural group, the person's current and expected environment, and conceptualized role categories. The types of roles and the ways the individual adapts to them are affected by that person's interests and goals. The assumption is that behavior is influenced by the environment, that areas of function are discrete and can be addressed separately, and that adaptive behavior is learned directly by experience in the expected environment. Purposeful activities of meaning to the individual are viewed as practical paths to learning skills and developing the abilities that form the basis of a life role like that of worker.

Acquisitional frames of reference utilize learning theories and behavioral approaches (Falk-Kessler, 1998; Mosey, 1996). Once a desired social role, such as that of worker, is prioritized, those task and interpersonal skills needed to maintain that role are acquired by practice and repetition in a reinforcing environment. It is assumed that individuals have a need to explore their environment and become competent, and the acquisitional models rely on client motivation and collaboration. There is an emphasis on doing; the person is aware and consciously learning; reality is stressed and, although activity may at first be simulated, as soon as possible there is a shift to natural activities.

In the Role Acquisition Frame of Reference, treatment to learn the adaptive behavior required by a social role would begin with task skills and interpersonal skills in the context of temporal adaptation. Behavioral change regarding social roles is acquired through activities that are designed to elicit the desired behavior. These learning activities would be of interest to the individual, would stimulate exploration and accomplishment, and would provide learning partners and role models.

EXPANDING ROLES OF OCCUPATIONAL THERAPISTS

The present trends in health care provide numerous opportunities for occupational therapists to creatively carve out new roles and perspectives. As psychotropic medications become more effective, the most disabling symptoms of **seriously and persistently mentally ill (SMI)** clients are being reduced, permitting their subsequent discharge from locked facilities back into their communities. It is the job of the **community support team** to assist these individuals in their reintegration back into community life by helping them identify and learn the skills necessary to survive. Among these are those needed for their new roles, such as that of worker.

But when is a person with SMI ready to return to work? And when the person experiences problems on a job, what factors need to be addressed? The occupational therapist, trained to perform task analysis in the field and to analyze the components that comprise functional performance, is able to analyze the factors that contribute to individual performance. The OTR can recommend and carry out targeted skill development for the client and can influence change in environmental factors for the severely mentally ill worker that may enhance the milieu for the rest of the workforce, disabled or not. The OTR providing employment supports is able to apply knowledge of the **Americans with Disabilities Act (1990)** to facilitate compliance in such areas as reasonable accommodations, job analysis, and identification of essential functions for jobs. People with histories of severe mental illness may avoid disclosure and subsequently miss out on important job accommodations through fear of stigma and discrimination. These fears are not unfounded. Employers rank their level of comfort in working with the mentally ill second to last of all different disability groups (U.S. Congress, 1994). Workers with severe mental illness benefit greatly from supports in all these areas. The needs of severely mentally ill clients who wish to enter the workforce have opened up a wide variety of opportunities for OTRs, who can utilize their unique practice skills in **supported employment (SE)** and education programs, assertive community treatment teams, and psychosocial clubhouses as service providers, program development consultants, and community-based advocates and educators.

Knowing Your Customers—New Alliances

In the current health care environment, high-quality, cost-effective service within the community is a priority. For the occupational therapist, providing service in a larger public arena can mean expanding one's definition of the customer. In this instance, customers include not only those who receive direct services, but also those who fund the services—and thus indirectly benefit. These customers can become important allies.

Clearly, the most important customers are the clients served and their family members and significant others. When clients value services, their message and active support carry weight in the clinic, community, and political arenas. Family members and significant others are also significant advocates (for further discussion see Chapter 2), representing a powerful voice about which services are critical to the health of their loved ones.

Internal allies. Intragency as well as interagency coordination often provides a vehicle for education within the provider community. Services that assist clients to attain functional outcomes, such as school or paid employment, demonstrate concretely to professional peers, administrators, policy makers, and community organizations the value of including occupational therapists in the multidisciplinary community team.

Community allies. The needs and concerns of the business community are important because it is this community group that holds and creates the jobs. A core role of the employment specialist is advocacy for the client with the employer. Additional services can include troubleshooting when symptoms interfere with job performance, analysis and recommendations to facilitate an optimal worksite environment, and collaboration on relationships with employer and co-workers. Suggestions regarding reasonable accommodations may include such areas as workstation setup, modification of schedules, assignment sharing, and need for targeted sick leave to manage therapy appointments. Employers in general avoid risk in hiring practices. Because entry-level and low-skill jobs routinely attract unreliable applicants, employers may be experienced with quirky, undependable, or slow workplace behaviors and used to spending extra time training many people with poor employment histories. Especially appealing to employers is knowing that they have a highly motivated job candidate who is supported by an employment specialist who will maintain contact with the employer, help with job skill training, facilitate good work habits, and assist in work adjustment and problem solving (Auerbach, 2001b; Marrone, Gandolfo, Gold, & Hoff, 1998).

IMPLEMENTATION OF OCCUPATIONAL THERAPY SERVICES

An occupational therapist is a facilitator at all levels of occupational therapy service and all phases of service implementation. As a facilitator, the occupational therapist's action and goals are directed by the original needs and interests expressed by clients.

Assessment

Current studies (Bond, Drake, Mueser, & Becker, 1997; Bond, 1998) have demonstrated that lengthy assessment followed by experience in treatment facility-based or transitional jobs only serves to prolong the pre-employment phase of treatment, unnecessarily delaying entry into paid, mainstream employment. Although clients are placed in various alternative work environments, such as treatment center-based jobs, sheltered employment, or transitional employment for many other reasons, including dealing with apprehension about loss of benefits, workplace anxiety, a stated client preference for a gradual approach into work, and unstable behaviors (Rogers, Anthony, Cohen, & Davies, 1997; Auerbach, 2001a), the benefits of using these types of graduated, step-wise entry into the workplace as useful means of assessing performance and predicting success have been largely discounted (Anthony, 1994; Anthony & Jansen, 1984). Instead, there has been a more recent focus on the advantages of supported employment, which places the individual in a job of that client's choice, then provides intensive supports, including on-the-job training and ongoing assessment in the actual workplace context for as long as the client needs it (Becker & Drake, 1993; Bond, 1998). There is significant evidence of the advantages of time-unlimited support and assessment in community-based, integrated employment, with this model of employment services, variously called Place-Then-Train, Choose-Get-Keep, and the **Individual Placement and Support (IPS) models** (Danley, Sciarappa, & MacDonald-Wilson, 1992; Drake, 1998). However, systems of care can be slow to change, especially when there is a need for reallocation of resources. So, at this time many mental health providers continue to refer clients to a variety of more traditional pre-employment experiences. Some of these placements are brokered by contract agencies offering rehabilitation services, which often are more or less separate from the treatment team. Clients are evaluated and assigned to different types of training jobs prior to receiving assistance with job search, placement, and support in mainstream employment (Auerbach, 2001a; Marrone, 1993). Among these types of experiences are the following:

- Sheltered employment: training and employment are limited to specific disability groups, including persons with developmental and psychiatric disabilities. Work is done in segregated environments on subcontracted jobs from outside industry (Bond, 1992). Payment is pro-rated according to productivity, with the center usually having a subminimum wage certificate. Sheltered settings have not proved to be an effective conduit to mainstream employment, but they do provide a work experience and a modified income to persons unable to perform in a regular, competitive work setting without intensive, continuing supervision.

- In-house jobs: these may include work-oriented day treatment programs and psychosocial rehabilitation clubhouses, such as Fountain House in New York, Thresholds in Chicago, or Towne House Creative Living Center in Oakland (Marrone, 1993). In these settings, the day activity is work, performed by both clients and staff. Staff both supervise and model appropriate workplace behaviors, teaching in the context of the job itself and also in more formalized skills training groups. Supported employment in community-based settings may also be offered in these programs after a specified period of time, in the form of assistance with job development, coaching, and continuing follow-along for a period of time.

- Transitional employment: this approach refers to "temporary community jobs employing clients under an arrangement between a psychosocial rehabilitation agency and a community employer" (Bond, 1992, p. 248). These jobs are established to be appropriate to the members' abilities and endurance, designed to help them adjust to work, enhance their self-confidence, and offer job experiences for their résumés (Bond, Drake, Mueser, & Becker, 1997).

Mental health treatment teams in acute settings such as hospitals, in longer-term settings such as locked facilities, day treatment, or behavioral health facilities, or in other longer-term settings such as outpatient and case management programs seek a definitive predictor of whether a given client will succeed in a job before they invest resources in that person's vocational rehabilitation. Despite differing opinions about clear-cut indicators of success, there are certain qualities that have been associated with positive outcomes in work-related rehabilitation efforts (Bond et al., 1997; Stauffer, 1986). We do know that persons with a work history are more likely to work again (Anthony, 1994; Anthony & Jansen, 1984). We have observed that clients' motivation to work plays a significant role in their job tenure, taking the form of their repeatedly seeking assistance to solve problems and in their general resilience (Auerbach, 2001b; Braitman et al., 1995). Also associated with success in the workplace is seeking entrance to a vocational program, ability to get along with others, level of self-esteem, and working in a job and an environment that the person likes (Anthony, 1994; Kirsh, 2000a; 2000b). Many studies demonstrate that the best clinical predictors of future work performance are ratings of a person's work adjustment skills made in a workshop setting or sheltered job site (Anthony & Jansen, 1984; Anthony, 1994). Assessment of work adjustment skills is a traditional area of expertise of the occupational therapist, and one that bears a closer look.

From the OT perspective, the usefulness of pre-employment evaluation has less to do with anticipating success or failure on the job than with supplying information for the mental health team members who will be providing the job supports. Once the mental health treatment providers—and this may include the outpatient therapist, case manager, occupational therapist, psychiatric rehabilitation counselor, job coach, or psychiatrist—know the client's deficits or weak areas, they are in a better position to anticipate difficulties in certain workplace situations, they can tailor support strategies with the client in advance, and, earlier in the process, they can offer problem-solving assistance to client and employer, before a small disturbance or issue on a job escalates into a big problem and the client is fired or quits.

What is the purpose of an initial assessment of performance? The OT is usually called in to determine competence in specific areas of daily life skills and to make a decision about the person's readiness for rehabilitation. There are several approaches to an initial occupational profile, including an unstructured or semi-structured interview (Auerbach, 2002; Page, 1999; Henry & Mallinson, 1999); a structured checklist of information, such as Mosey's survey of task skills (Mosey, 1996, p. 453); rating scales, such as Ethridge's Pre-vocational Evaluation of Rehabilitation Potential (Ethridge, 1968); work samples, such as the Valpar series, which are now generally seen as too time-consuming, with equivalent information available more readily in simple observation during clinic or workshop task performance; and cognitive assessments, such as the Allen Cognitive Level Test (Allen, Earhart, & Blue, 1992). Studies in the psychiatric rehabilitation literature for years have cited a particular rating scale, the Pre-Vocational Evaluation of Rehabilitation Potential developed by an occupational therapist (Ethridge, 1968) and considered a valid and reliable tool to assess work adjustment. This rating scale (Figure 21-2) is a 4-point scale: (1) very poor performance, (2) poor performance, (3) average or acceptable performance, and (4) excellent performance. Ethridge describes a score of 60 or above indicating good work adjustment and a score of below 60 indicating relatively poor work adjustment (p. 162).

Pre-Vocational Evaluation of Rehabilitation Potential

NAME _____
DATE _____
RATER _____
ASSIGNMENT _____

WORK SKILLS, HABITS, AND TOLERANCE

1. Interest, motivation or enthusiasm	Eager, absorbed Good or excellent	Acceptable Fair	Poor, Ambivalent Slow to interest	Little or none, Indifferent
2. Initiative, ability to initiate activity, energy output	Energetic, initiates jobs, absorbed	Adequate, applies self to job	Poor, slow to get started	Little or none, Can't start job
3. Ability to follow through, concentration, attention span	Attention good, Hard to mislead	Adequate attention, Satisfactory	Poor, needs reminding	Little or none, Distractible
4. Ability to take directions or authority, accepting of suggestions, response to controls	Good, adequate, Responds well	Accepting, tolerant, Responds to suggestions	Avoiding, openly defiant Debates suggestions	Poor, resentful, hostile, critical Resents authority
5. Quality of workmanship, neatness, accuracy, manual dexterity	Neat, exact, few mistakes, adequate	Passable, acceptable Improving skills	Poor, below average Untidy, errors	Inept, careless, slovenly
6. Quantity of work, production	Good, above average Considerable work	Average or acceptable, spasmodic	Below standard, Less than required	Little or none, Unacceptable
7. Attendance, punctuality, regularity	Regular, punctual, Stays overtime	Usually prompt, Fairly consistent	Unpredictable, often late, inconsistent	Irregular, late Habitual absence

SOCIALIZATION, ATTITUDE TOWARD OTHERS

1. Participation in social activities	Enjoys activities, Active participant	Goes regularly, some participation	Occasionally attends Little participation	Never participant Stays to himself
2. Verbalization, quantity and content	Appropriate, enjoys conversation Initiates discussions	Responds to conversation, No unusual speech	Chatters, often rambling —or— Underproductive	Talks constantly, confused, rambling —or— Doesn't talk
3. Aggressivity, hostility	None noticed, Appropriate	Occasional but no problems	Sometimes causes problems	Extremely high, Irritates others
4. Thoughtfulness, peer adjustment	Praises properly, Interested in others	Notices others and needs, shares	Doesn't share, indifferent	Belittles others, Non-sharing, taker

PERSONALITY CHARACTERISTICS

5. Ability to work with others, cooperativeness	Unable to adjust, Hostile, withdrawn Antagonizes others	Stubborn, distant Aloof, critical, Irritable	Quiet, but friendly Generally acceptable, fits in	Stimulates others, Active, friendly, Group participant
1. Unusual behavior or mannerisms	Hallucinates, gestures, bizarre	Occasionally noted, Can be controlled	Rare inappropriate behavior	Actions never unusual
2. Anxiety	Extremely high, Easily produced —or— Extremely low, Apathetic	Sensitive, often observed, Interferes with work	Moderately anxious, sometimes affects work	Casual, normal and appropriate
3. Judgment, dependability, responsibility	Irresponsible, inaccurate, oversteps authority	Needs reminding, Often inaccurate, Not dependable	Average, accepts responsibility Usually reliable	Sound in judgment Eager to advance
4. Frustration tolerance, self-control, emotional control	Verbal abuse, destructive, temper tantrums	Occasional poor control, moody	Mood seldom affects work, shows control	Very stable, well controlled

GENERAL OBSERVATIONS

1. Appearance	Slovenly, unkempt Inappropriate	Occasionally sloppy careless	Acceptable Usually presentable	Appropriate, well-groomed
2. Learning capacity, general intelligence	Slow or faulty Unable to learn	Slow to catch on, poor retention	Able to learn with instruction	Learns rapidly Remembers well
3. Knowledge of equipment, safety and shop policies	Needs help constantly, forgets procedures, hazard	Partial knowledge Some mistakes, a few accidents	Learns correct procedures, a safe worker	Can repair equipment, safe, protects others
4. Use of time	Dawdles, can't make up mind Unorganized	Wastes time, poor organization Slow at decisions	Usually on the job, Manages situations	Efficient, always busy, accurate and fast

Figure 21-2. Prevocational Evaluation of Rehabilitation Potential

The Program for Assertive Community Treatment, considered a model of the integration of employment and treatment services for persons with severe and persistent mental illness, initially assesses clients through a structured interview. Included are a work history and description of work interests, skills, and abilities; ratings of social functioning and psychological and illness factors, including a description of types of support needed; and relevant social-environmental factors, such as physical obstacles (e.g., transportation) or entitlement disincentives (Frey & Godfrey, 1991). As with the IPS model, PACT's vocational assessment is ongoing, with data gathered in the competitive work environment.

Occupational therapists use a variety of other tests, only some of which are designed by OTs. Examples of these are the Jacobs Prevocational Skills Assessment (Jacobs, 1991); the Bay Area Functional Performance Evaluation (BaFPE) (Bloomer & Lang, 1987); and a variety of tests to explore vocational interest areas, such as the California Occupational Preference Survey (COPS, 1971) or the Strong Interest Inventory (1994). In cases where there are mixed diagnoses, such as head injuries resulting in cognitive and physical deficits, it may be important to collaborate with practitioners in other service areas to evaluate functioning. Because OTs have a broad educational background covering neurological and physical dysfunction, their scope of practice covers other areas of disability and permits them to incorporate evaluation tools with a broader emphasis than psychosocial rehabilitation.

Figure 21-3 is an example of a client's self-report questionnaire used as the basis of a structured interview to develop an occupational profile. The information sought is comprehensive, covering all areas of occupation, only a part of which concerns work.

All in all, in deciding the type of assessment to use, it is helpful to consider the predicted length of stay in the treatment or vocational program, the purpose for the evaluation, and whether the client is self-selected for vocational services, that is, whether it is possible to gauge in advance the client's level of motivation.

Depending on the setting, the depth, extent, and value of vocational assessment can often be tailored to meet the needs of consumers at various levels of care. The process is often determined by the consumer's level of focus and expressed desire to consider work activity. The occupational therapist may find that, at the very least, this expressed interest can be an opening for dialogue and short-term interventions. Dialogue can be particularly useful when the identified barriers to working are related to disability management issues (e.g., medication compliance, self-medication with substances).

Note that the vocational counselor may be the same person as the occupational therapist. It is also likely that the occupational therapist may work in a consultative role. The choices and decisions made regarding the vocational plan of action are determined jointly by the client and the practitioner, often within the context of the treatment team. The client can choose to adopt or reject the recommendations of the practitioner. Service options can include job-seeking skills groups, time management and stress management skills training, social security benefits counseling, referral assistance to enter employment training programs

Date: _____
Team: _____
Case Manager: _____
ID#: _____

Occupational Profile

1. Client Information

Name _____ Date of Birth _____ Age _____

Address _____ Zip _____ Phone _____

Social Security No. _____ Marital Status _____

Where did you grow up?

Where is your family of origin now?

Describe your present living situation (type of housing and with whom):

Children's ages (if any):

Current source of income:

2. Education

Highest level of school completed:

Where: High School:

        College, Trade or Vocational School:

Do you have any degrees, licenses or certificates?
  Specify which type, date, and where received:

Have you ever had any special problems in school (e.g. learning disabilities, attention deficits)? Please describe:

Which were your favorite subjects?

Which were your least favorite subjects?

Do you plan to return to school? _____ Area of study? _____

3. Who in your household does these chores?

Grocery shopping: Laundry:
Cooking: Housecleaning:
Dishes: Bill paying:

Do you think the household tasks are shared in a fair way? _____

Figure 12-3. Sample Occupational Profile (adapted from Auerbach, 2002)

4. Work experience

Usual Occupation: _____

What are the last three jobs have you held (starting with the most recent):

Job Title	Dates of employment	Types of Duties	Reasons for leaving
a.			
b.			
c.			

Which was your favorite job of all you've done?

Which was your least favorite job?

What are your plans for returning to work?

What would you like to be doing a year from now?

Could you benefit from vocational counseling? _____

5. Individual activities, social and leisure time

List your special interests and hobbies:

_____

_____

What other things would you like to do in your spare time?

Do you like to read? What do you usually read? _____
Have you had any trouble concentrating lately?

_____

Do you generally spend your free time ❏ alone or ❏ with others
What kinds of things have you done with friends?

Figure 12-3. (continued)

6. Health and fitness

Have you ever participated in physical exercise ❑, active sports ❑, or have a fitness routine ❑?

Please describe:

What could you do to be more physically fit?

Do you have any physical problems that could prevent you from participating fully in such activities as bowling, stretching exercises, dance, movement, swimming, walking, etc.? (please describe)

❑ Blood pressure problems _____

❑ Back pain _____

❑ Cardiac or circulation problems _____

❑ Seizures _____

❑ Vision problems _____

❑ Joint Problems (e.g. arthritis) _____

❑ Other _____

Do you have a special diet? Please describe:

Do you feel best when you are active and productive? (please check ✓) ❑

   Or resting and unoccupied? ❑

7. Your typical day

List the activities in your daily routine (e.g. meals, work, recreation or leisure activities, therapy appointments or programs, housekeeping or child care responsibilities, shopping):

Morning:

(time you usually get up: _____)

(time you usually eat breakfast: _____)

_____

_____

(time you usually eat lunch: _____)

Afternoon:

_____

_____

(time you usually eat dinner: _____)

Evening:

_____

_____

(time you usually go to bed: _____)

Figure 12-3.   (continued)

8. Activities of Daily Living

Are you satisfied with how you are managing your daily self-care tasks?

I'm doing:	ok	not ok	Please explain
Eating well			
Food shopping			
Cooking meals or eating in restaurants			
Shopping for clothes and personal items			
Personal cleanliness and hygiene (e.g. teeth, hair, showering, laundry)			Teeth: Hair: Showers/baths: Shaving: Laundry:
Housekeeping (e.g. dusting, cleaning kitchen, bathroom, vacuuming)			
Money managing (e.g. budgeting, cashing checks, paying bills)			
Taking care of business (e.g. filling out forms, keeping appointments, etc.)			
Transportation (e.g. ❏ walking ❏ MUNI ❏ BART ❏ car ❏ bike)			
Ability to concentrate			

9. What would you like to be doing one year from now? (e.g. any changes in work, school, social life, leisure activities, other activities of daily living or areas of self-care?)

Figure 12-3. (continued)

or educational programs, and job development or work adjustment follow-along, depending on the desired goal.

Once the client is engaged in training or on the job, situational assessments are done to evaluate progress. These are done on the worksite while the person is performing the job or during telephone or in-person check-in before or after work. The following case illustration is an example of the evaluation process.

> ### CASE ILLUSTRATION: Charlotte—Occupational Therapy Evaluation
>
> *Charlotte is a 56-year-old female diagnosed with chronic paranoid schizophrenia who expressed interest in paid transitional work experience in the community. She was referred by a San Francisco mental health program to a vocational rehabilitation agency in San Francisco. Charlotte was specifically interested in the Clerical Program because her previous work history was in the secretarial field. After the initial intake interview, Charlotte was referred by the projects coordinator to occupational therapy for the vocational evaluation and assessment. The client was administered a battery of tasks designed to assess performance in specific work-related areas. Cognitive abilities, learning styles, strengths and limitations with respect to employment, social and communication skills, safety awareness, and special needs with respect to ability and disability were evaluated. Functional activities of daily living (ADL) skills, sensory perception and motor functioning, physical endurance, self-concept, and judgment were also assessed. A baseline for understanding the client's current skill level and work readiness was established to assist Charlotte, the occupational therapist, and the vocational counselors in determining appropriate job placement in the community.*
>
> *As a short-term goal, Charlotte wanted to receive clerical training and transitional work experience from the Clerical Program for approximately three to four hours per day, three days per week. Her long-term educational and vocational goals were to learn computer skills for data entry and to find a part-time clerical job in the community.*
>
> *From the assessment, it was determined that Charlotte had the following difficulties:*
>
> 1. *poor problem-solving skills*
> 2. *poor short-term memory*
> 3. *difficulty making decisions and self-correcting work*
> 4. *difficulty planning with foresight and accuracy*
> 5. *decreased activity tolerance (two hours)*
> 6. *need for increased time to learn new tasks*
> 7. *poor stress and frustration tolerance*
>
> *From the assessment, it was also determined that Charlotte had the following assets:*

1. *very motivated to work and to learn computer skills*
2. *previous work experience*
3. *clear, legible penmanship*
4. *able to initiate questions when needing clarification of instruction*
5. *strong sorting and filing skills*
6. *excellent telephone-answering skills*
7. *good self-care habits*
8. *daily living routines consistent with desired goals*

From the results of the assessment, the following functional requirements were identified:

1. *a very structured environment*
2. *clearly defined tasks*
3. *increased time to learn new tasks*
4. *both written and verbal instruction*
5. *compensatory techniques (e.g., lists)*
6. *feedback from supervisors and co-workers regarding task performance and decision making*
7. *opportunities to practice problem-solving behavior in familiar settings with familiar people and with simple tasks in simple situations*
8. *a break every two hours until activity tolerance increases*

After completing the Clerical Program five months later, Charlotte was placed in a paid transitional secretarial position at a human service agency. She did very well in her secretarial position and was referred to the job developer three months later to begin searching for permanent employment in the community.

Forms of Intervention

Client choices often determine the nature, timing, and context for occupational therapeutic interventions. The arena varies from the treatment or agency site to the community and the workplace. Regular assessment and/or intervention can occur at the training or work sites. The occupational therapist can often work with the training supervisors to adapt the training or work process.

Group or Individual Counseling. Counseling takes the form of problem solving as opposed to psychotherapeutic sessions. The stated objective is to support the individual in learning how to manage situations that arise within a day-to-day context. The focus is on the immediate situation, learning from the present moment, and developing personal resiliency for the future. The therapeutic value lies in consumer/client empowerment—empowering the client in his or her ability to make decisions, act on them, and learn from the experiences.

Problem solving occurs most often while assisting people to build interpersonal and communication skills. Often, uncertainty results from not knowing how to interpret an interaction. The cognitive stress from perceptions based on incomplete information or misinterpreted nonverbal cues is often the source of stress and difficulties in getting along with others.

People have greater motivation to take in new information and apply what they learn when they are concurrently engaged in work. The day-to-day issues can provide concrete incentives for addressing specific issues or to learn skills that relate directly to one's job or role.

The following case describes an example of an assertive community treatment (ACT)'s OT staff delivering first treatment center-based then community-based employment services to a client with co-occurring diagnoses.

CASE ILLUSTRATION: Mr. T.—A Gradualist Approach to Vocational Programming

Mr. T., a longtime client of a mental health day treatment center, was admitted to a newly formed assertive community treatment (ACT) program. He had an axis I diagnosis of psychotic disorder with delusions, secondary to a left arteri-ovenous malformation resection, that is, a brain injury after surgery to correct a cerebrovascular abnormality, which left him with neurological deficits, including recurrent episodes of paranoid delusions of religiosity. In addition, Mr. T. had right hemiparesis, expressive and some receptive aphasia, and a seizure disorder. Because of his difficulty with word-finding and his inability to grasp effectively with his right hand, it was very difficult to develop a job for him, and he worked in treatment center-based sheltered employment for several years.

Occupational Therapy

Initial evaluation of Mr. T's functional performance showed that because he was highly motivated to achieve and had a positive attitude toward task accomplishment, he was able to compensate for many impairments. He attempted whatever arts and crafts were offered in the Individual Projects OT group, participated fully in the Living Skills Class activities, began working on the Popcorn Project during prevocational OT groups, and regularly attended the Vocational Issues Group to fulfill his desire to work. Mr. T. eventually settled into one of the day treatment center's prevocational OT jobs working on a team that made and bagged popcorn to sell in the center.

Volunteer Employment

The next step for Mr. T. was a referral to the city's transitional volunteer center, where he was assigned to the Recreation and Parks Department as a volunteer in a short-term six-month job, watering plants in the nursery. OT staff helped him and his supervisor manage some of the problems he had, such as ways he could deal with how wet his feet were getting and how to adapt the watering can. In the past, leaving Mr. T. to struggle alone with these types of problems would precipitate suspicion and paranoia toward his boss or co-workers.

Transitional Employment

*After the time-limited job ended, OT staff referred Mr. T. to a vocational reha-
bilitation services agency that contracts with his county's Department of Community Mental Health Services to provide housing and jobs to its clients. Again,
this job was categorized as transitional, that is, a temporary training job owned
by the agency. Mr. T. was paid a minimum wage to mop, vacuum, and dust at
a support services hotel. Despite the limited mobility of his right lower extremity, Mr. T. was assigned to work on the stairs. He reported an inability to mop
the bathroom as the door kept shutting on him. OT staff made a site visit to
advocate that he have limited vacuuming assignments on stairs, and provided a
doorstop to keep the restroom door open for him. He was shown how to wrap
his affected hand around the mop and broom handles to stabilize the implement. He worked for over the allotted nine months on this assignment.*

*Despite this assistance, however, the vocational rehabilitation services staff
to which he had been referred determined that, although he had successfully
completed this limited-tenure transitional job, he was too slow to be productive
enough to compete for community-based jobs in integrated settings.*

Sheltered Employment

*The vocational rehabilitation services agency's job developer, an OTR, did not
think Mr. T. could be placed, and she recommended that he apply to the state
Department of Rehabilitation for training funds to send him to a sheltered
workshop. This organization gave him a packaging assignment with adapted
tools at subminimum wage. He worked at this job for over a year. However, the
sameness of the job eventually bored Mr. T., and he worried that his thoughts
were becoming morbid while working in this warehouse-like setting with other
mentally ill and developmentally disabled workers. Although OT staff persuad-
ed the owner to vary the work assignments, this intervention was not sufficient
to keep Mr. T. in the job. The tasks involved repetitive assembly of kits while
seated in a row of work stations, silent and isolated.*

Competitive, Community-Based, Integrated Employment

*An OT student next accompanied Mr. T. to a job fair advertised at the local fit-
ness center. The fitness center was looking for a part-time attendant for light
cleaning and to serve as a benign security presence in the locker room. Mr. T. was
highly motivated to move to a more stimulating work environment with regular
wages. The OT student accompanied him to the interviews, and provided the fitness center with information on the Private Industry Council (PIC), which offers
assistance to employers in qualifying for tax incentives, as well as the tax credit
forms for employers hiring disabled individuals who live in enterprise zones.*

*The fitness center employed Mr. T. and coached him through the training
phase with occupational therapy consultation. He required assistance to solve
simple logistical and equipment problems such as his needing a different handle length on the dustpan and larger rubber gloves for his hands. Because of*

Mr. T's aphasia, he had difficulty communicating his needs to his employer and understanding his employer's expectations and instructions. The OT student helped him solve problems with his supervisor regarding his initial need for frequent breaks, and developed a written checklist to help him organize a task and break routine. The client's psychosocial needs were addressed through problem-solving discussions regarding his misinterpretation of constructive criticism. He gradually learned that evaluation was not rejection or a potential firing, or that his work was not valued, but simply meant that he was to do things slightly differently. Further, the OT student educated the employer regarding the client's problem with recording his hours, as he had difficulty expressing numbers verbally and in writing because of his aphasia.

In the past, without this intensive outreach and support, Mr. T. would have succumbed to paranoia, and would have or did walk off the job or quit. The occupational therapy staff and students, with a grounding in both physical and psychosocial deficits, ability to do task analysis, and environmental modification at the job site, were prepared to help him manage work using both the gradualist and the direct entry approaches.

Money management skills. As individuals begin earning wages, money management and decision-making skills are developed concretely through learning how to calculate social security withholdings, report earnings, maintain records, and make decisions about increasing hours and jobs. Counseling and support are given throughout to assist the person to address the fears surrounding the loss of cash and medical benefits. Given the confusing nature of social security work incentives, it is only through continuous review of the information, support, and actual experience over time that a person can learn and gain confidence over money management. One example of a social security work incentive with which a client may need help in reporting is an Impairment Related Work Expense (IRWE). A person who has special needs in order to work may deduct these expenses from the earnings reported to the Social Security Administration. A person with a mental illness or cognitive impairments may need to pay for the assistance of a travel trainer to instruct in learning the route to work or with a **job coach** to train skills related to job duties.

When an individual on supplemental security income (SSI) reaches a point when he or she has set a specific employment objective and determined the specific equipment or training needs to achieve that goal, the occupational therapist can assist in developing a Plan for Achieving Self-Support (PASS) to set aside income funds for the long-term goal. An example of a PASS plan would be setting aside 10% of one's monthly wages over a year's time to pay for a computer, to be used to develop the person's career. This investment would lower the level of the person's income, and permit fewer dollars to be deducted from the individual's monthly social security checks.

The Ticket to Work program of the Social Security Administration is being slowly implemented nationally, and will increase the rehabilitation and vocational choices of people receiving assistance to get to work. It is not yet clear how this program will affect specific programs in the future. But it is certain that occupational therapists providing employment supports will benefit from keeping current on this program to better inform their clients and to be certain their services are of high quality so that they may qualify to be approved providers of these services (Social Security Administration, 2002). Again, the responsibility of decision making and choice returns to the client and is directly experienced as such.

Applying the skills in the community.   There are numerous opportunities to assist the client to practice communication skills, stress management, and organizational skills when the practitioner accompanies the client to outside community offices such as the local Social Security office, the local Employment Development Department office or hiring hall for job searches, the public library for vocational resources, the local community college campus or training site, or local neighborhoods or businesses to explore the types of job opportunities to be found there and to actually observe people at work. The occupational therapist can assist the client to anticipate questions and role-play the situation beforehand. After the visit, reviewing what happened reinforces learning and the client's sense of mastery. Regardless of the type of community-based activity, learning and adaptation are considered part of a growth process. Failure is reframed as a lesson learned to be added to one's stock of experience, reminding individuals that they are gaining their vocational maturity much in the same way that others have.

Interventions with the community.   As an advocate, educator, or consultant, the occupational therapist often works with several types of communities and groups. Such groups may include businesses and the organizations that support them, like the local chamber of commerce and Private Industry Council, consumer advocates, and other mental health and rehabilitation providers from either county or state and private sectors. The therapist can also practice the same concept of learning and adaptation for himself or herself when planning to work with community agencies, employers, and the local community at large.

It is often to the occupational therapist's benefit to research and identify the community or group audience with regard to values, attitudes, and culture. This can be part of a needs assessment done before the occupational therapist goes in to present information or education at a particular site. For instance, when working with an employment site, the workplace culture and practices can be identified and explored with the employees to facilitate the new employees' integration on the job as well as provide support services within or outside the workplace context (see Figure 21-4).

Interventions when the employer is involved.   Understanding the workplace culture assists to establish a dialogue with employers. An ideal situation would be an employer educated in the needs of mental health clients who would be receptive to hiring them as part of a diverse workforce and to providing the supports they might need. Employers of low-skill entry-level workers may have seen a range of performance and social behaviors in the past and found ways to draw out their best efforts. In developing an approach to informing the employer, it may be less helpful for the employer to understand all the dynamics of an individual's mental illness,

Community Mental Health	Local Community	Business Community
Consult/Educate Mental Health Providers Regarding:	Educate/Inform Members of the Community:	Consult/Educate Employers, Supervisors, Employees:
• Work readiness	• Mental illness	• ADA
• Program planning	• Support with	• Mental illness
• ADA	symptom	• Supervising employees
• System policy and	management	with mental illness
service design	• Resisting	• Staff education
• Supervision of	stigma	• Diversity awareness
consumer staff		

Types of forums for these interventions can be as follows:

Consult/Educate Mental Health Providers Regarding:	Educate/Inform Members of the Community:	Consult/Educate Employers, Supervisors, Employees:
• In-service	• Outreach	• Educational
presentations	• Community	• Sensitivity training
• Outreach	service education	• Community outreach

Figure 21-4. Types of Interventions within Different Communities

and offering a great deal of technical information may even alarm or intimidate the employer. Instead, the employment specialist can explore the workplace environment, talk with the employer or co-workers, and try to identify areas where a supportive intervention could ease stress and solve problems (Marrone et al., 1998). When a job is a good fit for the client, with shared values and a positive workplace culture, the employer, therapist, and client can form a team to analyze and resolve difficult situations (Kirsh, 2000a; 2000b). Many employers are unaware of how the Americans with Disabilities Act applies to such individuals. For an occupational therapist, adaptations made at the worksite are then considered reasonable accommodations for a qualified individual who can perform the essential functions of the job with certain modifications in either the job, the environment, or the supervisory process (Mancuso, 1993) (see Figure 21-5). Support is given to the employer throughout to address work issues that may arise. In the best-case scenario, an employer can appreciate certain accommodations as making good business sense for *all* employees. However, this does not always serve to eliminate the discrimination and stigma that an individual may fear or experience from others.

Interventions when the employer is not involved. When clients choose not to disclose their diagnoses, the decision must be respected and supportive interventions are done offsite. Coaching occurs in the preparation before and after

TYPES OF REASONABLE ACCOMMODATIONS

Modifications can be made to:

The Job	• Job sharing, trading duties between workers
Physical Environment	• Partitions
	• Rearranging/positioning location of work area in office
	• Changing fluorescent lighting
Assistive Aids or Technology	• Tape recorders
	• Day organizers
	• Handheld organizers (PDAs)
Schedule Modifications	• Change break times
	• Shift scheduled hours earlier/later
	• Work or paid/unpaid leave
Supervising Structure	• Additions or adaptations of supervision schedule/style
	• Mentor/buddy
	• Adapting mode of instruction/training
Policy and Work Culture	• Diversity training and education
	• Mental health days

Figure 21-5. Reasonable Accommodations

the job interview, on the telephone during working hours while on break, before or after work, and/or during lunch. Accommodations are rarely explicitly presented and often are worked out by the employee independently or with coaching.

Support takes whatever form the client perceives would be helpful, whether a peer support group, a peer counselor, a community group affiliation, a mental health agency affiliation or family and friends for therapeutic or socialization purposes.

The context of services. It is important to acknowledge that the extent, nature, and depth of occupational therapeutic intervention are driven, not only by customer choices and needs, but also by the setting in which the occupational therapist works. The variety of settings where occupational therapists work offer opportunities to develop programming to address varying levels of vocational and self-care needs of clients. Depending on the setting, the occupational therapist may focus on skills learning and building, skills application, or skills refinement and/or adaptation (see Figure 21-6).

CASE ILLUSTRATION: Lorelei—Direct Entry into Supported Employment

Lorelei is a 38-year-old female with a diagnosis of bipolar disorder mixed, recurrent, with psychotic features. Her residential counselor suggested that she apply for a deli position at a local supermarket, and, to her surprise, she was

Instrumental Activities of Daily Living Addressed Include:

- Money Management
- Transportation
- Stress Management
- Time Management
- Physical Health Self Care
- Communication Skills

Skills Learning and Building Can Begin within the Mental Health Community	Skills Application Can Occur in Vocational Settings	Skills Refinement Can Be Ongoing within the Mainstream Community
• Partial Hospitalization • ACT or case management programs	• Vocational Programs	• Community-Based Employment
• Day Treatment	• Volunteering	• Education
• Clubhouse Programs	• Transitional Employment Programs	

Figure 21-6.   Continuum for Occupational Therapy Assistance with Skills

hired. Her case manager at her **assertive community treatment (ACT)** program is an occupational therapist who regularly checks on her well-being on her job, and provides employment supports for Lorelei when she needs them. Because the ACT program offers long-term community support, these services are time unlimited. The two have worked on reality testing, anger management, problem-solving techniques, and assertive communications with her job supervisors, co-workers, and union representatives, including requesting reasonable accommodations for herself.

When she first started, Lorelei was thrilled to have a real community-based job in a regular integrated setting. However, issues arose that required some thinking-through. Lorelei had an excitable temperament and needed help in problem solving so that she could maintain control and achieve resolution of issues without blowing up or walking off the job. One of the OT/case manager's resources was a teaching technique found in the UCLA Social and Independent Living Skills Series, the problem-solving technique (UCLA, 1990), also described by Corrigan, Schade, and Liberman (1992). The client is assisted to understand the elements of the problem situation; a list of reasonable alternative solutions is developed and analyzed to determine feasibility; and the client decides which solution to try. Once the person has implemented the solution, the results are analyzed to determine their effectiveness. On several occasions, Lorelei had *been told to close down and clean the rotisserie too late in her shift, and, because this was a big, heavy job that took her a long time, she felt she was being set up to work extra unpaid time. Was her boss trying to indicate that she was too slow? Was he exploiting her? Lorelei was able to analyze the predicament with the OT/case manager, and eventually she decided to meet with her boss. She successfully negotiated extra time to complete the rotisserie cleanup to both their satisfaction and still be able to finish her shift on time.*

Another issue resulted in a more active OT/case manager intervention to assist her in disclosing her disability. Lorelei had been hired to work the swing shift at the deli; however, after a few months she was asked to work an A.M. shift one day, a swing shift the next, followed immediately by another A.M. shift. The result was an inadequate night's sleep between the swing shift and the next morning's A.M. shift. Lorelei's situation was delicate because her psychiatric condition, bipolar disorder, can be aggravated by irregular sleep patterns. The OT/case manager drafted a letter to the employer on the ACT program's letterhead stationery, which was co-signed by Lorelei's psychiatrist, requesting that she be allowed the reasonable accommodation of working the same shift throughout the work week to help prevent relapse. Her boss was understanding and readily agreed to this request.

When Lorelei moved to her next job as cashier at a drugstore, she was confronted with a new situation that required some on-site job coaching on the part of the OT/case manager. Lorelei was complaining of back strain, and the OT met with her for an on-site activity analysis at the drugstore, where she could observe Lorelei's work tasks firsthand. She was able to help Lorelei use back-saving biomechanics. First they worked on postural alignment. Then they practiced safe lifting techniques, first sliding the heavy purchases across the counter to be held close to her body before trying to lift them, as a way to reduce the torque on her back. These interventions readily cleared up her back strain, and she was successful in continuing the new job.

Job-related issues come up on a regular basis, and consistent support in her employment has helped Lorelei manage her symptoms, develop her problem-solving skills, and fully utilize all the resources she has available to her.

Summary

Occupational therapists who work in vocational rehabilitation may find themselves operating simultaneously within multiple arenas of service provision. Rather than considering it as a specialty, occupational therapy can be reframed to identify how services can directly contribute to a person's functional goals. Regardless of the number of arenas and where one stands in the system of care (see Figure 21-1), client choice can become both the central driving force and the compass for all aspects of service. The occupational therapist becomes primarily the navigator and facilitator.

Operating in a system of care requires continuous communication, negotiation, and adaptation. Such an arena is rich with experiences in which, much like the clients, occupational therapists can constantly challenge themselves to learn and adapt professionally in order to provide effective, evidence-based services.

To practice effectively in the community, many occupational therapists want to understand the total picture of health care and the community at large. Occupational therapy in work programming is not so much a specialty as it is a different, and perhaps renewed, commitment to reintegration of the severely mentally ill client into the community.

Review Questions

1. Name one occupational therapy frame of reference that closely reflects psychiatric rehabilitation's philosophy.
2. What are some unique contributions of the occupational therapist as a member of the community support team?
3. What types of assessment can an occupational therapist utilize in a work program?
4. What are some examples of workplace accommodations that may be available for workers with psychiatric disabilities?
5. How can the employment specialist help the worker make decisions about disclosure of disability to an employer?

References

Allen, C. K., Earhart, C. A., & Blue, T. (1992). Allen Cognitive Level Test, 1990. *Occupational therapy treatment goals for the physically and cognitively disabled.* Bethesda, MD: American Occupational Therapy Association.

Anthony, W. A. (1994). Characteristics of people with psychiatric disabilities that are predictive of entry into the rehabilitation process and successful employment. *Psychosocial Rehabilitation Journal, 17*(3), 3–13.

Anthony, W. A., & Jansen, M. A. (1984). Predicting the vocational capacity of the chronically mentally ill, research and policy implications. *American Psychologist, 39*(5), 537–544.

Anthony, W. A., & Liberman, R. P. (1992). Principles and practice of psychiatric rehabilitation. In A. P. Goldstein & L. Krasner (Series Eds.) & R. P. Liberman (Vol. Ed.), *General psychology series*: Vol. 166. *Handbook of psychiatric rehabilitation* (pp. 1–29). Boston: Allyn & Bacon.

Auerbach, E. (2001a). The individual placement and support model vs. the menu approach to supported employment: Where does occupational therapy fit in? *Occupational Therapy in Mental Health, 17*(2), 1–19.

Auerbach, E. (2001b). *The long term work experiences of persons with severe and persistent mental illness.* Unpublished master's thesis, San Jose State University, San Jose, CA.

Auerbach, E. (2002). *Occupational Profile.* Unpublished self-report questionnaire. (Available from Eileen Auerbach, Mission ACT, 2712 Mission Street, San Francisco, CA 94110; e-mail address: EenieA@aol.com.)

Becker, D. R., & Drake, R. E. (1993). *A working life: The individual placement and support (IPS) program.* Hanover: New Hampshire-Dartmouth Psychiatric Research Center.

Bloomer, J. S., & Lang, S. (1987). *Bay Area Functional Performance Evaluation (BaFPE).* Wayne, NJ: Maddak.

Bond, G. R. (1992). Vocational rehabilitation. In A. P. Goldstein & L. Krasner (Series Eds.) & R. P. Liberman (Vol. Ed.), *General psychology series*: Vol. 166. *Handbook of psychiatric rehabilitation* (pp. 244–275). Boston: Allyn & Bacon.

Bond, G. R. (1998). Principles of the individual placement and support model. *Psychiatric Rehabilitation Journal, 22*, 11–23.

Bond, G. R., Drake, R. E., Mueser, K. T., & Becker, D. R. (1997). An update on supported employment for people with severe mental illness. *Psychiatric Services, 48*(3), 335–345.

Braitman, A., Counts, P., Davenport, R., Zurlinden, B., Rogers, M., Clauss, J., Kulkarni, A., Kymla, J., & Montgomery, L. (1995). Comparison of barriers to employment for unemployed and employed clients in a case management program: An exploratory study. *Psychiatric Rehabilitation Journal, 19*(1), 3–8.

California Occupational Preference Survey (COPS). (1971). Educational and Industrial Testing Service, San Diego.

Corrigan, P. W., Schade, M. L., & Liberman, R. P. (1992). Social skills training. In A. P. Goldstein & L. Krasner (Series Eds.) & R. P. Liberman (Vol. Ed.), *General psychology series*: Vol. 166, *Handbook of psychiatric rehabilitation* (pp. 95–126). Boston: Allyn & Bacon.

Danley, K. S., Sciarappa, K., & MacDonald-Wilson, K. (1992). Choose-Get-Keep: A psychiatric rehabilitation approach to supported employment. In H. R. Lamb (Series Ed.) & R. P. Liberman (Vol. Ed.), *New directions for mental health services*: Vol. 53, *Effective psychiatric rehabilitation* (pp. 87–96). San Francisco: Jossey-Bass.

Drake, R. E. (1998). A brief history of the individual placement and support model. *Psychiatric Rehabilitation Journal, 22*, 3–7.

Ethridge, D. A. (1968). Pre-vocational assessment of rehabilitation potential of psychiatric patients. *American Journal of Occupational Therapy, 22*(3), 161–167.

Falk-Kessler, J. (1998). Occupational therapy models: Acquisitional frame of reference. In A. MacRae & E. Cara (Eds.), *Psychosocial occupational therapy in clinical practice* (pp. 115–119). Albany: Delmar.

Flexor, R. W., & Solomon, P. L. (1993). Introduction to psychiatric rehabilitation in practice. In R. W. Flexor & P. L. Solomon (Eds.), *Psychiatric rehabilitation in practice* (pp. xiii–xvii). Boston: Andover.

Frey, J. L., & Godfrey, M. (1991). A comprehensive clinical vocational assessment: The PACT approach. *Journal of Applied Rehabilitation Counseling, 22*(2), 25–28.

Henry, A. D., & Mallinson, T. (1999). The occupational performance history interview. In B. J. Hemphill-Pearson (Ed.), *Assessments in occupational therapy mental health: An integrative approach* (pp. 59–70). Thorofare, NJ: Slack.

Hunter, M. L. (1999). The prevocational assessment process in mental health occupational therapy. In B. J. Hemphill-Pearson (Ed.), *Assessments in occupational therapy mental health: An integrative approach* (pp. 109–115). Thorofare, NJ: Slack.

Jacobs, K. (1991). *Occupational therapy: Work-related programs & assessments* (2nd ed.). Boston: Little, Brown.

Kirsh, B. (2000a). Factors associated with employment for mental health consumers. *Psychiatric Rehabilitation Journal, 24*(1), 13–21.

Kirsh, B. (2000b). Organizational culture, climate and person-environment fit: Relationships with employment outcomes for mental health consumers. *Work, 14*, 109–122.

Lang, S. (1991). Perspectives—Work for psychiatrically disabled clients. In K. Jacobs (Ed.), *Work: A journal of prevention, assessment, and rehabilitation* (pp. 6–10). Boston: Andover.

Leavitt, R. T., & Spear, S. N. (1998). Cognitive assessments and work. *OT Practice, 3*(3), 35–38.

Mancuso, L. (1993). *Case studies on reasonable accommodations for workers with psychiatric disabilities.* Study funded by the Community Support Program at the Center for Mental Health Services of the U.S. Department of Health and Human Services, Substance Abuse and Mental Health Administration.

Marrone, J. (1993). Creating positive vocational outcomes for people with severe mental illness. *Psychosocial Rehabilitation Journal, 17*(2), 43–62.

Marrone, J., Gandolfo, C., Gold, M., & Hoff, D. (1998). Just doing it: Helping people with mental illness get good jobs. *Journal of Applied Rehabilitation Counseling, 29*(1), 37–48.

Mosey, A. C. (1996). *Psychosocial components of occupational therapy* (rev. ed.). Philadelphia: Lippincott-Raven.

Page, M. (1999). Interviewing as an assessment tool in occupational therapy. In B. J. Hemphill-Pearson (Ed.), *Assessments in occupational therapy mental health: An integrative approach* (pp. 19–39). Thorofare, NJ: Slack.

Rogers, E. S., Anthony, W. A., Cohen, M., & Davies, R. R. (1997). Prediction of vocational outcome based on clinical and demographic indicators among vocationally ready clients. *Community Mental Health Journal, 33*(2), 99–112.

Social Security Administration. (2002). The work site: Office of employment support programs. *Work Incentives.* Retrieved September 20, 2002, from http://www.ssa.gov/work/ResourcesToolkit/workincentives.html.

Stauffer, D. (1986). Predicting successful employment in the community for people with a history of chronic mental illness. *Occupational Therapy in Mental Health, 6*(2), 31–49.

Strong Interest Inventory. (1994). Palo Alto, CA: Stanford University Press.

UCLA Social & Independent Living Skills Series. (1990). Available from dissemination coordinator, Psychiatric Rehabilitation Consultants, PO Box 2867, Camarillo, CA 93011-2867, Phone: (805) 484-5663, Fax: (805) 484-0735. http://www.psychrehab.com/.

U.S. Congress. (1994, March). *Psychiatric disabilities, employment, and the Americans with Disabilities Act* (Office of Technology Assessment Report). Technology Assessment Board of the 103rd U.S. Congress.

U.S. Department of Justice, Civil Rights Division, Office on the Americans with Disabilities Act. (1990). *The Americans with Disabilities Act: Questions and Answers.*

Valpar International Corporation, P. O. Box 5767, Tucson, AZ 85703.

Suggested Reading

Anthony, W. A. (1994). Characteristics of people with psychiatric disabilities that are predictive of entry into the rehabilitation process and successful employment. *Psychosocial Rehabilitation Journal, 17*(13), 3–13.

Asher, I. E. (1996). *Occupational therapy evaluation tools: An annotated index* (2nd ed.). Bethesda, MD: American Occupational Therapy Association.

Bailey, E. L., Ricketts, S. K., Becker, D. R., Xai, H., & Drake, R. E. (1998). Do long term day treatment clients benefit from supported employment? *Psychiatric Rehabilitation Journal, 22,* 24–29.

Crist, P., & Stoffel, V. (1992). The Americans with Disabilities Act of 1990 and employees with mental impairments: Personal efficacy and the environment. *American Journal of Occupational Therapy, 46*(5), 434–443.

Harnois, G., & Gabriel, P. (2000). *Mental health and work: Impact, issues and good practices.* Geneva: World Health Organization (document WHO/MSD/MPS/00.2).

Harvey-Krefting, L. (1985). The concept of work in occupational therapy: A historical review. *American Journal of Occupational Therapy, 39,* 301–307.

Lang, S., & Cara, E. (1989). Vocational integration for the psychiatrically disabled. *Hospital and Community Psychiatry, 40*(9), 890–892.

Occupational therapy practice framework domain and process. (2002). Bethesda, MD: Author.

Torrey, W. C., Bebout, R., Kline, J., Becker, D. R., Alverson, M., & Drake, R. E. (1998). Practice guidelines for clinicians working in programs providing integrated vocational and clinical services for persons with severe mental disorders. *Psychiatric Rehabilitation Journal, 21*(4), 388–393.

Unger, K. (1990, Summer). Supported postsecondary education for people with mental illness. *American Rehabilitation,* 10–14.

CHAPTER 22

Case Management

Nancy Cooper, MS, OTR/L

Key Terms

advocacy
assertive community treatment
broker
client-directed services
conservator

deinstitutionalization
entitlements
in vivo
Medicaid
prodromal symptoms

Chapter Outline

Introduction

The traditional practice arena of most occupational therapists working with persons with serious mental illness has been the short-term, acute or long-term, locked institution. Day treatment, partial hospitalization, and prevocational training programs have provided additional domains as the **deinstitutionalization** movement of the 1950s set the stage for a new era of community practice. Since that time, treatment in the community has evolved from mirroring the medical model of the institution, with a focus on diagnosis and symptom reduction, to the development of innovative psychosocial rehabilitation programs. Case management, a model previously well established in nursing and social work with other needy populations, is one of these innovations. Occupational therapists facilitate adaptation through evaluation and training in functional living skill performance, which are "the very needs of a chronically mentally ill population" (Klasson, 1989, p. 85). With an emphasis on strengths and abilities and a focus on skill building, occupational therapists bring a unique and valuable perspective to case management for persons with serious mental illness in the community.

HISTORY OF CASE MANAGEMENT

In the mid-1950s, the development of phenothiazines, along with a new collective social conscience and concern for clients' civil rights and treatment costs, led to the release of large numbers of people with serious mental illness from state institutions into the community and to the expansion of community treatment programs. Initially, community treatment centers focused on, and adequately served, higher-functioning and less seriously ill individuals, but they were inadequate in both number and scope to address the needs of those with chronic serious mental illness. Significant numbers of treatment dropouts, with no mechanism or mandate for follow-up intervention, resulted in the "revolving door syndrome." The revolving door represents repeated returns to the hospital, as well as the formation in communities of the "mental health ghetto" (Platman, Dorgan, Gerhard, Mallam, & Spiliadis, 1982) as an alternative to the state hospital.

Recognizing the inadequacy of the response to these clients' needs and the fragmentation of services in the community, the U.S. Congress enacted the Community Mental Health Act of 1963. This act made continuous and coordinated service delivery in federally funded community mental health centers (CMHCs) a requirement. Services did become better coordinated at the CMHC level, but the responsibility for negotiating the service system and complying with treatment remained with the client. Moreover, the services continued to be directed toward persons with less severe illnesses and not toward those who had been released from the state hospitals. It was not until 1977, when the National Institute of Mental Health established the Community Support Program, that the needs of the most seriously mentally ill became an established focus of concern. Case management was introduced in the Community Support Program as one of the essential services required for this population. It was described as a way to facilitate access to the service system by designating a single individual or a team to be responsible for helping the client and for coordinating services to meet the client's needs and goals. In 1978, the Task Panel on Deinstitutionalization, Rehabilitation, and Long-Term Care of the President's Commission on Mental Health affirmed the use of individualized case management services in its recommendations (Robinson & Toff-Bergman, 1989).

Federal funding for case management became available in 1985 when the Omnibus Budget Reconciliation Act (OBRA) designated it as an optional benefit under **Medicaid**. OBRA defined case management as a service for assisting eligible persons to gain access to needed social, educational, medical, and other services. The act gave broad flexibility to individual states in determining how and to whom these services would be provided. The Consolidated Omnibus Reconciliation Act of 1986 (COBRA) designated individuals with severe mental illness as a target population under Medicaid. Later that same year, the U.S. Congress passed Public Law 99-660 requiring states to develop and implement comprehensive mental health plans. This law mandated the provision of case management services to all individuals with serious mental illness who receive substantial amounts of public funds or services and stipulated that implementation of case management services commence during fiscal year 1989. Because the vast majority of persons with serious mental illness are insured under Medicaid, Public Law 99-660 thus made case management services available to large numbers of seriously mentally ill persons who had previously had little appropriate or accessible community care.

MODELS OF MENTAL HEALTH CASE MANAGEMENT

Several models of case management have evolved out of a need to expand the initial **broker** functions that were identified as crucial for linking persons with serious mental illness to community services. Although there exists no precise operational definition of case management, general principles common to all models include identifying needs and facilitating access to community services, supporting continuity of care over time and across services, and matching the client's needs to the support provided (Harvey, 2003). It is generally agreed that the goals of all case management models are to reduce hospitalization, help the client remain in the least restrictive community setting possible, and maintain quality of life. In all models, a team or an individual case manager serves as a fixed point of responsibility, and in all but the broker model, services are provided **in vivo**. Resources for referral and service provision are found not just in the clinic or psychosocial rehabilitation program, but in the context of the larger community, such as the laundromat, bank, grocery store, church, library, or YMCA.

Case management lacks a specific disciplinary focus, being defined in terms of its functions rather than on the professional training of its practitioners (Bachrach, 1992). Case managers are drawn from many social and health service disciplines, including but not limited to psychology and psychiatry, social work, rehabilitation counseling, occupational therapy, and nursing. In 1991, the American Occupational Therapy Association (AOTA) recognized occupational therapy's role in the provision of case management services. Paraprofessionals and consumers also provide support with case management tasks; however, the need for clinical skills in assessment, engagement, therapeutic limit setting, and effective and appropriate referral requires these staff to work under the direction of professional clinical staff. When the case management model requires intensive direct clinical services, case managers should be professionally trained. The involvement of consumers in the provision of services and assistance to peers reinforces the principles of **client-directed services** and empowerment. Consumers are often able to advocate and support clients in ways that professional staff cannot, and they can also provide staff with additional insight into and awareness of some of the challenges of living with a mental illness.

In the United States, case management service models and guidelines vary as the individual states differ in their interpretation and implementation of federal mandates. In addition, models are chosen based on the availability of staff and community resources, as well as a particular organization's mission, funding, and philosophy of practice. The needs and resources of a large urban population vary significantly from those of a rural community; a small nonprofit organization may have a different organizational structure and philosophy of care than a large county mental health center.

While several terms have appeared in the literature to describe case management models of service, including such labels as the generalist case management model, standard case management, and cluster case management, six models have emerged as the most commonly described and reviewed (Mueser, Bond, Drake, & Resnick, 1998). These services can be viewed as existing on a continuum, with the model being distinguished primarily by caseload size and by the amount of direct clinical intervention by the case manager. It is important to remember that even among those models described in this chapter, there may be considerable overlap and blurring of boundaries.

The broker model is at one end of the continuum, and is primarily an administrative, office-based model in which the case manager assesses needs and makes referrals but provides no direct clinical service. This model does not require a case manager to act as a clinician or to have clinical skills. Caseload size varies considerably in this model, and can range from 50 to 150 clients. Clinical case management developed in response to the recognized need for the case manager to provide direct services and therefore to possess training and skills in areas such as psychotherapy and psychoeducation (Lamb, 1980; Kanter, 1989). Engagement, assessment, psychotherapy, living skills training, and psychoeducation are components of this model, and importance is placed on the collaborative nature of the client–case manager relationship. Caseload size may range from 30 to 50 clients, depending on such factors as client functional abilities, availability of community resources to augment direct service provision by the case manager, staff qualification, and risk level of the target population (Kanter, 1989; Mueser, Bond, Drake, & Resnick, 1998).

The strengths model of case management was developed in the early 1980s with a specific focus on identifying and maximizing client strengths, and obtaining the needed skills and/or resources to support community integration and improve quality of life (Rapp, 1994). The model is client–driven and strengths-oriented, and places importance on the client-case manager alliance as well as aggressive outreach to the community. A study by Stanard (1999) found this model effective in improving quality of life as well as vocational and educational outcomes, and also had a positive effect on the client's self-report of symptoms. Closely allied in theoretical principles is the rehabilitation model, which is also client-driven and attentive to client strengths, but emphasizes the identification and remediation of skill deficits in order to promote adaptation to the community and achievement of personal goals (Mueser et al., 1998). Caseload sizes vary from 20 to 30 clients, again related to factors such as client characteristics, staff qualifications, availability of community resources, and organizational structure and mission.

At the opposite end of the continuum are **assertive community treatment** (ACT) and intensive case management (ICM). Also described as "full support" models, these case management services are provided to clients with high rates of recidivism and/or more severe psychiatric impairments who may require assertive outreach to engage and remain in treatment. Developed in the 1970s by Stein and Test (1980; Thompson, Griffith, & Leaf, 1990) as an alternative to hospitalization, assertive community treatment programs are characterized by small caseloads, multidisciplinary team rather than single case manager responsibility, 24-hour coverage, time-unlimited service, and significant provision of in vivo outreach and direct skill training and service rather than referral. The distinction between ACT and ICM in the literature is not consistent, although some describe shared caseloads in ACT but not in ICM. The success of Stein and Test's original Program for Assertive Community Treatment (PACT) in reducing hospitalization and helping severely ill clients remain in the community with support has led to the development of AT teams across the country. Programs may vary slightly by location, staff composition, and agency service structure. Some ACT programs have caseloads of up to 20 while the original program's staff to client ratio was 1:10, and some have found 24-hour availability unnecessary.

The complex nature of case management service provision and the blurred boundaries and definitions of services are two factors that make research comparisons among the models difficult to design and interpret accurately. ACT and ICM models are the two most well researched and have proven success in achieving their goals when compared to other case management models. However, it is important in the search for the "best" case management model to ensure that the appropriate match is made between client need and service provided. In a study of consumer satisfaction with case management services, Tempier, Pawliuk, Perreault and Steiner (2002) found equivalent responses to clinical case management and ICM. Their conclusion is that this may be a result of service provision matching client level of functioning.

CASE MANAGEMENT SERVICE INTERVENTIONS

Case management service interventions typically include evaluation, service plan development, placement services, linkage and consultation, assistance in daily living skills, and emergency intervention. **Advocacy** is usually not a distinct service in itself but is frequently done in the course of a case manager's routine duties in the other areas.

Evaluation

The initial case management evaluation period is typically 30 days, during which it is desirable to gain as complete a picture as possible of the client's past and current functioning in order to develop an initial plan for services. The case manager must evaluate the client's status, needs, and goals in each of the following areas: mental health and substance abuse, physical health, financial status, housing, living skills, leisure, vocational and educational activities, and availability of a support system. Table 22-1 lists relevant topics to evaluate in each of these areas.

Table 22-1. Evaluation Data

Mental Health and Substance Use
- Brief psychiatric history: frequency and approximate number of hospitalizations, suicide ideation or attempts, assaultiveness, documented stressors or prodromal symptoms, typical patterns of decompensation, past treatment or services and results
- Current psychiatrist and medication regimen
- Compliance with medication and appointments or need for assistance
- Current or past alcohol or drug use and treatment, drug of choice, pattern of use or abuse

Physical Health
- Medical history, childhood illnesses or serious injury, learning disability
- Last physical examination and results, including tuberculosis test
- Ongoing medical problems requiring follow-up care or treatment
- Any indication of a current medical problem
- Date of last dental and vision examinations and results

Financial
- Amount and the source of income
- Need for assistance to receive the appropriate entitlements
- Name of representative payee, if any
- Bank accounts
- Current debts and monthly expenses

Legal Issues
- Current probation or parole
- Criminal history
- Outstanding warrants, fines, or restitution payments

(continues)

Table 22-1. (continued)

Housing
- Current place of residence and how long there
- Condition of living space
- Satisfaction with current housing
- Housing history, including successes and failures; client's preferences

Living Skills
- Money management
- Transportation
- Social and communication skills and habits
- Self-care and hygiene
- Time management
- Parenting
- Housekeeping and home management
- Community resource awareness
- Understanding of mental illness and relapse prevention
- Current leisure interests and activities, past sources of enjoyable activities
- Highest level of education completed, current educational goals
- Current and past volunteer or paid work experience, goals for work or vocational training

Support System
- Family available and nature of involvement with family members, frequency and type of contact
- Relationship with friends and neighbors
- Use of organized supports in the community such as a religious group or Alcoholics Anonymous

Client Strengths
- Personality traits, sense of humor
- Past successes, achievements
- Healthy or adaptive habits and routines
- Linkage with natural supports in environment such as family, church, AA

Because case management is designed to address the broad range of a client's needs for maintaining satisfactory and stable community living, the initial evaluation phase is critical in identifying existing resources, skills, and strengths, as well as service and support needs and skill deficits. Evaluation forms and procedures will vary with each facility. The overall goal of case management is to help maintain the client's quality of life in the least restrictive community environment possible; therefore, evaluation data should assist the case manager in identifying factors that may have resulted in either the client's successes or failures in the past.

Information should be gathered from a review of past records, interview and observation of the client, and interview of significant others in the client's environment, such as residential care operators, conservators, family members, and former treatment providers. Strict adherence to confidentiality laws is essential when seeking information from persons or facilities outside of the case manager's service agency.

Occupational therapists as case managers have a variety of pertinent assessment tools to supplement the evaluation process, particularly in the area of living skills. The Kohlman Evaluation of Living Skills, Bay Area Functional Performance Evaluation, Scorable Self-Care Evaluation, Activity Configuration, and the Allen Cognitive Level Evaluation are examples of instruments that may be helpful in gathering data on functional ability (see Chapter 17 for further information on evaluations and assessments). Because case management services are provided in vivo, there are many opportunities to observe the client, either formally or informally, functioning in his or her own environment. Interactions with retail clerks, roommates, and family or residential care staff; decoration and condition of living space; and the ability to perform housekeeping or money management tasks all provide direct feedback regarding social engagement and functional task performance. The Comprehensive Occupational Therapy Evaluation Scale is useful in organizing data gathered from these observations.

In most states, case management is a client-directed service, which means that interventions are made and service is provided primarily according to the client's stated needs and desires. Evaluation data provide information with which to help identify appropriate services, skills, and assistance for the client, but the case manager does not "do to" or "do for" him or her. Rather, the emphasis in case management is on "doing with" the client. Rather than being the problem solver, the case manager helps the client solve problems and seek solutions, thus helping him or her to gain skill as well as a sense of self-efficacy.

A component of the evaluation that underscores the client-directed nature of case management is the requirement for determining and documenting the client's level of satisfaction with various areas in his or her life. Client satisfaction is a subjective issue and must be considered in order to respect the client's individual choice and facilitate a successful outcome. It is important for the case manager to be aware of his or her own values and beliefs and not impose these on the client. For example, if the evaluation data indicates that a client has the living skills to function in his or her own apartment and has income sufficient for an available studio apartment or shared housing, it is nonetheless important to respect that client's wish should he or she choose to remain in a residential care facility (RCF). For many clients the RCF offers safety, socialization, and freedom from the stresses of homemaking responsibilities. Similarly, if a client is missing some teeth and Medicaid would pay for a bridge which would enhance his or her appearance and ability to eat a greater variety of foods, it is still essential to accept

EXPANDED ROLES FOR OCCUPATIONAL THERAPY

the client's decision to refuse that treatment. Reasons may range from delusions involving government implants in the bridgework to impatience with previously ill-fitting or repeatedly lost dental work. The case manager's role is to provide evaluation results to the client and to significant others, as appropriate. He or she should then discuss options and offer resources, which the client may choose to accept or decline. Exceptions to this are cases of the compromised health or safety of the client or others in his or her environment that may result in crisis intervention and emergency situations.

Concurrent with the initial evaluation phase is the period of engaging the client in case management services and beginning to establish trust. It is important that the client view case management as a help, and not a hindrance, and understand that it is a process through which to gain, and not lose, control over events and decisions in life. Depending on the client, this engagement process may be difficult and the development of trust may take months or never fully manifest. This is particularly true in the case of a client with a paranoid disorder. Similarly, an individual accustomed to the remote presence of a clinic-based therapist may not welcome a mobile, community-bound case manager. At its best, case management is a service that the client will welcome and he or she will be forthright in providing access to his or her life. Among the most challenging cases, however, is the client who appears paranoid, withdrawn, in denial of a mental illness, and resentful at what is perceived as an intrusion. Exercising clinical judgment is essential in these circumstances, and knowing when to terminate an interview or interaction can help establish trust. It is very important to respect the client's pace of interaction and gather as much information as possible without jeopardizing the relationship. A client is much more likely to allow access in the future to a case manager who is sensitive to his or her wishes and need for space and privacy from the beginning. Case management, by definition, is a long process, and evaluation is ongoing. Information not obtained within the first 30-day period may be accumulated later, as the relationship develops and as services are provided. Some guidelines for engaging the resistant client in case management services are:

- Make initial contacts brief.
- Meet with the client informally, for example, at his or her home or in a local coffee shop or park.
- Be clear about what case management is and how it will benefit the client.
- Be sure the client knows why and from whom you are obtaining information and that proper consent forms have been signed.
- Make it clear that you value the client's opinions and that he or she has input into the services received. Be sure to identify at least one issue of importance to the client.
- Respect the client's other activities and try to avoid scheduling visits that conflict with them.
- Allow the client to help determine future meeting times and places.

CASE ILLUSTRATION: Arturo—Initial Contact

Arturo is a 23-year-old male of Filipino descent who was referred to case management by the psychiatric hospital treatment staff because of a history of medication noncompliance and recent repeated hospitalizations. He was first hospitalized at age 18, during what was diagnosed as a manic episode, while he was a community college student: Arturo had parked his car on the freeway one night when he ran out of gas, and walked several miles to the airport. He was taken to the hospital by the police, who had been called by airport security to respond to Arturo's bizarre behavior in the airport terminal (involving kung fu–like moves, during which he claimed to be fighter Bruce Lee). Arturo has been on medication since that time, and he has been seeing a psychiatrist at a county outpatient mental health clinic. His diagnosis is bipolar affective disorder, mixed, with psychotic features. He has not resumed community college attendance. He lives with his parents and three older siblings in a single-family home. His parents have been reluctant to permit the intervention of mental health professionals. They tend not to seek help until Arturo becomes unmanageable, at which time his behavior often attracts the attention of the police.

Arturo was very engaging during the initial interview at his home. He signed consent forms to enable the case manager to obtain information from his father and sister Meg, who have assumed the primary liaison roles with mental health professionals. (Arturo's mother does not speak English.) The case manager observes Arturo's interactions with family members, talks with Arturo about his interests, and briefly discusses the effect of his illness on himself and his family. Arturo demonstrates no insight into his problems. He is unable to relate what led to his most recent hospitalization, and states that people "overreact" to him. He cannot name his current medications or dosages. When asked about specific past incidents leading to police involvement and hospitalization, Arturo laughs and says, "But I was only acting!" He does not associate stopping his medications with requiring hospitalization.

Arturo's medications are stored in a cabinet in the kitchen, where several outdated bottles are mixed in with current prescriptions. With the case manager's assistance and instruction, Arturo sorts through the bottles and safely disposes of the old medications by flushing the pills down the toilet. The case manager provides a pill organizer and helps Arturo distribute his medication into the individual compartments by daily dosages for a full week. This will lessen Arturo's confusion about the correct dosages and enable the case manager to monitor compliance by counting what remains of the current supply. In Arturo's presence, Meg provides the case manager with additional information about her brother's current and past functioning, including his occasional uncontrolled spending sprees. (Arturo's father is currently trying to clear up bills for expensive gold jewelry and a health club membership purchased by his son.) Arturo does not know his monthly income and cannot name any expenses he has other than buying an occasional soda from the local market. Arturo states that his father gives him small amounts of money "whenever I ask for it."

Most of the excessive spending has been the result of Arturo obtaining instant credit for purchases.

Service Plan Development

The service plan is the case management equivalent of the treatment plan as used in traditional inpatient or outpatient settings. It identifies the client's goals and objectives for a specified time period, typically a six-month time period, and it must be updated at least that often, or as necessary, as goals are achieved or are deemed inappropriate or unrealistic at any point during that period.

The format of the service plan varies, but generally it identifies the client's goals and the case management objectives and service activities for achieving each one. Because services are individualized, the number of goals appearing on the plan at any one time will vary. It is important to be realistic and set no more goals than can be accomplished within a given time period. It is preferable to state the client's goals in his or her own words. Objectives must be measurable, have projected timeframes, and be consistent with evaluation results and client goals. They should be realistic and broken down as necessary into tasks deemed achievable for the particular client.

Client service needs determined via the evaluation process may fall into two distinct categories: needs as a result of a skill deficit and those resulting from a resource deficit. For example, a client whose housing is jeopardized due to interpersonal conflicts may have limited available options for housing or may need to learn skills in communication and conflict resolution. Often a combination of both skill and resource deficits impedes a client's functioning, and it is the case manager's responsibility to help set goals and objectives to address the deficits.

In case management there is a great emphasis placed on the client's involvement in the goal-setting process. It is preferable, and often required, to have the client's signature on the completed plan to indicate acknowledgment of, and agreement with, the stated goals. This process is designed to ensure that the services are client directed and to promote individualized service planning. In this way an individual may experience a greater sense of responsibility for himself or herself, and participate actively in "doing" rather than "being done to."

In addition to involving the client in the planning process, it is advisable to identify appropriate family members or significant others to assist or support in achieving particular goals. Assigning appropriate responsibilities and facilitating healthy relationships with clearly defined boundaries and tasks promotes the development of an extended support system in the community. The development and maintenance of a comprehensive social support system in the community is often difficult for people with mental illness, and case managers may provide valuable assistance with support network expansion (Biegel, Tracy, & Corvo, 1994; Walsh, 1994). Adherence to confidentiality issues is crucial when actively enlisting others in the care of the client. The client must approve of the person's assistance or support, and the proper release forms must be signed and placed in the client's records. Table 22-2 contains examples of case management

Table 22-2. Sample Service Plan Components

Client's Goal	Measurable Objective	Service Activities	Significant Others' Assistance
"I want to live in my own apartment."	Lee will participate in living skills evaluation and training twice weekly for six months; he will also perform at least one task per week at home.	The case manager will provide living skills evaluation and training and monitor home task performance.	Lee's mother will remind him of training appointments, monitor home task performance, and provide feedback to the case manager.
"I need something to do with my time."	Juanita will volunteer at the Senior Center 10 hours per week for six months.	The case manager will link Juanita with the senior center and monitor attendance weekly via contact with the client and/or the volunteer coordinator.	The volunteer coordinator will train Juanita, meet with her weekly to provide feedback, and contact the case manager as needed.

goals and objectives, accompanying service activities, and the involvement needed from significant others.

CASE ILLUSTRATION: Arturo—Service Plan

Having gathered sufficient data from various sources to complete an initial evaluation, the case manager scheduled a meeting with Arturo to discuss his goals for the next six months. Arturo's sister Meg was present for the planning meeting, which was held at their home. Arturo expressed a desire to resume his education in computer-assisted design at the local community college. The case manager additionally introduced the issues of medication noncompliance and poor money management. Arturo was agreeable to having assistance with medication compliance but was offended by the case manager's characterization of his spending problem. He was initially unwilling to include the second item in the service plan but stated he was open to learning more about his income and expenses since his father currently handled all his money. The goal was written to address his lack of knowledge rather than his lack of control, a focus of which Arturo approved. Arturo also stated that he wanted to work on getting his own apartment. Although this was a reasonable and age-appropriate goal to the case manager, Meg explained that this is unacceptable in the Filipino culture, where "you stay with the family until you get married." For this reason, and because of the case manager's desire to gain the family's trust and cooperation, this goal was deferred. The case manager explained to Arturo that this might be a consideration for the future, after the current objectives had been achieved.

A service plan was developed, with Arturo and Meg's input and concurrence, to address the following objectives: community college attendance, medication compliance, and money management training.

Placement Services

Case management placement assistance may be defined as any support provided to the client in locating, obtaining, and maintaining a satisfactory living environment. This may include preplacement visits, negotiation of contracts and agreements, actual placement, and follow-up visits and monitoring.

Obtaining and maintaining stable, satisfactory community housing is a common goal for persons with serious mental illness. Unfortunately, unstable housing is often a chronic problem and is repeatedly addressed on service plans. Several factors that contribute to the disruption of housing are rehospitalization and the resultant loss of housing, a client's desire to move, eviction, lack of affordable housing alternatives in the community, a relapse that necessitates a move to a higher level of care, or progress that indicates a move to a lower level of care.

If a client is hospitalized for a brief, acute stay, housing usually is not disrupted, but long-term hospitalization (greater than 30 days) usually results in a loss of housing unless the client has the financial resources to pay for both rent and a hospital stay. Client **entitlements** are not adequate to provide for this, so most people are unable to retain housing during a serious relapse.

Clients obviously make decisions to move for many of the same reasons that persons without a mental illness decide to move. However, some of the reasons are related to difficulties resulting from their mental illness, such as unmanageable conflict with roommates, landlords, board and care staff, or neighbors; refusal or inability to accept and abide by established rules; and discomfort in the environment due to paranoia. A case manager may be able to intervene in all these situations and prevent the client's need to relocate.

A thorough knowledge and understanding of the available resources, including what a specific environment offers to the client and what it demands in return, is essential in order to assist with housing decisions and make appropriate placement referrals. Housing resources are usually identified by the amount and type of structure and support provided. Table 22-3 lists commonly available community housing options and gives a brief description of each. The table ranks resources from most to least restrictive, although there may be slight individual variations among programs in different geographic areas. Each program is a voluntary community placement and requires the client's concurrence with the decision, except in the case of placement decisions made by a **conservator**, who frequently has the authority to mandate placement and override the wishes of the client and the mental health treatment provider (although in some locales this authority is given to the treatment provider). Ideally, all individuals work together to reach agreement regarding placement decisions.

Table 22-3. Common Community Housing Options				
Type of Facility	Meals Provided	Medication Administered	On-Site Programming	On-Site Staff
Intermediate Care Facility	yes	yes	yes	yes
Residential Treatment Program	yes, with client participation	yes	yes	yes
Residential Care Facility	yes	yes	varies	yes
Boarding House	yes	no	no	manager
Homeless Shelter	varies	varies	varies	yes
Independent Living	no°	no°	no	no
Single-Room Occupancy (SRO) Hotel	no°°	no°	no	manager

°May be monitored by case manager via routine home visits.
°°May be set up by case manager or representative payee via voucher or charge account system at a local restaurant.

Placement issues may arise in several different ways, ranging from routine hospital discharge planning and placement to unexpected evictions. Routine or anticipated placements often follow a predictable pattern of assisting the client with identifying and exploring potential resources and then narrowing the choices to determine the best available. Whether dealing with the result of a hospital discharge back into the community or a client's voluntary decision to move from one community placement to another, the case manager usually follows these eight basic steps to secure alternative housing:

1. Discuss with the client which type of housing (of those types identified in Table 22-3) is desired or appropriate. Historical and current evaluation data, in conjunction with client preference, will guide this decision. Hopefully there will be concurrence on this issue and the client will be amenable to the case manager's suggestions based on the former's level of functioning. If the client is not amenable, discussion will need to focus on reaching agreement by providing the client with facts to support the case manager's recommendation.
2. Obtain or develop a list of local housing resources of that particular type. Depending on the type selected and the particular community, there may be several or very few from which to choose.
3. Assist the client with decision making regarding characteristics of places on that list. Desired geographic area, physical environment and surroundings, coed versus single-sex, house rules and restrictions, cultural or ethnic

background of owners or staff, cost, and current vacancy all must be considered. A case manager's familiarity with resources and sensitivity to the client's needs and preferences are invaluable in this phase. Some clients may want to reside with people of a common cultural background, while others may want to avoid a particular race or culture due to personal biases or delusional beliefs. Alternately, a client may place great emphasis on food and the quality of the meals provided, and a case manager's awareness of a facility's reputation in that regard is helpful. Some clients may want to be near family members, which may rule out certain geographic areas. Others may want to live close to parks, shopping areas, day treatment or vocational programs, or specific bus lines.

4. Determine which of the available resources fits the criteria that are important to the client.
5. Select two or three places to visit and schedule interviews.
6. Assist the client with the interview if needed or desired and with evaluating the pros and cons of each facility in order to promote decision-making skills. Clients have varying abilities and methods of approaching decisions. Some are very impulsive and will accept the first placement opportunity presented; others will be ambivalent about all options and have difficulty settling upon any placement decision. The amount and type of assistance the case manager provides will vary depending on the client's needs and skills. Some clients are quite familiar with community resources and procedures for obtaining housing, while others will need guidance and support through each step of the process. As a way to encourage independence, the case manager may provide a client with a selected list of residential care facilities and assign him or her the task of scheduling two interviews. Training in how to use the classified ads to find an apartment and assistance in identifying appropriate questions to ask by telephone and during the interview are other ways of building skills and promoting autonomy. It is often helpful to role-play the interview and application process, either in a group setting or on a one-on-one basis.
7. Once a decision has been reached, the case manager or client must notify the facility landlord or manager and ensure that all follow-up requirements of the application process are completed.
8. Assist the client with making the move or securing the resources necessary to move personal possessions into the new residence.

Engaging in routine follow-up and monitoring of a new placement allows the case manager to be proactive, dealing with issues as they arise in order to avoid potential problems. The frequency and type of monitoring is highly individualized. A client with a long history of placement failures who is newly discharged to a residential care facility after a lengthy period of hospitalization may benefit from daily contact initially. This contact may be either face-to-face or by telephone and may include an additional weekly check-in with facility staff. Clients who have been stable in the community for some time may require weekly or monthly monitoring with the frequency to be increased or decreased as changing situations warrant.

If two or more of the case manager's clients share housing, particularly in a supported independent living situation, house meetings are an effective and efficient way of monitoring placement. A house meeting gives the case manager an opportunity to address any current issues among the roommates as well as to provide living skills training, assess the living environment, and facilitate social gatherings. It is also an opportunity to organize and perform major group chores such as yard work or spring cleaning. Common issues that arise in shared housing situations are interpersonal conflicts, inequitable sharing of household chores, and difficulties in dealing with roommates' psychiatric symptoms. In many supported independent living situations, house meetings are led by facility staff and the case manager then acts as a liaison to the staff and to the individual client in addressing these issues.

Sudden evictions and other housing emergencies can be stressful for the client, and in these instances, a knowledge of housing regulations and tenants' rights is essential. State and federal housing regulations protect persons from sudden eviction without cause. For example, in California there must be a minimum of three days' notice provided with just cause, which must include an option for correction of the violation, which would then enable the tenant to remain. A 30-day notice is required for an eviction without cause. State and federal laws also protect an individual from discrimination based on mental illness or source of income. However, depending on the severity of the threat and the precipitating factors, an eviction due to verbal or physical assaultiveness by the client may necessitate immediate removal from the environment and referral to intermediate care or acute hospitalization.

The key to successful placement is finding a good match between client and housing. Factors that enhance the likelihood of successful client placement and housing stability include the following:

1. familiarity with the client's placement history and coping skills
2. thorough knowledge of community housing resources
3. a trusting relationship with the client and respect for client choice
4. knowledge of housing laws pertaining to people with disability
5. skills in crisis intervention, conflict resolution, negotiation, and advocacy
6. routine monitoring of placement

CASE ILLUSTRATION: Janice—Placement

Janice is a 34-year-old female, diagnosed with schizophrenia, paranoid type, currently staying at an intermediate care facility (ICF) after a two-week acute hospitalization. Prior to her hospitalization, Janice had been living with a roommate in a two-bedroom, supported, independent living situation. Her case manager had been addressing medication compliance and living skills training through weekly home visits. Janice had recently been refusing her medication,

*with a resulting deterioration in self-care skills and increasing psychotic symp-
toms. Janice was hospitalized one afternoon after the police were called to her
apartment complex. She had been at home watching a soap opera when she
became convinced that she was involved in the television events and ran outside, agitated and crying that she had just committed a murder on a carousel.
Neighbors called the police, who took Janice to emergency psychiatric services,
where she was subsequently hospitalized.*

*A conference was held to coordinate plans prior to Janice's discharge from
the ICF. Janice became angry when told by her case manager that she could not
return to her apartment and blamed the problems she encountered on her former roommate. She did not recall her behavior or the events prior to her acute
hospitalization and demonstrated no insight into her difficulties in maintaining
independent living despite receiving ongoing support and assistance from the
case manager. Janice insisted on getting her own apartment, despite the ICF
staff and case manager's recommendation of a residential care facility placement. Janice does not have a conservator.*

*With further discussion among Janice, her case manager, and the ICF treat-
ment staff, a compromise was reached whereby Janice agreed to enter a three-
month residential treatment program to focus on independent living skills, with
the ultimate goal of obtaining her own apartment upon successful completion of
the program.*

Linkage and Consultation

Linkage and consultation in case management may be defined as the identification and pursuit of community resources necessary and appropriate to implement the service plan. This includes, but is not limited to, interagency and
intraagency consultation and referral, and communication with the client's family and significant others. The purpose of linkage and consultation activities (as
shown in Figure 22-1) is to coordinate and monitor service delivery to ensure the
client's access and to facilitate continuity of care. These activities help prevent the
client from "falling through the cracks," which was characteristic of traditional
community mental health services.

The case manager links a client or consults with another resource whenever
information or a service is needed outside what the former has or can directly
provide. A case manager also provides linkage whenever there is information to
relay that may facilitate service delivery or enhance continuity of care for the
client. Linkage or consultation may be done in the client's presence or on behalf
of the client.

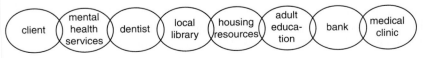

Figure 22-1.   Linkage with Community Resources

As a member of a multidisciplinary team, a case manager may perform intra-agency linkage by scheduling an appointment for the client with the team psychiatrist (for medication problems) or the psychotherapist (for counseling). A client may be referred to a weekly substance abuse group facilitated by another team member. Likewise, the case manager may consult with other team members to gain or provide information regarding any of these issues if direct client linkage is not deemed necessary.

Interagency linkage and consultation and communication outside of the case management agency require a consideration of confidentiality laws if the client is identified by name as a recipient of mental health services. Often, however, information can be obtained or referrals can be made without such identification. For example, making a dentist appointment for a client or inquiring about volunteer opportunities available at a local museum does not require that the client be identified as mentally ill. Referral to a program specifically targeted for persons with mental illness will identify the client as mentally ill, so in this case the case manager must have the client sign the appropriate consent forms before the referral is made. A case manager may also make direct referrals to the client for independent follow-up, such as a recommendation to attend a local Alcoholics Anonymous meeting.

Making appropriate and timely referral depends on accurate and ongoing assessment and planning with the client as well as a clear understanding of the services provided by a particular agency. A client who states that he or she wants a job may or may not have realistic ideas about what he or she is able to do. Prevocational evaluation and training by the case manager may help the client identify areas of strength and weakness, gain needed skills, and identify interests in preparation for employment. Based on those results, a decision may be made to seek volunteer work, a sheltered workshop, a vocational training program, or competitive employment.

Knowing the purpose and the parameters of an agency is essential in determining its suitability for a client's needs. For example, a vocational rehabilitation program designed for a client's placement in competitive community employment would not be a suitable referral for a client whose goal is to work in a sheltered workshop. Community resources need not be targeted specifically for the mentally ill in order to be useful and appropriate for a client's needs. When using resources available to the general population, a client may or may not choose to disclose his or her diagnosis of mental illness. The case manager may assist with this decision, discussing and role-playing the range of potential consequences of this disclosure and how to deal with them. Individuals or agencies unfamiliar with mental illness or the mental health system may require or request specific information. This is usually a good opportunity to advocate and enhance awareness of the needs and potential contributions of persons with mental illness in the community. Table 22-4 lists some possible community resources and suggested indications for referral or consultation with them. (See Appendix B for further information.)

Once a resource has been identified as potentially appropriate, a client will need varying degrees of assistance to be linked with that resource. It is important

Table 22-4. Community Resources for Linkage and Consultation

Resource	Available Services
Churches, religious organizations	Support, volunteer work opportunities
Visiting Nurses Association, American Diabetes Association, Planned Parenthood, services for the deaf or blind, psychologists	Medical support, consultation, education, and testing; peer support; volunteer work opportunities
Adult education, community college, YMCA	Low-cost educational opportunities, leisure activities
Alcoholics Anonymous, cultural centers, gay community centers	Peer support and education
Food bank, beauty college	Low-cost products and services
Senior center, nursing home	Volunteer opportunities
State Department of Rehabilitation	Vocational evaluation and training
County housing authority, Housing for Independent People	Low-cost housing opportunities

to allow the client as much freedom and autonomy as possible, providing support as needed and withdrawing it as tolerated to promote client empowerment and ensure a successful referral. For some clients, merely providing the agency name and phone number or address will be sufficient for them to follow through and make the contact successfully. Other clients may require that the referral be made on their behalf and that they then be accompanied and assisted with an application and intake process or a doctor's visit or lab test. For example, a client with a strong fear of having blood drawn may benefit from the comforting presence of a trusted case manager. A client making an initial visit to a doctor's office may have difficulty filling out the necessary intake forms without assistance due to reading problems or an inability to accurately recall medical history. Some programs or facilities may want to limit a case manager's involvement, particularly if it is a mental health program designed for client independence. The usual steps in making a referral to link a client with services are shown in Figure 22-2.

Once a referral has been made, it is important to facilitate continuity of care via regular contact with the appropriate resource person or agency. As with monitoring after-placement, the frequency and type of consultation and communication will depend on the client and the resource to which referral has been made. Some agencies will want close communication to share information; others will want to be more autonomous. For example, a probation officer may want weekly telephone or written contact to verify a client's court-mandated compliance with mental health treatment, but it would probably not be advisable to make weekly contact with a client's supervisor in competitive employment unless a previous agreement had been made, among the supervisor, client, and case manager, to do so. For a client placed in an inpatient program, important information can be mutually shared about medication history, compliance with the program, family issues, and discharge plans.

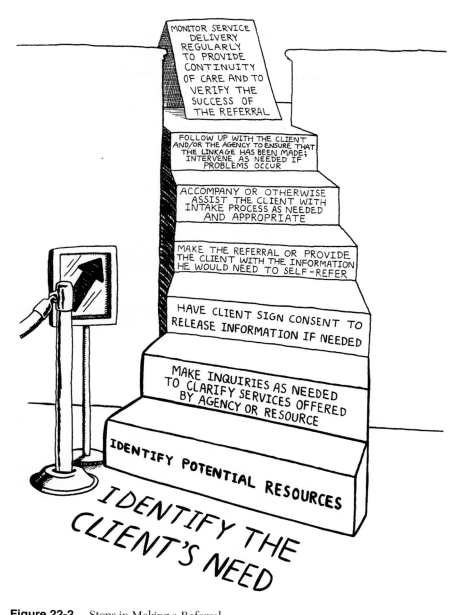

Figure 22-2. Steps in Making a Referral

It is helpful to develop a resource book, keeping notes or a log of particularly helpful or knowledgeable resources in the community. Developing a positive working relationship with other agencies helps ensure open lines of communication regarding your client, provides good-role modeling for the client, and enhances the probability of success of future referrals. The case manager will encounter particularly sensitive dentists, doctors, and agencies and want to recommend them. Likewise, insensitive or otherwise inappropriate resources may be encountered, to which the case manager will want to avoid further referrals. It is important to get the client's feedback regarding the referral experience, such as how he or she was treated. The client and case manager may identify stigma, unresponsiveness, poor communication, and resultant poor continuity of care. Accompanying the client whenever necessary or appropriate helps the case manager obtain direct experience with the program staff. Some staff will be more openly communicative with the case manager than others, and more willing to assist the client. Encountering undesirable situations provides an opportunity for the case manager to intervene to attempt to rectify a situation, offer in-service education, advocate for the client as needed to obtain service, or seek another resource if these efforts are not effective.

CASE ILLUSTRATION: Robert—Linkage

Robert is a 34-year-old male with a diagnosis of schizophrenia, undifferentiated type, who lives in a residential care facility. Robert had been complaining of vomiting after meals but described no other symptoms. He was not disturbed about his condition but rather accepted it as a consequence, he explained, of being "still connected to my mother's womb." The case manager consulted with staff at the RCF, who confirmed that Robert occasionally vomited after meals and that no other signs of illness are present. Despite his nonchalance about his symptoms, Robert was willing to see a doctor at his case manager's recommendation.

The case manager scheduled an appointment with a family practice physician and accompanied Robert to the clinic. During the interview and examination in the physician's office, Robert became annoyed as he agitatedly insisted to the physician that "there's a piece of my mother's womb in there." The case manager informed the doctor of Robert's rapid eating habits, ongoing pattern of experiencing a single episode of vomiting shortly after meals, and previous report to her that "it feels like something's stuck in there." The doctor ordered an upper gastrointestinal (GI) series and scheduled a return appointment. The case manager reviewed the preexamination instructions with Robert and the RCF staff and left a written copy with them. She accompanied Robert to the hospital x-ray department to ensure compliance with the test and then accompanied him back to the clinic for the follow-up appointment. The doctor diagnosed a mild hiatal hernia, prescribed Tagamet, and advised Robert regarding his pace of eating and positioning after mealtime. The case manager discussed the results with the RCF staff and monitored adherence to follow-up treatment to ensure a resolution of the problem.

Daily Living Skills Development

The development of daily living skills involves the direct provision of assistance or training in those skills needed for successful community living. This is the occupational therapist's area of expertise. As case manager, the OT provides this direct service to clients and, as a member of a multidisciplinary team, serves as a resource for the provision of this service to other clients. The range of skills requiring support or training is as broad as that addressed in the initial evaluation, that is, any skill the client needs and wants to develop or enhance to aid in successful community living. Daily living skills includes the wide range of activities such as money management, grooming and hygiene, social skills, time management, leisure skills, health, safety, and relapse prevention, housekeeping, laundry and clothing management, nutrition, meal planning and preparation, transportation and use of community resources, coping and stress management, decision making and problem solving, and prevocational issues.

A case management service agency following strictly a brokerage model (acting merely as a broker of services rather than a direct provider) may not be as effective in promoting client growth and skill development as full-service, multidisciplinary teams, which provide brokerage in conjunction with direct service. Daily living skills training can be very effective at the case management level. Persons with serious mental illness often demonstrate concrete thought processes and extreme passivity, and they may have difficulty generalizing learning and transferring skills learned in one setting to another living environment (Morrison & Bellack, 1984). Recidivism from day treatment or other traditional outpatient settings is a common problem. Skills may not be adequately maintained over time, as periods of unstable functioning, possibly accompanied by acute hospitalization and a move to a higher level of care, often result in a deterioration in skill functioning. In addition, skills training in the client's own environment facilitates integration into the neighborhood. The case manager who works with the client over time in his or her own environment is ideally suited to train, reinforce, or support existing skills as applied to the current environment and to help monitor and maintain skill performance. Liberman et al. (1998; 2002) describe the value of community case managers in facilitating generalization of skills in clinic-based training sessions, as they monitor and help clients practice new tasks in their own environments.

Occupational therapy principles and techniques of living skills training and assistance in the community do not differ from those used in a clinic or inpatient setting. The use of task analysis and graded activities enables the client to experience success at each level, and gradually decreasing the support and assistance empowers the client as he or she gains independence in a particular skill area. Skills training may be done on a one-on-one or group basis. Some activities are more conducive to groups, such as meal planning and preparation or communication and social skills training. Others are more effective with individual instruction and support, such as grocery shopping, money management, and laundry. Some tasks may initially be taught and discussed in a group setting and then practiced and monitored on an individual basis. It is often effective to encourage peer support and have more experienced clients provide support and assistance to those learning a new skill. This is a way of empowering and reinforcing higher-functioning clients while encouraging socialization and peer support-building.

Living skills training in the community does differ in some respects: the length of time available to work with a client is greater than in most institutional settings, there is more opportunity to work with clients on an individual basis, and the amount of control over the environment is less. For example, a case manager may be unprepared for a rude or impatient bank teller, the angry or fearful reactions of other shoppers to a client's delusional speech, or the client's slowness in writing out a check at the register. A cooking activity held in a well-stocked, readily accessible, and fully equipped OT clinic kitchen is much more predictable than one planned in a client's apartment, as a client living on a limited budget may consider items such as measuring spoons or a loaf pan to be an unnecessary extravagance. These situations offer the opportunity for creative adaptation and problem solving and give the therapist a glimpse of the obstacles encountered and values held by the client. It is important to make living skills training both culturally and economically relevant.

Daily living skills training and assistance in case management may range from initial task instruction to periodic monitoring of successful task performance. For example, the occupational therapist may begin living skills training by teaching a client to perform various housecleaning tasks. When the client is able to perform the tasks independently, case management support may then advance to helping the client develop a household chore checklist and monitoring adherence to that list. Tasks begun on a training level ideally will progress to maintenance and monitoring levels as competence increases and the client becomes empowered to assume more responsibility. In one-on-one training situations it is often effective to do a task with the client. This lessens the stress on the client of being watched while performing a new task and helps promote a relationship of trust and mutual problem solving. Figure 22-3 shows a client doing a daily activity with a case manager.

CASE ILLUSTRATION: Jim—Living Skill Development

Jim is a 32-year-old male who has been stable in a residential care facility (RCF) in the community for almost one year. He was diagnosed with a schizophrenic disorder, paranoid type. His case manager has provided home visits to monitor placement and has worked with Jim to try to engage him in structured daily activity. Recently, Jim has expressed to his case manager a desire to live in his own apartment, complaining that the other residents in the home "are always asking me for money and cigarettes because they know I always have some."

Jim has many strengths that suggest he would be a good candidate for independent living, including good money management skills, family support, a one-year history of medication compliance, ability to keep his living space clean and neat, an established routine for doing his own laundry, experience with the local bus system, and knowledge of community resources. However, interview, task observation, and administration of the Kohlman Evaluation of Living Skills test

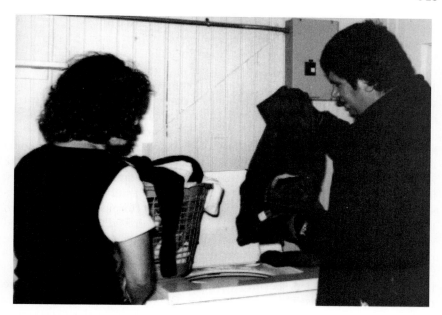

Figure 22-3. Living Skills Training in a Client's Home

enables the case manager to identify several skill deficits: lack of skill in meal planning, shopping, and food preparation tasks; lack of skill in kitchen- and bathroom-cleaning tasks; lack of work or leisure activity involvement; difficulty setting limits; and limited social contact.

The case manager began Jim's living skills training with housecleaning, meal planning, nutrition, food storage, kitchen safety, and price comparison activities at the RCF and at a local supermarket. The RCF staff allowed Jim to help with some of the simple food preparation and cleaning tasks. The case manager arranged a "pot luck" lunch at the home of two other clients, and Jim participated in group meal planning, shopping, food preparation, and cleaning for that event.

Living skills training continued after Jim moved into a studio apartment. The case manager facilitated the transition by helping Jim explore local resources, such as the closest bank and supermarket, and by assisting him with using the new laundry facilities at the apartment complex. She also accompanied him on grocery shopping trips until he was able to complete the task on his own. Initially, home visits were made twice weekly to monitor and reinforce successful performance of housecleaning, meal planning, and preparation tasks.

Emergency Intervention

Emergency intervention may be defined as a quick, unplanned response at the onset of a crisis situation to solve a problem or facilitate the client's access to other needed services. The goal is to maintain, to the greatest possible extent, the client's status as a functioning community member. Often a crisis is determined by the severity of the client's response to an incident or situation. What is perceived as a threat or is stressful for one client may not be a stressor for another. Moreover, the crisis may be brought to the attention of the case manager by a telephone call from the client or a significant other person, or it may be discovered in the course of a routine case management appointment or home visit.

Clinical judgment guides the case manager's response to a crisis. An emergency related to the client's physical health and safety may require a trip to the hospital emergency room or doctor's office or the application of simple emergency first aid. A housing crisis may involve promoting conflict resolution among roommates, arranging a temporary respite placement, or obtaining the services of a repair person to see that emergency household maintenance is performed. A crisis in which the client shows signs of psychiatric relapse may be resolved by an unscheduled visit with the psychiatrist for medication adjustment along with close monitoring until the client restabilizes, or it may require an emergency hospitalization.

The case manager who works with a client over an extended period of time will become aware of stressors specific to that client and often be able to recognize **prodromal symptoms**. There are clients for whom any change in residence is stressful and therefore must be monitored carefully and provided with extra support during those transition periods. Some clients are vulnerable to environmental stressors such as storms, fires, and earthquakes. Some will react strongly to changes in a structured daily routine, money problems, changes in support staff, arguments with significant others in their lives, or a serious illness of their own, a family member, or their residential care operator. Drug or alcohol abuse, noncompliance with the prescribed medication regimen, or any change in the medication prescription may precipitate relapse. Prodromal symptoms include any alteration in the client's typical behavior, such as the rate, volume, or content of speech; style of dress; or sleep or activity pattern.

Clients have different ways of responding to a case manager's intervention during a period of relapse, which will depend on the relapse stage and on client-specific traits and patterns characteristic of relapse. Some individuals will welcome the support and comfort of a familiar and trusted person in a stressful and unstable period, but others will resent the intrusion, be suspicious of motives and intentions, and be resistant to any intervention, particularly if they suspect it will lead to hospitalization. It is always advantageous to recognize prodromal symptoms and intervene before a full-blown relapse occurs and hospitalization is required, which underscores the value of routine monitoring via regularly scheduled case management contacts.

As in any inpatient setting, it is important for the case manager to be aware of safety issues in the community. The case manager who feels that his or her safety or the safety of the client is jeopardized at any time during a community visit should leave the environment immediately to obtain adequate help. Because of the sensitivity and unpredictability of relapse situations, it is advisable to take another staff member or ensure that others are around when making a contact in which you suspect the client may be unstable. In a particularly volatile situation, it may be appropriate or necessary to have the police make an initial check or meet the case manager at the client's home. Most police departments have a "welfare check" policy through which they will go to a home if there is concern regarding the well-being of a resident, and they will always respond to a report of potential danger in the community. Because of the long relationship a case manager will usually have established with a client, including prior experience with his or her specific relapse patterns, should the police need to be involved, the case manager should be available to advise them how best to approach and communicate with the client.

Agency policies and state regulations for hospitalizing a client against his or her will vary. Some clients will cooperate with the process and demonstrate insight, awareness of their need, and a willingness to be admitted, but others may need to be restrained for their own safety and must be transported via police car or ambulance.

CASE ILLUSTRATION: Beth—Emergency Intervention

Beth is a 35-year-old female, diagnosed with schizoaffective disorder, who lives with her boyfriend, Mark, and their 2-year-old son, Jason. Beth's case manager received a telephone call one morning from Mark, who told her that Beth was "up all night changing clothes, and now she's mad at me and talking weird." When questioned, he reported that Beth had not eaten since the previous morning and that he had not seen her take her medication since that time. Beth's angry verbalizations were audible in the background. She refused to come to the telephone.

The case manager, who was familiar with Beth's pattern of rapid relapse, enlisted the assistance of another team member for a home visit involving a probable hospitalization. (Beth had never been assaultive, but an extra staff person is nonetheless helpful for support in a crisis situation.) At the home, the case manager found Beth dressed bizarrely, with heavier makeup than usual and black nail polish carelessly applied. She was agitated and pacing; her speech was rapid, pressured, and tangential and was coupled with hostile glares and accusations. She called Mark "Hitler" and shouted at the case manager, "You're all made of wax and you're going to die in the nuclear meltdown." She made no appropriate responses to her case manager's attempts to talk with her.

The case manager told Beth that she had to go to the hospital and reminded her that it was hard for her to take care of Jason when she was feeling like this. Beth made no verbal acknowledgment of the case manager's statements and rather continued her pacing, stopping occasionally to stare at the two staff members and make a bizarre accusation. While the case manager talked with Beth, her team member wrote a hold order for an involuntary 72-hour commitment to psychiatric emergency services, citing Beth as gravely disabled due to acute psychotic symptoms and her recent lack of sleep and food intake. Mark drove Beth to the hospital, accompanied by the case manager. Beth continued her tirade but offered no resistance. The other team member met them at the hospital, where the written hold order was given to the hospital staff and Beth was admitted for evaluation.

THE CLIENT–CASE MANAGER RELATIONSHIP

There has been considerable research and discussion regarding case management service provision, including its definition, its methods, and its effects (Ziguras, Stuart, & Jackson, 2002). One aspect of this research is the case management relationship itself, as distinct from the service (Walsh, 2000). This relationship may be a strong factor in the success or failure of any particular intervention; it has been described as being as strong an effector of change as the intervention itself (Harris & Bergman, 1987).

In 1978, the Task Panel on Deinstitutionalization, Rehabilitation and Long-Term Care of the President's Commission on Mental Health described the case manager as someone "remaining in extended contact with the individual and acting as friend and advocate if required and desired by him or her" (Platman et al., 1982, p. 308). Case managers have been described as "travel guides" (Kanter, 1989, p. 362) and "life coaches" (Robinson & Toff-Bergman, 1989, p. 42). In a study of case management support, Baker and Weiss (1984) found that case managers viewed their clients as "individuals to work with rather than individuals to treat" (p. 926). Clients participating in that study described their case managers as persons who provide advice and support similar to that of an older brother or sister. While their therapists and psychiatrists seemed distant, they felt that their case managers established a "peer-like friendliness" (p. 926). The relationship was described by the clients as comfortable, nonthreatening, and respectful. They felt they were taken seriously, were worthy of attention, and were less vulnerable because there was "someone to rely on when things get rocky" (p. 927).

A client–case manager relationship has challenges and benefits that may differ from those of a treatment relationship established in a hospital or traditional outpatient program. In these settings an individual is treated for a time-limited period in a specific environment with a focus on more narrowly defined objectives, while in case management, boundaries and roles are less clearly defined and contained as a case manager works with a client over time and across a spectrum of environments and experiences and through periods of crisis and stability.

There may be challenges in setting limits with a client who considers the case manager a friend and with family members who expect or want more from the case manager than is realistically possible. There are challenges in being consistent and continually modeling behavior that may encourage positive growth in the client. There are challenges in providing the needed assistance without creating excessive dependency and to intervening for the safety and well-being of a client at times when he or she may view the case manager's action as intrusive and controlling. There may be challenges to the case manager in attending to personal needs when the needs of the clients seem vaster and far more serious in comparison. Challenges such as these can be managed with time, experience, and awareness, as well as through open communication and problem solving with team members, peers, and supervisors. Lamb (1979; 1986) addressed many of these issues, and Carl Rogers's characteristics of a helping relationship are beneficial in establishing professional guidelines for authenticity, consistency, and facilitation of positive client growth (Rogers, 1989).

The challenges of being a case manager for persons with serious mental illness are balanced with the benefits. A case manager may derive a sense of professional pride in being able to establish and maintain a trusting relationship with individuals who have been slow to trust; and there is gratification in discovering that along with the dark side of mental illness, the sufferer usually has an enjoyable, bright side as well. There is a shared journey of discovery and joy as a determined case manager and client work together to help the client move into a first apartment, accomplish a new and difficult task, take a risk, or negotiate a bureaucratic system to get needs met. There will be a growing sense of competence as the case manager gets to know the clients and becomes able to recognize or even anticipate problems and to intervene successfully to prevent hospitalization. Case management services, when provided sensitively and effectively, can be the lifeline that helps a client remain a part of the larger community. By facilitating the gradual development of more effective habits of living and dealing with chronic illness, the case manager provides an opportunity for clients to finally feel at home in the community after years of rotating through the "revolving door."

Summary

Case management is a community treatment method designed to provide continuity of care for persons with serious and persistent mental illness. Its goals are to reduce hospitalization, maintain the client in the community in a minimally restrictive setting, and help maintain the client's quality of life. Unlike traditional mental health treatment, case management services are provided in vivo and are of unlimited duration.

Case management service components typically include evaluation, planning, placement, linkage and consultation, daily living skills assistance, and emergency intervention. Researchers who have studied the client–case manager relationship have described the unique qualities that make it a powerful effector of change, and which are distinct from the actual services provided. Working as case manager, with a professional focus on enhancing functional daily living skills and facilitating adaptation to disability, the occupational therapist plays a key role in achieving the goals of case management. With this support and assistance, individuals with serious and persistent mental illness can live far more satisfactory and meaningful lives in the community than were available in the institutions from which many of them came.

Review Questions

1. The following is a list of community mental health service activities. Indicate which are case management functions and explain your reasons.
   a. counseling a client regarding grief issues
   b. referring a client to Planned Parenthood for birth control education
   c. helping a client find a job
   d. evaluating a client's social skills
2. What are the three main goals of case management?
3. Discuss ways of engaging a treatment-resistant client in case management services.
4. What is meant by the phrase *client-directed services*?
5. Discuss reasons why living skills training for people with serious mental illness may be particularly effective at the case management level. How does training in the community differ from training in the institution?
6. Discuss safety precautions that may be taken when dealing with a crisis situation in the community.
7. In the case illustration about Beth, what are some of her prodromal symptoms?
8. The National Alliance for the Mentally Ill has actively supported the development of Assertive Community Treatment teams nationwide. How is ACT different from the earlier broker, clinical, or strengths case management models?

References

Bachrach, L. (1992). Case management revisited. *Hospital and Community Psychiatry, 43*, 209–210.

Baker, F., & Weiss, R. S. (1984). The nature of case manager support. *Hospital and Community Psychiatry, 35*, 925–928.

Biegel, D. E., Tracy, E. M., & Corvo, K. N. (1994). Strengthening social networks: Intervention strategies for mental health case managers. *Health and Social Work, 19*, 206–216.

Harris, M., & Bergman, H. C. (1987). Case management with the chronically mentally ill: A clinical perspective. *American Journal of Orthopsychiatry, 57*, 296–302.

Harvey, C. A. (2003). The configuration of mental health services to facilitate care for people with schizophrenia. *Medical Journal of Australia, 178*(9), S49–S52.

Kanter, J. (1989). Clinical case management: Definition, principles, components. *Hospital and Community Psychiatry, 40*, 361–368.

Klasson, E. M. (1989). A model of the occupational therapist as case manager: Two case studies of chronic schizophrenic patients living in the community. *Occupational Therapy in Mental Health, 9*(1), 63–90.

Lamb, H. R. (1979). Staff burnout in work with long-term patients. *Hospital and Community Psychiatry, 30*, 396–398.

Lamb, H. R. (1980). Therapist-case managers: More than brokers of services. *Hospital and Community Psychiatry, 31*, 762–764.

Lamb, H. R. (1986). Some reflections on treating schizophrenics. *Archives of General Psychiatry, 43*, 1007–1011.

Liberman, R. L., Glynn, S., Blair, K. E., Ross, D., & Marder, S. R. (2002). In vivo amplified skills training: Promoting generalization of independent living skills for clients with schizophrenia. *Psychiatry, 65*(2), 137–155.

Liberman, R. L., Wallace, C. J., Blackwell, G., Kopelwicz, A., Vaccaro, J. V., & Mintz, J. (1998). Skills training versus psychosocial occupational therapy for persons with persistent schizophrenia. *Psychiatry, 155*(8), 1087–1091.

Morrison, R. L., & Bellack, A. S. (1984). Social skills training. In A. S. Bellack (Ed.), *Schizophrenia: Treatment, management, and rehabilitation* (pp. 247–279). New York: Grune & Stratton.

Mueser, K. T., Bond, G. R., Drake, R. E., & Resnick, S. G. (1998). Models of community care for severe mental illness: A review of research on case management. *Schizophrenia Bulletin, 24*(1), 37–74.

Platman, S. R., Dorgan, R. E., Gerhard, R. S., Mallam, K. E., & Spiliadis, S. S. (1982). Case management of the mentally disabled. *Journal of Public Health Policy, 3*, 302–314.

Rapp, C. A. (1994). Theory, principles and methods of the strengths model of case management. In M. Harris & H. Bergman (Eds.), *Case management: Theory and practice*. Washington, DC: American Psychiatric Press.

Robinson, G., & Toff-Bergman, G. (1989). *Choices in case management: Current knowledge and practice for mental health programs*. Washington, DC: Mental Health Policy Research Center.

Rogers, C. R. (1989). The characteristics of a helping relationship. In H. Kirschenbaum & V. L. Henderson (Eds.), *The Carl Rogers reader* (pp. 108–126). New York: Houghton Mifflin.

Stanard, R. P. (1999). The effect of training in a strengths model of case management on clients outcome in a community mental health center. *Community Mental Health Journal, 35*(2), 169–179.

Stein, L. I., & Test, M. A. (1980). Alternative to mental hospital treatment. *Archives of General Psychiatry, 37*, 392–397.

Tempier, R., Pawliuk, N., Perrault, M., & Steiner, W. (2002). Satisfaction with clinical case management services of patients with long-term psychosis. *Community Mental Health Journal, 38*(1), 51–59.

Thompson, K. S., Griffith, E. E. H., & Leaf, P. J. (1990). A historical model of the Madison model of community care. *Hospital and Community Psychiatry, 41*, 625–634.

Walsh, J. (1994). The social networks of seriously mentally ill persons receiving case management services. *Journal of Case Management, 3*, 27–35.

Walsh, J. (2000). *Clinical case management with persons having mental illness: A relationship-based perspective*. Belmont, CA: Wadsworth.

Ziguras, S. J., Stuart, G. W., & Jackson, A. C. (2002). Assessing the evidence on case management. *British Journal of Psychiatry, 181*, 17–21.

Suggested Reading

Adams, R. (1990). The role of occupational therapists in community mental health. *Mental Health Special Interest Section Newsletter, 13* (1), 1–2.

Chamberlain, R., & Rapp, C. A. (1991). A decade of case management support: A methodological review of outcome research. *Community Mental Health Journal, 27*, 171–188.

Dass, R., & Gorman, P. (1985). *How can I help?* New York: Knopf.

Estroff, S. (1981). *Making it crazy: An ethnography of psychiatric clients in an American community*. Berkeley: University of California Press.

McGurrin, M. C., & Worley, N. (1993). Evaluation of intensive case management for seriously and persistently mentally ill persons. *Journal of Case Management, 2*, 59–65.

Mercier, C., & Racine, G. (1995). Case management with homeless women: A descriptive study. *Community Mental Health Journal, 31*, 25–37.

Moeller, P. (1991). The occupational therapist as case manager in community mental health. *Mental Health Special Interest Section Newsletter, 14*(2), 4–5.

Olfson, M. (1990). Assertive community treatment: An evaluation of the experimental evidence. *Hospital and Community Psychiatry, 41*, 634–641.

Quinlivan, R., Hough, R., Crowell, A., Beach, C., Hofstetter, R., & Kenworthy, K. (1995). Service utilization and costs of care for severely mentally ill clients in an intensive management program. *Psychiatric Services, 46*, 365–371.

Skinner, P. C. (1995). The role of the family in the strengths model of psychiatric community case management. *Kansas Nurse, 70*, 3–4.

Witheridge, T. F. (1989). The assertive community treatment worker: An emerging role and its implications for professional training. *Hospital and Community Psychiatry, 40*, 620–624.

PART VIII

Clinically Related Roles

Many changes have occurred in clinical practice in all fields since the first edition of this textbook. Notably, fieldwork supervision and demonstration of positive outcomes of intervention have become essential in all clinical practices, including occupational therapy practice. Accordingly, there has been an abundance of information regarding supervision and demonstration of effectiveness.

Both supervision (Chapter 23) and outcome evidence (Chapter 24) are particularly important in mental health. The terms *psycho* and *social* mean treating both psychological and social issues. They direct occupational therapists to intervene in what the practice framework terms client factors of internal and interpersonal motivation. Intervention in internal and interpersonal dynamics requires one's best sense of therapeutic self-in-relationship and an understanding of what works best for whom and regarding those client factors that are not so readily apparent. Therefore, fieldwork supervision with an expert clinician is crucial to a reflective and reasoned practice, and evidence of outcomes is crucial to successful and good practice.

Fieldwork Supervision in the Mental Health Setting

Elizabeth Cara, PhD, OTR/L, MFT

Key Terms

eclectic
interpersonal
intrapersonal
mode

parallel process
style
supervision

Chapter Outline

Introduction

This chapter focuses on the fieldwork experience and the process of **supervision** during fieldwork. Because it emphasizes the fieldwork experience, a discussion of how to supervise other employees in the mental health setting is not included. However, since the chapter delineates useful models and practical approaches, the information should also be useful for general supervision in the mental health setting.

The American Occupational Therapy Association ([AOTA], 1988, 1996; Privott, 1998) states that the purpose of fieldwork is to provide the opportunity to integrate academic knowledge with applied skills at progressively higher levels of performance and responsibility. The student is able to test firsthand what was learned in school and to refine skills while interacting with clients and staff under the "supervision of qualified personnel." In Level II fieldwork, the qualified personnel must be a registered occupational therapist with at least one year of experience. The person responsible for the day-to-day training is considered a fieldwork educator (also known as a clinical educator, fieldwork supervisor, or student supervisor). In this chapter the terms are used interchangeably. All designate the person responsible for the day-to-day supervision of the student (as opposed to the person who may be the fieldwork coordinator and has primarily administrative duties).

The American Occupational Therapy Association defines supervision as

a process in which two or more people participate in a joint effort to promote, establish, maintain, and or elevate a level of performance and service. Supervision is a mutual undertaking between the supervisor and the supervisee that fosters growth and development; assures appropriate utilization of training and potential; encourages creativity and innovation; and provides guidance, support, encouragement, and respect while working toward a goal. (1994, p. 1045)

This chapter will discuss, for those new to the role, the tools needed to assume the role of fieldwork supervisor and ways in which the process can be made smoother for individuals in both the supervisor and supervisee positions. In an attempt to offer a comprehensive view of supervision, different models that address particular aspects of the supervision process in occupational therapy and other fields will be presented. It is hoped that supervisors and supervisees can adapt this broad view for their specific experience and mental health setting.

In occupational therapy as well as other professions, supervision is a valuable aspect of training. The fieldwork experience is also important because it may influence graduates' selection of the field in which they are going to practice as well as where one is first employed (Andersen, 2002). In most health professions, supervision is mandated and is recognized as a learning situation. A good relationship between the supervisor and supervisee is valued or, indeed, essential, and the emphasis is on the role, rather than the techniques, of the supervisor (Christie, Joyce, & Moeller, 1985; Gillfillan, 2001; Loganbill, Hardy, & Delworth, 1982; Noelle, 2003). Despite these common assumptions, there is little formal training given prior to promoting someone to the role of supervisor, and it is expected that:

- Training will be a somewhat smooth process.
- The supervisor will successfully guide the process.
- The supervisee will successfully become a competent occupational therapist.
- Quality occupational therapy will be promoted.
- Professional development of the involved individuals will be enhanced.

A supervisee may experience the same ups and downs and the same anxieties or worry about adequacy and competency that students experience during the academic process. A fieldwork educator may question her or his skills and competency to facilitate the training process and may also experience anxiety and confusion. However, ultimately both supervisor and supervisee expect that the "learner" will successfully "pass" through the training on the way to becoming a professional and that the supervisor will successfully guide the process.

Perhaps the practical fieldwork process can be viewed as similar to the academic process. Learning is acquired in a nonlinear manner and the course does not always seem smooth. Think back on your academic learning career, whether for the past four or more years or the last few years specifically in occupational therapy. Was the process as smooth as you expected? Was it linear or was it an up-and-down pattern of certainty and confusion? Did you approach graduation in a step-by-step process in which each step was clear or did you sometimes stumble, or miss a step—or take two at a time?

As you read this chapter keep in mind that fieldwork education and training, and supervision as one aspect of it, can be seen as a metaphor for the entire learning process. Thus, it is difficult to predict how each step will be taken.

DIMENSIONS OF FIELDWORK EDUCATION AND SUPERVISION

Supervision is an aspect of training that includes four elements: the supervisor, the supervisee, the relationship, and the context or environment (Frum & Opacich, 1987; Loganbill, Hardy, & Delworth, 1982). Within the mental health arena specifically, supervision is "an intensive, interpersonal focused, one-to-one relationship in which one person is designated to facilitate the development of therapeutic competence in the other person . . . [It is] a master apprentice approach" (Loganbill, Hardy, & Delworth, 1982, p. 4).

The Supervisor

The supervisor is a licensed or registered professional with a minimum of one year of clinical experience who assumes authority for the student's education. The supervisor is responsible for setting, encouraging, and evaluating the standard of work performed by the supervisee (AOTA, 1994). The fieldwork supervisor's responsibilities include:

- Providing an adequate orientation to the site and to its policies and procedures
- Assigning clients to the student
- Supervising the provision of services, including oral reports and documentation
- Evaluating the skills and knowledge level of the student
- Meeting with the student regularly to provide guidance and review performance
- Using the fieldwork performance evaluation at midpoint and termination (AOTA, 1988)

In addition, the supervisor assumes responsibility for the supervisee's client caseload and is responsible, not only for the supervised person's development into a professional in clinical practice, but also for the outcome of client interventions. Bradley and Gould (2000) have suggested that the primary role of the supervisor is to teach the student and therefore the primary commitment should be to the student while monitoring the client's welfare. Therefore, the supervisor assumes multiple roles (Munroe, 1988), serving as a coach, model, guide, teacher, organizer, and clinician all in one. The personality, roles, styles, and skills of the supervisor are dimensions that have been researched and are considered important to the supervision process (Bradley, & Gould, 2000; Sumerall, Barke, Timmons, Oehlert, Lopez, & Trent, 1998; Vidlak, 2002).

The Supervisee

The supervisee is the student who is learning to practice. The supervisee will assume a caseload and learn clinical practice, including the skills of relating therapeutically, choosing and applying interventions correctly, communicating and documenting information accurately, and becoming a team member. Standards (AOTA, 1988) ask that students experience roles of service management and research in addition to direct care. The supervisee thus learns the multiple roles of the professional. The assistance or guidance of another experienced professional is integral to the process of professionalization. The supervisees' preferences regarding the supervisor and relationship and the supervisees' experiences (Greer, 2002; Hantoot, 2000; Ramos-Sanchez, Esnil, Goodwin, Riggs, Touster, Wright, et al., 2002) have been researched and are considered important to the supervision process (Henderson, Cawyer, Stringer, & Watkins, 1999; Sumerall et al., 1998). Also, the emotions (Hahn, 2001; Foullette & Batten, 2000: Yourman, 2003) and reflective capacity (Peyton, 2002) have been explored and are considered essential to the supervision process and client treatment.

The Relationship

The interaction of the supervisee and supervisor constitutes a relationship. The relationship developed between the two is recognized as an important and influencing component of the supervision process (Ladany, Lehrman-Waterman, Molinaro, & Wolgast, 1999; Nelson & Friedlander, 2001; Nelson, Gray, Friedlander, Ladany, & Walker, 2001). In occupational therapy, the relationship is not emphasized as much as in some other professions, such as psychotherapy. However, the nature of the relationship, participation therein, and the opportunity it affords to work out communication and personality differences are recognized by supervisors as an important element in learning. (See Chapter 18 for a discussion of this text's viewpoint concerning relationships.)

The Environment

The environment in which the supervision and training takes place is recognized as having an impact on the supervision process (Dougher, 2001; Trant, 2001; Gilfillan, 2001; Walker & Cooper, 1993). The environment can include the physical setting, the people and rules of the organization, and the relationships of the staff. All these elements form the culture of the organization, which is the unique way in which it operates.

The context in which the fieldwork is experienced also influences the process. The context of fieldwork is educational; in this case, learning how to apply knowledge in a practical setting. Therefore, educational goals and objectives for the experience defined by the fieldwork site, the academic institution of the student, and the professional organization (AOTA) will necessarily delineate the broad parameters in which the experience occurs (Privott, 1998b).

THEORETICAL MODELS OF SUPERVISION

Traditional psychotherapy professions have presented models for supervision that have been based in their theoretical orientation. However, concepts of supervision have an **eclectic** background, having been developed from various professions and theories (Bradley & Gould, 2001). Occupational therapy has also adopted ideas of supervision from various professions and theories. Concepts also have emerged in a trial-and-error way from the actual training of therapists. Each field has maintained a specific emphasis.

Psychoanalytic

The concept of supervision began to develop in the 1920s with the acceptance of psychoanalysis. Psychoanalysis, or psychoanalytic therapy, goes much further than other theoretical practices in emphasizing the **intrapersonal** aspects of training and supervision. In fact, the dynamics of supervision and therapy are considered a rich process akin to an artistic weaving, in which students learn how the process of therapy is intertwined with an individual's personality and tendencies to respond. A perspective from this theory that sheds light on the occupational therapy supervisory process is that of the supervisor as a master who joins the student therapist in a rite of passage (Meerlo, 1952, cited in Loganbill, Hardy, & Delworth, 1982). Additionally, the psychoanalytic literature describes a developmental process of various stages through which the supervisee travels; hence the term **parallel process** (Hora, 1957) comes from this field. In this developmental process, the therapist identifies with the client and then elicits emotions in the supervisor that he or she experienced with the client. Although occupational therapy supervision is not often conducted utilizing this concept, it is applicable to the mental health setting.

Occupational therapy and psychoanalytic supervision differ in that psychoanalytic therapy does not allow for as much variability in, or emphasis on, learning style and developmental level of learning as occupational therapy supervision does.

Humanistic

"Facilitative" supervision (Leddick & Bernard, 1980) was originally addressed by Carl Rogers, who discussed a program of experiences that gave trainees an opportunity to model the empathy and unconditional positive regard of the therapist/supervisor. The supervisor was to provide a model of behavior so that supervisees could learn by example. The assumption was that the supervisor would be an excellent therapist/counselor. Later research was contradictory regarding which methods (modeling, personal growth, or didactic training) were more useful and whether the supervisory relationship was similar to, or different from, the counseling relationship.

Occupational therapy supervision is similar to humanistic supervision in that occupational therapy supervisors traditionally emphasize role modeling, mentoring, and positive reassurance.

Behavioral

Behavioral therapy stresses learning theory. Trainees learn behaviors from skilled therapists through role modeling and coaching. They learn goal setting—identifying and selecting appropriate learning techniques—in behavioral terms. That is, supervision includes instruction in various behavioral techniques.

Occupational therapy supervision is similar to behavioral therapy supervision in the sense that traditional supervision stresses instruction in techniques and goal setting and recognizes the supervisor role as that of a coach.

Developmental

Developmental models assume that development proceeds in a chronological, hierarchical, sequential pattern. Development proceeds through identifiable stages, each stage of learning increases in complexity, and each stage must be experienced prior to further development in the next stage. Developmental theories may describe development in a specific area, such as the cognitive, moral, intellectual, sexual, or personality aspects of a person. A knowledge of developmental levels can aid in designing and fostering learning experiences specific to each stage.

Supervision in the area of cognitive development has been explicated in the occupational therapy literature and will be described in the next section, "Practical Models and Methods of Supervision."

Consistencies in Supervision

Aspects of different models have been blended and represent what is commonly recognized by most professions as supervision. Some consistencies that cross boundaries are (Cara, 2000; Leddick & Bernard, 1980; Privott, 1998b):

1. Supervision is seen as a learning, "professionalizing" situation.
2. A good relationship between supervisor and supervisee is valued.
3. The role of the supervisor as coach and competent person has been emphasized rather than specific supervisory techniques.

PRACTICAL MODELS AND METHODS OF SUPERVISION

Useful developmental approaches for supervision have been conceptualized in occupational therapy and in counseling psychology, although currently the psychology literature on supervision emphasizes dimensions of supervision that can fit broadly into the categorizations (discussed above) of the supervisor, the supervisee, the supervisory relationship, and the environment. That is, different aspects of the supervision process are explored, such as the supervisor-supervisee relationship and its impact on client treatment; the effect of the supervisor's personality, such as attractiveness or sensitivity, or of the supervisory style, such as supportive or directive on the process of supervision (Sumerall et al., 1998) and on the progress of the supervisee; how events in the supervision process or the personality characteristics of the supervisor influence the supervisee; or the willingness of the supervisee to disclose an accurate picture of his or her work and how this accuracy influences the supervision and the client treatment.

Although dimensions of supervision have been emphasized, many supervisors may find models of supervision as helpful guides in understanding the process that fieldwork students may go through. These models may guide how supervisors think about their students' skills, how they might talk about clients and cases, the timing of specific interventions in supervision, and the expectations they may have of their fieldwork students.

Occupational Therapy

Schwartz (1984) proposed a method of supervision based on a synthesis of developmental (meaning that skills and knowledge are acquired in a sequential and hierarchical manner) models of personality that are correlated with learning experiences. Her model emphasizes the supervisor (importance of the approach) and supervisee (particularly cognitive and personality style). Table 23-1 shows ego stages, or individuals' ways of knowing, that are pertinent to occupational therapy clinical education. Ways of knowing are then correlated to student behavior and perceptions and interventions are suggested according to developmental levels

Table 23-1. Loevinger's Ego Stages Pertinent to Occupational Therapy Clinical Education

Ego Stage	Character Development	Inter-personal Style	Cognitive Style	What is Knowledge	The Learning Process
Level 3	Conformity to external rules, guilt for breaking rules.	Belonging, superficial niceness.	Conceptual simplicity, stereotypes.	Necessary information in order to achieve the desired end. Takes the form of right or wrong, good or bad.	Revelation of truth by an expert authority; if conflict between ideas is perceived, one element is dismissed as incorrect.
Level 3/4	Differentiation of norms, goals.	Aware of relation to group, helping.	Multiplicity.	Information to be applied to situational problems, possibility of several correct solutions.	Student questions information received from the expert authority and tries to align with own view.
Level 4	Self-evaluated standards, self-criticism, guilt for consequences, long-term goals and ideals.	Intensive, responsible, mutual, concern for communication.	Conceptual complexity.	Skill in problem solving.	Discovery of solutions through logical analysis, multiple views acknowledged but simplicity sought.

Source: Schwartz (1984), p. 395, Table 1.

(see Table 23-2 for one method of supervision). In an effort to move away from negative images and convey the concept of strengths, potential problems have been conceptualized instead in terms of levels. Behavior that is typical of occupational therapy students in fieldwork, as well as student perceptions of the learning process and suggestions for supervisory interventions, are described for each level.

The observation of behavior in the clinic and in the supervision process enables the supervisor to discern the supervisee's stage of development. Expectations can then be established based on a student's **interpersonal** cognitive style and sense of self at each stage of development. Hypotheses can thus be formed and checked concerning the supervisee's view of the learning process.

Table 23-2. A Method for Clinical Supervision

Student Group	Teaching Approach	Supervision Sessions	Administrative Instructions	Counseling Intervention
Conscientious (Stage Level 3)	Assume student sees supervisor as "authority" and expert. Present information; show how several solutions can work. Lead toward student identification of problems, solutions.	Structure, with clear description of expectations. Make assignments to think about, bring to next meeting.	Delineate rules. Expect student to follow. Show disapproval if student does not.	Student desires acceptance, wants things to go well. Student will be upset with problems and look to supervisor for answers. Lead student to join supervisor in seeking answers.
Explorer (Stage Level 3/4)	Assume student in process of developing own system of problem solving. Discuss how student's view is worthwhile, problematic. Lead student toward accepting multiple viewpoints. Encourage exploration with clearly defined limits.	Negotiate: explain supervisor expectations, seek student input. Lead, but allow some flexibility in goals.	Delineate rules. Expect student will not follow if rules conflict with own ideas. Discuss implications if student chooses to follow low own inclination.	Student will be dogmatic and upset when things do not work according to plan. Lead student to see several ways to be effective. Support student through confusion.
Achiever (Stage Level 4)	Assume student has developed systems of beliefs, problem solving. Challenge ideas. Discuss implications. Lead toward greater analytic competence in problem solving. Encourage exploration with feedback.	Discuss supervisor expectations and student's. Collaborate on discussing best method to achieve goals.	Delineate rules. Discuss origins where appropriate. Expect student to seek exceptions. Explain when supervisor can/cannot be flexible.	Student will be hypercritical of failures. Help student see when guilt is appropriate, when student is exceeding reasonable limit of responsibility.

Source: Schwartz (1984), p. 395, Table 2.

Once the supervisor has gained some understanding of students' behavior or a reasonable expectation of what their behavior may mean, he or she can then plan and implement specific approaches. The supervisor's role is that of model and evaluator and involves teaching, counseling, and instruction. The student's role is to learn through doing and by analyzing and critiquing his or her behavior within the supervisory sessions.

Analysis of cognitive levels and interventions. The developmental levels are posited as guides and not as rigid classifications. An individual does not always fit neatly into one level, particularly since this represents a combination of areas of development. However, the developmental model suggests patterns of learning and, therefore, clear methods of clinical supervision. (The levels noted are most typical of supervisees. It is assumed that knowledge in previous levels has been acquired by the time individuals begin fieldwork.)

Level 3. Conscientious students usually obey rules without questioning because they wish to belong to a group and to gain approval from peers and authority figures. They have limited self-awareness and find it difficult to entertain many solutions to a problem, so they may personalize criticism. This group views the supervisor as the expert, which means that students do not realize or trust their own ability to elicit solutions. They will need assurance and an understanding of the separation of personal from professional worth. Structured questioning should elicit successful problem solving, and follow-up assignments should be given.

Level 3/4. In the explorer group, thinking becomes more complex. The individual is able to see more possibilities and alternatives, and self-reflective ability increases. There is a conflict between wanting to stand out yet not wanting to stand outside the group. Although thinking is more complex, beliefs are stated in a dogmatic way. Explorers may fail to incorporate feedback with which they do not agree, and they may challenge the rules. The supervisor should engage in comparing the student's own view with the professional judgment of others. The explorer group consists of students who are developing their own problem-solving techniques, which means that a discussion of alternative solutions may ensue. The discussion should be limited and not provide so much information as to overwhelm supervisees.

Level 4. Achievers are able to accept and utilize multiple strategies. Students are able to follow standards of performance in an individualistic way yet may still be hypercritical. The achiever group can define problems and solutions; therefore, an approach that will critique and analyze the solutions is useful. An analytical discussion of why and how solutions were arrived at can be useful. Also indicated is instruction in how new information can be accommodated or assimilated with previous knowledge.

CASE ILLUSTRATION: Darren, Cordelia, and Tabetha— The Developmental Stages

Darren and Cordelia had started their internship at the same time. They came from the same school, where they had been friends and worked on group proj-

ects together. As interns, they were joined by Tabetha, a student from a different school. Darren was a conscientious (level 3) student. He was quiet and rarely asked questions, but he listened intently to his supervisor and took notes during the supervisory sessions. He initially observed his supervisor's treatment. After each session, his supervisor carefully broke down her treatment in a step-by-step fashion and, for each step, explained what she was doing and why. She regularly provided Darren with a list of questions posed as treatment hypotheses regarding the treatment sessions. Dareen then would return to the next session and discuss his understanding of the hypotheses. His supervisor provided specific answers regarding his hypotheses, reassured him that his reasoning was sound, and thanked him for his earnest work.

Cordelia preferred to try out treatment right away. She was an explorer (level 3/4), who was more comfortable discussing alternatives in which she was involved. Her supervisor began a treatment and invited Cordelia to assist. She then pointed out one or two steps she had observed and elicited alternative ways of treatment from Cordelia.

Tabetha was an achiever (level 4), who also preferred to experience treatment right away. In fact, she had arrived early to observe treatment before the formal internship began. In supervisory sessions, she reported what she had learned from her observations and what she might add to the treatment. She then reported how the treatment session had turned out, what her strengths and weaknesses were, what she might change, and the reasons why the session had turned out the way it had. She requested permission to do a research project that she had been thinking about before starting the internship. Darren, Cordelia, and Tabetha eventually designed their own peer supervision group. Although the interns were at different developmental levels, their supervisors were able to incorporate their levels of learning into the supervisory process. Moreover, the three were eventually able to help each other in the learning process.

Counseling Psychology Model

This model mainly addresses the supervisee and explains the process he or she may go through. It also emphasizes the relationship's ability to help the student progress successfully through the learning process. The model is explained in some length here because:

- Training in occupational therapy supervision is based on it (Frum & Opacich, 1987).
- It is the model most cited in the supervision process literature.
- It specifically focuses on affect and the emotional process that may occur in supervision.

The counseling psychology model was influenced by the developmental stage theorists (primarily Erik Erikson and Margaret Mahler). Both indicate optimism and trust in the adaptive capacities of human beings, and both encourage the emergence of qualities such as competence and a sense of personal and professional identity. Erikson discusses "potential crises," meaning periods of vulnerability and heightened potential. The supervisor can be aware of these crises in the supervisee's development and make appropriate interventions. In Erikson's developmental model, identity is central in development. The training process is one in which the central task of the student is to acquire a professional identity. Mahler emphasizes separation and autonomy. The supervisee not only is learning how to disengage from those on whom he or she has relied, such as teachers and classes, but is also learning how to become independent in thinking and behavior. Figure 23-1 shows a three-stage model of stagnation, confusion, and integration with key issues for each stage (Loganbill, Hardy, & Delworth, 1982). It appears that students pass through and revisit different stages in the supervisory process. Moreover, they must grapple and struggle with the themes in each stage before reaching an emotional understanding that allows them to progress to the next stage. You will recognize some of the behavior, styles and thinking as similar to the occupational therapy model. An in-depth description of the stages of supervision can be found in Table 23-3.

Stage I—Stagnation.   In the stage of stagnation, the beginning supervisee is usually unaware, naively, of any difficulties or important issues in supervision. For the more experienced student, this is characterized more by feeling stuck or experiencing blind spots. Usually there is a naive sense of security and stability, and there may be some simplistic, black-and-white thinking or inability to define the

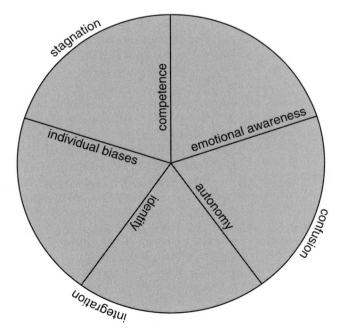

Figure 23-1.   The Three-Stage Developmental Model

Adapted from Loganbill et al. (1992).

Table 23-3. Stages of Supervision

	Supervisee's Process	External Attitude	Internal Attitude	Attitude toward Supervisor
Stagnation	Unaware Stuck Blind spots Over- or under-estimates skills	Narrow, rigid, linear thinking and uncreative problem solving	Low self-concept or false sense of well-being	Idealizing or indifferent

Implications for practice: Caution against independence and responsibility, explain intricacies of practice, make few demands for advanced knowledge, give reassurance, show tolerance. Do not personalize.

	Supervisee's Process	External Attitude	Internal Attitude	Attitude toward Supervisor
Confusion	Erratic Confusion Conflict	Less rigid Inadequate problem solving	Unsure Fluctuate between incompetent and able	Disappointed and angry that supervisor does not have all the answers

Implications for practice: A nondefensive attitude and ability to identify problems and emotions and discuss them. Validate realistic portrait of the supervisee. Do not join in the turbulence.

	Supervisee's Process	External Attitude	Internal Attitude	Attitude toward Supervisor
Integration	Intellectual understanding Flexibility Stability	Understanding Acceptance of therapeutic situation	More realistic Acceptance of strengths and weaknesses, more confidence	More realistic and independent

Implications for practice: The supervisee can take much more responsibility for supervision, treatment, and learning. There is a consolidation of knowledge and probably less need for structured supervision. The supervisor, while still providing feedback, can enlist supervisees in reviewing what they find important in treatment, what they have learned, and what they must still develop.

nuances of interventions. The student may be particularly uninsightful regarding his or her skills in practice. Typically, supervisees overestimate their skills or, conversely, believe that they have none or have not learned enough to prepare them for this endeavor.

Attitudes toward the world and environment can be characterized by very narrow and/or rigid thinking. With the more experienced student, this may be confined to a specific issue in practice. Usually, thinking is linear and uncreative and problem solving is narrow. Often the supervisee may accurately recognize problems in practice but offer a solution that is too narrow to be realistic.

Attitudes toward the self are usually characterized by a low self-concept and dependency on the supervisor as the source of new learning or by a lack of awareness leading to a false sense of well-being that is not based on actual behavior. Usually the attitude toward the supervisor is one of idealizing him or her as an omniscient and omnipotent figure or being indifferent to the supervisor and considering him or her somewhat irrelevant. Although this stage may seem somewhat negative by the supervisor, it can be characterized as one in which the supervisee is passively learning and constituting an identity that will aid in the next, turbulent stages.

Implications for practice. This is a difficult stage for the supervisor, who should resist the temptation to give the supervisee too much early independence and responsibility. This stage demands an explanation of the intricacies of practice without too many demands for advanced knowledge. The supervisor should provide reassurance and understanding concerning the student's positive interventions. To cope with a defiant attitude, the supervisor must understand and tolerate both the tendency to idealize and that to be indifferent. In other words, supervisors should enjoy being admired and not deny their knowledge. They must tolerate indifference and not personalize behavior.

CASE ILLUSTRATION: Darren, Cordelia, and Tabetha— Stage 1, Stagnation

After the initial two weeks, Darren and Tabetha showed indications that they were in the stagnation stage, though they expressed it differently. Darren wanted to continue to observe and discuss treatment and planned interventions that were just like his supervisor's. He felt that he could never know as much as she and he wondered if he could pass the internship. Tabetha asked if she could have her own caseload and did not think that she needed more than weekly supervision. She was not sure whether her supervisor really provided the best interventions.

Stage 2—Confusion. Stage 2 is one of confusion. This represents a marked shift from the first stage, which can occur abruptly or gradually. It is often marked by instability; erratic fluctuations in emotions, thoughts, and practice; confusion; and, sometimes, conflict. The supervisee no longer is guided by, or guarded about, beliefs about the self, others, and solutions. His or her attitude toward treatment or the setting is less characterized by rigid thinking, though solutions to problems seem inadequate and may be impossible. However, the supervisee will recognize that something is amiss.

Generally, the attitude toward the self reflects the basis of this stage. Supervisees' attitudes fluctuate between a sense of self as inadequate and incompetent and a sense of being expert and able. The supervisee may know that she or he possesses some valuable skills or competencies yet be unsure that the skills will be useful in the context of practice. Students are also unsure whether their competencies are perceived by others.

Due to confusion and still-narrow thinking, the supervisee may continue to look to the supervisor for answers; however, the student will recognize that the supervisor does not have all the answers. Anger and disappointment may result. The supervisee may still idealize the supervisor and think he or she is deliberately withholding answers, or the supervisor may be viewed as incompetent or inadequate. Perhaps this is the source of the apparent contradiction in students' report that they perceive supervisors poorly while at the same time labeling their overall experience as good. Obviously, this stage may be difficult for the supervisor as well as the supervisee.

Implications for practice. The supervisor must recognize and understand the particular stage and the emotions that characterize it and not take any display of disappointment or anger personally. Naming the problem and emotions and being able to discuss them in a nondefensive way will go a long way toward helping a student move through this stage.

The supervisor should validate a realistic portrayal of the student and resist joining in the erratic self-evaluation. It is important to resist the temptation to overvalue yet nevertheless maintain a realistic, reassuring viewpoint of the supervisee as an occupational therapist. The value of this stage is in giving up former rigid, narrow beliefs and experiencing the opportunity to gain new ideas, perspectives, and skills. It is important for the supervisor to:

- Remain objective
- Remain unperturbed by the panic or turbulence that the supervisee may be experiencing
- Be able to recognize and verbalize what is happening for the supervisee

The supervisor can help the student remain aware that out of confusion come knowledge and learning.

CASE ILLUSTRATION: Darren, Cordelia, and Tabetha—Stage 2, Confusion

After about five weeks, just prior to her midterm evaluation, Cordelia, who was usually talkative, became quiet and almost surly. She failed to attend two supervision sessions, claiming that her clients needed that treatment time. She revealed to Darren and Tabetha that she was not sure if any treatment in mental health was valuable or whether people really did get better. She was disappointed in her supervision and thought that her supervisor might be "testing" her before the midterm evaluation. A client who was paranoid and who, she believed, did not like her, stopped coming to Cordelia's vocational group. Cordelia began to feel better after her supervisor explained how students might feel at that stage and emphasized that her concerns were normal. She also became more aware of how her attitude affected her behavior with clients.

Stage 3—Integration. Stage 3 is characterized by integration, cognitive understanding, flexibility, and personal stability. The supervisee grasps and understands important issues for supervision. Usually supervisees can realistically assess their strengths and weakness without interference from their emotions and are able to grasp what skills need to be polished and integrated in treatment.

The supervisees' attitude toward the environment is less rigid and idealistic or extreme, and they now have a cognitive understanding of the therapeutic situation. There is acceptance and a sense of direction for the future. An individual's attitude toward the self is characterized by a more realistic view and an acceptance of both strengths and weakness. There is a sense of confidence that growth will continue, and the attitude toward the supervisor also becomes more realistic. The supervisor is now seen as a person who has strengths and weakness. The student is able to take more responsibility for the supervisory sessions and agenda, usually becoming more independent of the supervisor at this stage. This is a stable period with much flexibility and potential for further growth.

Implications for practice.   The supervisee can take much more responsibility for supervision, treatment, and learning. There is a consolidation and probably less need for structured supervision. The supervisor, while still providing feedback, can enlist the supervisee in reviewing what is important in treatment, what he or she has learned, and what can still be developed.

CASE ILLUSTRATION: Darren, Cordelia, and Tabetha—Stage 3, Integration

In their peer supervision group held prior to their last weeks of the internship, Darren, Cordelia, and Tabetha discussed what they had learned and what they hoped for the future. They realized that their final project, in which they had developed a community outreach group that would be taken over by clients, was valued and desired by both staff and clients. They felt proud that they had been able to contribute.

The interns realized that although they were not sure whether they were advanced enough to work independently in mental health, they had acquired some good skills. They began to understand how their responses, attitudes, and behavior could affect clients; Cordelia had particularly learned this during stage 2. They appreciated what they had learned from their supervisor and other staff and were also able to differentiate what they could do best and less well. They realized that working in mental health is like an interesting dance between client and therapist; if they each listened to different music they would be unable to follow each other, but when they were hearing the same tune, treatment progressed more easily. They felt secure in their knowledge and identity as occupational therapists, and they had some ideas about the similarities and differences in their own and other mental health professions.

Themes in the stages.   Within these stages, certain themes, or issues, of competence, emotional awareness, autonomy, identity, and respect for individual differences for beginning professionals may appear. The issues may not necessarily appear in sequential order, and they tend to continually resurface.

Competence.   Competence means the ability to use skills and knowledge to carry out an appropriate treatment plan. Most often, this entails the student's ability to translate intellectual knowledge learned in a classroom to the practice or clinical situation. Usually, this is a core issue in stage 1, or in the beginning of training, because the supervisee does not have a repertoire of skills. In stage 2 she may realize that she does not yet have the adequate skills and may feel frustrated. In stage 3 the supervisee may have an understanding and integration of skills and techniques that she can use for a variety of clients and situations.

In the case illustration, Darren, Cordelia, and Tabetha displayed issues of competence in each stage. Darren was most questioning of his ability in stage 1, Cordelia felt frustrated in stage 2, and all three had realistically integrated their skills and knowledge during stage 3.

Emotional awareness.   Emotional awareness is important in the psychosocial arena because it relates to an ability to be aware of how one affects, and is affected by, client responses, behavior, and style (see Chapter 1 for more information). This awareness of personal reactions and attitudes toward a client is particularly useful for formulating impressions and directing interventions in the psychiatric arena.

In stage 1, supervisees may often be unaware of personal feelings toward clients or themselves. They may particularly deny anger, frustration, inadequacy, and attraction to, or from, clients. Supervisees finding their own way during the beginning of training most likely cannot risk revealing personal emotions. Moreover, beginning therapists may still carry the impression that they should always be "nice," thereby being unable to accept emotions considered "not nice" in either themselves or clients. The shunned feelings may then be expressed in inappropriate ways and at the wrong times in treatment. In stage 2, an awareness of feelings may occur but may be frightening or unacceptable. Stage 3 recognizes a newfound sense of acceptance and control that emotions and thoughts regarding clients can be distinguished from behavior.

The supervisor should name the feelings for the supervisee and accept them or explain their importance. Alternately, the supervisor should assure the supervisee they are natural feelings in this situation and that it would be unnatural not to have them.

While in stage 2, Cordelia had been most unaware of her feelings. After reassurance from her supervisor, however, she became able to accept them. In stage 3, she still wondered whether her feelings were important but was able to acknowledge and discuss with her supervisor concerns regarding her behavior toward clients.

Autonomy.   Students may have the sense that they are merely a reflection of all the books they have read, and the theories and teachers they have experienced. They may doubt that they can be effective. Supervisees may have a shaky self-concept and difficulty thinking of themselves as responsible occupational therapists.

In stage 1 the supervisee may be overdependent on the supervisor, seeing him or her as a magician who has all the right answers. The supervisee may want specific "how to" answers or to be told the "right way" to handle clients. Sometimes students are experiencing the unawareness characteristic of this period and so may disregard advice or information from the supervisor.

In stage 2, the supervisee may alternate between dependency and independence. This may be manifested by relying on the supervisor to have the right answer or, alternatively, countering suggestions or assuming that the supervisor's suggestions are one's own ideas. In stage 3, supervisees may recognize areas in which they are functioning autonomously and be able to realistically and unashamedly accept those areas in which they should rely on the supervisor for more assistance.

This issue will usually show up in the context of interpersonal supervision. The supervisor may be overburdened with the responsibility of providing the correct answer and may become annoyed with the pressure to do so, or he or she may feel unneeded by a student who naively feels too independent early in practice. The supervisor may feel chaotically pulled one way and then another. The supervisee may not be quite sure how to act in this tumultuous period of alternation between overreliance and no reliance. Again, the supervisor can weather these issues by not taking personally any actions by the supervisee and by naming and validating the behavior.

Darren initially displayed this issue in stage 1. However, by the middle of the fieldwork period he had become more confident in his ability to work independently. He thanked his supervisor for gently facilitating his independence through her concrete interventions and suggestions.

Identity. The theme of identity may appear as the student struggles to assume a theoretical identity or discern which theory works best. The supervisee may be caught in a conflict of learning one theory while practicing with therapists who use another. In stage 1, the student may not understand how the theory relates to her or his practice and clients. In stage 2, there may be confusion and a sense of trying out different theories or a resistance to learning new theories. In stage 3, the supervisee usually has some sense of how theory relates to clients and which theory seems most appropriate.

Supervisors should consistently help the supervisee integrate theory with practice and explain how the theory relates specifically to clients and the occupational therapy department as a whole. Students may also benefit from projects in which they can research theories and their usefulness for the population with which they are working.

In the case illustration, Darren and Cordelia had learned a specific theory for mental health treatment. They were able to use it throughout the treatment, and were pleased that their supervisor followed the same theory. Tabetha had not learned a specific theory for mental health treatment and initially felt skeptical about having to follow one. However, she gradually came to appreciate its use in the mental health setting. Her final project discussed the theory more in depth.

Individual biases. The theme of individual biases arises because of the negative stereotypes associated with many people with mental disabilities and because of the fear, on the part of society in general, of those stereotypes. Particularly in mental health, one must separate out behaviors that are maladaptive and need change from aspects of the person, which need to be respected.

In stage 1, bias may be manifested in cases where the supervisee criticizes clients yet is unaware of any disrespect. In stage 2, supervisees may find themselves avoiding or dreading contact with a client but be unaware why or, conversely, may find themselves overly controlling in their behavior toward clients and interacting in a demeaning, authoritative way that leaves little room for client autonomy. In the third stage, supervisees will be aware of their biases and prejudices and will hopefully strive, through self-education, to become familiar with different cultural patterns and the effect of symptoms on behavior.

Supervisors should remark on criticisms and authoritative interactions, elicit how the supervisee thinks and feels toward the clients, and discuss the fact that emotions experienced in this context are part of working with clients and thus are natural. Discussing client behavior as a result of, or in the context of, the mental illness rather than as behavior that is deliberately and willfully chosen is often helpful for the beginning therapist who is still learning the difference.

All three students initially were fearful of people with mental disabilities; specifically, they secretly believed them to be unpredictably violent, hopeless, and, maybe, lacking in discipline. They were able to discuss these attitudes with their supervisor, who tolerated the attitudes while at the same time questioning them. The students were shocked when they saw some of the symptoms of the different mental disorders about which they had read. At the same time, they were aware of how the people with whom they worked had thoughts, hopes, desires, dreams, frustrations, and struggles with many of the same issues as they had. Darren, Cordelia, and Tabetha finished their fieldwork with a new sense of respect for the clients' struggles to cope with their disorders and abilities to do many things independently in spite of the disorders.

Learning Styles Approach

A useful model in supervision is based on the experiential learning approach of Kolb (1976; 1984) and Kolb, Rubin, and McIntyre (1979). Experiential learning is considered a cyclical process perceiving and processing (Torrance & Rockenstein, 1988), and the effective learner relies equally on four different learning modes or strategies (Figure 23-2). For example, a **mode** could represent a style of clinical reasoning.

The effective learner is able to flexibly use all of these approaches and experiences for learning, but most people emphasize just one or two of the strategies and do not recognize that they use them exclusively. Consequently, they might not be able to learn effectively in situations or with people who do not include their modes or rely on a different **style**.

The Learning Style Inventory (LSI) (Kolb, 1976) measures relative emphasis on the four learning modes and provides two combination scores, or styles, that indicate the extent to which an individual emphasizes abstractness over concreteness (AC-CE) and active experimentation over reflection (AE-RO) (see

Learning Modes

Concrete Experience (CE) involving oneself fully, openly and without bias in new experiences

is the basis for

Reflection Observation (RO), the ability to reflect on and observe these experiences from many perspectives

these observations are assimilated into a "theory" using

Abstract Conceptualization (AC), the ability to create concepts that integrate observations into logically sound theories

and then to use these theories for

Active Experimentation (AE) or the ability to use hypotheses that serve as guides to create new experiences. (Kolb et al., 1979)

Learning Styles

Divergers (RO/CE) perceive information in a concrete manner, process it reflectively and can generalize from it.

Assimilators (AC/RO) take in information abstractly, begin with an idea and process it reflectively. They watch and think.

Convergers (AC/AE) take in information abstractly and actively process it through experimentation.

Accommodators (AE/CE) take in information concretely and process it actively through doing. (Torrance & Rockenstein, 1988)

Figure 23-2. Experiential Learning Modes and Styles

Table 23-4 for a description of the various learning modes and styles). Divergers perceive information in a concrete manner, process it reflectively, and can generalize from it. Assimilators take in information abstractly, begin with an idea, and process it reflectively; they watch and think. Convergers take in information abstractly and actively process it through experimentation. Accommodators take in information concretely and process it actively through doing (Torrance & Rockenstein, 1988).

Matching modes and styles. For the supervisee, knowing the modes and style of learning that she or he emphasizes will provide an understanding of personal strengths and limitations. Modes and styles that are used can be emphasized in treatment, and less used modes and styles can be identified, learned, and practiced.

The setting and organization can be analyzed to assess the opportunities that exist for the supervisee's learning style; the supervisee can be placed in activities that match her or his style. Opportunities and learning experiences can be designed that appeal to specific styles.

An assessment of the supervisor's style offers an opportunity to match supervisory interactions. It provides an ongoing basis of mutual understanding that may consistently be referred to throughout a fieldwork experience. It also provides a safe and nonthreatening context in which to discuss more personal aspects of self.

Table 23-4. Learning Modes and Styles

Learning Modes

	Concrete Experience	Reflective Observation	Abstract Conceptualization	Active Experimentation
Approach to Learning	Experience-based approach to learning, relies on "feeling" judgments	Tentative, impartial, reflective approach to learning	Analytic approach to learning relies on logical thinking, rational evaluation	Active, "doing" approach to learning; relies on experimentation
Learn Best by	Specific examples in which one can become involved. Treat each situation as unique case	Situation that allows for role of impartial observer rather than participant	Authority-directed, impersonal situations that emphasize theory and systematic analysis	Engagement with activities that test one's own knowledge and ability
Emphasize	People oriented	Introverts	Orientation toward things and symbols	Extroverts
Learn Least by	Theoretical approaches	Doing without thinking	Unstructured, or "discovery," approaches/ simulations	Passive learning situations

Learning Styles

Accommodator (AE/CE)	Diverger (RO/CE)	Assimilator (AC/RO)	Converger (AC/AE)
Ability to carry out plans, action oriented	Imaginative ability, good at generating ideas, brainstorming	Ability to create theoretical models	Good at practical application of ideas
Likes new experiences, "risk-taker," intuitive, trial-and-error style	Can view a situation from many perspectives	Inductive reasoning	Likes a single answer to a problem
Adapts to immediate circumstances	Emotional, interested in people	Concepts over people Less concerned with practical application of theory	Less emotional, less interested in people

CASE ILLUSTRATION: Darren, Cordelia, and Tabetha— A Learning Styles Approach

Modes

Concrete Experience (CE): involving oneself fully, openly, and without bias in new experiences.

Reflection Observation (RO): the ability to reflect on, and observe, experiences from many perspectives.

Abstract Conceptualization (AC): the ability to create concepts that integrate observations into logically sound theories.

Active Experimentation (AE): the ability to use hypotheses that serve as guides to create new experiences.

Styles

Accommodator (AE/CE): take in information concretely, process it actively through doing.

Diverger (RO/CE): take in information concretely, process it by reflection and generalizing.

Assimilator (AC/RO): take in information abstractly with an idea, process it by reflection. Watch and think.

Converger (AC/AE): take in information abstractly, process it actively through experimentation.

Darren's modes of learning were reflective observation (RO) and abstract conceptualization (AC). His style was that of the assimilator. *Cordelia emphasized modes of abstract conceptualization (AC) and concrete experience (CE). Her style of learning was the* accommodator. *Tabetha's preferred modes were abstract experimentation (AE) and concrete experience (CE). Her preferred style was as a* converger. *When they began their internship, all three interns filled out the LSI. They were then able to decide which groups and treatment approaches would most likely to interest them and which would most likely be difficult. With their supervisor's help, they were able to select which aspects of the program would match their styles, and therefore, where they would start. They also agreed on which aspects might be less of a match and therefore saved their involvement in these for later in the fieldwork.*

Their supervisor's learning style was diverger, *and her preferred modes were RO and CE. Since her preferred style was different than that of the students, all four anticipated how they might think or work differently and how the supervisor's expectations might evolve. She went through the Fieldwork Performance Evaluation (AOTA, 1988) to clarify specifically what behavior she expected. Whenever there were snags or confusion in their supervision, they were able to reflect back to their learning styles. They had fun throughout their fieldwork reflecting on their behavior and validating or disproving the validity of the learning styles for themselves. They appreciated that their supervisor made her expectations clear and at the same time listened to their thoughts and feelings before suggesting interventions.*

MAXIMIZING LEARNING—BENEFITING FROM SUPERVISION

As a fieldwork student, you can use different ways of learning to maximize your experience and to benefit most from supervision. Ways of maximizing learning during fieldwork are listed in Table 23-5 and elaborated in the following sections of this chapter.

Emotional Learning

Most individuals about to embark into fieldwork are excited, apprehensive, and willing to do all that they can to maximize the experience. Often the tendency is to find more academic texts or technical material to read. While seeking out

Table 23-5. Guidelines for Maximizing Learning during Fieldwork

Emotional	Intellectual	Interpersonal	Professional
Read narratives and personal stories of mental illness	Review academic material	Ask for help	Take initiative
Anticipate emotional issues and stages of fieldwork		Communicate expectations responsibly in supervision	Become familiar with your setting
Know your learning style	Plan a progressive program of involvement according to your learning style	Discuss learning style in supervision	Time management—plan a daily schedule and routine and use time effectively and flexibly
Self-reflection		Remain open and genuine and communicate with awareness	Schedule regular supervision time
Recognize when the work setting touches off personal issues		Communicate in supervision or with other staff when the work setting influences personal issues	Communicate in supervision when the work setting influences personal issues

information is always a good idea, certain information can be more useful for the fieldwork experience in mental health. Specifically, any texts that are personal stories or narratives that could broaden an understanding of people, of people with mental disabilities, or of oneself will help maximize the experience.

This chapter has highlighted a model that delineated emotional stages and issues, many of which will be encountered. A knowledge of the stages and understanding of the issues that might be most pertinent to yourself can help in anticipating potential personal "snags" in the process. Alerting the supervisor in advance to problems or anxieties that might arise will help both the supervisor and supervisee to flow through troublesome spots. This chapter also highlighted a model based on learning styles. Knowing your learning style in advance and alerting the supervisor to it may also anticipate, and possibly avoid, misunderstandings. You can anticipate in advance which experiences at your fieldwork site may match your learning style and therefore will be easiest to participate in, and which experiences will not match and therefore may be more difficult. Together, you and your supervisor could plan a step-by-step, progressive program starting with involvement in experiences that may be more comfortable and then attempting those that may be more difficult. Together, you and the supervisor can solve anticipated problems in advance.

Knowing yourself, your possible emotional stages, and your learning style will assist in maximizing a successful fieldwork experience. However, expressing your emotional interior and learning style in a direct, honest, and genuine manner with the ability to be self-reflective is also essential. In general, the more aware, open, and willing an individual is to communicate responsibly, the more the fieldwork and supervisory relationship will develop smoothly and the fewer problems will arise. With self-awareness and responsible communication, conflicts and disagreements can be avoided or resolved with mutual satisfaction.

Learning about Expectations

Fieldwork sites must clearly identify expectations of the fieldwork experience (AOTA, 1988; Privott, 1998b). Therefore, students should be aware of, and ready to discuss, expectations at the outset of fieldwork. Expectations should be written and can be in the form of objectives specific to each category of the Fieldwork Performance Report (AOTA, 1988); guidelines outlining goals to be achieved during certain time periods; guidelines, dates, and formats of any assignments; and criteria for professional behavior at that center. The expectations should be verbally discussed and can be referred to during the experience. The early discussion of expectations is a good time to discuss strengths and weaknesses, interests, learning style, goals, and expectations.

Intellectual and Interpersonal Learning

Generally, now is the time to utilize material learned from academic classes, and to go back and look at it. Keep in mind a rule that never will fail; ask for help whenever there is the slightest doubt or question, provided taking the initiative to find the answer has failed. Take the time to familiarize yourself with your setting.

This means finding out where things are kept and what is available. Ask if you are unsure of the use of some equipment.

Plan a daily schedule and learn the day-to-day routine as quickly as possible. Observe other therapists to learn their successful treatment techniques and personal approach. Choose one whose style you can emulate. Make sure that regular time is scheduled with your supervisor and that appointments are always kept. If you are not getting enough feedback, or need to be observed more times, let your supervisor know.

Sometimes, how ideas and emotions are conveyed makes a difference. Take the time to read a few books concerning responsible communication. Remember that in mental health settings, issues and problems with which clients are dealing may touch off issues and problems that you are struggling with yourself. It is not normal in a mental health setting to deny emotions due to personal problems that may be uncovered or raised by client contact. It is normal to use your supervisory relationship to make sense of those emotions and plan the best way to personally handle them and use them in service of the client.

Professional Learning

Professional behaviors will be expected during the fieldwork experience. Behaviors of a professional are (AOTA, 1988; Privott, 1998b):

- Responsibility, such as initiative in learning and using resources, dependability in routine work, and punctuality
- Organizational skills, such as planning and carrying out daily responsibilities in a timely manner
- Flexibility, such as knowing how to use time effectively when changes in treatment or schedules occur
- Commitment to the department and profession

THE TRANSITION TO FIELDWORK EDUCATOR OR SUPERVISOR

The transition to fieldwork educator is an important change in professional identity. Although there has been much preparation for developing clinical skills, there is less preparation for using supervisory skills. In addition, there are no rituals or rites of passage, such as passing the registry exam that indicates the transition from student to professional, to facilitate the role transition from clinician to supervisor.

In spite of this, supervisors informally use different experiences to assume their new role. *As a trainee,* the supervisee has had "hands-on" experience in supervision. Trainees have had a variety of role models, and the orientation of previous supervisors will influence their own style. *As a clinician,* the new supervisor has developed clinical competence in assessing and treating clients' needs and judging when to intervene. These skills can be useful in a supervisor relationship. The new supervisor has experience as a *colleague*, responding to, and interacting with, other professionals. In classrooms, they have taken clinical seminars where they have nondefensively assessed their strengths and weaknesses, provided and received feedback. New supervisors can generalize from their rich experiences to support their transition.

Skills of the Fieldwork Educator or Supervisor

Supervisor attitudes or values and skill development have not been highly researched in the psychology literature (Vidlak, 2003) and also are not a popular topic in the occupational therapy literature (for example, *Willard and Spackman's* 10th edition [2003] does not mention the topic of fieldwork, and it is not a concern in the Occupational Therapy Practice Framework [2002]). Nevertheless, there are important skills that a fieldwork educator should develop, particularly in view of the many studies in the psychology literature that validate what students perceive and want in a supervisor and supervisory relationship. Also, more recent studies document the existence of negative events or negative supervision that may be harmful to the student (see this chapter's section, Dimensions of Fieldwork Education and Supervision, for the citations and Lew, 2003).

Useful skills and values that are necessary in the fieldwork educator for the specific task of supervision particularly in mental health environments are:

- Ability to listen purposively (Gillfillan, 2001) more than talk (Fleck, 2001)
- Positive regard (Bradley & Gould, 2000)
- Trust and mutuality
- Warmth and genuineness
- Emotional neutrality (Gillfillan, 2001) and acceptance
- Interpersonal sensitivity (Nelson & Friedlander, 2001)
- Supportiveness, particularly in the early stages of fieldwork II (Ramos-Sanchez et al., 2002) or in fieldwork I (Cara, 2000; Summerall et al., 1998)
- Self-awareness and the capacity for self-reflection
- Self-disclosure and the capacity to know when to self-disclose (Noelle, 2002)
- Ethics, particularly keeping confidentiality (Ladany et al., 1999)
- Guidance in difficult cases or clinical dilemmas (Shanfield, Heterly, & Matthews, 2001)
- Integrity and ruthless honesty
- Sympathy for the student process and personal concerns (Shanfield, Heterly, & Matthews, 2001)
- Provision of adequate time and attention to the supervisee (Trant, 2001)
- Ability to "own conflicts" and to resolve conflicts (Nelson & Friedlander, 2001)

- Ability to at least understand, if not work with, different perspectives (Ladany et. al., 1999) (although this is usually a skill required of a student!).

Role of the Fieldwork Educator or Supervisor in Mental Health

The supervisor has multiple roles:

- Maintaining a contract with the academic setting and communicating with the academic fieldwork supervisor
- Facilitating the development of clinical competence through skill and knowledge development, particularly the clinical reasoning process
- Facilitating professional growth in attitude and performance in the supervisee
- Shepherding the supervisee through a training process that includes standards, expectations, and evaluation
- Introducing the supervisee to the people and culture of the department and the overall setting
- Being a role model of a professional and clinically competent occupational therapist
- Being alert to the differences and conflicts that may arise in the supervisory relationship

Perhaps the most important emphasis in occupational therapy is on the supervisor's role of clinical educator. Accordingly, the role of educator and the model the educator uses also dictate the important task of teaching clinical reasoning, discussed in the next section, along with the roles of manager, teacher, mentor, guide, and coach. The last role is important specifically in a mental health setting, where therapists emphasize being sensitive to the nuances of interpersonal relationships and often urge clients to be aware of emotions that may arise. Being able to openly discuss or focus on emotions and differences, and communicating expectations clearly may be crucial to patients needs (Frum & Opacich, 1987).

Hopefully, the new supervisor will use the models presented in this chapter to assess the supervisory process and will further explore each of its dimensions. For example, using the Learning Style Inventory will allow a supervisor and a supervisee to recognize interpersonal differences in learning and expectations that may occur in the supervisory relationship. Knowing a student's learning style will enable both the supervisor and supervisee to assess the opportunities for learning that exist at the setting and perhaps to anticipate how the setting may be lacking in experiences that match the student's learning style. Knowing the counseling psychology developmental stages may enable the supervisor to better understand and to validate the student's emotions and behavior as they relate to the stages and critical issues. The supervisor and student can both learn and anticipate the ebb and flow of the fieldwork experience. Knowing the cognitive developmental model may enable the supervisor to design specific interventions and to use specific language in the supervision process. Knowing the various dimensions of supervision that have been researched in other literature will enable fieldwork educators to expand their repertoire of skills, understand students' needs and behaviors, and tailor the supervisory relationship and expectations to each individual student.

Tasks of the Fieldwork Educator or Supervisor

The tasks of supervision in a mental health setting are: (1) prearrival responsibilities, (2) orientation, (3) on-site assignments, (4) evaluating student performance, (5) developing fieldwork objectives, and (6) conducting supervision (Kolodner, Wiener & Frum, 1989) including teaching the clinical reasoning process (Cara, 2000; Privott, 1998c). The fieldwork tasks can be adapted for any supervision process. (The skills roles and tasks of the fieldwork educator are listed in Table 23-6).

Prearrival responsibilities.   The responsibilities of the fieldwork educator include:

- Working with the academic fieldwork coordinator to coordinate scheduling and gathering relevant information concerning the student
- Developing fieldwork objectives
- Developing a fieldwork manual

Orientation.   Orientation includes written and verbal information and orientation sessions during the beginning two weeks of the fieldwork experience. The information should orient the student to the facility, department, and community, if necessary, and explain how the facility and its separate elements and departments operate together. Different sessions conducted by different departments can be planned in advance.

On-site assignments.   Many centers have a schedule of weekly assignments that taper off after the midpoint evaluation. Many have special onetime assignments such as case studies, literature reviews, and projects. Some require students to visit other sites and to assess other delivery systems. It is highly recommended that supervisors collaborate and develop an assignment with the student, and if any projects are assigned, that only one, comprehensive assignment be required. The purpose of fieldwork education is for the student to develop as a professional and apply knowledge that has been already learned. Weekly assignments (unless necessary for certain individuals) may have the effect of keeping the fieldwork learner in a "student" performance mode and derail him or her from the business of learning to be a clinician.

Student evaluations.   The student's performance should be evaluated formally at least twice, usually at the midpoint and at the completion of the fieldwork, using the official AOTA Fieldwork Performance Report (FWPR). It is recommended that the supervisor carefully go through the form with the student during the beginning two weeks of the fieldwork. At that time the supervisor can

Table 23-6.	Skills, roles and Tasks of the Fieldworker Educator	
Skills	*Roles*	*Tasks*
Purposive listening	Contract with academic setting	Coordinate scheduling, develop objectives and a manual
Positive regard toward student	Facilitating clinical competence and professional growth	Ongoing observation and evaluation and supervision
Trust and mutuality		
Warmth and genuineness	Shepherding student through fieldwork	On-site assignments
Emotional neutrality	Introducing student to setting	Orientation
Acceptance		Consistent clinical and professional behavior
Interpersonal sensitivity	Role model	
Support	Being alert to supervisory relationship	Ongoing observation and communication, ongoing training
Self-awareness and self-reflection		
Self-disclosure		
Ethics and keeping confidentiality		
Guidance in dilemmas		
Integrity and ruthless honesty		
Sympathy		
Adequate time		
Own and resolve conflicts		
Understand different perspectives		

delineate those areas that are emphasized, any biases that the supervisor maintains about the performance areas, and expectations regarding the specific behaviors that are evaluated. The supervisor should inform the supervisee of what is considered to be ideal communication and the expectations for performance of those skills at different points in the fieldwork.

Ongoing evaluation should take place throughout the fieldwork experience. Specific instances should be cited in giving feedback to the student, and a representative sample of work behavior and performance should be gathered in order to evaluate. Regular observations are recommended, particularly observations that are made immediate to a situation or behavior (AOTA, 1988).

Fieldwork objectives. These are written statements that specify the minimal level of performance that should be attained. Although these may be verbally communicated they should be written and available for current and potential students. Objectives usually specify competency in assessment and evaluation, implementing treatment, effective written and oral communication, and the demonstration of professional characteristics (AOTA, 1988).

Supervision. Supervisory tasks are divided into categories of skill development, personal growth, and evaluation. An implicit goal of fieldwork training is to learn how a clinician thinks, that is, how a clinician reasons in the clinic (Cohn, 1989; Privott, 1998c) and helpful ways of teaching clinical reasoning are explicated in the field (Neidstadt, 1996). In fact, clinical reasoning may be the very process by which students learn skills and acquire a professional identity. (See Chapter 18 for further information regarding clinical reasoning.) Personal growth is crucial in a mental health setting. Recognizing one's own behavior and how it is influenced by clients' responses will assist supervisees to better deal with clients' own interpersonal and intrapersonal struggles. Supervisors' acceptance and interpretation of client interactions and of a supervisee's reactions and behavior with clients facilitate both personal growth and clinical competence. Overall, the supervisor should have firsthand information about the student's strengths and weaknesses that is compiled from frequent observations of performance. The firsthand knowledge should be communicated regularly to help the supervisee to learn. Feedback should be constructive, timed as close to the occurrence as possible, and based on behavior.

Supervisory training.   There are various methods of learning how to be a supervisor. In addition to the resources listed in this chapter, it is recommended that individuals attend workshops and training at state, regional, and national conferences, belong to fieldwork councils associated with university programs, and seek consultation and training from academics who specialize in fieldwork supervision training. One study found that "supervisors who had participated in a practicum class on supervision, a combined practicum/didactic class on supervision, or had received supervision of his/her provision had significantly higher scores on supervisor development than those supervisors who had not" (Vidlak, 2002, p. 3029).

TRENDS AND RECOMMENDATIONS

Various trends in the psychological literature of the past five years indicate directions for occupational therapy fieldwork and research into fieldwork. Primary attention has been paid to the roles of the supervisor and supervisee. The role of the fieldwork educator indicates that students prefer the skills of support, warmth, genuineness, integrity, ethical behavior, and ability to own and resolve conflicts (Bradley & Gould, 2001; Shanfield, Hetherly, & Matthews, 2001). The literature suggests that fieldwork educators can learn these facilitative skills in a variety of ways through classes, conferences, clinical councils, or purchasing consultation (Vidlak, 2002).

More attention has been paid to students' experiences in supervision The role of the fieldwork student indicates that students who can be more reflective can develop advanced skills and trust in their own experiences as a guide to delivering occupational therapy (Peyton, 2002). Positive outcomes indicate that there is a role for emotion (Hahn, 2001; Foullette & Batten, 2000), the expression of emotion (Yourman, 2003), and self-disclosure in the supervision relationship (Ladany & Walker, 2003). Unfortunately, there are many more articles documenting negative supervisory experiences (Greer, 2002; Ladany et al., 1999; Nelson et al., 2001;

Nelson & Friedlander, 2001; Ramos-Sanchez et al., 2002; Trant, 2001). In some cases the experiences were harmful to students. One study in occupational therapy has indicated that negative experiences also happen in fieldwork (Lew, 2003).

Fewer studies have explored experimental programs for supervision; however, some innovations suggest programs that might be established in occupational therapy. For example, supervision groups (Altfeld, 1999; Oegren, Apelman, & Klawitter, 2001) and use of video supervision (Sorlie, Gammon, Bergvik, & Sexton, 1999) appeared successful. Also, a one-session introduction to supervision appeared helpful for residents (Whitman, 2001) and a three-hour training for practicum students appeared to increase self-efficacy and decrease anxiety (Cara, 2000).

Pressing practice, training, and research needs identified for psychotherapy supervision (Watkins, 1998) can equally apply to occupational therapy. The practice and training needs include more training in how to supervise, and the development of supervision manuals. The research needs include valid and reliable measurements, more rigorous research designs, a multimethod and rater longitudinal focus, and replication studies.

Summary

Supervision is valued in most health professions, particularly mental health settings. Supervisors and supervisees often have different expectations of supervision. Students look more for instruction, while supervisors emphasize the interaction and relationship. The goal of the supervisee is often to learn techniques. The supervisor's goal is to help an individual become a professional.

There are four components influencing supervision: the supervisor, the supervisee, the relationship and the interaction of the two, and the environment or setting. Supervision is a dynamic process among these components. Theoretical models of supervision have been developed from the psychoanalytic, behavioral, humanistic, and developmental schools. Supervision usually involves an eclectic blend of techniques from all of these models. An occupational therapy developmental model emphasizes the supervisee and supervisor components. A counseling psychology model emphasizes the process the supervisee goes through and the supervisory relationship. A learning styles approach emphasizes the supervisee and the setting. Students can prepare for their role in fieldwork. The transition to the role of supervisor is supported by a variety of experiences. Supervisors can learn a variety of skills, roles, and tasks.

Review Questions

1. Describe the elements or components of supervision.
2. What have the theoretical models contributed to supervision? Which has contributed most to occupational therapy?
3. What are the similarities of the developmental models?
4. How can the learning styles contribute to supervision?

5. Of the three students in the examples and case studies, with whom are you most similar, and why? What are experiences that might be easy and those that might be difficult for you during your fieldwork experience?

References

Altfeld, D. A. (1999). An experiential group model for psychotherapy supervision. *International Journal of Group Psychotherapy, 49*(2), 237–254.

American Occupational Therapy Association (AOTA). (1991). *Self-Paced instruction for clinical education and supervision [SPICES]: An instructional guide for clinical educators and supervisors.* Rockville, MD: Author.

American Occupational Therapy Association. (1994). Guide for supervision of occupational therapy personnel. *American Journal of Occupational Therapy, 48*, 11.

American Occupational Therapy Association. (1996). Purpose and value of occupational therapy fieldwork education. *American Journal of Occupational Therapy, 50*, 10:845.

American Occupational Therapy Association. Commission on Education. (1988). *Fieldwork experience manual for academic fieldwork coordinators, fieldwork supervisors and students.* Rockville, MD: Author.

Andersen, S. O. (2002). Fieldwork: A road to employment. *Occupational Therapy in Health Care, 16*(1), 37–43.

Bradley, L., & Gould, L. J. (2000). Psychotherapy-based models of counselor supervision. In L. Bradley & N. Ladany (Eds.), *Counselor supervision: Principles, process, and practice* (pp. 147–180). New York: Brunner-Routledge.

Cara, E. D. (200). *The effects of a prepracticum educational module on self-efficacy, self-esteem, anxiety, and performance.* Unpublished doctoral dissertation. The Fielding Institute, Santa Barbara, CA.

Cohn, E. S. (1989). Fieldwork education: Shaping a foundation for clinical reasoning. A. *American Journal of Occupational Therapy, 43*, 240–244.

Christie, B. A., Joyce, P., & Moeller, P. L. (1985). Fieldwork experience, Part II: The supervisor's dilemma. *American Journal of Occupational Therapy, 39*(10), 675–681.

Dougher, M. K. (2001). *Multiple concurrent supervision: The impact on case conceptualization.* Dissertation Abstracts International, 61(12-B), 6702, UMI AAI9997137.

Fleck, S. (2001). Fifty-five years of supervision. In R. Balsam (Ed.), *Psychodynamic psychotherapy: The supervisory process* (pp. 3–23). Madison, CT: International Universities Press.

Foullette, V., & Batten, S. (2000). The role of emotion in psychotherapy supervision: A contextual behavioral analysis. *Cognitive and Behavioral Practice, 7*(3), 306–312.

Frum, D., & Opacich, K. (1987). *Supervision: Development of therapeutic competence.* Rockville, MD: AOTA.

Gillfillan, S. (2001). On teaching the role of neutrality in listening within the era of managed care. In R. Balsam (Ed.), *Psychodynamic psychotherapy: The supervisory process* (pp. 229–247). Madison, WI: International Universities Press.

Greer, J. A. (2002). Where to turn for help: Responses to inadequate clinical supervision. *Clinical Supervisor, 21*(1), 135–143.

Hahn, W. K. (2001). The experience of shame in psychotherapy supervision. *Psychotherapy: Theory, Research, Practice, and Training, 38*(3), 272–282.

Hantoot, M. S. (2000). Lying in psychotherapy supervision: Why residents say one thing and do another. *Academic Psychiatry, 24*(4), 179–187.

Henderson, C. E., Cawyer, C. S., & Watkins, Jr., C. E. (1999). A comparison of student and supervisor perceptions of effective practicum supervision. *Clinical Supervisor, 18*(1) 47–74.

Hora, T. (1957). Contribution to the phenomenology of the supervisory process. *American Journal of Psychotherapy, 11*, 769–773.

Kautzmann, L. N. (1987). Perceptions of the purpose of level I fieldwork. *American Journal of Occupational Therapy, 41*(9), 595–600.

Kolb, D. (1976). Learning Style Inventory technical manual. Boston: McBer.

Kolb, D. (1984). *Experiential learning: Experience as the source of learning and development*. Englewood Cliffs, NJ: Prentice-Hall.

Kolb, D., Rubin, I., & McIntyre, J. (Eds.). (1979). *Organizational psychology: An experiential approach* (3rd ed.). Englewood Cliffs, NJ: Prentice-Hall.

Kolodner, E., Wiener, W., & Frum, D. (1989). *Models for mental health fieldwork*. Rockville, MD: AOTA.

Ladany, N., Lehrman-Waterman, D., Molinaro, M., & Wolgast, B. (1999). Psychotherapy supervisor ethical practices: Adherence to guidelines, the supervisory working alliance, and supervisee satisfaction. *Counseling Psychologist, 27*(3), 443–475.

Ladanay, N., & Walker, J. (2003). Supervision self-disclosure: Balancing the uncontrollable narcissist with the indomitable altruist. *Journal of Clinical Psychology, 59*(5), 611–621.

Leddick, G., & Bernard, J. (1980, March). The history of supervision: A critical review. *Counselor Education and Supervision*, pp. 187–196.

Lew, N. (2003). *Negative Fieldwork experiences in occupational therapy*. Unpublished master's project. San Jose State University, San Jose, CA.

Loganbill, C. R., Hardy, E. V., & Delworth, U. (1982). Supervision: A conceptual model. *Counseling Psychologist, 10*(1), 3–42.

Meerlo, J. A. (1952). Some psychological processes in supervision of therapists. *American Journal of Psychotherapy, 6*, 467–470.

Munroe, H. (1988). Modes of operation in clinical supervision: How clinical supervisors perceive themselves. *British Journal of Occupational Therapy, 51*(10), 338–343.

Neistadt, M. (1996). Teaching strategies for the development of clinical reasoning. *American Journal of Occupational Therapy, 50*, 676–684.

Nelson, M. L., & Friedlander, M. L. (2001). A close look at conflictual supervisory relationships: The trainee's perspective. *Journal of Counseling Psychology, 48*(4), 384–395.

Nelson, M. L., Gray, L. A., Friedlander, M. L., Ladany, N., & Walker, J. A. (2001). Toward relationship-centered supervision: Reply to Veach (2001) and Ellis (2001). *Journal of Counseling Psychology, 48*(4), 407–409.

Noelle, M. (2003). Self-report in supervision: Positive and negative slants. *Clinical Supervisor, 21*(1), 125–134.

Oegren, M. L., Apelman, A., & Klawitter, M. (2001). The group in psychotherapy supervision. *Clinical Supervisor, 20*(2), 147–175.

Peyton, E. A. (2002). *Reflecting on the therapeutic relationship: A qualitative study of trainees' experiences in learning a relational treatment modality*. Dissertation Abstracts International, 63(6B), 3020, UMI AAI3056998.

Privott, C. R. (1998a). In C. Privott (Ed.), *The fieldwork anthology: A classic research and practice collection* (pp. xi–xii). Bethesda, MD: American Occupational Therapy Association.

Privott, C. R. (1998b). *The fieldwork anthology: A classic research and practice collection*. Bethesda, MD: American Occupational Therapy Association.

Privott, C. R. (1998c). Learning styles and clinical reasoning. In C. R. Privott (Ed.), *The fieldwork anthology: A classic research and practice Collection* (p. 2, section 1). Bethesda, MD: American Occupational Therapy Association.

Ramos-Sanchez, L., Esnil, E., Goodwin, A., Riggs, S., Touster, L. O., Wright, L. K., et al. (2002). Negative supervisory events: Effects on supervision and supervisory alliance. *Professional Psychology: Research and Practice, 33*(2), 197–202.

Schwartz, K. B. (1984). An approach to supervision of occupational therapy students. *American Journal of Occupational Therapy, 38*, 1033–1037.

Shanfield, S. B., Hetherly, V. V., & Matthews, K. L. (2001). Excellent supervision: The residents' perspective. *Journal of Psychotherapy, Practice, and Research, 10*(1), 23–27.

Sorlie, T., Gammon, D., Bergvik, S., & Sexton, H. (1999). Psychotherapy supervision face to face and by videoconferencing: A comparative study. *British Journal of Psychotherapy, 15*(4), 452–462.

Still, J. R. (1982). Mini-councils: A solution to fieldwork supervision. *American Journal of Occupational Therapy, 36*, 390–394.

Sumerall, S. W., Barke, C. R., Timmons, P. L., Oehlert, M. E., Lopez, S. J., & Trent, D. D. (1998). The adaptive counseling and therapy model and supervision of mental health care. *Clinical supervisor, 17*(2), 171–176.

Torrance, E., & Rockenstein, Z. (1988). Styles of thinking and creativity. In R. Schmeck (Ed.), *Learning styles and learning strategies* (pp. 275–290). New York: Plenum.

Trant, R. P. (2001). Elements and outcome of school psychologist internship supervision: A retrospective study. *Dissertation Abstracts International 61*(9–A): 3477, IS 0419–4209.

Vidlak, N. (2002). *Identifying important factors in supervisor development: An examination of supervisor experience, training, and attributes.* Dissertation Abstracts International, 63(6B), UMI AA13055295.

Walker, C., & Cooper, F. M. (1993). Fieldwork education: To charge or not to charge. *British Journal of Occupational Therapy, 56*(2), 51–54.

Watkins, C. Edward, Jr. (1998). Psychotherapy supervision in the 21st century: Some pressing needs and impressing possibilities. *Journal of Psychotherapy, Practice, and Research, 7*(2), 93–101.

Whitman, S. M. (2001). Teaching residents to use supervison effectively. *Academic Psychiatry, 25*(3), 143–1467.

Yourman, D. B. (2003). Trainee disclosure in psychotherapy supervision: The impact of shame. *Journal of Clinical Psychology, 59*(5), 601–609.

Suggested Reading and Other Resources

Amerantes, J. (1994). *Supervisory styles of practicing occupational therapists.* Unpublished manuscript, San Jose State University.

Cara, E. (1994, May). *Ways of supervision: The Learning Styles Inventory.* Workshop presented at the San Jose State University Fieldwork Council.

Cara, E., & Schwartz, K. (1992, October). *Reflections on clinical supervision: What works, what doesn't.* Workshop presented at the Occupational Therapy Association of California, Los Angeles.

Cohn, E., & Frum, D. (1988). The issue is: Fieldwork supervision: More education is warranted. *American Journal of Occupational Therapy, 42*(5), 325–327.

Kasar, J., & Clark, E. N. (2000). *Developing professional behaviors.* Thorofare, NJ: Slack.

Lewin, J. E., & Reed, C. A. (1998). *Creative problem solving in occupational therapy.* Philadelphia: Lippincott.

Mitchell, M., & Kampfe, C. (1990). Coping strategies used by occupational therapy students during fieldwork: An exploratory study. *American Journal of Occupational Therapy, 44*(6), 543–549.

Palladino, J., & Jeffries, R. N. (2000). *The occupational therapy manual for assessing professional skills.* Philadelphia: F. A. Davis.

Scott, S., Wells, S., & Hanebrink, S. (1997). *Educating college students with disabilities: What academic fieldwork coordinators need to know.* Bethesda, MD: American Occupational Therapy Association.

Sladyk, K. (2002). *The successful occupational therapy fieldwork student.* Thorofare, NJ: Slack.

Stafford, E. (1986). Relationship between occupational therapy student learning styles and clinic performance. *American Journal of Occupational Therapy, 40*(1), 34–39.

Swinehart, S., & Meyers, S. (1993). Level I fieldwork: Creating a positive experience. *American Journal of Occupational Therapy, 47*(1), 68–73.

Vidlak, N. (2002). Identifying important factors in supervisor development: An examination of supervisor experience, training, and attributes. *Dissertation Abstracts International,* 63(6B), UMI AA13055295.

Wells, S. A., & Hanebrink, S. (1998). *A guide to reasonable accommodations for occupational therapy practitioners with disabilities: Fieldwork to employment.* Bethesda, MD: American Occupational Therapy Association.

CHAPTER 24

Demonstrating Effectiveness in Occupational Therapy

Anne MacRae, PhD, OTR/L

Key Terms

collaboration
efficacy
evidence based practice

hypothesis
networking
research

Chapter Outline

Introduction
Communication
Evidence-based Practice
Documentation
    Types of Documentation
    Documentation Review
Research
    Collaborative Research
    Methods

Promotion
Presentation and Publication
Summary

Introduction

The philosophy of occupational therapy is, on the surface, so simple that it tends to be taken for granted. However, the relationship between occupation and health has profound significance, and it is our responsibility to fully explore all facets of occupational therapy. A core concept of occupational therapy philosophy is the belief that occupation plays an important role in the maintenance and improvement of mental as well as physical health. This philosophy is thoroughly discussed in Chapter 3 but can also be identified throughout this book, even though the clinical presentations and treatment environments are quite diverse. In a study conducted by Moll and Cook (1997) occupational therapists identified many client-related benefits of engagement in occupation for people with mental illness. These included "skill development; impairment reduction; self-awareness; positive self concept; interaction or connection with others; healthy, balanced routines; pleasure; and enhancement of occupational role performance" (p. 662). Although these beliefs about occupation are at the core of practice and anecdotal support abounds, the focus on gathering, documenting, and disseminating scientific evidence regarding the **efficacy** of occupational therapy (OT) interventions is a recent phenomenon.

The foremost outcome of occupational therapy services is the development, improvement, or restoration of occupation with OT intervention directed toward "engagement in occupation to support participation" (Occupational Therapy Practice Framework, 2002, p. 614). In mental health settings, the specific functional outcomes encompass the entire range of performance areas, including activities of daily living, productive activities, and leisure activities. Many people, even with serious and persistent mental illness, can accomplish substantial goals within these areas with observable behavioral change. However, in some cases the outcome of occupational therapy is subtle and may take considerable time. In this era of cost containment, it is essential that occupational therapists be able to articulate such outcomes and demonstrate the need for skilled interventions. It is also critical for occupational therapists to understand the context or environment of treatment in order to develop realistic goals (see Chapter 2). For example, in acute psychiatric settings, it is often not possible to achieve substantial change in functional performance. However, occupational therapy facilitates the stabilization process of acute episodes, allowing the client to benefit from follow-up treatment. Activities in acute care are often enabling precursors to improved function. In some cases, acute care treatment must be viewed as part of a treatment continuum, where the outcome of the acute care treatment only constitutes the initial part of the process.

The documentation of functional outcomes in mental health OT is sometimes problematic because of the cyclical and sometimes chronic nature of many mental illnesses. Continued structure and support provided by occupational therapy contributes to the prevention of relapse and maintenance of function, particularly in the community. This may be accomplished through consultation as well as training and supervision of nonprofessionals; however, although conclusive evidence is lacking, the clinical skills and experience of an occupational therapist are invaluable in the continuity of care. **Research** on the cost-effectiveness of direct clinical services of occupational therapy versus consultative services is urgently needed.

There is a direct link in the ability to provide effective occupational therapy and the professional competence of OT practitioners. Ensuring continued competency and professional development is the ultimate responsibility of the individual occupational therapist (Fawcett & Strickland, 1998; Youngstrom, 1998), but professional associations provide guidance and support through continuing education opportunities, as well as the publication of standards of practice and codes of ethics. The American Occupational Therapy Association (AOTA) also provides an on-line professional development tool for clinicians to assess, develop, and document a professional development plan (AOTA, 2003).

In a client-centered occupational therapy practice, competence implies much more than technical proficiency. Occupational therapy addresses all areas of an individual's occupational functioning in context, therefore, professional competence must be broad based. "We understand that competence means aptitude, proficiency and experience, as well as personal fitness to undertake the tasks and responsibilities that are assigned to professional occupational therapists. These pertain to ethical practice, appropriate public representation of what professional organizations stand for, and action with respect to civil, political, economic, social and cultural rights if deemed necessary" (Watson, 2002, p. 8).

COMMUNICATION

All avenues of efficacy demonstration begin with the ability to articulate the philosophical principles and professional identity of occupational therapy. In other words, in order to show the effectiveness of OT, occupational therapists must be able to clearly express their beliefs and values in both oral and written communication. In their day-to-day lives, occupational therapists have many opportunities to share these principles. In a health care setting, the occupational therapist will routinely represent the profession to clients, other health care professionals, administrators, and family members. This representation may be an informal conversation in a hallway or a presentation at a team or family meeting or case conference. However, in order for that sharing to be effective, the occupational therapist must have strong, confident communication skills and the ability to adapt the communication to the needs and level of understanding of others. Figure 24-1 suggests strategies for successful communication in these situations.

Descriptions of occupational therapy will vary depending on who is receiving the information and for what purpose. However, all descriptions should show a clear professional identity with identifiable goals. The recipient of the information should be able to identify the uniqueness of occupational therapy and what the occupational therapist has to offer.

Remember audience and purpose
  identify philosophical premise of treatment within the institution
  know expectations of meeting
  use shared, understandable language
Know yourself
  identify your own personal strengths and weaknesses as appropriate
  share desires for further development
  delegate and clarify roles within the OT department
Listen to others
  add, rather than duplicate, information
  be familiar with training and background of other professionals
  avoid "turf wars"
Structure Presentation
  use consistent format (based on predefined role)
  avoid repetitive or obvious information
  summarize data (technical competence and justification of services)
  interpret data (clinical competence)
Consult as needed
  refer audience to additional resources or documentation
  offer in-service education
  provide written protocols

Figure 24-1.   Strategies for Successful Clinical Communication

EVIDENCE-BASED PRACTICE

The occupational therapy profession throughout the world has recognized the need for the establishment of **evidence-based practice**. Literature on its definitions, purpose, and need as well as specific articles on how to locate and apply evidence in practice can be found in every major occupational therapy journal. Among the leaders in publishing about evidence-based practice are Tickle-Degnen (2000; 2001; 2002), Law and Baum (1998) and Lloyd-Smith (1997; 1999). For the purposes of this chapter, a brief outline of evidence-based practice is provided. However, the reader is urged to explore the plethora of original literature (including but not limited to the references cited in this chapter) in order to fully understand the implications of evidence-based practice.

The concept of evidence-based practice began within the medical model, and occupational therapists are justifiably concerned about over-identification with medical models to define OT practice. The need for outcome studies and establishing efficacy of treatment is very real, but the concern is that traditional scientific research and medically oriented methods of establishing efficacy may not really address the realities of occupational therapy intervention. In order to address this issue, the Canadian Association of Occupational Therapists (CAOT, 1999) presented a unique definition of evidence-based occupational therapy as follows: "The client-centered enablement of occupation based on client infor-mation and a critical review of relevant research, expert consensus and past expe-rience" (p. 3).

The cornerstone of evidence-based practice is the utilization of systemic analy-sis of the existing literature. However, using the CAOT definition, one must go beyond the published research material and utilize information provided by the client (personal narratives, subjective reports, goal setting) as well as identify spe-cific expertise of the practitioner (knowledge, training, experience, theory base).

In order for occupational therapy clinicians to engage in evidence-based prac-tice, skills must be developed in data retrieval (particularly from electronic sources) as well as in clinical reasoning and critical analysis. In her Eleanor Clark Slagle Lecture (1962), Mary Reilly foretold the need for these skills long before the current emphasis on evidence-based practice. "Criticism stings a profession into a new and more demanding formulation of purpose . . . A disciplined person in either the sciences or the professions uses critical thinking as a personal tool of reality testing and problem solving" (p. 2). Yerxa (influenced by Reilly in her early years of practice) implores occupational therapists to not settle for being bio-medical technicians but to develop into detectives who search "for new ideas that will support clinical practice and enable the profession to achieve its potential contribution to humankind" (2000, p. 192).

DOCUMENTATION

Therapists often cite documentation as their least favorite job responsibility. Often it is considered a "waste of time" or meaningless paperwork. However, it serves several legal and ethical functions. Moreover, if documentation is done properly, it can be a valuable tool for increasing interdisciplinary communication and therapeutic effectiveness as well as provide a vehicle for client and profes-sional advocacy. According to the American Occupational Therapy Association (AOTA) (Kohlman Thompson & Foto, 1995), the purpose of documentation is to:

1. provide a chronological record of the consumer's condition, which details the complete course of therapeutic intervention.
2. facilitate communication among professionals who contribute to consumers' care.
3. provide an objective basis to determine the appropriateness, effectiveness, and necessity of therapeutic intervention.
4. reflect the practitioner's reasoning.

Documentation in mental health settings poses some difficulties because "psy-chiatric problems are often complex due to individual variables not specific to a diagnostic category" (Menenberg, 1995, p. 140). Care must be taken to provide clear and concise documentation while maintaining a holistic approach and recog-nizing the interrelated complexities of the individual and the environment. As dis-cussed in Chapter 2, concepts of mental illness are value laden and presentation of psychiatric symptoms is at least partially culturally determined. Clinicians who are not sensitive to diversity or who are not insightful about their own personal biases will often negatively show this in their documentation. A study conducted by Mohr and Noone (1997) found that psychiatric nurses often report "on patients in judgmental and unflattering ways" (p. 325). Client-centered mental health practitioners, including occupational therapists, must carefully and accurately document functional deficits without personal judgment.

Types of Documentation

There is tremendous variation in the forms and amount of documentation found in occupational therapy practice. However, recommended procedure includes an evaluation summary, a treatment plan, progress notes, and a discharge summary. This is typically, but not uniformly, required for reimbursement and/or institution accreditation.

Evaluation summary.   The evaluation summary can be as little as a few handwritten lines in a chart or a lengthy typed report sent to outside parties. Essentially, an evaluation summary should include an assessment of the client's assets and deficits based on the overall evaluation process, including the results of any or all of the following: observation, interview, informal and formal assessments (nonstandardized and standardized tests), and previous chart history. Often, health care facilities have their own evaluation forms with information relevant to the treatment provided in the particular setting. In these cases, the summary is usually provided in a short narrative at the end of the form. The evaluation summary is crucial because it provides the baseline data by which the success or failure of treatment is measured.

Treatment plan.   Some treatment plans are written in the form of behavioral objectives, others are simply an added note to the evaluation form or first progress note. In some settings the actual treatment plan is only written on a form for reimbursement purposes. For example, Medicare requires a form known as a Plan of Treatment (POT). Regardless of format, all treatment plans should contain goals that realistically can be obtained in the particular setting and typical treatment timeframe and should clearly represent the domain of occupational therapy. If treatment is to last for more than a couple of sessions, goals should be broken down into short- and long-term.

Long-term goals are developed by establishing with the client the functional level he or she can achieve by discharge. However, in many cases, short-term goals are needed to reach the long-term goals. For example, the client's long-term goal may be to "return home and participate independently in daily activities again." Two short-term goals, then, could be, "client will shower and dress in clean clothing daily, independently, within one week"; and, "client will plan and cook one meal of choice with minimum assistance from the occupational therapist within three treatment sessions." Long-term goals may be similar to major life changes, such as working in a paid job for 20 hours per week for two months, while short-term goals may be those steps in the process, such as exploring work options, participating in volunteer work or in vocational groups, and writing a resume.

Table 24-1. Elements and Sample of a Behavioral Objective

Example: Given participation in the daily grooming group, within one week, the client will start to comb her hair without reminders prior to attending the group.

Element		
Performance (observable behavior)	Criterion (measure)	Condition (intervention)
Example		
independent hair combing	prior to group within one week	daily grooming group

Developing behavioral objectives for goals is desirable because the results are measurable and observable, thereby allowing the therapist to document the outcome of treatment accurately. Table 24-1 lists the elements of a behavioral objective and gives an example.

Progress notes. The various forms of progress notes include narratives (often called progress notes), Subjective-Objective-Assessment-Plan (SOAP) notes, Problem-Oriented Record (POR) notes, and checklists. It may be required, at least for reimbursement purposes, to chart a note following every treatment. Institutional protocol generally dictates the type of notes expected. Regardless of the type, it is expected that the professional service rendered will be stated and that an assessment of the individual's progress toward established goals will be noted.

Discharge summary. The purpose of the discharge summary is to assess the overall treatment process by stating the intervention provided, the goals met and not met (and rationale), and recommendations. Discharge summaries are, all too often, a single line at the end of the last treatment note. This is unfortunate because if the client goes on to receive other treatment, a well-written discharge summary can be invaluable to the new treatment team. Mechanisms should be established in every health care setting to facilitate the continuity of a client's care by providing appropriate information. For example, it is not uncommon for a client to transfer from an acute care hospital to a long-term facility or a day treatment center. If discharge summaries were provided at each stage of intervention, treatment could be more time efficient. Discharge summaries are often the only contact the occupational therapist may have with other professionals. Therefore, the summary can be a powerful tool for promoting occupational therapy services as well as providing input into a client's long-term care.

Documentation Review

Skill in documentation comes primarily from practice, but even an experienced therapist can fall into bad habits. A consistent critique of documentation is necessary to ensure quality. Furthermore, reviewing documentation (one's own and others) is a valuable learning tool for improving documentation skills. Documentation review is facilitated by asking the questions presented in Figure 24-2.

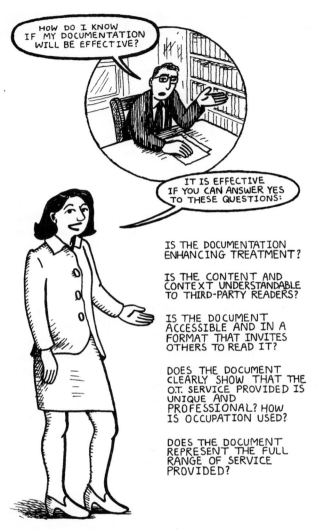

Figure 24-2.   Self-Review Questions for Quality Documentation

Treatment enhancement.   Is the documentation enhancing treatment? Well-written documentation can help a therapist provide excellence in treatment as long as the descriptions are complete, with clearly stated objectives and an accurate representation of performance, strengths, and deficits. The data recorded should also follow a logical sequence, and it should be evident how a client proceeded from point A to point B and what the next step should be. In other words, a new therapist should be able to take over treatment and proceed without repeating evaluations or treatments. In addition, documentation should not be laborious or redundant, as this robs valuable treatment time.

Understandable content.   Is the content understandable to third-party readers? People who read (or should read) documentation include all members of the treatment team (medical doctors, nurses, other therapists), as well as quality assurance reviewers, clerks, and insurance providers. The content of the documentation must be clear to people with various levels and types of training. Most important, the written words must be able to tell a story on their own without the benefit of knowing the client, setting, or situation.

Legibility.   Is the document accessible and in a format that invites others to read it? Probably the most common mistake made in documentation is illegibility. However, even if one's penmanship is readable, it is of little value if the note is poorly organized or filled with grammar and spelling errors. Furthermore, in this high-tech age, the format, or "packaging," is becoming more important. An evaluation or discharge summary that is well designed with clear subtitles and professional format is much more likely to be read. Another problem with notes is accessibility. That is, can the reader find the occupational therapy documentation? All charting should be placed in a clearly marked chart or subsection of a larger chart. Sometimes it is necessary to establish methods to call attention to documentation. For example, therapists may leave a note or phone message for a referring physicians, thanking them for the referral and stating that an evaluation has been completed and that they should refer to the appropriate section of the chart. If the referring physician or other interested professional is not on site, then an offer to mail the information (particularly the discharge summary) can be made, providing the necessary legal consent forms have been signed by the client.

A recent trend in documentation is to computerize all entries. Studies on computerized documentation have shown an increase in completeness, accuracy, and legibility of documentation, with a majority of participants in these studies reporting increased efficiency in both finding and recording documentation (Tan & Isaacks, 1999; Tang, LaRosa, & Gorden, 1999).

Professional service.   Does the document clearly show that the OT service provided is unique and professional? Duplication of service and nonprofessional service are two common reasons for reimbursement denial and may lead to the occupational therapist being replaced in a job by a less expensive service. Charting should reflect the particular service offered. If the intervention is generic or likely to be provided by someone else, it is unlikely that it will be valued or reimbursed. For example, clients may need someone to give them a shower, write letters for them, or take them for a walk. These may be very real needs but should not be the focus of occupational therapy or the subsequent documentation. When the necessity of such tasks consistently interferes with meeting the established goals, the therapist can make appropriate professional referrals or train nonprofessionals to perform such tasks. On the other hand, there are situations when a task such as giving someone a shower with maximum assistance is a prelude for meeting a goal of independence in showering. In such cases, evidence that the treatment is rehabilitative rather than maintenance is required. A plan for gradation of the activity with a realistic timeline should be included in the documentation. Subsequent notes should also reflect the progress in the task. The best way to ensure that documentation reflects a unique and professional service is for occupational therapists to have a clear concept of their roles and responsibilities.

Full range of service. Does the document represent the full range of service provided? Occupational therapists perform many functions. However, therapists sometimes fall into the habit of charting only treatment they perceive as reimbursable and desirable to their employers (Pierre, 2001). For example, in one treatment session, a therapist may evaluate a person's money management skills and explore new leisure activities. The tendency in many settings would be to chart only the evaluation because it is more likely to be reimbursed. The problem with this approach to documentation is that it devalues many important aspects of occupational therapy and confounds any research attempts made to determine the range, frequency, and effectiveness of OT. Certainly it is a professional responsibility to perform reimbursable service. However, it is not necessary to forfeit the integrity of occupational therapy in the process.

RESEARCH

Even for therapists who do not choose to conduct research themselves, it is essential for all practitioners to have a working knowledge of research designs and principles in order to be competent consumers of research. It is not possible in this chapter to provide an exhaustive overview of research design and methodology, and readers are urged to consult research texts as needed. Among the ones that are commonly used in occupational therapy are Bailey (1997), Creswell, (2002), Fowler (2002), Guba & Lincoln (1985), Moustakas (2000), Seidman (1998), and DePoy and Gitlin (1998).

Research is absolutely essential in the field of occupational therapy for several reasons. For one, all health care professionals, including occupational therapists, are currently being pressured by the economic market to "prove" the effectiveness of their techniques and interventions. While the need for outcome or efficacy studies is indisputable, occupational therapy also needs to continue developing its philosophical and theoretical basis, which usually implies a need for more exploratory methodologies. Both kinds of research should be encouraged in the field, and both have relevance to clinicians.

There appears to be a general consensus that occupational therapists should engage in clinically oriented research, especially outcome studies, and that the overall level of productivity in research must be increased. However, occupational therapists still seem resistant to engaging in research. As more occupational therapists receive advanced degrees, the sophistication of the research and the willingness to engage in it are increasing, but it is still necessary to increase the productivity of all occupational therapy clinicians. In a study conducted by Colborn, she concluded that "practitioners can be successfully involved in research given favorable conditions in the clinical work environment, as well as through a variety of educational and learning experiences" (1993, p. 699). It is important to remember that the basis of most clinical research is composed of the interview, treatment interventions, and observation, which are skills already incorporated into clinical practice. However, new technological trends may assist researchers. The most significant change in the production of research and collection of data is the advent of the computer. New technology can be tremendously useful in accessing literature and other resources, and it can be used to create a database for multipurpose analysis. However, the technology also requires that the researcher develop a whole new set of skills, including a knowledge of hardware and software, to manage the technology. As Renwick stated: "Computerized databases can facilitate several types of occupational therapy research. The value and usefulness of any database, however, is dependent on how well it has been designed" (1991, p. 827). (See Appendix B for related resources.)

The analysis of already existing literature was previously discussed as being the cornerstone of evidence-based practice. However, it can also be viewed as a type of clinical research. According to Bailey, "Research is any activity undertaken to increase our knowledge; it is the systematic investigation of a problem, issue, or question. This may mean reviewing all of the literature on a given topic and drawing new conclusions about that topic" (1997, p. xxi). An example of this technique is a study conducted by Henry and Coster (1996) in which the authors reviewed outcome studies in the psychiatric literature. Their purpose was to determine predictors of functional outcome among adolescents and young adults with psychotic disorders. The findings showed that premorbid functioning is the most consistent indicator of functional outcome. They therefore concluded that occupational therapists have a definitive role with this population especially in programs designed to "strengthen competence, coping skills, and social supports" (1996, p. 177).

Collaborative Research

Collaborative research is a common practice among experienced researchers, but it also has advantages for clinicians who feel they lack the necessary skills or resources to conduct research independently. **Collaboration** is especially helpful when an inexperienced researcher teams up with a mentor. A study conducted by Taylor and Mitchell "showed a strong belief in the importance of research in the profession, yet minimal involvement in research due to limited time, money, and skill. The role of collaborator with experienced researchers was rated as highly desirable" (1990, p. 350). DePoy and Gallagher (1990) suggest that an ideal collaborative team may consist of a clinician and an educator who is experienced in research methodology. Bloomer (1995) further suggests that student fieldwork is an ideal time to engage in collaborative research, citing both the high educational value to the student and the importance of the already existing relationship between the university and the clinical community.

Another form of collaboration involves the recipient of services in the actual research design. Current day mental health practice is consumer oriented and there is a trend to include clients in the entire range of clinical, educational and research activities. Clark, Scott, and Krupa describe using this methodology in a study of client satisfaction. They concluded that "involving clients in all aspects of planning, including clinical decision-making, programme development and evaluation, and research must become a priority in order that occupational therapy remain meaningful to clients, and their treatment" (1993, p. 197).

In addition to collaboration between academics and clinicians and between clinicians and clients, there are several models of clinical team research available to occupational therapists that offer some of the same benefits as collaboration with educators.

Unidisciplinary research. Unidisciplinary research is undertaken by a team of people from the same field, such as occupational therapy, but may involve several different settings. This is an especially helpful design for occupational therapy outcome studies. Wilma West described this strategy and stated, "I feel strongly that our best hope for such documentation, with numbers that will have significance, lies in the collaborative studies that link together therapists using the same treatment strategies for patients with the same conditions" (1990, p. 10).

Multidisciplinary research. Multidisciplinary research is conducted with two or more representatives of different disciplines; however, each researcher retains his or her professional identity and generally collects data independently. An example of such a study may be a program evaluation wherein each discipline is responsible for collecting data for a certain piece of an overall program. This may include results of assessments from all the involved disciplines.

Interdisciplinary research. Interdisciplinary research implies that researchers from different disciplines are studying the same phenomenon but each from a unique perspective. For example, researchers studying the social climate on a hospital unit or interactions within a group would use the same format for observation and record keeping, but the clinical insights would be based on the philosophy and training of each researcher. This type of study can yield a very rich description and understanding of the phenomenon, providing it is well coordinated. An added benefit of this type of study is that each member of the team has the opportunity to learn about each other's skills and perspectives.

Transdisciplinary research. Transdisciplinary research involves multiple researchers studying the same topic and engaging in the same tasks with no regard to professional identity. For example, a group of researchers may all be interested in a single symptom, such as hallucinations, or a condition, such as homelessness. All the researchers use the same research tool. Although there is considerable role blurring in these situations and the research does not particularly show the efficacy of any single discipline, it may result in unique information about the phenomenon itself. In addition, the opportunity to work equally with an experienced team of researchers benefits occupational therapy by increasing the disciplines' knowledge base and increasing visibility of the profession in published reports. Another perceived benefit is that generally, while they are being conducted, these types of studies are viewed as client focused, whereby individual professional biases and attempts for the researcher to be self-serving are minimized.

Methods

Table 24-2 provides examples of clinical research methods, but readers are also urged to explore them and other methods through additional sources. Within

Table 24-2. Examples of Clinical Research Methods

Type	Use
Retrospective chart review and computerized databases	The basis of extensive data collection
Case studies	May be exploratory or used to examine clinical outcomes. Case studies have different designs such as descriptive or quantitatively analyzed, single subject
Specifically designed assessment tools	Clinical outcome studies or program review
Predetermined assessments	Clinical outcome studies or to establish reliability and validity of the assessment
Interview	May be transcribed and analyzed in different ways, using a phenomenological methodology or a more quantitative style, such as content analysis
Observation	The clinical basis for many types of data collection. Participant observation is usually used in ethnographic research

each of these methods there are many variations. For example, life history and narrative research are specific types of case studies that have recently been introduced into the occupational therapy literature. These methods are significant for occupational therapy because they "provide the therapist with a view of the client's daily occupations, routines, family member relationships, sociocultural influences, and the effects of these factors on the delivery of occupational therapy services" (Larson & Fanchiang, 1996, p. 247).

An example of a specifically designed assessment tool is goal attainment scaling, as described by Ottenbacher and Cusnick (1990). This tool is "a flexible evaluation methodology that can address the documentation and accountability concerns facing health care providers. Perhaps, most important, goal attainment scaling is a method that is practice based and practitioner oriented" (p. 524).

Several recent research studies found in the occupational therapy literature related to mental health have focused on the reliability and validity of psychiatric OT assessment tools (Evans & Salim, 1992; Pan & Fisher, 1994; Penny, Mueser, & North, 1995; Brown, Tollefson, Dunn, Cromwell, & Filion, 2001; Kielhofner, Mallinson, Forsyth, & Lai, 2001). These are especially significant in this era when the profession must clearly demonstrate the value of occupational therapy in mental health care.

Although specific methods are not covered in this chapter, a discussion of general categories of methodologies is also in order. Typically, methodologies are considered either qualitative or quantitative in nature. However, many research designs can incorporate both quantitative and qualitative analysis.

Quantitative research. Quantitative research involves many methods, but the most recognized form is the experimental method. In actuality, however, occupational therapy researchers rarely use a true experimental design. The limitations of the traditional experiment in clinical situations has been well documented in the OT literature (Ottenbacher, 1983; Ottenbacher & York, 1994). The limitations most often addressed include the difficulty of finding a suitable control group and the financial strain in a clinical environment. The researchers who support the use of quantitative methods generally seem to believe that true experiments are always desirable but not always feasible. Therefore, many studies conducted in occupational therapy use adapted designs, often involving a single subject.

There are a number of different designs used in single-study research, but most single-subject designs begin with a baseline phase where data is gathered on a subject's level of functioning without any treatment being provided.

Single-subject designs are more practical than traditional experiments for the clinician-researcher. They are less expensive to perform and generally require less time to complete. However, the limitations and concerns when using experimental methods with human beings as subjects also apply to single-subject designs. The most important consideration involves the ethical issues involved in withholding treatment during baseline periods. Another concern using experimental methods, including single-subject designs, is the level of therapist bias in data collection and interpretation. An automatic conflict will arise when a therapist attempts to use an experimental method, as the objectivity of the researcher is supposedly essential to the success of the method, however, critics of the experimental method state that researcher objectivity is impossible, and all researchers must acknowledge this in their designs.

The single-subject case study is a preferred method in mental health occupational therapy as it can "tap into and document the 'insider's experience and perceptions of engaging in occupations" (Legault & Rebeiro, 2001, p. 90). Another benefit of single-subject design is the ability to use preexisting and ongoing clinical documentation, thereby allowing the busy clinician the opportunity to actively engage in research (Joshi, 2000; Bray & Rebeiro, 1998).

Qualitative research. Qualitative research differs philosophically from quantitative research. "The goal of quantitative methodology is to arrive at proof; therefore, it employs hypothesis testing. The goal of qualitative methodology is to provide evidence for an account of some aspect of the social world. Therefore, it employs a heuristic strategy of generating explanations, weighing evidence, and revising explanations to match new evidence" (Kielhofner, 1982, p. 71). Quantitative research is generally designed to test a specific **hypothesis**; qualitative research is meant to be a discovery or exploratory process in the development of theories. Therefore, if the objective of clinical research in occupational therapy is to demonstrate the efficacy of specific treatment techniques, qualitative research is probably not appropriate. However, qualitative research does have its place in clinical research. Often what is needed in clinical studies is richer, more complete clinical descriptions in order to refine and appropriately use quantitative studies at a later date.

Unlike in quantitative research, it is not necessary for a researcher to have a sophisticated knowledge of statistics in order to utilize any of the qualitative designs. However, it is a mistake to assume that qualitative research is less difficult.

> Most seasoned researchers agree that the methods and rules for qualitative research, if done well, are more difficult to follow than procedures for randomization of groups to treatments and controls, counterbalancing and blinding research designs, and some of the other techniques common to quantitative research. (Philips & Pierson, 1982, p. 168)

In summary, qualitative research is used to gather data for detailed descriptions of situations, events, people, and observed behavior. It is especially appropriate for research into areas where little is known or understood about the phenomenon to be studied or the concepts involved are not easily reduced to numerical values.

Both quantitative and qualitative research designs have their place in clinical settings, and each has specific benefits and limitations. Furthermore, it seems quite obvious that the choice of designs should be based on the particular subject to be studied. However, it is also obvious that researchers make decisions regarding design for a multitude of reasons having nothing to do with the research question. The considerations most often cited include ease of publication, prestige, funding, and (perceived) ease of analysis, as well as a simple lack of knowledge regarding possible research designs. In clinical professions, particularly developing ones such as occupational therapy, it is vitally important that the choice of research design be based on a thorough understanding of the characteristics of each design.

PROMOTION

Promotion is often negatively thought of as a self-serving mechanism of "selling" oneself. However, promotion is necessary to ensure that significant contributions are known and available to the people who may benefit from the services. How this is accomplished is varied, but all occupational therapists share the responsibility of promoting the profession and should be versed in a variety of communication techniques, including multimedia.

At the 1992 AOTA National Conference in Houston, Texas, Lang, Kannenberg, and Brinson identified a number of ways in which occupational therapists can promote occupational therapy in mental health. Figure 24-3 is made up of suggestions based on their presentation. In addition to these suggestions, which are primarily geared toward practicing clinicians, it should be noted that the universities' programs and professional associations also have major roles in the promotion of occupational therapy in mental health.

A serious mistake often made by well-meaning promoters is attempting to undermine the integrity and skills of other professionals. The promotion of

Communicate

Formulate a clear, simple definition of occupational therapy.
Write an article about occupational therapy for an agency newsletter.
Offer to hold an event sponsored by a nonprofit mental health agency.
Place visual media about the OT process and outcomes in the workplace.
Provide clients with pamphlets about OT in mental health.
Emphasize something about OT in business cards and stationery.

Educate others

Take a physician or other health care provider to lunch.
Volunteer to speak at a community center.
Mentor an OT student who shows a special interest in mental health.
Provide ongoing in-service training for new employees and interns.
Write letters to the editors of newspapers and magazines in response to
    health-related articles.
Write nondefensive, helpful letters to media personnel who misrepresent
    occupational therapy.
Speak at your local school district at a career day.

Educate yourself

Attend continuing education classes.
Tour other facilities that have occupational therapy.
Read the mental health professional literature, both within and outside
    occupational therapy.

Participate

Join your local, state, and national professional organizations.
Consider membership in non-OT organizations with shared interests.
Meet with representatives of the government, insurance companies, and
    legal agencies involved with mental health.
Collaborate with a consumer-oriented group on community-oriented
    projects.
Support and encourage occupational therapists who are pioneering
    programming in nontraditional areas.

Have a positive attitude

Make sure you are not talking down to people.
Convey enthusiasm about mental health to students and interns.
Remember that first impressions count.
Do not be defensive.
Display a positive, energetic, open, and nonjudgmental attitude.
Do not be apologetic about practicing psychiatric occupational therapy.

Figure 24-3. Simple Things You Can Do to Promote Occupational Therapy in
                 Mental Health

Adapted from Lang et al., 1992.

occupational therapy does not need to be accomplished by competition, and in fact, that approach is often counterproductive. Health care professionals quite often work in teams, and health care delivery improves significantly when the team has open lines of communication, is well coordinated, and is based on mutual respect and understanding of each other's roles. Interprofessional colleagues are an underutilized resource and can be powerful allies for promotion, providing we, as occupational therapists, are willing to advocate for them in a client-centered fashion.

"If interdisciplinary teams are to more effectively address the occupational and other needs of those living with mental illness" Fossey (2001) recommends "improved opportunities for dialogue through shared education and professional development, informed dialogue about balancing generic, specialist and nonprofessional roles in service delivery, as well as inclusion of consumers and carers in these dialogues" (p. 232).

If one keeps in mind that the purpose of promotion is ultimately to provide the best client service possible, then cooperation among the disciplines is optimum. One way to facilitate such cooperation is by forming interdisciplinary coalitions among service providers and agencies for the purposes of **networking**. According to Hurff, Lowe, Ho, and Hoffman, "the process of networking has extended and strengthened our individual professional efforts. A wealth of ideas has emerged from our relationships with one another" (1990, p. 430). Hurff and colleagues state that networking is especially needed in response to the trend toward community- rather than hospital-based treatment. They also report that through their networking efforts "they extended the role of occupational therapy into nontraditional settings" (p. 424). Networks among mental health occupational therapists and interdisciplinary mental health coalitions are currently operating in several regions of the United States. Among them is the Psychiatric Occupational Therapy Action Coalition (POTAC) of the San Francisco Bay area in California. Members of this group are involved with projects such as lobbying for mental health resources, research and publication, advocacy, program development, education, and publicity (Dressler & MacRae, 1998).

PRESENTATION AND PUBLICATION

The culmination of the demonstration of effectiveness involves disseminating the information that has been gathered. Without presentations and publications, any knowledge and insights gained through documentation, research, and promotion will, at best, only be meaningful on a local level. Too often, valuable clinical information does not get shared, creating a situation whereby occupational therapists are constantly "reinventing the wheel."

Presentations are typically given at conferences, which may be local, regional, national, or international. Formats also range from posters, papers, and workshops to symposiums, seminars, roundtables, and institutes. The choice of type of presentation depends on the level of skill and experience of the presenter, the depth of the information to be presented, and the type of information. For example, a poster can relay much visual information quickly but cannot provide a significant depth of process and theory. Posters are also limited in the scope of information that can be presented. Some presentations require an experiential or interactive component that does not fit well with a usual paper presentation format. These are more appropriate for workshops.

Another decision that applies to both presentations and publications is choosing the audience. There are advantages and disadvantages with each choice, and potential presenters should think carefully about their goals. Intraprofessional presentations and publications are essential to the growth and continuing education of occupational therapy, but there are also advantages to going outside the profession to share with others. Occupational therapists should consider publications and conferences of other related fields or interdisciplinary arenas. In the field of mental health, there is also an increasing number of journals and conferences sponsored by nonprofessional groups such as the National Alliance for the Mentally Ill (NAMI), which are geared toward client and family advocacy. These arenas provide excellent opportunities for occupational therapists to share their expertise and learn from others.

Publication can be an intimidating process for the novice. Many of the same suggestions for collaborative research apply to the publication process. It is especially helpful to have a mentor if this is a first attempt at publishing a paper. Figure 24-4 provides guidelines for the publication process.

Summary

Clear definitions and descriptions of occupational therapy services are essential for professional survival in these difficult times. This chapter provided guidelines for occupational therapists to articulate, document, research, and promote the profession of occupational therapy. In order to complete the process of demonstrating effectiveness, it is essential that occupational therapists present and publish the results of these efforts. Diligence is necessary to ensure that the unique and valuable contributions of occupational therapy to the field of mental health are recognized. "As a profession, we are increasingly confident about what occupational therapy is and how to communicate this to others. However, the future holds many challenges both within and external to the profession" (Lindquist & Unsworth, 1999, p. 28). Betty Yerxa (2003) described her hopes for the future of occupational therapy with the following statement:

> To serve humankind well will require that occupational therapy practitioners learn much more about people as agents, in their own environments, engaged in daily occupations . . . Only then will practitioners fulfill the profession's commitment to people with chronic impairments and ensure that their humanistic values are actualized in the practice of occupational therapy for a new millennium. (2003, p. 979)

In 1984 (p. 34), Lela Llorens also provided a vision for the future of OT that remains only partially fulfilled today.

Getting Started
  pick a topic
  choose a journal
  determine authorship (single author versus joint authorship; primary and
    secondary authors)
  write an outline
  seek advice
  contact the editor

Clinically Oriented Topics
  evaluation procedures
  application of theory
  specific techniques of treatment
  unique aspects of a treatment setting
  OT role (traditional and nontraditional)
  peripheral topics (controversies and politics)

Components of Publishable Papers
  statement of the issue or problem
  background
  critical review of the literature
  data — statistical and descriptive
  case study and other types of examples
  graphics: tables, charts, figures, photographs
  discussion and recommendations

Article Submission
  author guidelines
  hard copy and computer disk (sometimes requested by editor)
  time line
  rejection, revision, acceptance

Figure 24-4.   Guidelines for the Publication Process

- It is time for commitment to the science of occupational therapy and to the verification of occupational therapy theory.
- It is time for commitment to understanding and articulating the clinical reasoning process.
- It is time for commitment to the ownership of the meaning of occupation and activity, and the responsibility to explain the phenomena.
- It is time for commitment to unity of the profession.
- It is time for commitment to proactive professional management and publicly claiming the legacy of health through occupation.
- It is time for commitment to the habilitation and rehabilitation of clients in both clinical and community settings and to the quality of life beyond the role of medicine in the client's care.

- It is time for commitment to bridging the gap between the level of knowledge, theory, development, and practice as a vital part of our heritage.
- It is time for commitment to our belief in the poetry and value of the commonplace.

Review Questions

1. What skills does an occupational therapist need to engage in evidence-based practice?
2. How can occupational therapists enhance the effectiveness of their documentation?
3. What are the barriers for clinicians conducting research?
4. What skills does an occupational therapist need to effectively promote occupational therapy?
5. What are the pros and cons of collaboration in research and publication?

References

American Occupational Therapy Association. (2003). *Professional development tool.* Bethesda, MD: AOTA.

Bailey, D. (1997). *Research for the health professional* (2nd ed.). Philadelphia: F. A. Davis.

Bloomer, J. (1995). Applied research during fieldwork: Interdisciplinary collaboration between universities and clinics. *American Journal of Occupational Therapy, 49,* 207–213.

Bray, K., & Rebeiro, K. L. (1998). The light at the end of my tunnel. In *Outcomes that matter* (p. 65). Toronto: Canadian Occupational Therapy Foundation.

Brown, C., Tollefson, N., Dunn, W., Cromwell, R., & Filion, D. (2001). The adult sensory profile: Measuring patterns of sensory processing. *American Journal of Occupational Therapy, 55*(1): 75–82.

Canadian Association of Occupational Therapists (CAOT), the Association of Canadian Occupational Therapy University Programs (ACOTUP), the Association of Canadian Occupational Therapy Regulatory Organizations (ACOTRO), and the Presidents' Advisory Committee (PAC). (1999). *Joint position statement on evidence-based occupational therapy.* CAOT.

Clark, C., Scott, E., & Krupa, T. (1993). Involving clients in programme evaluation and research: A new methodology for occupational therapy. *Canadian Journal of Occupational Therapy, 60*(4), 192–199.

Colborn, A. (1993). Combining practice and research. *American Journal of Occupational Therapy, 47,* 693–703.

Creswell, J. W. (2002). *Research design: Qualitative, quantitative, and mixed methods approaches* (2nd ed.). Newbury Park, CA: Sage.

Depoy, E., & Gallagher, C. (1990). Steps in collaborative research between clinicians and faculty. *American Journal of Occupational Therapy, 44*(1), 55–59.

DePoy, E., & Gitlin, L. N. (1998). *Introduction to research: Understanding and applying multiple strategies.* St. Louis, MO: Mosby.

Dressler, J., & MacRae, A. (1998). Advocacy, partnerships, and client centered practice. *Occupational Therapy in Mental Health, 14*(1/2), 35–43.

Evans, J., & Salim, A. (1992). A cross-cultural test of the validity of occupational therapy assessments with patients with schizophrenia. *American Journal of Occupational Therapy, 46,* 685–695.

Fawcett, L. C., & Strickland, zL.R. (1998). Accountability and competence: Occupational therapy practitioner perceptions. *American Journal of Occupational Therapy, 52*(9), 737–743.

Fossey, E. (2001). Effective interdisciplinary teamwork: An occupational therapy perspective. *Australasian Psychiatry, 9*(3), 232–235.

Fowler, F. (2002). *Survey research methods.* Newbury Park, CA: Sage.

Guba, E., & Lincoln, Y. S. (1985). *Naturalistic inquiry.* Newbury Park, CA: Sage.

Henry, A., & Coster, W. (1996). Predictors of functional outcome among adolescents and young adults with psychotic disorders. *American Journal of Occupational Therapy, 50,* 171–181.

Hurff, J., Lowe, H., Ho, B., & Hoffman, N. (1990). Networking: A successful linkage for community occupational therapy. *American Journal of Occupational Therapy, 44,* 424–430.

Joshi, A. S. (2000). Single-system design: An effective strategy for evaluating clinical change. *British Journal of Occupational Therapy, 63*(6), 283–287.

Kielhofner, G. (1982). Qualitative research: Part I: Paradigmatic grounds and issues of reliability and validity. *Occupational Therapy Journal of Research, 2*(2), 67–79.

Kielhofner, G., Mallinson, T., Forsyth, K., & Lai, J. (2001). Psychometric properties of the second version of the Occupational Performance History Interview (OPHI-II). *American Journal of Occupational Therapy, 55*(3), 260–267.

Kohlman Thompson, L., & Foto, M. (1995). *Elements of clinical documentation.* Bethesda, MD: American Occupational Therapy Association (AOTA).

Lang, S., Kannenberg, K., & Brinson, M. (1992). *50 simple things you can do to promote occupational therapy in mental health.* American Occupational Therapy Association.

Larson, E., & Fanchiang, S. (1996). Nationally speaking—Life history and narrative research: Generating a humanistic knowledge base for occupational therapy. *American Journal of Occupational Therapy, 50,* 247–250.

Law, M., & Baum, C. (1998). Special edition on evidence-based practice. *Canadian Journal of Occupational Therapy, 65*(3), 131.

Legault, E., & Rebeiro, K. L. (2001). Occupation as means to mental health: A single case study. *American Journal of Occupational Therapy, 55*(1), 90–96.

Lindquist, B., & Unsworth, C. (1999). Commentary: Occupational therapy—reflections on the state of the art. *World Federation of Occupational Therapists (WFOT) Bulletin, 39,* 26–30.

Llorens, L. (1984). Changing balance: Environment and individual. *American Journal of Occupational Therapy, 38*(1), 29–34.

Lloyd-Smith, W. (1997). Evidence-based practice and occupational therapy. *British Journal of Occupational Therapy, 60*(11), 474–478.

Lloyd-Smith, W. (1999). Building on the evidence: Changing times, changing practice. *British Journal of Therapy & Rehabilitation, 6*(6), 266–267.

Menenberg, S. R. (1995). Standards of care in documentation of psychiatric nursing care. *Clinical Nurse Specialist, 99*(3), 140–142.

Miles, M. B., & Huberman, A. M. (1994). *Qualitative data analysis: An expanded sourcebook* (2nd ed.). Newbury Park, CA: Sage.

Mohr, W. K., & Noone, M. J. (1997). Deconstructing progress notes in psychiatric settings. *Archives of Psychiatric Nursing, 119*(6), 325–331.

Moll, A., & Cook, J. V. (1997). Doing in mental health practice: Therapists' beliefs about why it works. *American Journal of Occupational Therapy, 51*(8), 662–670.

Moustakas, C. E. (2000). *Phenomenological research methods.* Newbury Park, CA: Sage.

Occupational Therapy Practice Framework: Domain and Process. (2002). *American Journal of Occupational Therapy, 56*(6), 614–639.

Ottenbacher, K. (1983). Quantitative reviewing: The literature review as scientific inquiry. *American Journal of Occupational Therapy, 37,* 313–319.

Ottenbacher, K., & Cusnick, A. (1990). Goal attainment scaling as a method of clinical service evaluation. *American Journal of Occupational Therapy, 44,* 519–525.

Ottenbacher, K., & York, J. (1984). Strategies for evaluating clinical change: Implication for practice and research. *American Journal of Occupational Therapy, 38,* 647–659.

Pan, A., & Fisher, A. (1994). The assessment of motor and process skills of persons with psychiatric disorders. *American Journal of Occupational Therapy, 48,* 775–782.

Penny, N., Mueser, C., & North, C. T. (1995). The Allen Cognitive Level Test and social competence in adult psychiatric patients. *American Journal of Occupational Therapy, 49,* 420–427.

Philips, B., & Pierson, W. (1982). Qualitative research on occupational therapy. *Occupational Therapy Journal of Research, 2*(3), 165–170.

Pierre, B. L. (2001). Occupational therapy as documented in patients' records—part III. Valued but not documented. Underground practice in the context of professional written communication. *Scandinavian Journal of Occupational Therapy, 8*(4), 174–183.

Reilly, M. (1962). Occupational therapy can be one of the great ideas of 20th century medicine. *American Journal of Occupational Therapy, 16*, 1–9.

Renwick, R. (1991). A model for database design. *American Journal of Occupational Therapy, 45*(9), 827–832.

Seidman, I. (1998). *Interviewing as qualitative research: A guide for researchers in education and the social sciences* (2nd ed.). New York: Teacher's College Press.

Tan, R. S., & Isaacks, S. (1999). Computerized records and quality of care. *Annals of Long Term Care, 7*(9), 348–353.

Tang, P. C., LaRosa, M. P., & Gorden, S. M. (1999). Use of computer-based records, completeness of documentation, and appropriateness of documented clinical decisions. *Journal of the American Medical Informatics Association, 6*(3), 245–251.

Taylor, E., & Mitchell, M. (1990). Research attitudes and activities of occupational therapy clinicians. *American Journal of Occupational Therapy, 44*, 350–355.

Tickle-Degnen, L. (2002). Client-centered practice, therapeutic relationship, and the use of research evidence. *American Journal of Occupational Therapy, 56*(4), 470–474.

Tickle-Degnen, L. (2001). Evidence-based practice forum. Choosing books to guide evidence-based practice. *American Journal of Occupational Therapy, 55*(1), 109–110.

Tickle-Degnen, L. (2000). Evidence-based practice forum: Gathering current research evidence to enhance clinical reasoning. *American Journal of Occupational Therapy, 54*(1), 102–105.

Watson, R. M. (2002). Competence: A transformative approach. *World Federation of Occupational Therapists (WFOT) Bulletin, 45*, 7–11.

West, W. (1990). Perspectives on the past and future, Part 2. *American Journal of Occupational Therapy, 44*(1), 9–10.

Yerxa, E. (2003). Dreams, decisions, and directions for occupational therapy in the millennium of occupation. In E. B. Crepeau, E. S. Cohen, & B. A. B. Shell (Eds.). *Willard and Spackman's occupational therapy* (10th ed.). Philadelphia: Lippincott Williams & Wilkins.

Yerxa, E. (2000). Confessions of an occupational therapist who became a detective. *British Journal of Occupational Therapy, 63*(5), 192–199.

Youngstrom, M. (1998). Evolving competence in the practitioner role. *American Journal of Occupational Therapy, 52*(9), 716–720.

Suggested Reading

Alsop, A. (1997). Evidence-based practice and continuing professional development. *British Journal of Occupational Therapy, 60*(11), 503–508.

Acquaviva, J. (1998). *Effective documentation for occupational therapy* (2nd ed.). Bethesda, MD: American Occupational Therapy Association (AOTA).

Barnard, S. (2001). *Writing, speaking and communication skills for health professionals*. New Haven, CT: Yale University Press.

Dubouloz, C. J., Egan, M., Vallerand, J., & von Zweck, C. (1999). Occupational therapists' perceptions of evidence-based practice. *American Journal of Occupational Therapy, 53*(5), 445–453.

Eakin, P. (1997). The Casson Memorial Lecture 1997: Shifting the balance—evidence-based practice. *British Journal of Occupational Therapy, 60*(7), 290–294.

Egan, M., Dubouloz, C., von Zweck, C., & Vallerand, J. (1998). The client-centred evidence-based practice of occupational therapy. *Canadian Journal of Occupational Therapy, 65*(3), 136–143.

Errington, E., & Robertson, L. (1998). Promoting staff development in occupational therapy: A reflective group approach. *British Journal of Occupational Therapy, 61*(11), 497–503.

Grossman, J. (1998). Continuing competence in the health professions. *American Journal of Occupational Therapy, 52*(9), 709–715.

Kettenbach, G. (1995). *Writing SOAP notes* (2nd ed.). Philadelphia: F. A. Davis.

Nardi, P. M. (2002). *Doing survey research: A guide to quantitative research methods.* Boston: Allyn & Bacon.

Ogles, B. M., Lambert, M. J., & Masters, K. S. (1996). *Assessing outcome in clinical practice.* Newton, MA: Allyn & Bacon.

Parham, D. (1987). Toward professionalism: The reflective therapist. *American Journal of Occupational Therapy, 41,* 555–561.

Peloquin, S. M. (2002). Reclaiming the vision of reaching for heart as well as hands. *American Journal of Occupational Therapy, 56,* 517–526.

Richards, S. B., Richards, R. Y., Ramasamy, R., Taylor, R. L., & Richards, S. (1998). *Single-subject research: Application in educational and clinical settings.* Belmont, CA: Wadsworth.

Salvatori, P., Baptiste, S., & Ward, M. (2000). Development of a tool to measure clinical competence in occupational therapy: A pilot study. *Canadian Journal of Occupational Therapy, 67*(1), 51–60.

Schon, D. (1983). *The reflective practitioner: How professionals think in action.* New York: Basic.

Yin, R. K. (2002). *Case study research: Design and methods.* Newbury Park, CA: Sage.

Psychopharmacology for the Occupational Therapist

Anne MacRae, PhD, OTR/L

Introduction

Although various herbs and other culturally based treatments have existed for millennia in certain parts of the world, drug therapy for mental illness as we know it today did not emerge as a viable treatment option until the 1950s with the introduction of the antipsychotic, chlorpromazine (Thorazine). It is difficult to imagine treatment for severe mental illness without medication, and the advent of these drugs greatly reduced the need for restraints, isolation, and other harsh and ineffective treatments. It is therefore understandable how these drugs came to be viewed as a panacea. However, the passage of time has shown that psychotropic medication is not a cure or without negative consequences.

Psychotropic medication is now the most common form of treatment for many mental illnesses and new, more effective medications are being formulated every year. However, pharmaceuticals rarely work in isolation to control all of the symptoms and deficits found in persons with mental illness; drug therapy should be viewed as one facet of a comprehensive, interdisciplinary treatment approach. All team members must be aware of both the therapeutic and adverse effects of drug therapy. Although occupational therapists do not prescribe medication, the OT focus on function (doing) provides an ideal perspective from which to observe the effectiveness of the medication regime and work with both the team and the client to establish an individualized and optimum plan of treatment.

Psychopharmacology is not an exact science and although there are suggested uses and dosages for each drug, prescribing physicians must also take into account a client's individual physical characteristics. These include age, weight, and gender, as well as extenuating circumstances such as the safety of the medication for women of childbearing age or those individuals with systemic diseases, especially those with hepatic or renal dysfunction. Even with such knowledge, there are known differences in how an individual may react to a particular medication so a thorough personal and family medication history is needed. In addition, knowledge of all of the current symptoms the client is experiencing must be taken into account. For example, many of the typical antipsychotic medications target the positive symptoms of hallucinations and delusions. However, if the client also displays cognitive deficits such as poor memory or time disorientation, an injectable and/or long-lasting medication may be the first choice. The social and environmental context of the client must also be recognized. Insurance or other reimbursement to pay for medications may be a factor in the choice of prescriptions as well as the physical environment. For example, homeless clients may not have access to regularly scheduled food or even sufficient water and would be at increased risk of side effects with some medications. They also might have a difficult time with the close medical monitoring required with some psychotropic medications.

This appendix provides information about the common classifications of psychotropic medications, adverse effects, and suggested occupational therapy and team interventions. It is not intended to be the sole source of information for the occupational therapist. Readers are urged to consult the suggested reading and resources found in this appendix, as well as recent journal articles. Psychopharmacology is a rapidly evolving field and all members of the mental health treatment team are ethically responsible to stay apprised of changes that will affect their clients. Table A-1 lists the trade and generic names of commonly prescribed medications and their use in the treatment of mental illness. The list is not exhaustive and further explanation of the drug classifications follows the table.

ANTIPSYCHOTIC MEDICATIONS

Antipsychotic medication is viewed as either "typical" or as belonging to a newer group of drugs referred to as the "atypical" antipsychotics. Conventional or typical antipsychotic medications generally target the positive or psychotic symptoms of an illness such as hallucinations, delusions, and bizarre behavior as well as agitation. However, they do little or nothing to control the negative symptoms, such as anhedonia and avolition, commonly found in disorders such as schizophrenia. Typical antipsychotics are primarily dopamine antagonists whereas the atypical medications are serotonin-dopamine antagonists. Individuals may respond differently to each of these medications (hence the great number of them) and there are also differences in when they are best used. For example, Haldol is a fast-acting drug that is often used for sedation in acute psychotic episodes. Prolixin can be time released and therefore given in injection form at

Table A-1. Generic and Trade Names of Commonly Prescribed Psychotropic Medications.

Antipsychotic medications	Antidepressant medications	Antianxiety medications	Mood-stabilizing medications
"Typical" antipsychotics	*Tricyclic compounds*	*Benzodiazepines*	*Valproates*
haloperidol (Haldol)	amitriptyline (Elavil, Endap)	lorazepam (Ativan)	Valproic Acid (Depakene)
loxapine (Loxitane)	clomipramine (Anafranil)	diazepam (Valium)	Divalproex (Depakote)
thioridazine (Mellaril)	desipramine (Norpramin)	clonazepam (Klonopin)	Also used for seizure disorders and the prevention of migraine headaches
thiothixene (Navane)	doxepin (Adapin, Sinequan)	triazolam (Halcion)	
fluphenazine (Prolixin)	imipramine (Tofranil)	alprazolam (Xanax)	
Trifuoperazine (Stelazine)		temazepam (Restoril)	*Lithium*
Chlorpromazine (Thorazine)	*Other*	sertraline (Zoloft)	(Eskalith, Lithobid, Lithonate)
Perphenazine (Trilafon)	bupropion (Wellbutrin)		The most widely used mood stabilizers
	Sometimes used in conjunction with SSRI's		
	trazodone (Desyrel)		
	Also used for panic disorder and obsessive-compulsive disorder		
"Atypical" antipsychotics	*Selective serotonin reuptake inhibitors (SSRI)*	*Other*	*Other*
clozapine (Clozeril)	Flouxetine (Prozac, Sarafem)	Busipirone (BuSpar)	carbamazepine (Tegretol)
ziprasidone (Geodon)	paroxetine (Paxil)	Unlike the benzodiazepines, there is a low risk of abuse	Used for treatment of acute mania as well as a mood stabilizer
rispiradone (Risperdal)			
quetiapine (Seroquel)			
olanzapine (Zyprexa)			

Table A-2.   Medication-Induced Movement Disorders

Acute Dystonia	Acute muscular rigidity, especially in the neck, tongue, face, and back. Subacute symptoms include subjective reports of tongue "thickness" or difficulty swallowing. May impair speaking or breathing.
Neuroleptic Malignant Syndrome	An acute and severe muscular rigidity and elevated temperature with the possibility of dysphagia, tachycardia, diaphoresis, confusion, and elevated blood pressure. May be fatal.
(Neuroleptic-induced) Parkinsonism	Characterized by rigidity, tremor, masked facies, stooped posture, shuffling gait, drooling. If severe, it can develop into akinesia.
Akathesia	Characterized by restlessness, agitation, inability to sit or stand still, pacing. Subjectively described as an intensely unpleasant need to move.
Tardive Dyskinesia	Involuntary choreiform, athetoid or rhythmic movements involving the tongue, jaw, trunk, or extremities. Symptoms may be worsened by stress and are particularly severe in the older adult.

approximately three-week intervals. This is especially helpful for clients with memory or other cognitive deficits.

The atypical antipsychotic agents are generally considered to be more effective than conventional or "typical" antipsychotic medications in individuals with treatment-resistant schizophrenia (schizophrenia that has not responded to other drugs). Also the risk of tardive dyskinesia (a movement disorder) is lower with the atypical agents. However, because of the potential development of a serious blood disorder, agranulocytosis (loss of the white blood cells that fight infection), clients who are on medications such as Clozeril (clozapine) must have a blood test every one or two weeks. The inconvenience and cost of blood tests and the medication itself can make maintenance on clozapine difficult for many people. Clozapine and other atypical agents, however, continue to be the drugs of choice for people with treatment-resistant schizophrenia. Each antipsychotic medication has a unique therapeutic effect profile and the adverse effects of antipsychotic medications are many and varied (see Tables A-2 and A-3) but in general the newer atypical antipsychotics are better tolerated than older medications.

ANTIDEPRESSANT MEDICATION

All of the antidepressant medications take three to four weeks to bring about significant change in symptoms. During this time, the client may be at especially high risk of suicide and may require careful monitoring. The tricyclic medications themselves can cause death by either accidental or deliberate overdose, but other means of suicide, including the ingestion of additional drugs, must also be considered.

Table A-3. Interventions for Medication Management

Reason	Description	Interventions
Delusions or beliefs of potential harm	Paranoid delusions may include fears of poisoning or other physical damage. However, clients also may refuse medication based on nonpathological belief systems grounded in their socio-cultural and religious upbringing.	Trust building—Clients who have a solid therapeutic relationship with someone in the system are less likely to think they will come to harm. Correcting misinformation—Erroneous beliefs such as an individual's fear of becoming a "drug addict" can be addressed through education.
Admission of illness	Denial is a common reaction to the onset of severe, especially chronic, illness. With psychiatric disorders, there are the added problems of dealing with social stigma and the possible presence of thought disorder.	Create an accepting environment—Rather than attempting to "convince" someone of his or her illness, it is important to convey that individuals are accepted for who they are. Peer counseling—Often clients can benefit from hearing about the personal experience of others. Education—The realities of the illness may not be as frightening as the assumptions. It is important for clients to know that many people are able to live satisfying and productive lives with the presence of a mental illness.
Side effects	Many side effects disappear or decrease with time. However, others must be tolerated or managed.	Medical interventions—May include switching medications or reducing dosages as well as adding additional medications. Educational techniques (individual or group) for medication management—May include instruction in nutrition (increasing fluid and fiber, decreasing caffeine); avoidance of direct sunlight (sunscreen, outing schedule, hats, etc.); regulation of sleep and exercise as well as relaxation techniques.

(continues)

Table A-3. (continued)		
Reason	*Description*	*Interventions*
Cognitive deficits	Deficits may include poor memory, confusion, poor time orientation, concrete thinking, poor organizational skills	Medical intervention—Simplify regime by decreasing dosages per day and using long-acting agents. Supervision—Health care staff or appropriately instructed caregivers. Memory and orientation strategies—Reminder notes, pill organizers, schedules.
Perceived loss of freedom	Complaints of restrictive monitoring and dislike of precautions, including recommendations to avoid caffeine or alcohol as well as the necessity for remaining on a schedule and reporting to the clinic for follow-up lab work.	Education—Clients are more likely to adhere to recommendations if they understand the consequences of avoiding advice. Change of medication—Choice may be for a medication with limited side effects or precautions even if it is considered less effective than alternatives. Adaptation of daily living—Helping client switch to decaffeinated nonalcoholic beverages, use of calendar, day planner, and/or clock and visual reminders.

The SSRIs as well as Wellbutrin and Desyrel are usually the treatment of choice because they are considered to be much safer than the tricyclics. However, for reasons yet unknown the particular effect of any antidepressant medication is highly variable. Clients may need to have medications changed several times before the safest and most effective treatment is determined.

There is also much debate as to how long an individual should remain on antidepressant medication. For a single episode, it is generally recommended that the client remain on the prescribed medication for at least six months. For recurrent episodes, the recommendation is to remain on medication for at least as long as the duration of the previous episode. However, many sources suggest a course of at least five years and some individuals remain on medication for life.

ANTIANXIETY MEDICATIONS

The benzodiazapines have been used in the treatment of anxiety disorders for several generations. However, they are not universally effective and there is a high incidence of abuse and developed tolerance. They are best reserved for short-term use as in acute stress disorder. Buspirone is much safer than the benzodiazapines, but it takes much longer to significantly change symptoms, so it is sometimes recommended for clients to use both medications simultaneously and then taper off the benzodiazapines. Although not considered in the anxiolytic (antianxiety) category, the SSRIs are now frequently used to treat anxiety disorders, including panic disorder, obsessive compulsive disorder, and post-traumatic stress disorder.

MOOD-STABILIZING MEDICATIONS

Lithium is considered the most effective drug of choice for prophylaxis of both depressive and manic episodes, although it is probably more effective in decreasing manic episodes. It takes several weeks for Lithium to achieve therapeutic levels in the body so additional medication is usually needed for acute manic episodes. Lithium maintenance is long-term, often for life, and is known to have negative effects on the heart and kidneys. The therapeutic levels for lithium are close to toxic levels so regular blood work to determine concentration is recommended.

Valproate may be administered in isolation or in conjunction with lithium. It is more effective than lithium for rapid cycling bipolar disorders but less effective in preventing the recurrence of depression. Both lithium and valproate may cause adverse gastrointestinal symptoms such as nausea. Tegretol may also be administered in conjunction with lithium and/or valproate and is effective for acute manic episodes. However, it is not considered as effective as lithium for prevention of either depressive or manic episodes.

SIDE EFFECTS AND ADVERSE REACTIONS

The systemic side effects associated with psychotropic medication are highly variable but can include the autonomic nervous system symptoms of dry mouth, stuffy nose, irregular heartbeat, fainting, dizziness, sedation, constipation, blurred vision, and difficulty in urination, as well as pigmentary changes and photosensitivity. Symptoms often disappear after the first few weeks of treatment, but persistent problems may require a change in medication. Adverse reactions also include medication-induced movement disorders. These are described in Table A-2. Treatment of movement disorders typically consists of changing medications and dosages as well as prescribing additional medication such as Cogentin, Akineton, Artane, or Benadryl to control symptoms; however, these medications are ineffective for tardive dyskinesia. Medication-induced movement disorders may constitute a medical emergency, therefore, it is essential that all health care providers, including occupational therapists, observe for early symptoms of these disorders and communicate observations to the team immediately.

OCCUPATIONAL THERAPY AND TEAM INTERVENTIONS

The medication problem that is most often cited by health professionals is noncompliance. However, in a client-centered model of practice (and legally in many cases), a client does have the right to refuse to take prescribed medications. A client-centered clinician must attempt to understand the resistance from the client's perspective. Table A-3 lists commonly cited reasons for refusal or inability to take medication and some techniques that may help the individual adhere to prescribed treatment. However, the ultimate choice remains the client's and that must be respected.

Summary

Psychopharmaceuticals offer an important strategy for the treatment of many mental illnesses; however, they are not without their problems and clinicians must work closely with each other and the client to ensure the optimum individual medication regime.

Resources (also see Web sites listed in Appendix B)

Albers, L., Hahn, R. K., Reist, C. (2003). *Handbook of psychiatric drugs, 2004 edition*. Irvine, CA.: Current Clinical Strategies.
Physican's Desk Reference. (2003). Montvale, NJ: Thomson Healthcare
Sadock, B. J., Sadock, V. A. (2003). *Kaplan and Sadock's synopsis of psychiatry: Behavioral sciences, clinical psychiatry*. Philadelphia: Lippincott Williams & Wilkins.

Resources

The organizations and Web sites listed in this appendix offer continuing education to the occupational therapist as well as resources for clients and families. Students will also find a wealth of relevant information to augment their learning. This list is not inclusive of all resources available; however, many of the Web sites included here contain additional links. Every effort has been made to ensure that the information is current at the time of publication.

Advocacy and Client/Family Support

Anxiety Disorders Association of America (ADAA)	8730 Georgia Avenue, Suite 600 Silver Spring, MD 20910 http://www.adaa.org/ Main # (240) 485-1001
Canadian Mental Health Association	8 King Street East, Suite 810 Toronto, ON M5C 1B5 http://www.cmha.ca/ (416) 484-7750
Depression and Bipolar Support Alliance	730 North Franklin, Suite 501 Chicago, IL 60610-7224 http://www.DBSalliance.org (800) 826-3632
National Alliance for the Mentally Ill (NAMI)	Colonial Place Three 2107 Wilson Blvd., Suite 300 Arlington, VA 22201-3042 http://www.nami.org (703) 524-7600 (800) 950-NAMI (6264)

National Mental Health Association

2001 N. Beauregard Street, 12th Floor
Alexandria, VA 22311
http://www.nmha.org/
(703) 684-7722

National Mental Health Consumer
Self-Help Clearinghouse

http://www.mhselfhelp.org/
(Internet only—Provides links to many
other organizations)

Assessment (Occupational Therapy)

AMPS Project International (Assessment
of Motor and Process Skills)

http://www.ampsintl.com/

Canadian Occupational Performance
Measure (COPM)

http://www.caot.ca/copm/

Claudia Allen's OT Page
(Allen's Cognitive Levels)

http://www.allen-cognitive-levels.com/

The Model of Human Occupation
Clearinghouse

http://www.uic.edu/ahp/OT/MOHOC/

Brain Injury

Brain Injury Association of America

105 North Alfred Street
Alexandria, VA 22314
http://www.biausa.org
(800) 444-6443

Centre for Neuro Skills (Traumatic
Brain Injury Resource Guide)

2658 Mt. Vernon Avenue
Bakersfield, CA 93306
http://www.neuroskills.com
(800) 922-4994

National Resource Center for
Traumatic Brain Injury

Virginia Commonwealth University
Richmond, VA 23284
http://www.neuro.pmr.vcu.edu
(804) 828-0100

Perspectives Network, Inc.

PO Box 121012
W. Melbourne, FL 32912-1012
http://tbi.org

Children and Adolescents

The American Academy of Child and
Adolescent Psychiatry

3615 Wisconsin Ave., N.W.,
Washington, DC 20016-3007
http://www.aacap.org
(202) 966-7300

Federation of Families for Children's
Mental Health

1101 King Street, Suite 420
Alexandria, VA 22314
http://www.ffcmh.org
(703) 684-7710

Cultural and International Concerns

Diversity, Healing, and Health Care

On Lok Senior Health and the Stanford
Geriatric Education Center
http://www.gasi.org/diversity.htm

United Nations

UN Headquarters
First Avenue at 46th Street
New York, NY 10017
http://www.un.org/

United States Census

http://www.census.gov/

World Federation of Occupational
Therapists (WFOT)

WFOT Secretariat
PO Box 30
Forrestfield, Western Australia
Australia 6058
http://www.wfot.org.au

World Health Organization
(Includes links for the International
Classification of Function [ICF]

WHO Headquarters
Avenue Appia 20
1211 Geneva 27
Switzerland
http://www.who.int/
(+ 41 22) 791 21 11
e-mail inf@who.int

Environment

Adaptive Environments

374 Congress Street, Suite 301
Boston, MA 02210
http://www.adaptenv.org/
(617) 695-1225
e-mail: info@AdaptiveEnvironments.org

The American Horticultural Therapy
Association

909 York Street
Denver, CO 80206
http://www.ahta.org/
(800) 634-1603

Delta Society - Health Benefits of
Animals

Delta Society
580 Naches Avenue SW Suite 101
Renton, WA 98055-2297
http://www.deltasociety.org/
(425) 226-7357

Legal Issues

Bazelon Center for Mental Health Law

1101 15th Street, NW, Suite 1212
Washington, DC 20005
http://www.Bazelon.org/
(202) 467-5730

Department of U.S. Justice ADA
(Americans with Disabilities Act)
homepage

U.S. Department of Justice
950 Pennsylvania Avenue, NW
Civil Rights Division
Disability Rights Section - NYAV
Washington, DC 20530
http://www.ada.gov
(202) 467-5730

Mental Health (General Information)

Boston University Center for Psychiatric
Rehabilitation

940 Commonwealth Avenue West
Boston, MA 02215
http://www.bu.edu/cpr/p
(617) 353-3549

Internet Mental Health

http://www.mentalhealth.com/

National Electronic Library for Mental
Health (UK)

http://www.nelmh.org/

National Institute of Mental Health
(NIMH)

Office of Communications
6001 Executive Boulevard, Room 8184,
MSC 9663
Bethesda, MD 20892-9663
http://www.nimh.nih.gov
(866) 615-NIMH (6464)
e-mail: nimhinfo@nih.gov

Older Adults

Alzheimer's Association

225 North Michigan Avenue
Suite 1700
Chicago, IL 60601-7633
http://www.alz.org/
(800) 272-3900
(312) 335-8700

National Institute on Aging (NIA)

Building 31, Room 5C27
31 Center Drive, MSC 2292
Bethesda, MD 20892
http://www.nia.nih.gov/
(301) 496-1752

Pain Management

American Academy of Pain Management

13947 Mono Way #A
Sonora, CA 95370
http://www.aapainmanage.org/
(209) 533-9744

American Chronic Pain Association

PO Box 850
Rocklin, CA 95677
http://www.theacpa.org/
(800) 533-3231

The National Foundation for the
Treatment of Pain

P.O. Box 70045
Houston, Texas 77270-0045
http://www.paincare.org/
(713) 862-9332

Pharmacology

The American College of
Neuropsychopharmacology (ACNP)

http://www.acnp.org/

PDR (Physician's Desk Reference) Health

http://www.pdrhealth.com

Research and Evidence-based Practice

Cochrane Collaboration

http://www.cochrane.org/

OTseeker

OTseeker Project Manager
Department of Occupational Therapy
The University of Queensland
Brisbane QLD 4072
Australia
www.otseeker.com
61 7 3365 6174

Substance Abuse

Alanon

1600 Corporate Landing Parkway
Virginia Beach, VA 23454-5
http://www.al-anon.org
WSO@al-anon.org

Alcoholics Anonymous

Grand Central Station
PO Box 459
New York, NY 10163
http://www.alcoholics-anonymous.org

Narcotics Anonymous

PO Box 9999
Van Nuys, CA 91409
(818) 773-9999
Fax (818) 700-0700
http://www.na.org/

National Association for Children of
Alcoholics

11426 Rockville Pike, Suite 100
Rockville, MD 20852
http://www.nacoa.net
(888) 55-4COAS
(301) 468-0985

Substance Abuse and Mental Health
Services Administration (SAMHSA)

Substance Abuse and Mental Health
Services Administration, Room 12-105
Parklawn Building
5600 Fishers Lane
Rockville, MD 20857
http://www.samhsa.gov/

Work-related

Employment Intervention
Demonstration Program (EIDP)

UIC Mental Health Services Research
    Program
104 South Michigan Avenue, Suite 900
Chicago, IL 60603
http://www.psych.uic.edu/eidp/
(312) 422-8180

Job Accommodation Network

918 Chestnut Ridge Road, Suite 1
Morgantown, WV 26506-6080
(800) ADA-WORK
http://www.jan.wvu.edu/

National Business Group on Health

http://www.wbgh.com/

U.S. Equal Employment Opportunity
Commission (U.S. EEOC)

1801 "L" Street, NW
Washington, DC 20507
http://www.eeoc.gov/
ADA Helpline (800) 669-4000

Glossary

Abstract thinking—the ability to critically reason using analytical methods to infer relationships between differing ideas and to filter irrelevant data from relevant data.

Acting out—expression of thoughts and feelings through maladaptive behavior instead of recognizing and verbalizing thoughts and feelings.

Activity demands—demands that may be influencing performance skills and patterns.

Activity group—one whose content focuses on activity, emphasizes occupation, and addresses occupational performance components or skills to aid in occupational performance.

Adaptation—adjustment to one's disability.

Adjudication—the multistep process of coming to a judicial decision or sentence by going through criminal court proceedings.

Adjustment—in the context of this book it means adjustment to life with a physical disability.

Adolescent—the period of life from puberty to maturity terminating at the age of majority.

Advocacy—speaking or writing in support of someone or something such as the rights of persons with mental illness.

Affecting unstability—lack of control over emotions or mental state.

Aging in place—intervention theory that promotes allowing the aging to live in the environment they are most comfortable and familiar with and for the best care possible to be provided in this location.

Allopathic—refers to the tradition of medicine practiced in the West.

Americans with Disabilities Act (1990)—a federal law that provides for equal access and opportunity to all qualified individuals with disabilities in the areas of employment (Title I), equal access to public services (Title II), physical access to public facilities and transportation (Title III), and communications (Title IV) (EEOC, U.S. Department of Justice, 1991).

Analgesics—refers to the class of drugs that relieve pain.

Analysis of occupational performance—a way to determine what a client wants and needs to do and what the barriers might be to obtaining these goals.

Anosognosia—refers to a cognitive impairment of persons with frontal lobe damage that inhibits them from recognizing deficits in cognition, perception, or mobility.

Assertive community treatment (ACT)—a form of "full-support" therapy that is characterized by small caseloads, a multidisciplinary team rather than single case manager responsibility, 24-hour coverage, time-unlimited service, significant provision of in vivo outreach, and direct skill training.

Assessment—a number of tools and methods used to determine a client's disability or disorder and also used to determine a path of treatment for a client.

Autogenic training—a relaxation program that teaches people to respond physically and mentally to their own verbal commands.

Ayurvedic—the traditional medical practices of India.

Benzodiazapenes—a group of medications that act as sedatives and are commonly used for treatment of anxiety.

Biopsychosocial focus—the theoretical paradigm that aims to provide the most comprehensive understanding of the development of normal and abnormal behavior by exploring the interaction among biological, psychological, and social influences on behavior.

Broker—a person, group, or entity crucial to linking persons with serious mental illness to community services.

Chronic pain—pain that is constant.

Client factors—factors in a client's personal life that may be influencing performance skills and patterns.

Client-driven services—coming from a social rehabilitation perspective. Services are often considered in the language of the client and what the client wants in terms of treatment and support. The goals of treatment are stated in the client's words, and treatment must meet these goals with relevant treatment and service plans. The client is the customer and drives the service sector.

Clinical reasoning—refers to forms of reasoning that the occupational therapist uses to always guide methods and interpersonal strategies used in practice in collaboration with the client.

Cognitive deficits—a broad range of impairments, including but not limited to actual intelligence. In schizophrenia, the common cognitive deficits include poor judgment and reasoning, impulsivity, lim-

ited ability to abstract, and delayed processing time.

Collaboration—working together. This implies a greater amount of active interaction than cooperation, which may merely mean not interfering with each other. There is an expectation that people working in collaboration are helping each other produce an end or reach a common goal.

Commitment—court-ordered consignment to a mental institution.

Community support team—support given by many members of a community to a client with serious and persistent mental illness.

Competency model—model developed for educational use that, when applied to the mentally ill, offers a positive approach for working with the family.

Comprehensive evaluation—refers to evaluations that are designed to gather a complete contextually specific understanding of the client's occupational performance needs, strengths, abilities, and preferences.

Compulsions—repetitive and deliberate actions intended to diminish obsessions.

Confabulation—a behavioral reaction to memory loss in which the client fills in memory gaps with inappropriate words or fabricated details, often in great detail.

Conservator—the person legally designated to make decisions regarding medical issues, legal matters, housing, and finances for an individual with a mental illness. The primary purpose of appointing a conservator is to protect the client from abuse or exploitation.

Consistency—the routine, reliable aspects of treatment that develop trust and reliance in the human and nonhuman environment.

Consumer/client empowerment—the client, not the service providers, makes all decisions and directs the process.

Consumers' movement—refers to patients/clients/consumers of mental health services who meet for support, education, and advocacy. They are organized in most communities and are advocates of research and humane treatment.

Contexts—the situations in which a client lives or is involved in.

Conversion—a predominant psychic mechanism in which an unconscious fear, wish, or conflict is transformed into physical pain, thus providing an avenue for psychological release.

Coping strategies—strategies developed alone or through professional intervention that enable a disabled person to better cope with his or her circumstances.

Cultural blindness—choosing not to recognize cultural differences in others.

Culture-bound syndromes—manifestations of mental illness unique to a particular cultural group.

Curative occupations—a course designed to educate institution attendants in occupations for those with mental illness.

Cyclothymia—a *DSM-IV* diagnosis that includes symptoms of mania, but is considered less severe than bipolar disorder.

Decisional balance—using different types of exercises to articulate pros and cons of current drug use.

Decompensation—the process whereby an individual with a mental illness loses the ability to maintain normal or appropriate compensatory functions; the individual loses touch with reality.

Deinstitutionalization—the process that released large numbers of persons with mental illness from state institutions into the community.

Dementia—a medical condition of deteriorated mentality often accompanied by emotional apathy and identified by the presence of multiple cognitive defects.

Demotivational syndrome—lack of interest and apathy toward previous occupations or events often resulting from frontal lobe damage.

Depersonalization—feelings of unreality.

Depression—a clinical term, ambiguous in general use; used to refer to a mood, a symptom, and a disease entity. As a symptom, it could be replaced with sadness. The use of the term may be restricted to a syndrome or disorder.

Derealization—feeling detached from one's surroundings.

Diagnosis—the result of a process of elimination in which a disorder is identified by meeting very specific criteria, including demographic information such as age, as well as range, severity, and duration of symptoms.

Diffuse axonal injury—an injury resulting from the tearing and shearing of the axons of the nerve fibers throughout the brain due to the bouncing of the brain within the skull. The injury is not visible through brain imaging.

Dimensions—a hierarchy of lower-order personality traits that are organized into higher-orders categories such as neuroreoticism or extraversion.

Disinhibition—a condition resulting from frontal lobe damage causing a client to lose the ability to filter or screen behavior, often resulting in inappropriate language or actions.

DSM—the *Diagnostic and Statistical Manual of Mental Disorders* published by the American Psychiatric Association (APA). The third edition, known as *DSM-III*, was published in 1980 and contained a significantly different multiaxial format from earlier editions, allowing for more complete diagnostic descriptions. The current edition, the *DSM-IV*, was published in 1994 and continues to use a multiaxial format.

Dual diagnosis—a situation in which a person has two distinct diagnoses that require different treatment. Often applied to individuals diagnosed with both mental illness and substance abuse. The term may be used to refer to the presence of a psychiatric condition concurrent with a physical disability or illness.

Dynamic—a way of interacting between or among people; generally applied to a pattern of relating that is not explicitly or consciously acknowledged.

Dynamical systems theory—the view that new and unpredictable states of organization arise spontaneously within a system when sufficient energy flows through it.

Dysfunction—a deficit in the ability to perform tasks. It is often a result of effects of symptoms but there is not always a direct correlation. Occupational therapists view these deficits in a function/dysfunction continuum in the realm of occupational performance that includes work, leisure, and self-care activities.

Dysthymia—a *DSM-IV* diagnosis that includes symptoms of major depression, but is considered less severe than major depression.

Eclectic—generally, made up of the best elements selected from a variety of sources. Used to refer to theorists and practitioners who do not adhere to any one system of beliefs, but who select and utilize what they consider to be the best elements of many different theories in their attempts to understand and treat aberrant behavior and psychological dysfunction.

Efficacy—effectiveness, or the power to produce effects or intended results.

Ego strength—a psychoanalytic term that has become a popular term for the ability to accurately and appropriately deal with reality adaptively, such as through the use of coping skills.

Ego-syntonic—not disturbing to the ego; generally applied to disordered traits or patterns that would usually be disturbing.

Elder abuse—the physical, emotional, or sexual abuse of the elderly in their own home or in nursing care facilities.

Electroconvulsive therapy (ECT)—a form of treatment for mental disorders, particularly depression, by the induction of unconsciousness and convulsions through the use of electric current applied to the brain.

Enabling—behaviors, usually practiced by family and friends, that inadvertently reinforce the destructive habits of the substance abuser.

Entitlements—comprehensive term used to describe government programs such as Medicaid and Medicare.

Evidence-based practice—an occupational therapy approach utilizing systemic analysis of the existing professional literature as well as the client's personal narra-

tive and the identification of the specific expertise of the practitioner.

Feng-Shui—a Chinese art form that is concerned with how energies of the environment interact with individuals and their dwellings.

Forensics—the science that deals with the interface between the practice of medicine and the law. Forensics may be limited to the interface between mental illness and the criminal justice system.

FRAMES—an acronym that guides motivational interviewing and includes Feedback, Responsibility, Advice, a Menu of alternate change options, Empathy, and Self-efficacy.

General systems theory—the view that the universe is a whole composed of interconnected parts and that all phenomena belong to this larger whole and share similar properties.

Generalization—the utilization of cognitive and functional skills from a variety of different environments.

Geriatric—branch of medicine that deals with the problem and diseases of old age.

Glasgow Coma Scale (GCS)—a scale used to evaluate the client's level of consciousness at the scene of an accident or afterward.

Group—two or more people who have a consciousness that they are a group. An intentional gathering of people for the purpose of change.

Group content—activity carried out in the group; what is said in the group. It can be verbal or nonverbal.

Group dynamics—the forces that influence the relationships of members and influence the group outcome.

Group norms—standards, either implicit or explicit, verbalized or unstated, that are often developed by a group leader or based on group interaction.

Group process—how the work of the group is carried out, including how participants relate to each other, who talks to whom, how tasks are accomplished and how decisions are made, and how therapy is undertaken; patterns or stages that groups usually go through.

Group protocol—a description of a group, including its purpose, goals, content, structure, logistics, who would and would not benefit by participation in it, and referral process.

Group structure—the way in which the activity is presented, the directions, procedures, techniques, and time arrangements, and the way in which membership is organized.

Habit training—the development of cultural, personal, and occupational habits in the client with mental illness.

"Hardwired"—an expression originating in computer science that designates an innate biological structure.

Harm reduction—the use of alternate strategies that might lessen the potential negative impact of substance misuse.

Hierarchical—a term used in the context of relationships referring to the fact that no single aspect is considered to be at the core of successful occupational performance.

HIV—Human Immunodeficiency Virus; the causative agent of a syndrome characterized by a progressive, gradual, irreversible, and disabling deterioration of the human immune system, which renders the host susceptible to a wide range of opportunistic infections and other clinical syndromes. HIV disease is any stage of the disease caused by infection with HIV, including AIDS.

Hypothesis—a logical assumption, reasonable guess, or educated conjecture that gives direction to research.

ICF—*International Classification of Functioning, Disability, and Health* published by the World Health Organization.

Identified patient (ip)—a term used to indicate the individual within the family system for whom the family is seeking treatment.

In vivo—a Latin term referring to any treatment or intervention that occurs within a client's natural environment ("in real life"), rather than in the artificial or simulated environment of a hospital, clinic, or laboratory setting.

Incarceration—confinement in a jail, prison, or forensic state hospital.

Individual Placement and Support (IPS) model—a model of employment services.

Individuation—the process by which the developing child comes to recognize himself or herself as distinct from parent(s) and the surrounding environment; may also be used to refer to the process of becoming a unique individual.

Initiation—refers to the ability to begin an activity at an appropriate time to accomplish a goal.

Interpersonal—referring to external psychological processes, usually observable in an interaction between two or more people.

Intersubjective process—a condition where the occupational therapist is more reflective, self-aware, and insightful in the therapeutic process.

Intrapersonal—referring to the internal psychological processes and experience of a person. It is not observable and can be understood only through the explanation of the person.

Jail—a correctional facility where individuals are confined while awaiting trial, or a correctional facility where those with a sentence of one year or less are confined.

Job coaching—a service whereby assistance is given in any or all of the phases of the supported employment (SE) approach, for example, skills training, job modifications, employee/employer interventions, and ongoing support.

Lapse—a slip back into substance abuse or other undesirable behavior.

Latency age—between the ages of about 5 and 12. In Freudian theory, the stage when both sexual and aggressive drives and impulses are latent, or hidden and subdued.

Least restrictive environment—environment with the optimum balance of individual freedoms and supervision where the client can function.

Life satisfaction—a person's satisfaction with the circumstances of her or his life. Life satisfaction is not necessarily correlated with the severity of a physical disability.

Lifestyle redesign—an intervention model that promotes quality of life in well elders.

Mania—a mood that is elevated, expansive, or irritable. Associated symptoms are hyperactivity, pressured speech, flight of ideas, diminished need for sleep, grandiosity, distractibility, short attention span, and extremely poor judgment in interpersonal and social areas.

Medicaid—the federal health insurance program for low-income U.S. residents.

Medicare—a government-sponsored health care payment program, primarily for those over 65 years of age.

Melancholia—as an emotional symptom, it is detachment, alienation, sadness, apathy, and dejection. Formerly used as a clinical term to describe the mental disorder of depression.

Memory—the ability to store and recall thoughts. This ability is crucial to acquiring new information and is highly influential on everyday functioning.

Mentor—a wise and trusted counselor, instructor, guide, coach, or advisor.

Mode—method, approach, strategy, or procedure for learning.

Monochronic (M-time)—view of time as linear and as a commodity, as something that can be saved or lost.

Mood—emotional state that usually colors one's whole psychological life.

Moral treatment—a system of treatment for those with mental illness consisting of humanitarian and therapeutic approaches to illness and characterized by kindness and respect for the client.

Moxibustion—an alternative medical practice from Asia employing cauterization and counter-irritation to treat disease.

National Alliance for the Mentally Ill (NAMI)—national support and advocacy group for the mentally ill.

Negative symptoms—absent or decreased emotional and behavioral repertoire. Includes flat affect, alogia (poverty of speech), avolition (poor initiation of activities and/or inability to sustain goal-directed activities), and anhedonia or hypohedonia (inability or decreased ability to experience pleasure).

Networking—the process by which individuals and agencies link together for the purposes of sharing information, providing support, and working toward a common goal.

Neurasthenia—term used by psychiatrists to refer to nervous conditions such as hysteria, hypochondria, depression, compulsive behavior, and anxiety.

Neurobiological—term used to describe the nervous system.

Neuroplasticity—the ability of the brain to reorganize alternate neuronal pathways to compensate for damaged areas.

Obsessions—intrusive ideas, images, thoughts, and impulses that persist.

Occupational alienation—a loss of meaning that was once associated with performance.

Occupational deprivation—loss of once important occupations necessary for a satisfying life.

Occupational profile—profile intended to provide an understanding of the client's occupational history and experiences, patterns of daily living, interests, values, and needs.

Opioids—refers to brain chemicals that act as natural painkillers, commonly known as endorphins.

Outcome evaluation—refers to the process of tracking the specific changes that interventions are making in the lives of the clients being served.

Parallel process—refers to the dynamic between patient and therapist, and between therapist and clinical supervisor; the therapist identifies with the patient and then elicits emotions in the supervisor that he or she has experienced with the patient.

Parallel task group—one in which individuals work on individual tasks in the presence of others, but not necessarily with the others.

Performance in areas of occupation—how a client performs in certain areas of occupational therapy.

Performance patterns—habitual or routine patterns of behavior related to daily life activities.

Performance skills—what one does (such as concentrate), not what one has (such as feelings); include motor, process, and communication skills.

Perseveration—refers to the inability to disengage from an activity and reengage in other activities.

Personality—style of relating, coping, behaving, thinking, and feeling. A concept that represents a network of traits that persist over a lifetime.

Personhood skills—a term used to describe skills that depend on personal traits acquired through a combination of temperament and experience.

Polychronic (P-time)—cyclical and unscheduled time, typically a natural rhythm where several things can happen at once and is not controlled by human beings.

Polyculturalism—state of identifying oneself as a member of several different cultural backgrounds.

Positive symptoms—the active symptoms of psychotic disorders, including delusions and hallucinations as well as disorganized speech and behavior.

Post-traumatic amnesia—short- or long-term memory deficits resulting from concussion or other brain trauma.

Preferred defense structure—those defenses preferred by a particular individual, in addition to other skills, abilities, and strategies, to form the basis for psychological survival.

Prevocational services—services that provide structured activities that assist individuals to learn basic self-care skills, habits, and routines critical to developing work behaviors.

Prison—a correctional facility where sentences in excess of one year are served.

Prodromal symptoms—those that typically appear prior to onset of a psychiatric disorder or relapse.

Proxemics—an aspect of culture that refers to people's use and comfort with personal and social space.

Psychiatric rehabilitation—the use of various interdisciplinary interventions aimed at restoring function and role performance. The goal is to assist people with severe mental disabilities to function at their highest potential, in their environment of choice, with the least amount of professional support necessary.

Psychoanalysis—psychiatric treatment developed by Freud that proposed psychological problems arise in individuals as a result of unconscious conflicts over past events, especially of a sexual nature.

Psychobiological—approach to treatment of mental illness that takes into account an individual's performance and occupational history as well as the biological and neurological data.

Psychodynamic—aspect of a therapeutic process in which change is brought about primarily by talking and reflecting on one's thoughts and actions, and by a therapist's or group leader's interpretations. It assumes an unconscious process.

Psychoeducational—aspect of a therapeutic process in which change is brought about by learning or through education, usually about a psychological topic. There is a clear objective to teach specific information or techniques.

Psychogenic—originating in the mind or in mental processes.

Psychopathology—from the Greek, meaning "the study of mind or brain disease." It refers to the study and classification of symptoms; can characterize a condition as a mental disorder.

Psychopharmacology—the science of how drugs effect psychomotor behavior and emotional states.

Psychosis—significant impairment of reality testing and daily functioning due to the presence of positive symptoms.

Psychotropic—a descriptor for an agent, usually a prescribed drug, that directly affects the actions of the brain.

Quality of life—a term difficult to define in the medical literature but generally meaning a concept broader than health or disease and consisting of such characteristics as good mobility, social relations, self-esteem, independent living, and other daily living factors.

Rancho Los Amigos Levels of Cognitive Functioning—a common rating scale used to assist an interdisciplinary assessment and treatment team in determining a client's cognitive, behavioral, and functional status following brain injury.

Recovery—a process of active sobriety maintenance through using support such as AA (Alcoholics Anonymous) groups, increasing awareness of use patterns, and active relapse prevention planning.

Redirection—verbal tactic used in therapy with children to provide structure.

Referential thinking—ideas of reference, or the feeling that casual incidents and events have an unusual or particular meaning specific to the person.

Relapse—a return to a former drug-centered lifestyle.

Reliability—the dependability and accuracy of assessment scales.

Research—systematic and careful investigation that requires gathering and analyzing of data in order to establish facts and principles, or add to a general body of knowledge.

Risk reduction—prevention programs where groups or individuals are identified at being at high risk for developing substance use disorders.

Role Acquisition Frame of Reference—a frame of reference used in occupational therapy concerned with the learning of social roles required of the individual in an expected environment.

Schizophrenogenic mother—now outdated term applied during the 1950s and 1960s to mothers of children who had mental illness. It was thought that the environment and, more specifically, the parenting in which one grew up was the cause of mental illness.

Screening evaluation—screening intended to provide an initial indication of a person's need for services.

Self-concept—refers to an individual's own conception of his or her life.

Self-help—refers to an individual's motivation to participate in his or her own mental health and empowerment.

Seriously and persistently mentally ill (SMI)—persons suffering the most severe forms of mental or physical disorder.

Somatic—a term used to describe concerns or conditions relating to the body as opposed to the realm of the psyche.

Splitting—a psychoanalytic concept, considered a defense, that causes an individual to perceive people as either all good or all bad and be unable to acknowledge both negative and positive features in one person. Resulting behavior may correlate with destabilizing relationships among staff members.

Standard drink measure—a screening method used to determine alcohol abuse.

Strategies—refers to the tangible tools that are often readily identified or observed in practice.

Structure—providing a form and design for treatment.

Style—inclination to use the same adaptive strategies in various situations. A stable, consistent approach to attending, perceiving and thinking. Cognitive style or orientation.

Supervision—a process in which two or more people make a joint effort to promote, establish, maintain, and /or elevate a level of performance and service.

Supported education—similar to supported employment (SE), assisting a person to develop the community resources needed to pursue his or her educational and career goals.

Supported employment (SE)—an approach grounded in psychiatric/psychosocial rehabilitation that assists a person to choose, get, and keep a job. It is often referred to as the Choose, Get, Keep approach.

Symptom—a subjective experience of the individual, such as what he or she may feel, do, or think. It is different from a sign, which is the objective finding of a medical practitioner.

Synthetic eclecticism—integrating concepts and principles from various theoretical paradigms to develop a more comprehensive understanding of a client's presenting problems.

Technical eclecticism—using therapeutic tools, techniques, and strategies from various theoretical paradigms in order to better meet the needs of individual clients.

Techniques—refers to the tangible tools that are often readily identified or observed in practice.

Temperament—an individual's unique intellectual and emotional makeup.

Tic—any stereotyped movement or vocalization that is sudden, nonrhythmic, rapid, and repeated.

Time-out—a therapeutic intervention that is based on behavior modification involving a person's removal from a problematic situation and removal of positive reinforcers following the behavior that is to be extinguished.

TM/CAM—traditional medicine (TM) means the approach to medicine primarily practiced within one's own culture while complementary and alternative medicine (CAM) is typically viewed as health care techniques and treatments not compatible with Western medical practices.

Tolerance—the biological mechanism whereby greater amounts of an abused substance are required to produce the same/desired physiological and psychological effects of intoxication.

Traits—distinguishing characteristics of one's personal nature. A person can respond to a particular situation in a particular way. When the response occurs in a variety of situations it becomes a habit. A group of response habits that form a repetitive way of psychological functioning or relating to the environment can be classified as a trait.

Transitional services—services provided to young people as they move from school to work or from adolescence to young adulthood.

Treatment team—a team may be composed of some or all of the following: psychiatrist, psychologist, psychiatric nurse, social worker or therapist, case manager, occupational therapist, psychiatric nurse, psychiatric technician, recreational therapist, and, more recently, family members.

Universal design—the design of products and environments usable by all people without the use of adaptation or specialized design.

Validity—degree to which data are correct or true.

Vasodilatation—expansion of the blood vessels especially small arteries.

Well elderly—healthy and active older persons.

Withdrawal—the development of a substance-specific syndrome due to the cessation of (or reduction in) substance use that has been heavy and prolonged.

Work programming—the focused application of occupational therapy principles, knowledge, and skills to assist people to work productively and resume culturally valued roles in their community. The term *work* is any productive activity, paid or nonpaid, that is valued and seen as contributing to the community.

Index